We dedicate this handbook to our patients, whose unwavering courage in the face of adversity inspires us to be better physicians and human beings.

CONTENTS

POCKET NOTEBOOK

Pocket ONCOLOGY

Third Edition

Edited by

NOURA CHOUDHURY, MD
Assistant Attending, Thoracic Oncology & Early Drug Development Services
Memorial Sloan Kettering Cancer Center
New York, New York

YONINA R. MURCIANO-GOROFF, MSC, DPHIL, MD
Instructor, Early Drug Development Service
Memorial Sloan Kettering Cancer Center
New York, New York

Advisors

ALEXANDER DRILON, MD
Chief, Early Drug Development Service
Memorial Sloan Kettering Cancer Center
New York, New York

NEIL VASAN, MD, PHD
Assistant Attending Physician
Breast Medicine Service
Memorial Sloan Kettering Cancer Center
New York, New York

Wolters Kluwer

Philadelphia • Baltimore • New York • London
Buenos Aires • Hong Kong • Sydney • Tokyo

Acquisitions Editor: Nicole Dernoski
Development Editor: Eric McDermott
Editorial Coordinator: Vinoth Ezhumalai
Marketing Manager: Kirsten Watrud
Production Project Manager: Catherine Ott
Manager of Graphic Arts and Design: Stephen Druding
Manufacturing Coordinator: Beth Welsh
Prepress Vendor: Aptara, Inc.

Third edition

9 8 7 6 5 4 3 2 1

Printed in China

Library of Congress Cataloging-in-Publication Data available upon request

ISBN: 978-1-9751-9081-1

shop.lww.com

CCS0822

CONTRIBUTORS

SECTION EDITORS

Omar Abdel-Wahab, MD
Director, MSK Center for Hematologic Malignancies
Department of Medicine
Memorial Sloan Kettering Cancer Center
New York, New York

Duaa H. Al-Rawi, MD, PhD
Fellow, Medical Oncology
Department of Medicine
Memorial Sloan Kettering Cancer Center
Manhattan, New York

Viswatej Avutu, MD
Assistant Attending
Department of Medicine
Memorial Sloan Kettering Cancer Center
New York, New York

Lauren Baker Banks, MD, PhD
Fellow, Medical Oncology
Department of Medicine
Memorial Sloan Kettering Cancer Center
New York, New York

Marilia Bernardes, MD
Fellow, Infectious Diseases
Department of Medicine
Memorial Sloan Kettering Cancer Center
New York, New York

Alexander P. Boardman, MD
Fellow, Hematology and Oncology
Department of Medicine
Memorial Sloan Kettering Cancer Center
New York, New York

Laura Boucai, MD
Associate Professor of Medicine, Endocrinology
Department of Medicine
Memorial Sloan Kettering Cancer Center
New York, New York

Bharat Burman, MD, PhD
Fellow, Medical Oncology
Department of Medicine
Memorial Sloan Kettering Cancer Center
New York, New York

Mario D. Caldararo, MD, MS
Fellow, Infectious Diseases
Department of Medicine
Memorial Sloan Kettering Cancer Center
New York, New York

Maria Carlo, MD
Assistant Attending
Department of Medicine
Memorial Sloan Kettering Cancer Center
New York, New York

Elizabeth Anne Coffee, MD
Fellow, Neuro-Oncology
Department of Neurology
Memorial Sloan Kettering Cancer Center
New York, New York

Maria Diaz, MD
Fellow, Neuro-Oncology
Department of Neurology
Memorial Sloan Kettering Cancer Center
New York, New York

Lara Dunn, MD
Assistant Attending
Department of Medicine
Memorial Sloan Kettering Cancer Center
New York, New York

Kevin B. Elmore, MD
Fellow, Neuro-Oncology
Department of Neurology
Memorial Sloan Kettering Cancer Center
New York, New York

Dan Feng, MD, PhD
Fellow, Hematology and Oncology
Department of Medicine
Memorial Sloan Kettering Cancer Center
New York, New York

Cesar J. Figueroa Ortiz, MD, MPH
Infectious Diseases Attending
Department of Medicine
Memorial Sloan Kettering Cancer Center
New York, New York

Allyson Flower, MD
Assistant Attending
Department of Pediatrics
Memorial Sloan Kettering Cancer Center
New York, New York

Christina Fong, MD
Fellow, Pediatric Hematology/Oncology
Department of Pediatrics
Memorial Sloan Kettering Cancer Center
New York, New York

Devika Gajria, MD, MPH
Attending Physician
Breast Medicine Service
Memorial Sloan Kettering Cancer Center
New York, New York

Eliza B. Geer, MD
Medical Director, Multidisciplinary Pituitary and Skull Base Tumor Center
Department of Medicine and Neurosurgery
Memorial Sloan Kettering Cancer Center
New York, New York

Mark Blaine Geyer, MD
Assistant Attending
Leukemia Service and Cell Therapy Service
Department of Medicine
Memorial Sloan-Kettering Cancer Center
New York, New York

Daniel Gomez, MD, MBA
Director, Thoracic Radiation Oncology
Vice Chair of Clinical Operations, Department of Radiation Oncology
Memorial Sloan Kettering Cancer Care Center
New York, New York

Jennifer Gorelov, AGNP-BC, MSN, OCN
Nurse Practitioner
Nursing
Memorial Sloan Kettering Cancer Center
New York, New York

Yonina R. Murciano-Goroff, MSc, DPhil, MD
Instructor, Early Drug Development Service
Memorial Sloan Kettering Cancer Center
New York, New York

An Thi Nhat Ho, MD
Fellow, Interventional Pulmonary
Department of Medicine
Memorial Sloan Kettering Cancer Center
New York, New York

Malin Hultcrantz, MD, PhD
Attending Physician
Myeloma Service, Department of Medicine
Memorial Sloan Kettering Cancer Center
New York, New York

Tony El Jabbour, MD
Fellow, Molecular Genetic Pathology
Department of Pathology
Memorial Sloan Kettering Cancer Center
New York, New York

Niamh M. Keegan, MB, BCH, BAO
Fellow, Medical Oncology
Department of Medicine
Memorial Sloan Kettering Cancer Center
New York, New York

Amber C. King, PharmD, BCOP
Clinical Pharmacy Specialist III
Pharmacy, Clinical Programs
Memorial Sloan Kettering Cancer Center
New York, New York

Mark G. Kris, MD
Attending Physician
Department of Medicine
Memorial Sloan Kettering Cancer Center
New York, New York

Matthew R. Kudelka, MD, PhD
Fellow, Medical Oncology
Department of Medicine
Memorial Sloan Kettering Cancer Center
New York, New York

Josiah D. Land, PharmD, BCOP
Clinical Pharmacy Specialist
Department of Pharmacy
Memorial Sloan Kettering Cancer Center
New York, New York

Emily S. Lebow, MD
Resident Physician
Department of Radiation Oncology
Memorial Sloan Kettering Cancer Center
New York, New York

Jay S. Lee, MD
Fellow, Complex General Surgical Oncology
Department of Surgery
Memorial Sloan Kettering Cancer Center
New York, New York

Alexander M. Lesokhin, MD
Associate Attending Physician
Department of Medicine
Memorial Sloan Kettering Cancer Center
New York, New York

Melissa Amy Lumish, MD
Fellow, Medical Oncology
Department of Medicine
Memorial Sloan Kettering Cancer Center
New York, New York

Jia Luo, MD
Fellow, Medical Oncology
Department of Medicine
Memorial Sloan Kettering Cancer Center
New York, New York

Lauren Martino, MSN, RN
Fertility Nurse Specialist
Memorial Sloan Kettering Cancer Center
New York, New York

Matthew Matasar, MD, MS
Director, MSK Bergen
Department of Medicine
Memorial Sloan Kettering Cancer Center
New York, New York & Montvale, New Jersey

Varun Narendra, MD, PhD
Fellow, Hematology and Medical Oncology
Department of Medicine
Memorial Sloan Kettering Cancer Center
New York, New York

Mariam T. Nawas, MD
Chief Fellow, Hematology
Department of Medicine
Memorial Sloan Kettering Cancer Center
New York, New York

Ryan Q. Notti, MD, PhD
Fellow, Medical Oncology
Department of Medicine
Memorial Sloan Kettering Cancer Center
New York, New York

Juan C. Osorio, MD
Fellow, Medical Oncology
Department of Medicine
Memorial Sloan Kettering Cancer Center
New York, New York

Rekha Parameswaran, MD
Attending
Hematology Service
Memorial Sloan Kettering Cancer Center
New York, New York

Sandeep S. Raj, MD
Fellow, Hematology and Oncology
Department of Medicine
Memorial Sloan Kettering Cancer Center
New York, New York

Ezra Rosen, MD, PhD
Assistant Professor of Medical Oncology
Department of Medicine
Memorial Sloan Kettering Cancer Center
New York, New York

Maria Rubinstein, MD
Assistant Attending, Gynecologic Medical Oncology
Department of Medicine
Memorial Sloan Kettering Cancer Center
New York, New York

Anton Safonov, MD
Fellow, Medical Oncology
Department of Medicine
Memorial Sloan Kettering Cancer Center
New York, New York

Jennifer A. Salant, MD
Director, Pediatric Advanced Care Team
Department of Pediatrics
Weill Cornell Medicine
Fellow, Hospice and Palliative Medicine
Memorial Sloan Kettering Cancer Center
New York, New York

Leonard Saltz, MD
Attending Physician and Member
Department of Medicine
Memorial Sloan Kettering Cancer Center
New York, New York

Alison Schram, MD
Assistant Attending Physician
Department of Medicine
Memorial Sloan Kettering Cancer Center
New York, New York

Michael Scordo, MD
Assistant Attending, Adult Bone Marrow Transplant Service, Cellular Therapy Service
Department of Medicine
Memorial Sloan Kettering Cancer Center
New York, New York

Monika K. Shah, MD
Deputy Physician-in-Chief, Education and Faculty Affairs
Memorial Sloan Kettering Cancer Center
New York, New York

Stacy Stabler, MD, PhD
Associate Attending, Supportive Care
Department of Medicine
Memorial Sloan Kettering Cancer Center
New York, New York

Zsofia K. Stadler, MD
Clinic Director, Clinical Genetics Service
Gastrointestinal Oncology, Associate Attending Physician
Department of Medicine
Memorial Sloan Kettering Cancer Center
New York, New York

Maximilian Stahl, MD
Chief Fellow, Hematology
Department of Medicine
Memorial Sloan Kettering Cancer Center
New York, New York

Robert Stuver, MD
Fellow, Medical Oncology and Hematology
Lymphoma Division
Memorial Sloan Kettering Cancer Center
New York, New York

Martin S. Tallman, MD
Chief, Leukemia Service
Memorial Sloan Kettering Cancer Center
New York, New York

William D. Tap, MD
Chief, Sarcoma Medical Oncology Service
Co-Director of AYA Program
Department of Medicine
Memorial Sloan Kettering Cancer Center
New York, New York

Santosha A. Vardhana, MD, PhD
Assistant Professor
Medicine, Lymphoma Service
Memorial Sloan Kettering Cancer Center
New York, New York

Vibhor Wadhwa, MD
Fellow, Interventional Radiology
Department of Radiology
Weill Cornell Medical Center
Memorial Sloan Kettering Cancer Center
New York, New York

Julian A. Waksal, MD
Chief Resident
Department of Medicine
Memorial Sloan Kettering Cancer Center
New York, New York

Beatriz Wills, MD
Chief Fellow, Hematology
Department of Medicine
Memorial Sloan Kettering Cancer Center
New York, New York

Xiaodi Wu, MD, PhD
Fellow, Medical Oncology
Department of Medicine
Memorial Sloan Kettering Cancer Center
New York, New York

CONTRIBUTING AUTHORS

Ghassan K. Abou-Alfa, MD, MBA
Professor
Department of Medicine
Memorial Sloan Kettering Cancer Center
New York, New York

Tarik Al-Bermani, MD
Chief Resident
Department of Medicine
Memorial Sloan Kettering Cancer Center
New York, New York

Dean Bajorin, MD, FACP
Attending Physician and Member, Memorial Hospital
Department of Medicine
Memorial Sloan Kettering Cancer Center
New York, New York

Ryma Benayed, MS, PhD
Associate Attending
Department of Pathology
Memorial Sloan Kettering Cancer Center
New York, New York

Julia Glade Bender, MD
Vice Chair for Clinical Research; Member, Memorial Hospital
Department of Pediatrics
Memorial Sloan Kettering Cancer Center
New York, New York

Victoria Blinder, MD, MSc
Associate Attending
Department of Psychiatry
Department of Medicine
Memorial Sloan Kettering Cancer Center
New York, New York

Jessie Bourcier, MD
Research Fellow
Omar Abdel-Wahab Lab—Human Oncology and Pathogenesis Program
Memorial Sloan Kettering Cancer Center
New York, New York

Kelsey Breen, MS, MSc
Senior Genetic Counselor
Department of Medicine
Memorial Sloan Kettering Cancer Center
New York, New York

Alexandra Budhai, MD
Attending Physician
Laboratory Medicine
Memorial Sloan Kettering Cancer Center
New York, New York

Michael J. Buege, PharmD
Clinical Pharmacy Specialist
Department of Pharmacy
Memorial Sloan Kettering Cancer Center
New York, New York

Sheng F. Cai, MD, PhD
Assistant Attending
Department of Medicine, Leukemia Service
Memorial Sloan Kettering Cancer Center
New York, New York

María I. Cancio, MD
Assistant Professor
Department of Pediatrics
Memorial Sloan Kettering Cancer Center
New York, New York

Fiorella Iglesias Cardenas, MD, MS
Assistant Attending
Department of Pediatrics
Memorial Sloan Kettering Cancer Center
New York, New York

Andrea Cercek, MD
Associate Attending Physician
Department of Gastrointestinal Oncology
Memorial Sloan Kettering Cancer Center
New York, New York

Jason E. Chan, MD, PhD
Instructor, Sarcoma Medical Oncology Service
Department of Medicine
Memorial Sloan Kettering Cancer Center
New York, New York

Paul Chapman, MD
Attending Physician, Melanoma Service
Department of Medicine
Memorial Sloan Kettering Cancer Center
New York, New York

Mohit Chawla, MD, FCCP
Chief
Pulmonary Service, Department of Medicine
Memorial Sloan Kettering Cancer Center
New York, New York

Martin. S. Chin, MD
Attending Psychiatrist
Department of Psychiatry and Behavioral Sciences
Memorial Sloan Kettering Cancer Center
New York, New York

Christina Cho, MD
Assistant Attending
Department of Medicine
Memorial Sloan Kettering Cancer Center
New York, New York

Philip Choi, MD, PhD
Fellow, Medical Oncology and Hematology
Department of Medicine
Memorial Sloan Kettering Cancer Center
New York, New York

Noura Choudhury, MD
Assistant Attending, Thoracic Oncology & Early Drug Development Services
Memorial Sloan Kettering Cancer Center
New York, New York

Christopher H. Crane, MD
Attending
Department of Radiation Oncology
Memorial Sloan Kettering Cancer Center
New York, New York

Michael I. D'Angelica, MD, FACS
Attending, Department of Surgery
Director, Hepatopancreatobiliary Fellowship Program
Director, Surgical Oncology Fellowship Program
Vice Chair, Education
Memorial Sloan Kettering Cancer Center
New York, New York

Chau Dang, MD
Medical Director
Department of Medicine
Memorial Sloan Kettering Cancer Center
West Harrison, New York

Nicole Daukshus, PharmD
Pediatric Hematology/Oncology Clinical Pharmacy Specialist
Department of Pharmacy
Memorial Sloan Kettering Cancer Center
New York, New York

Susan Ehrenkranz De Wolf, MD
Instructor
Department of Medicine
Memorial Sloan Kettering Cancer Center
New York, New York

Melanie Degliuomini, MD
Fellow Physician
Department of Pediatrics
Memorial Sloan Kettering Cancer Center
New York, New York

Anjali Varma Desai, MD, MSCE
Attending Physician, Supportive Care and Hospital Medicine Services
Department of Medicine
Memorial Sloan Kettering Cancer Center
New York, New York

Joshua Z. Drago, MD
Assistant Attending Physician
Breast Medicine Service
Memorial Sloan Kettering Cancer Center
New York, New York

Ira J. Dunkel, MD
Attending Pediatric Oncologist
Department of Pediatrics
Memorial Sloan Kettering Cancer Center
New York, New York

Stephen Eng, PharmD, BCOP
Bone Marrow Transplant Clinical Pharmacy Specialist
Department of Pharmacy
Memorial Sloan Kettering Cancer Center
New York, New York

Zachary Epstein-Peterson, MD
Assistant Attending
Department of Medicine
Lymphoma Service, Division of Hematologic Malignancies
Memorial Sloan Kettering Cancer Center
New York, New York

Maly Fenelus, MD, MPH
Medical Director, Clinical Hemostasis and Coagulation Laboratory
Laboratory Medicine
Memorial Sloan Kettering Cancer Center
New York, New York

Emanuela Ferraro, MD
Fellow, Clinical Research
Breast Medicine Service
Memorial Sloan Kettering Cancer Center
New York, New York

Olga T. Filippova, MD, MSc
Fellow, Gynecology Service
Department of Surgery
Memorial Sloan Kettering Cancer Center
New York, New York

Kelly N. Fitzgerald, MD
Fellow, Medical Oncology
Department of Medicine
Memorial Sloan Kettering Cancer Center
New York, New York

Michael B. Foote, MD
Fellow, Medical Oncology and Hematology
Memorial Sloan Kettering Cancer Center
New York, New York

Samantha Francis, MD
Assistant Attending
Medicine/Supportive Care
Memorial Sloan Kettering Cancer Center
New York, New York

Samuel Freedman, MD
Assistant Attending
Hospital Medicine
Memorial Sloan Kettering Cancer Center
New York, New York

Samuel A. Funt, MD
Assistant Attending
Department of Medicine, Division of Genitourinary Oncology
Memorial Sloan Kettering Cancer Center
New York, New York

Karuna Ganesh, MD, PhD
Assistant Member and Attending Physician
Molecular Pharmacology Program, Sloan Kettering Institute and Gastrointestinal Oncology Service
Department of Medicine
Memorial Sloan Kettering Cancer Center
New York, New York

Aaron D. Goldberg, MD, PhD
Assistant Attending Physician
Leukemia Service, Department of Medicine
Memorial Sloan Kettering Cancer Center
New York, New York

Sushmita Gordhandas, MD
Fellow, Gynecologic Oncology
Department of Surgery
Memorial Sloan Kettering Cancer Center
New York, New York

Rachel N. Grisham, MD
Associate Attending, Gynecologic Medical Oncology
Department of Medicine
Memorial Sloan Kettering Cancer Center
New York, New York

Christian Grommes, MD
Attending Physician
Department of Neurology
Memorial Sloan Kettering Cancer Center
New York, New York

Ayca Gucalp, MD
Assistant Attending Physician
Breast Medicine Service, Department of Medicine
Memorial Sloan Kettering Cancer Center
New York, New York

Brendan J. Guercio, MD
Fellow, Hematology-Oncology
Memorial Sloan Kettering Cancer Center
New York, New York

Jillian Gutierrez, PharmD, BCOP
Bone Marrow Transplant Clinical Pharmacy Specialist
Department of Pharmacy
Memorial Sloan Kettering Cancer Center
New York, New York

Allan Halpern, MD, MSc
Chief
Dermatology Service
Associate Vice Chairman
Department of Medicine
Memorial Sloan Kettering Cancer Center
New York, New York

Benjamin Herzberg, MD
Chief Fellow, Medical Oncology
Department of Medicine
Memorial Sloan Kettering Cancer Center
New York, New York

Daniel S. Higginson, MD
Assistant Member
Department of Radiation Oncology
Memorial Sloan Kettering Cancer Center
New York, New York

Alan L. Ho, MD, PhD
Associate Member
Department of Medicine
Memorial Sloan Kettering Cancer Center
New York, New York

Steven Horwitz, MD
Member and Attending Physician
Department of Medicine
Memorial Sloan Kettering Cancer Center
New York, New York

Zahra Hudda, MD
Fellow, Pediatric Hematology-Oncology
Memorial Sloan Kettering Cancer Center
New York, New York

Andrew D. Hunter, MD/MPH
Fellow, Hospice and Pallative Medicine
Memorial Sloan Kettering Cancer Center
New York, New York

Brandon S. Imber, MD, MA
Assistant Attending Radiation Oncologist
Department of Radiation Oncology
Memorial Sloan Kettering Cancer Center
New York, New York

Priya Jaisinghani, MD
Fellow, Endocrinology
Endocrinology, Diabetes & Metabolism/Internal Medicine
New York Presbyterian-Weill Cornell
Memorial Sloan Kettering Cancer Center
New York, New York

Yelena Y. Janjigian, MD
Associate Professor and Chief of Gastrointestinal Oncology Service
Department of Medicine
Memorial Sloan Kettering Cancer Center
New York, New York

Karan Jatwani, MBBS, MD
Fellow, Hospice and Palliative Medicine
Department of Medicine
Memorial Sloan Kettering Cancer Center
New York, New York

Hyeyoung Erin Jeun, MD
Fellow, Hospice and Palliative Medicine
Memorial Sloan Kettering Cancer Center
New York, New York

Erel Joffe, MD
Assistant Attending
Lymphoma Service, Department of Medicine
Memorial Sloan Kettering Cancer Center
New York, New York

Thomas J. Kaley, MD
Associate Attending
Department of Neurology
Memorial Sloan Kettering Cancer Center
New York, New York

Yugandhara Kate, MD
Fellow, Hospice and Palliative Medicine
Memorial Sloan Kettering Cancer Center
New York, New York

Jonathan Kentley, MBBS, MSC, MRCP (UK)
Research Associate
Department of Dermatology
Memorial Sloan Kettering Cancer Center
New York, New York

Michael Kinnaman, MD
Instructor
Department of Pediatrics
Memorial Sloan Kettering Cancer Center
New York, New York

Christopher A. Klebanoff, MD
Assistant Member and Attending Physician
Human Oncology and Pathogenesis Program, Immuno-Oncology Section
Memorial Sloan Kettering Cancer Center
New York, New York

David Knorr, MD, PhD, MSc
Assistant Attending Physician
Department of Medicine
Memorial Sloan Kettering Cancer Center
New York, New York

Anita Kumar, MD
Assistant Attending, Medical Site Director
Department of Medical Oncology
Memorial Sloan Kettering Cancer Center
New York, New York & Basking Ridge, New Jersey

Alyce M. Kuo, BS
Medical Student
Dermatology Service, Department of Medicine
Memorial Sloan Kettering Cancer Center
New York, New York

Andreana Kwon, MD
Assistant Attending, Clinical Professor
Department of Medicine, Department of Emergency Medicine
Memorial Sloan Kettering Cancer Center
New York, New York

Mario Lacouture, MD
Director, Oncodermatology
Department of Dermatology
Memorial Sloan Kettering Cancer Center
New York, New York

Shilpa S. Lad, MD, MS
Fellow, Psycho-Oncology
Department of Psychiatry
Memorial Sloan Kettering Cancer Center
New York, New York

W. Victoria Lai, MD
Assistant Professor
Department of Medicine
Memorial Sloan Kettering Cancer Center
New York, New York

Madhavi Lakkaraja, MD, MPH
Fellow, Pediatric Hematology Oncology
Memorial Sloan Kettering Cancer Center
New York, New York

Heather Landau, MD, PhD
Assistant Professor
Department of Medicine
Memorial Sloan Kettering Cancer Center
New York, New York

Michael Lattanzi, MD
Fellow, Medical Oncology
Department of Medicine
Memorial Sloan Kettering Cancer Center
New York, New York

Yonit Lavin, MD, PhD
Fellow, Medical Oncology
Department of Medicine
Memorial Sloan Kettering Cancer Center
New York, New York

Chung-Han Lee, MD, PhD
Assistant Attending Physician
Department of Medicine
Genitourinary Oncology Service
Memorial Sloan Kettering Cancer Center
New York, New York

Robert P. Lee, MD
Section Head, Section of Interventional Pulmonology
Pulmonary Service, Department of Medicine
Memorial Sloan Kettering Cancer Center
New York, New York

Ross Levine, MD
Chief, Molecular Cancer Medicine Service
Human Oncology Pathogenesis Program
Memorial Sloan Kettering Cancer Center
New York, New York

Andréa LeVoir, PharmD
Clinical Pharmacy Specialist, Lymphoma
Department of Pharmacy
Memorial Sloan Kettering Cancer Center
New York, New York

Dazhi Liu, PharmD, BCOP
Clinical Pharmacy Specialist
Department of Pharmacy
Memorial Sloan Kettering Cancer Center
New York, New York

Sydney X. Lu, MD, PhD
Assistant Attending Physician
Department of Medicine
Memorial Sloan Kettering Cancer Center
New York, New York

Jennifer Ma, MD
Radiation Oncology Resident Physician
Department of Radiation Oncology
Memorial Sloan Kettering Cancer Center
New York, New York

Kylee Maclachlan, BSc, MBChB, PhD
Postdoctoral Researcher
Memorial Sloan Kettering Cancer Center
New York, New York

Simon Mantha, MD, MPH
Attending Physician
Hematology Service, Department of Medicine
Memorial Sloan Kettering Cancer Center
New York, New York

Michelangelo Marasco, MD, PhD
Research Scholar
Molecular Pharmacology Program
Sloan Kettering Institute
Memorial Sloan Kettering Cancer Center
New York, New York

Salvador Alonso Martinez, MD
Clinical Fellow
Department of Medicine
Memorial Sloan Kettering Cancer Center
New York, New York

Peter Maslak, MD
Chief, Immunology Laboratory Service
Pathology and Laboratory Medicine
Memorial Sloan Kettering Cancer Center
New York, New York

Anthony Rocco Mato, MD
Director, CLL Program
Department of Medicine
Memorial Sloan Kettering Cancer Center
New York, New York

Michael J. Mauro, MD
Leader, Myeloproliferative Neoplasms Program
Leukemia Service, Department of Medicine
Memorial Sloan Kettering Cancer Center
New York, New York

Sheila S. McThenia, MD
Fellow, Pediatric Hematoloy Oncology
Department of Pediatrics
Memorial Sloan Kettering Cancer Center
New York, New York

Scott Millman, MD, PhD
Instructor, Leukemia Service
Memorial Sloan Kettering Cancer Center
New York, New York

Abhinita S. Mohanty, MS
Senior Computational Biologist I
Department of Pathology
Memorial Sloan Kettering Cancer Centre
New York, New York

Jodi Mones, MD
Associate Attending Physician
Department of Medicine
Memorial Sloan Kettering Cancer Center
New York, New York

Natalie Moryl, MD
Attending
Addiction, Hospice and Palliative Care
Supportive Care Service, Department of Medicine
Memorial Sloan Kettering Cancer Center
New York, New York

Alison Moskowitz, MD
Associate Attending
Department of Medicine
Memorial Sloan Kettering Cancer Center
New York, New York

Lea A. Moukarzel, MD
Fellow
Department of Surgery, Gynecology
Memorial Sloan Kettering Cancer Center
New York, New York

Ryan Moy, MD, PhD
Fellow, Medical Oncology
Department of Medicine
Memorial Sloan Kettering Cancer Center
New York, New York

Samyukta Mullangi, MD, MBA
Fellow, Medical Oncology
Department of Medicine
Memorial Sloan Kettering Cancer Center
New York, New York

Sapir Nachum, MD
Resident Physician
Memorial Sloan Kettering Cancer Center
New York, New York

Benjamin Alexander Nacev, MD, PhD
Assistant Attending Physician
Department of Medicine
Memorial Sloan Kettering Cancer Center
New York, New York

Ariela Noy, MD
Attending Physician, Lymphoma Service
Memorial Sloan Kettering Cancer Center
New York, New York

Roisin E. O'Cearbhaill, MD
Medical Oncologist
Department of Medicine
Memorial Sloan Kettering Cancer Center
New York, New York

Michael Offin, MD
Assistant Attending, Thoracic Oncology Service
Department of Medicine
Memorial Sloan Kettering Cancer Center
New York, New York

Eileen M. O'Reilly, MD
Attending Physician, Professor of Medicine
Department of Medicine, Gastrointestinal Oncology Service
Memorial Sloan Kettering Cancer Center
New York, New York

Michael V. Ortiz, MD
Assistant Attending
Department of Pediatrics
Memorial Sloan Kettering Cancer Center
New York, New York

Terry Pak, PharmD
Pharmacist
Department of Pharmacy
Memorial Sloan Kettering Cancer Center
New York, New York

M. Lia Palomba, MD
Member and Attending Physician
Department of Medicine
Memorial Sloan Kettering Cancer Center
New York, New York

Jae H. Park, MD
Associate Attending Physician
Department of Medicine, Leukemia Service & Cellular Therapeutics Service
Memorial Sloan Kettering Cancer Center
New York, New York

Tim Peterson, PharmD, BCOP
Clinical Pharmacy Specialist
Department of Pharmacy
Memorial Sloan Kettering Cancer Center
New York, New York

Morgan Pines, MD
Fellow, Pediatric Hematology-Oncology
Department of Pediatrics
Memorial Sloan Kettering Cancer Center
New York, New York

Ioannis Politikos, MD
Assistant Attending
Adult Bone Marrow Transplant Service
Memorial Sloan-Kettering Cancer Center
New York, New York

Michael Postow, MD
Chief, Melanoma Service
Department of Medicine
Memorial Sloan Kettering Cancer Center
New York, New York

Simon N. Powell, MD, PhD
Chair
Department of Radiation Oncology
Memorial Sloan Kettering Cancer Center
New York, New York

David Qualls, MD
Fellow, Hematology and Oncology
Department of Medicine
Memorial Sloan Kettering Cancer Center
New York, New York

Nitya Raj, MD
Assistant Attending Physician
Department of Medicine
Memorial Sloan Kettering Cancer Center
New York, New York

Raajit K. Rampal, MD, PhD
Associate Member
Leukemia Service
Memorial Sloan Kettering Cancer Center
New York, New York

Diane Reidy-Lagunes, BS, MS, MD
Oncologist
Department of Medicine
Associate Deputy Physician-in-Chief, Regional Care Network
President, MSK Medical Staff
Memorial Sloan Kettering Cancer Center
New York, New York

Samantha N. Reiss, PharmD, BCOP
Clinical Pharmacy Specialist
Memorial Sloan Kettering Cancer Center
New York, New York

Gregory J. Riely, MD, PhD
Attending
Department of Medicine
Memorial Sloan Kettering Cancer Center
New York, New York

Carly Rosemore, MD
Fellow, Pediatric Hematology/Oncology
Department of Pediatrics
Memorial Sloan Kettering Cancer Center
New York, New York

Barry S. Rosenstein, PhD
Professor of Radiation Oncology and Genetics & Genomic Science
Icahn School of Medicine at Mount Sinai
Course Director, Radiation and Cancer Biology
Memorial Sloan Kettering Cancer Center
New York, New York

Jaclyn Rosenzweig, MD
Fellow, Pediatric Hematology/Oncology
Department of Pediatrics
Memorial Sloan Kettering Cancer Center
New York, New York

Sameer Farouk Sait, MBBS
Instructor
Department of Pediatrics
Memorial Sloan Kettering Cancer Center
New York, New York

Reggie T. Saldivar, MD
Associate Program Director, Hospice and Palliative Medicine Fellowship
Assistant Attending
Memorial Sloan Kettering Cancer Center
New York, New York

Gilles Salles, MD, PhD
Chief, Lymphoma Service
Department of Medicine
Memorial Sloan Kettering Cancer Center
New York, New York

Ernesto Santos, MD
Attending Physician
Interventional Radiology Service, Department of Radiology
Memorial Sloan Kettering Cancer Center
New York, New York

Patricia Mae G. Santos, MD, MS
Resident Physician
Department of Radiation Oncology
Memorial Sloan Kettering Cancer Center
New York, New York

Howard I. Scher, MD
D. Wayne Calloway Chair in Urologic Oncology
Head, Biomarker Development Program
Office of the Physician in Chief
Member and Attending Physician
Genitourinary Oncology Service, Department of Medicine
Memorial Sloan Kettering Cancer Center
New York, New York

Adam J. Schoenfeld, MD
Assistant Attending
Department of Medicine
Memorial Sloan Kettering Cancer Center
New York, New York

Joshua D. Schoenfeld, MD, PhD
Fellow, Medical Oncology
Department of Medicine
Memorial Sloan Kettering Cancer Center
New York, New York

Ramy Sedhom, MD
Fellow, Hospice and Palliative Medicine
Memorial Sloan Kettering Cancer Center
New York, New York

Neil H. Segal, MD, PhD
Associate Attending
Gastrointestinal Oncology Service, Department of Medicine
New York, New York

Varun Shah, MD
Fellow
Interventional Pulmonology—Pulmonary Medicine
Memorial Sloan Kettering Cancer Center
New York, New York

Sanam Shahid, MD
Fellow, Pediatric Hematology/Oncology
Department of Pediatrics
Memorial Sloan Kettering Cancer Center
New York, New York

Armin Shahrokni, MD, MPH
Associate Attending
Department of Medicine
Memorial Sloan Kettering Cancer Center
New York, New York

Anupriya Singhal, MD, PhD
Fellow, Medical Oncology
Department of Medicine
Memorial Sloan Kettering Cancer Center
New York, New York

Emily Slotkin, MD
Assistant Attending, Pediatric Sarcoma Service
Department of Pediatrics
Memorial Sloan Kettering Cancer Center
New York, New York

Melody Smith, MD, MS
Assistant Attending
Adult Blood & Marrow Stem Cell Transplantation Service, Department of Medicine
Memorial Sloan Kettering Cancer Center
New York, New York

James W. Smithy, MD, MHS
Fellow, Medical Oncology
Department of Medicine
Memorial Sloan Kettering Cancer Center
New York, New York

Krisoula H. Spatz, PharmD
Clinical Pharmacy Specialist
Department of Pediatric Oncology
Memorial Sloan Kettering Cancer Center
New York, New York

Barbara Spitzer, MD
Assistant Attending, Transplantation and Cellular Therapy Service
Department of Pediatrics
Memorial Sloan Kettering Cancer Center
New York, New York

Robert Stanley, MD, PhD
Fellow, Oncology
Department of Medicine
Memorial Sloan Kettering Cancer Center
New York, New York

Jessica Stiefel, MD, MS
Assistant Attending
Department of Pediatrics
Memorial Sloan Kettering Cancer Center
New York, New York

Aaron James Stonestrom, MD, PhD
Fellow, Hematology & Medical Oncology
Department of Medicine
Memorial Sloan Kettering Cancer Center
New York, New York

Maria Luisa Sulis, MD
Member, Attending physician
Department of Pediatrics
Memorial Sloan Kettering Cancer Center
New York, New York

Neil K. Taunk, MD, MSCTS
Assistant Professor
Radiation Oncology
University of Pennsylvania
Philadelphia, Pennsylvania

William P. Tew, MD
Attending
Clinical Director
Gynecologic Oncology Service
Department of Medicine
Memorial Sloan Kettering Cancer Center
New York, New York

Meghan C. Thompson, MD
Fellow, Hematology & Medical Oncology
Department of Medicine
Memorial Sloan Kettering Cancer Center
New York, New York

Katherine Thornton, MD
Associate Attending, Medical Oncology
Department of Medicine
Memorial Sloan Kettering Cancer Center
New York, New York

Tiffany A. Traina, MD
Vice Chair, Oncology Care
Breast Medicine Service, Department of Medicine
Memorial Sloan Kettering Cancer Center
New York, New York

Alexandre G. Troullioud Lucas, MD, MSc
Fellow, Pediatric Hematology/Oncology
Department of Pediatrics
Memorial Sloan Kettering Cancer Center
New York, New York

Grashma Vadakkel, PharmD, BCOP
Bone Marrow Transplant Clinical Pharmacy Specialist
Bone Marrow Transplant
Memorial Sloan Kettering Cancer Center
New York, New York

Anna M. Varghese, MD
Assistant Attending
Department of Medicine
Division of Solid Tumor Oncology, Gastrointestinal Oncology Service
Memorial Sloan Kettering Cancer Center
New York, New York

Maya Viavant, MD
Chief Resident
Department of Medicine
Memorial Sloan Kettering Cancer Center
New York, New York

Andrew Vickers, PhD
Attending Research Methodologist
Epidemiology and Biostatistics
Memorial Sloan Kettering Cancer Center
New York, New York

Martin H. Voss, MD
Clinical Director, Genitourinary Oncology Service
Department of Medicine
Memorial Sloan Kettering Cancer Center
New York, New York

Alice Chia-chi Wei, MD, MSc, FRCSC, FACS
Associate Attending Surgeon
Department of Surgery
Memorial Sloan Kettering Cancer Center
New York, New York

Taylor M. Weis, PharmD
Clinical Pharmacist Specialist—Leukemia
Department of Pharmacy
Memorial Sloan Kettering Cancer Center
New York, New York

N. Ari Wijetunga, MD, PhD, MS
Resident
Department of Radiation Oncology
Memorial Sloan Kettering Cancer Center
New York, New York

Jessica A. Wilcox, MD
Assistant Attending
Department of Neurology
Memorial Sloan Kettering Cancer Center
New York, New York

Cy R. Wilkins, MD
Assistant Attending Physician—Hematology Service
Department of Medicine
Memorial Sloan Kettering Cancer Center
New York, New York

Rona Yaeger, MD
Associate Attending Physician
Department of Medicine
Memorial Sloan Kettering Cancer Center
New York, New York

Yoshiya (Josh) Yamada, MD, FRCPC
Attending Radiation Oncologist
Department of Radiation Oncology
Memorial Sloan Kettering Cancer Center
New York, New York

William A. Zammarrelli III, MD
Fellow, Gynecologic Oncology
Department of Surgery
Memorial Sloan Kettering Cancer Center
New York, New York

Marjorie G. Zauderer, MD, MS, FACP
Associate Attending and Co-Director of MSK Mesothelioma Program
Memorial Sloan Kettering Cancer Center
New York, New York

Michael J. Zelefsky, MD, FASTRO
Professor of Radiation Oncology
Department of Radiation Oncology
Memorial Sloan Kettering Cancer Center
New York, New York

Binbin Zheng-Lin, MD, MSc
Chief Medical Resident
Department of Medicine
Memorial Sloan Kettering Cancer Center
New York, New York

Etay Ziv, MD, PhD
Assistant Attending
Department of Radiology
Memorial Sloan Kettering Cancer Center
New York, New York

FOREWORD

This is the third edition of the *Pocket Oncology*. The prior editions have proven to be highly successful. Since there have been significant advances particularly in the areas of immuno-oncology and precision medicine over the past several years, we wanted to keep *Pocket Oncology* fresh. The authors of the chapters are top-notch cancer specialists from Memorial Sloan Kettering Cancer Center and as in the first and second editions our experts are often partnered with our outstanding trainees. *Pocket Oncology* is intended to provide a concise, practical reference for trainees and clinicians in the fields of medical oncology and hematology. It spans a wide range of topics critical to the care of patients across the spectrum of cancer types and stages. It is intended to be a succinct and practical resource that enables clinicians to find essential information quickly and efficiently. We hope you find the handbook to be a valued resource that helps you care for patients.

Deb Schrag, MD, MPH
Chair, Department of Medicine
Memorial Sloan Kettering Cancer Center

PREFACE

It is with great enthusiasm that we introduce the third edition of *Pocket Oncology*. Since the release of the second edition, both the field of oncology and the world at large have changed dramatically, with a cascade of new drug approvals, expansion of precision medicine and immuno-oncology, and of course, the COVID-19 pandemic. This latest edition of *Pocket Oncology* reflects these updates while maintaining the conciseness and brevity that characterize the *Pocket Medicine* series.

Several new sections have been added to this updated edition, including an entirely new section dedicated to pediatric oncology. In recognition of the multidisciplinary teams needed to care for patients with cancer, we have also incorporated new sections on the principles of surgical oncology, interventional radiology, and interventional pulmonology. Finally, new material on telemedicine and COVID-19 provide guidance on how the COVID-19 pandemic has altered the delivery of oncologic care. Beyond new content, each disease section has been thoroughly reviewed and updated by a team of experts at Memorial Sloan Kettering Cancer Center to reflect cancer care in 2022.

As with prior editions, we have organized this handbook into 29 thematic sections that cover the breadth of hematology and oncology for both adults and children. The handbook is further subdivided into short chapters covering specific diseases or concepts, with tables and figures included within each spread for quick reference. We have also incorporated a section of clinically essential color photos and appendices.

Cancer is too complex a disease to attempt to summarize in a handbook of any size. Clinical decision making and a nuanced understanding of the field certainly require additional reading and consultation. *Pocket Oncology* is only intended to be a quick reference and educational guide, providing useful information and general context until more definitive resources such as the primary literature can be consulted. It is not a substitute for good clinical judgment nor intended to influence clinical decisions.

Pocket Oncology was composed with an emphasis on information that general oncology providers and providers in training might find important. Each chapter was written by a resident, fellow, or pharmacist, and subsequently reviewed by an attending faculty member for accuracy and completeness. We are grateful for the efforts of all the contributors at Memorial Sloan Kettering Cancer Center who have made this handbook possible.

Should you have any comments or suggestions, please feel free to contact us through the publisher. We hope that you will find this edition of *Pocket Oncology* useful!

NOURA CHOUDHURY AND YONINA R. MURCIANO-GOROFF, EDITORS

CANCER EPIDEMIOLOGY

Cancer epidemiology research methods

- **Epidemiology:** Study of distribution, determinants, & outcomes of CA at a population level; applies public health or policy perspective, rather than the perspective of an individual pt
- **"Efficacy":** Tx demonstrates an effect, often in a clinical trial, vs. **"effectiveness":** Effect in "real-world," at the population level
- **Observational studies:** Cross-sectional, cohort, & case-control
- **Experimental studies:** Individual-based vs. community-based
- Epidemiology research can include analyses of patterns of care, comparative outcomes, cost-effectiveness, & healthcare disparities
  - A classic study showed women w/ breast CA who are uninsured or on Medicaid had a higher risk of death compared to women w/ private insurance (*NEJM* 1993;329:326)
- **Molecular & genetic epidemiology:** Identification of biomarkers & genetic features linked to CA susceptibility

Cancer cases & deaths

U.S. cancer incidence trends 2003–2017 (*ACS Cancer Facts & Figures* 2021)

- CA is the 2nd leading cause of death in the United States, incidence ↑ w/ aging population
- Higher overall mortality in non-Hispanic black > non-Hispanic white > American Indian/Alaska Native > Hispanic > Asian/Pacific Islander
- Overall ↑ breast & uterine CA cases d/t ↓ fertility rate & ↑ body wt
- Lung CA cases ↓ twice as fast in men compared to women d/t decline in smoking
- Overall ↓ in colorectal CA cases, but ↑ in adults <65 y
- Liver CA incidence stabilized in men but ↑ in women d/t ↑ HCV infxn (opioid epidemic)
- Overall ↓ in prostate CA d/t ↓ in PSA screening, but ↑ in distant-stage prostate CA
- ↑ in CA of kidney, pancreas, melanoma, oral cavity, & pharynx CA incidence (in non-Hispanic Whites)
- ↑ mortality in CA of uterine corpus, oral cavity, pharynx, & pancreas

Figure 1-1 2021 estimates for leading sites of new cancer cases and deaths in the United States. (Adapted with permission, *ACS Facts & Figures* 2021.)

Estimated New Cases

Males			Females		
Prostate	248,530	26%	Breast	281,550	30%
Lung & bronchus	119,100	12%	Lung & bronchus	116,660	13%
Colon & rectum	79,520	8%	Colon & rectum	69,980	8%
Urinary bladder	64,280	7%	Uterine corpus	66,570	7%
Melanoma of the skin	62,260	6%	Melanoma of the skin	43,850	5%
Kidney & renal pelvis	48,780	5%	Non-Hodgkin lymphoma	35,930	4%
Non-Hodgkin lymphoma	45,630	5%	Thyroid	32,130	3%
Oral cavity & pharynx	38,800	4%	Pancreas	28,480	3%
Leukemia	35,530	4%	Kidney & renal pelvis	27,300	3%
Pancreas	31,950	3%	Leukemia	25,560	3%
All Sites	**970,250**	**100%**	**All Sites**	**927,910**	**100%**

Estimated Deaths

Males			Females		
Lung & bronchus	69,410	22%	Lung & bronchus	62,470	22%
Prostate	34,130	11%	Breast	43,600	15%
Colon & rectum	28,520	9%	Colon & rectum	24,460	8%
Pancreas	25,270	8%	Pancreas	22,950	8%
Liver & intrahepatic bile duct	20,300	6%	Ovary	22,950	5%
Leukemia	13,900	4%	Uterine corpus	12,940	4%
Esophagus	12,410	4%	Liver & intrahepatic bile duct	9,930	3%
Urinary bladder	12,260	4%	Leukemia	9,760	3%
Non-Hodgkin lymphoma	12,170	4%	Non-Hodgkin lymphoma	8,550	3%
Brain & other nervous system	10,500	3%	Brain & other nervous system	8,100	3%
All Sites	**319,420**	**100%**	**All Sites**	**289,150**	**100%**

Global cancer epidemiology

- **Temporal trends:** (1) CA incidence is ↑ in the developing world d/t ↑ longevity & growing adoption of Western diet, physical inactivity, & tobacco use; (2) ↓ incidence of CAs d/t infectious etiologies (stomach, liver, uterine, cervix)
- **Environmental factors** that contribute to geographic distribution of CA, eg, higher incidence of infxn-related CAs (stomach, liver, cervical) in Sub-Saharan Africa,

East Asia, & Central Asia; higher stomach CA rates in East Asia & Central/Eastern Europe d/t diets high in salt & processed foods, low in fresh fruits & vegetables
- **Migration studies:** Japanese-Americans in California have lower rates of gastric CA compared to Japanese people in Japan but higher rates than non-Japanese California residents (*Cancer* 1965;18:656)

Etiologic agents in cancer

Agent	Cancer(s)
Tobacco:	
• Causes 30% of all CA deaths, up to 40% in men in some Southern states • Overall ↓ in smoking prevalence, less in those w/ low levels of education • In 1950, the 1st large study published linking smoking & lung CA (*BMJ* 1950;2:739; *JAMA* 1950;143:329) • Tobacco-related carcinogens → covalent bonds formed w/ DNA → DNA adducts → miscoding → mts	Lung, larynx, nasal, oral cavity, esophagus, liver, pancreas, cervix, bladder, kidney, leukemia, stomach, & colorectal Smokeless tobacco: Oral, esophageal, pancreas E-cigarettes (vaping): Long-term risks not yet known
Infectious:	
HCV	Liver, NHL
HBV	Liver
EBV	Burkitt lymphoma, nasopharynx, Hodgkin lymphoma, stomach
HHV-8	Kaposi sarcoma, pulm effusion lymphoma, Castleman dz
HPV	Anogenital, cervix, oral cavity
Merkel cell polyomavirus (MCV)	Merkel cell carcinoma
JC virus	PML
HTLV-1	Adult T-cell leukemia/lymphoma
HIV-associated	Kaposi sarcoma, cervix, various NHL
H. Pylori	Stomach, gastric MALT lymphoma
Schistosomiasis	Bladder (squamous cell)
Liver flukes (*Clonorchis sinensis*)	Cholangiocarcinoma
Inflammation:	
Reflux esophagitis	Barrett esophagitis → esophageal CA
Liver cirrhosis	Liver CA
Chronic pancreatitis	Pancreas CA
Chemical Factors:	
Asbestos, silica	Lung, mesothelioma
Radon, nickel dust, arsenic, chromium	Lung
Aromatic amines	Bladder
Cadmium	Prostate
Benzene	Leukemia
Aflatoxin	Liver
Estrogen (HRT)	Breast, endometrial
Androgen	Prostate
Immunosuppressants	NHL
Chemotherapy (alkylating agent, platinum, anthracycline)	MDS, leukemia
Physical Factors:	
RT	MDS, leukemia, breast, thyroid, GI
Radiation (Chernobyl, atomic bomb)	Thyroid, leukemia, other solid tumors
UV light	Skin CAs
Lifestyle Factors:	
Obesity	Esophagus, endometrium, kidney, liver, gallbladder, stomach, multiple myeloma, pancreas, colorectal, breast, thyroid
EtOH	Oral cavity, esophagus, liver, colorectal, breast
Smoked, salted, pickled foods	Stomach
Red meat	Colorectal

CANCER PREVENTION & SCREENING

General principles

- 1° **CA prevention:** To **reduce CA incidence** & mortality, eg, smoking cessation, sun avoidance, cancer virus vaccination, chemoprevention
- 2° **CA prevention:** To **identify asx CA** w/ goal of earlier interventions & mortality reduction. Most CA screening is 2° prevention
- Various guidelines (USPSTF, NCCN, ACS, ASCO, etc.) differ

Breast cancer

- 1° **prevention:**
  - **Surgery:** See "Cancer Genetics section"
  - **Chemoprevention:**
    - For postmenopausal women, use aromatase inhibitors (anastrozole, exemestane), raloxifene, tamoxifen to reduce incidence of breast CA (DXA prior to aromatase inhibitor). In premenopausal women, avoid aromatase inhibitors (*JCO* 2019;37:33)
    - Who should be treated?
      - ASCO: For women ≥35 y: h/o atypical hyperplasia or LCIS, chest wall RT <30 y, est. 5-y risk of breast CA ≥3% (NCI BCRAT calc), est. 10-y risk ≥5% (IBIS calc), or RR ≥4× avg person 40–44 y or ≥2× in 45–69 y
      - USPSTF: Offer to prescribe to women ≥35 y who are at ↑ risk of breast CA & at low risk for adverse effects (does not define risk factors)
    - Some risks: Tamoxifen/raloxifene a/w ↑ thromboembolic events. Tamoxifen w/ ↑ risk of endometrial CA (*JAMA* 2019;322(9):868)
  - **Lifestyle modification:** EtOH, smoking, obesity ↑ risk. Exercise likely to ↓ risk
- **Rec screening for avg-risk women** (for high-risk women, see "Cancer Genetics section"). Individualized approach (screening guidelines vary)
  - NCCN: Annual MMG for women 40–74 y. 75 y+ continue annual screening if life expectancy >10 y (*"Breast Cancer Screening and Diagnosis," NCCN Guidelines® Version 1.2021*)
  - ACS: Ages 40–44 can offer annual MMG, 45–54 annual MMG, 55+ biennial or annual MMGs, continue until life expectancy <10 y (ACS 2021)
  - USPSTF: Can offer biennial MMG 40–50 y. For women 50–74 y, biennial MMG. Insufficient evidence for screening in women 75 y+ (*USPSTF 2016 Guidelines*)
  - Tomosynthesis can decrease call-back rates & improve CA detection; not available at all centers; currently being studied to assess for mortality benefit
  - Dense breast tissue: MMG has lower sensitivity in this setting but currently insufficient evidence to recommend supplemental imaging
- **Annual MRI:** For *BRCA* mt carriers > age 25 (adjunct to annual MMG), untested 1st-degree relatives of *BRCA* mt carriers (>25 y), Li–Fraumeni syndrome, *PTEN*, & Bannayan–Riley–Ruvalcaba syndromes, lifetime risk of ≥20% using risk assessment models, h/o chest RT 10–30 y
- **U/S:** Not routinely rec for screening

Cervical cancer

- **Vaccination:** Directed at HPV subtypes (16 & 18 responsible for 70% of cervical CA, 31, 33, 45, 52, & 56 responsible for 20%); rec by ACIP for everyone 11–12 y (as early as 9 y), catch-up through 26 y; individualized for >26 y
  - **9-valent HPV vaccine** (Gardasil® 9): Protects against high-risk HPV subtypes, incl. 6, 11, 16, 18, 31, 33, 45, 52, 56 (quadrivalent; bivalent no longer in the United States)
    - Prevents 97% of high-grade **cervical, vulvar, or vaginal dz** related to the 9 HPV types in the vaccine in pts neg for these HPV subtypes prior to vaccination (*NEJM* 2015;372:711)
    - Efficacy in preventing **anal** SIL 2/2 the relevant HPV vaccine subtypes was 78% in HPV-naive men (50% overall) (*NEJM* 2011;365(17):1576)
    - Granted approval for prevention of **oropharyngeal** dz based on effectiveness against anogenital dz
    - Continued protection for at least 10 y
- **Screening methods:** Cytologic methods (liquid-based cytology more common than pap smears); HPV DNA testing for high-risk subtypes often used as co-testing
  - No formal guidelines on screening for **anal** lesions (trials currently in progress—ANCHOR study). Some groups suggest HIV-infected MSM
- **Age at screening initiation:** Begin screening at age 21 even if not sexually active, even if received HPV vaccine (other oncogenic HPV subtypes); avoid screening if younger than 21 y as cervical CA is rare & overtreatment can lead to complications

- **Screening frequency:** q3y w/ cytology alone for ages 21–29, more frequently if immunocompromised (eg, HIV-infected), h/o cervical dysplasia/CA, in utero DES exposure; for age 30–65, q5y cytology + HPV DNA co-testing (preferred) or cytology alone q3y
- **Discontinue screening if:** S/p total hysterectomy for benign dz & no residual cervix (& no h/o CIN 2 or higher for at least 20 y); intact cervix, age >65 (if adequate neg prior results: 3 consecutive neg cytology results or 2 consecutive neg co-test results w/in past 10 y)

Colon cancer

- **Prevention in familial syndromes:** See "Cancer Genetics section"
- **Prevention:** Polypectomy, removal of adenomatous polyps; USPSTF: Adults 50–59 y w/ ≥10% CVD risk, rec low-dose aspirin for 1° prevention of CVD, CRC if low bleeding risk—must take for 10 y (*Ann Intern Med* 2016;164:836)
- **Screening modalities:** Colonoscopy; flexible sigmoidoscopy; CT colonography: All capable of detecting CA as well as precancerous adenomas; stool-based tests: Detect CA but not adenomas. **Follow abnl stool test results w/ full colonoscopy**
  For avg-risk pt, use of structural exam vs. high-sensitivity stool-based test depends on pt preference

Screening Recommendations for Individuals at Average Risk*	
Colonoscopy (preferred)	q10y
Flexible sigmoidoscopy	q5y (*NEJM* 2012;366:2345) ± immunohistochemical (IHC) testing at 3 y
Stool-based (guaiac, IHC or DNA-based)	Annually (guaiac or IHC) or q3y (DNA-based), consider w/ flex sigmoidoscopy q10y
CT colonography	No consensus, but q5y may be sufficient; note may see extracolonic findings of unclear significance

*Age ≥45; no personal h/o adenoma, CRC, inflammatory bowel dz; no family h/o CRC.

- **When to begin screening**
  - **Avg risk:** 45 y (ACS, ACG), 50 y (USPSTF) until 75 y (75–85 y individualized approach)
  - **1st-degree relative w/ CRC <50 y or 1st-degree relatives w/ CRC at any age:** Age 40 or 10 y before earliest dx of 1st-degree relative, whichever first
  - **1st-degree relative w/ CRC aged ≥50:** Age 45 or 10 y before earliest dx, whichever 1st
  - **1st-degree relative w/ advanced adenoma(s):** Age 45 or at age of onset of relative, whichever 1st
- **Screening intervals:** Shorter than q10y if:
  - + Family hx; suboptimal colonoscopy (poor bowel prep); sx; adenomatous or villous polyps removed during prior colonoscopy

Prostate cancer

- **SELECT trial:** Selenium & vitamin E do not prevent prostate CA (*JAMA* 2011;306(14):1549)
- **PSA testing:** Controversial; early detection may not correlate w/ improved survival, as most prostate CA low-grade, lack of stratification by risk; some risks of screening: False (+) leading to prostate biopsy, overdiagnosis, & overtreatment w/ complications such as incontinence & erectile dysfunction
  - **ERSPC trial:** Reduction in prostate CA-specific but not all-cause mortality from screening (PSA on avg q4y); 1,410 men needed to be screened to prevent 1 death
  - The decision to undergo PSA testing should be individualized—PSA velocity not rec
  - ACS: Discussion on screening at 50 y (avg risk), 45 y (African Americans, 1st-degree relative w/ prostate CA <65 y), 40 y (>1 1st-degree relative w/ prostate CA <65 y)
- **No consensus regarding testing:** Consider age, life expectancy, family hx, risks, & benefits a/w early detection, & tx of prostate CA

Lung cancer

- **Smoking cessation:** Most effective prevention, dose–response relationship of smoking to risk of lung CA
- **Annual low-dose helical CT:** Cumulative rate ratio for death from lung CA at 10 y: 0.67 women, 0.76 men (*NEJM* 2020;382:503)
- **Current recommendations:** Annual LDCT for current smokers or former smokers <15 y since cessation (age 50–80 w/ 20 py smoking hx); discontinue when person stops smoking for 15 y

TELE-ONCOLOGY

General principles

- **Telemedicine:** Use of telecommunications technologies to synchronously deliver care remotely in real time. Telephone communications, email, & video chat technology can deliver care asynchronously
- **Tele-oncology:** The application of telemedicine specifically for the dx, tx, monitoring, & supportive care of pts w/ CA or CA-related conditions
- **Context for growth:** COVID-19 pandemic highlighted importance of telemedicine as a tool for delivering care to pts w/ CA
- "Virtual" visits grew exponentially in spring 2020 during nation-wide quarantine
- Stafford Act invocation and national emergency declaration March 2020: Temporarily incr. reimbursement for telemedicine interactions that were previously restricted
- Remote care likely to remain permanent in some aspects of outpt oncology care

Potential Applications
Initial visit consultations
Follow-up visits
E-Consultations (asynchronous communication b/w healthcare providers)
Toxicity monitoring & mgmt
Post–stem cell transplant surveillance
Care for rural pts w/ limited access to care
Palliative care consultations
Clinical trials (FDA 2021. https://www.fda.gov/media/136238/download)

Considerations

Benefits	Limitations
Incr. access to tertiary care facilities or centers of excellence (*Annu Rev Public Health* 2021;42:463-481)	Access to broadband Internet
Incr. pt convenience & possibly satisfaction (*Ann Fam Med* 2017;15(3):225)	Pt concerns about privacy w/ communication over 3rd party software
Decr. visit burden (*BMJ Open* 2017;7(8):e016242)	Difficulty establishing close pt–provider relationship
Possible reduction in financial toxicity of CA care (*Med J Aust* 2013;199(6):414)	Unclear effect on pt & provider satisfaction
Decr. exposure to healthcare setting associated pathogens	Interstate licensure limitations
Improved access to clinical trials (*Stroke* 2010;41(3):566)	Widening care disparities through language barriers
Incr. exposure to subspecialty care (*Health Affairs* 2014;33(2):336)	Home crowding & lack of privacy Medical malpractice insurance coverage

Administrative hurdles

- **Reimbursement:**
  - Emergency CMS reimbursement for interstate telehealth services expired (CMS.gov). Some intrastate telehealth services are covered, but varies from state to state (CMS.gov)
- **State licensing:** Physicians limited to providing care for pts physically located w/in the state of their medical license, even via telehealth
- **Medical malpractice:** Lack of clarity on malpractice coverage for telehealth, particularly interstate telehealth
- **Documentation:**
  - Obtain & document pt consent for virtual visits
  - Include pt & physician location & audio/visual system used
  - Include CMS level of complexity for each visit
  - Include appropriate limited physical exam components that can be conducted via video (eg, general appearance)
  - Real-time (synchronous) video of visit or recording of phone call is not required to be saved; asynchronous communications (incl. videos or photos) must be stored according to state regulations

PHASE I CLINICAL TRIALS

Phase 0 trials

- Administration of single or several doses (<7 d), often subtherapeutic, of the study drug to a small number of subjects for correlation w/ biomarkers/imaging & gathering of preliminary data on PK & PD; gives no significant data on safety or efficacy

Phase I trials

- Often the initial phase of human experimentation
  - **When to perform:** Novel drug or combination & promising preclinical data
  - **Primary objectives:** Identify drug tox, MTD, schedule, & RP2D
  - **Secondary objectives:** Describe PK/PD, biomarkers, & response rate
  - **Population:** Historically adv CA w/ no std tx options left → now more inclusive of less heavily pretreated pts, good PS, & end-organ fxn, heterogeneous tumor types, may select pts based on genetic abnormality or tumor antigen-HLA type (basket trial)
  - **Starting dose:** Dose chosen to treat 1st cohort based on animal studies, commonly 1/10 of mouse LD_{10} or STD_{10} (dose resulting in death or severe tox of 10% of mice)

Definition of Terms	
CTCAE	Standard rating for severity of tox: Grade 0 (none), 1 (mild), 2 (moderate), 3 (severe), 4 (life-threatening), 5 (fatal)
Dose-limiting tox (DLT)	Unacceptable tox early in tx (eg, C1) that limits further dose escalation, protocol-specific (typically ≥G3 non-heme or ≥G4 heme tox)
Maximum tolerated dose (MTD)	Highest-dose level at which a defined proportion of pts (often ≤33%) experience a DLT
Target tox level	Typically 20–33%, max probability of DLT considered acceptable
Recommended phase II dose (RP2D)	Dose recommended for subsequent phase II trials: Often **MTD or 1 dose level below MTD** (Note: tox after C1 may lead to exploration of alternative dosing or schedule → RP2D)
Biologically effective dose	Dose at which the target is sufficiently inhibited to generate efficacy
Dose–tox curve	Reflects relationship b/w dose & probability of tox for a specific drug
PK	Relationship b/w time following drug admin & plasma concentration, "what body does to drug": Absorption, distribution, metabolism, & excretion; several PK levels taken along study course (Note: Drug–drug & food interactions important to consider)
PD	Drug effects on host, "what drug does to body," incl. tumor & nl tissue; uses biomarker endpoints from tumor &/or nl tissue (ie, skin bx, hair follicles, etc.)
Therapeutic index	Dose required to produce critical tox divided by dose yielding defined antitumor effect

Adapted from *J Natl Cancer Inst* 2009;101:708.

Types of phase I designs *(ASCO Educational Book 41. 2021, e133)*

- **Rule-based designs**
  Examples: Standard 3+3, rolling 6, & accelerated titration dose escalation
  Traditional phase I designs w/ no prior assumptions of dose–tox curve → dose escalation & reduction that are easily implemented w/o need for special mathematical software → MTD based on current dose level & does not incorporate all DLT data
- **Model-based designs**
  Examples: Continual reassessment method (CRM), mCRM, BLRM
  Statistical models that start w/ initial dose–tox curve → model modified by tox experienced by pts on trial → MTD estimated w/ confidence interval & incorporates all DLT data
- **Model-assisted designs**
  Examples: Bayesian optimal interval (BOIN), modified toxicity probability interval (mTPI)
  An attempt to use both predetermined algorithms of rule-based design & statistical models from model-based designs

Traditional 3+3

- Classic phase I clinical trial design where pts are treated initially **in cohorts of 3s** at escalating dose levels, dose-level escalation or deescalation may follow **modified**

Fibonacci sequence: 100% → 67% → 50% → 40% → 33%, intra-pt dose escalation is not historically allowed (contemporary protocols may allow for previously cleared dose levels)

3+3 Design Based on Number of Patients Experiencing DLT per Cohort			
Cohort	**Dose Escalate** (↑ to next higher dose level)	**Expand Cohort** (↑ cohort by 3 pts)	**Dose Deescalate** (↓ to next lower-dose level)
3 pts	0 DLTs	1 DLT	≥2 DLTs
6 pts (expanded)	1 DLT	N/A	≥2/6 DLTs

- MTD definition = Highest-dose level at which ≤33% experience a DLT
- **Advantages:** Relatively simple to implement, multiple pts at each dose level providing more info on PK inter-pt variability per dose level
- **Pitfalls:** Dose escalation is slow, many pts treated at subtherapeutic doses, information from prev dose levels not incorporated into RP2D determination

Accelerated titration (*JNCI* 1997;89:1138)

- Affords rapid initial dose escalation. Wide variety of designs. Intra-pt dose escalation permitted in some designs. Potentially appropriate for drugs w/ wide therapeutic index
- **Design example:** Initial dose-escalation phase w/ single-pt cohorts, dose is doubled until defined stopping rule is hit (eg, drug-related tox ≥G2) → reverts to 3+3 design w/ lower-dose increments b/w cohorts
- MTD can be estimated using all tox data collected during trial or using 3+3 rules
- **Advantages:** Reduces number of pts treated at subtherapeutic doses. Designs w/ intra-pt dose escalation afford tx at higher & potentially more effective doses
- **Pitfalls:** Requires acute tox. Intra-pt dose escalation may mask or falsely attribute cumulative/delayed tox. Aggressive & may expose more pts to higher doses

Continual reassessment method (*Biometrics* 1990;46:33; *JNCI* 2009;101:708)

- **Bayesian approach:** Starts w/ defined acceptable probability of DLT (20–33%), 1–3 pts selected per cohort, starts at dose thought to be close to MTD
- **Design:** Mathematical model for dose–tox curve continuously modified w/ each pt → dose is escalated & deescalated accordingly (next pt treated at new estimated dose close to MTD) → trial stopped if prespecified condition met (eg, 6 pts tx at same dose) or precision in probability of DLT at estimated MTD level is achieved
- **Modified CRM:** Starts at lower dose, escalate 1 dose level at a time but not if last pt had DLT
- **Advantages:** Uses all available data, rapid escalation, thought to provide more precise MTD estimate
- **Pitfalls:** Requires intensive statistical assistance & starting dose/tox assumptions

Other model-based designs (*Biometrics* 2000;56:1177; *JNCI* 2009;101:708)

- **Time-to-event CRM:** Subjects weighted for time observed & model adjusted for late-onset tox; **EffTox & TriCRM:** Incorporate both efficacy & tox

Predicting survival on phase I trials

Royal Marsden Prognostic Score						
Variable	LDH		Albumin, mg/dL		Site of mets	
	<ULN	>ULN	<3.5	>3.5	0–2	>2
Score	0	1	0	1	0	1

JCO 2009;27:2692.

Higher score = worse prognosis

Score	**Median OS (wk)**
0–1	33
2–3	15.7

Emerging issues in phase I clinical trials

- Tox & efficacy of novel agents (targeted Rx, IO) may not be dose dependent → movement toward more rational dose selection (use of BED)

Expansion cohorts

- Add'l pts enrolled after RP2D. Called phase Ib (escalation is phase Ia)
- Objectives: confirm safety of RP2D, prelim efficacy, confirm PK/PD, explore biomarkers

Combination trials

Common approaches include:

(1) Holding 1 dose constant & escalating the other
(2) Viewing each combination as a "dose" & ordering these

PHASE II AND III CLINICAL TRIALS

Definition of Common Statistical Terms Used in Clinical Trials	
Historical controls	Pt previously treated (or not) used as standard for comparison to pt treated in current experimental design
Null hypothesis	Hypothesis that there is no association b/w the intervention & outcome variable
Alternative hypothesis	Hypothesis that there is an effect of the intervention on the outcome variable
Sidedness	2-Sided: Testing for significance of association in **either** direction (better **or** worse, α-split b/w both sides) 1-Sided: Testing for significance of association in 1 direction (better or not, worse or not; full α allotted to 1 side)
Type I error (α)	FP, error of rejecting null when it is actually true
Type II error (β)	FN, error of not rejecting null when it is actually false
Estimate of effect (eg, HR, OR, RR)	Magnitude of effect of the intervention on outcome of interest
p-Value	The probability that the data would be equal to or more extreme than what is observed, while the null hypothesis is true
Intent to treat (ITT)	Endpoint analysis incl. all pts as originally allocated after randomization (regardless of having received tx)
Per-protocol (PP)	Endpoint analysis incl. only those pts who completed the tx to which they were allocated

See limits of P-value: *The American Statistician* 2016;70:129; *NEJM* 2019;381:285.

Common Phase II and III Cancer Trial Endpoints	
OS (overall survival)	Time from study entry/randomization to death from any cause
DFS (dz-free survival)	Time from study entry/randomization to tumor recurrence or death from any cause
PFS (progression-free survival)	Time from study entry/randomization to objective tumor progression or death (assumes deaths are related to progression)
ORR (objective response rate)	Proportion of pts w/ dz reduction of prespecified amount (such as RECIST for solid tumors, ELN criteria for AML, etc.)
Sx endpoints (pt-reported outcomes aka PROs)	Subjective measure of pt sx & fxn (like QOL). Typically used in phase III trials

See *Clinical Trial Endpoints for the Approval of Cancer Drugs & Biologics, FDA-2005-D-0225.*

Phase II trials

- **Primary objectives:** To test antitumor efficacy in a defined clinical setting
- **Secondary objectives:** Usually multiple 2° safety & efficacy endpoints. Statistics & samples size are not built around these but tailored exclusively to the 1° objective
- **Choice of primary endpoint is critical**, most commonly **ORR or PFS**
- **Historical data** guides projection of what standard arm is likely to achieve
- Variations include **combination of phase I/II** which sequence dose determination followed by efficacy assessment & **combination phase II/III** which sequence signal exploration in a smaller cohort to justify immediate expansion to a large, randomized trial comparing to standard control. Both attempt to optimize pace of a registration strategy

Types of phase II designs (*Clin Can Res* 2010;16(6):1764)

- **Single arm**
  - **Single-stage:** All pts enrolled in 1 stage & evaluated for clinical endpoints Generally, no early termination rules except for instances of unacceptable tox
  - 2-Stage: Early termination rule for inefficacy can be triggered after completion of the 1st stage per prespecified efficacy threshold (eg, Simon optimal 2-stage design, Gehan design); if stage 1 goal met, 2nd stage continues accrual to achieve full sample size

Randomized designs

- Noncomparative randomized: Multiple experimental arms, each compared to historical control; essentially, multiple phase II studies, run in parallel
- Comparative:
  - Selection "Pick the Winner": Multi-arm trial w/ each arm compared to control & not powered to compare b/w arms → most efficacious arm evaluated in phase III

- Randomized phase II: Compares investigational to a standard. Requires larger sample size but reduces bias compared to single arm/historical control comparison; thus, can provide stronger signal to justify subsequent phase III effort
- Randomized discontinuation: All pts treated w/ study agent followed by double-blind randomization in pts w/ SD to continuation of study agent vs. placebo
- Useful to determine if continued benefit present

Phase III trials

- Aim is to challenge an approved standard w/ a novel tx or approach
- **Large number** of pts, requires multi-institutional recruitment to reach accrual goals
- **Population:** Single CA type w/ well-defined eligibility criteria

Operational aspects of phase III trials

- **Outcome measurement:** See common endpoints above
  - **Co-primary outcomes:** Used when demonstration of effect on ≥2 outcomes is needed to establish clinical benefit; requires "splitting" of α across the 1° outcomes as all separate endpoints must be statistically significant. Large sample size needed to ↓ error
  - **Composite outcome:** Composed of multiple outcomes, may provide greater power (more events), but each outcome must be of equal importance
  - **Multiple primary outcomes:** Achievement of any 1 of multiple outcomes is sufficient to reject the null hypothesis of no effect, creates multiplicity problem (↑ type I error), many methods to address (eg, hierarchical: Test certain endpoints 1st, only test subsequent endpoints if 1st endpoint significant)
- **Randomization:** Assures baseline characteristics that could confound observed associations are distributed equally among tx groups
  - **Stratified random allocation:** Randomization incorporates an algorithm that ascertains even distribution across groups based on certain prespecified variables (eg, known risk factors for dz, prior lines of therapy, geographical region)
  - **Permuted blocked allocation:** Designed to ensure equal distribution among study groups, randomization performed in "blocks" of predetermined size; used in small trials to achieve small gain in power
  - **Unequal allocation:** Eg, 2:1 design to make trial more attractive to pts; requires larger sample size but affords a larger experience w/ investigational regimen
  - **Crossover:** Pts can enter alternative tx arm at POD (ie, pt receiving placebo offered access to tx arm). May confound OS (*Ann Oncol* 2018;29:1079)
- **Blinding:** ↓ postrandomization source of bias, such as biased outcome assessment; types include 1-sided (pt blinded) vs. double-blinding (physician & pt blinded)
  - **Interim analysis:** Sequential data analysis at prespecified timepoints; enables early termination for futility or confirmed efficacy; typically performed by **Data Monitoring Committees** (DMCs): Independent group of experts who are not study investigators

Types of phase III trials

- **Superiority:** Seeks to show intervention is **superior** to the control (standard of care, placebo, observation) for the outcome of interest
- **Noninferiority:** Seeks to show intervention is **not worse** than control (1-sided hypothesis; goal is to accept alternative hypothesis of no difference); based on **noninferiority margin:** Largest acceptable difference b/w test drug & comparator; study seeks to confirm that the CI of the comparator to standard tx (HR, RR, etc.) is below this threshold in its entirety; sample size generally > superiority
- **Equivalence:** Seeks to show intervention is **not worse & not superior** (2-sided hypothesis); defines smallest difference of practical clinical significance then designs trial w/ power to accept the null hypothesis of no difference; requires large sample

Phase IV trials

- Post-FDA approval, investigation of risk/benefit, efficacy, tox, subpop effect

Adaptive trial designs

- Allow for preplanned trial modifications based on accumulating data as the trial progresses, such as adaptive randomization (eg, see *BMC Medicine* 2018;16:29)
- **Adaptative tx arms:** Prospectively planned modifications to tx arms based on comparative interim results, such as terminating arms early
- **Biomarker-guided adaptation:** Often initiated in broad pop & then adapts strategy w/in a biomarker defined subgroup (eg, adapting tx strategy in pts w/o response but limiting further study to biomarker + pts only) (*JCO* 2012;30:3304)
- **Adaptive randomization:** Many formats; allows for adaptation of randomization & stratification strategy based on early findings (*JNCI* 2019;111:1255)
- **Umbrella trials:** Creates central infrastructure to screen & identify pts, usually of a single tumor type, then test several interventions simultaneously in subtrials

BIOMARKER DEVELOPMENT

Biomarker definition

"A defined characteristic that is measured as an indicator of nl biologic processes, pathogenic processes, or biologic responses to an exposure or intervention, incl. therapeutic interventions; may include molecular, histologic, radiographic, or physiologic characteristics; not a measure of how an individual feels, functions, or survives" (FDA–NIH Biomarker Working Group 2016, https://www.ncbi.nlm.nih.gov/books/NBK326791/)

Types of biomarkers (FDA–NIH Biomarker Working Group 2016)

- **Susceptibility/risk:** Indicates potential for developing dz in currently unaffected pts; guides preventive strategies; may be useful for clinical trial enrichment
- **Prognostic:** Indicates ↑ risk of future clinical event, dz recurrence, or progression in pts w/ dz; measured at baseline usually independent of interventions/drugs, but may include background tx; useful in assessing chance of specified outcomes
- **Diagnostic:** Detects or confirms presence of dz or identifies dz subtype; diagnostic classification may have prognostic or predictive implications
- **Monitoring:** Used for serial assessment of dz status or burden or for evidence of exposure
- **Predictive:** Identifies pts more likely to have favorable response to a tx or exposure; useful in selecting tx & stratifying pts for trials
- **Pharmacodynamic/response:** Assesses biologic response after tx or exposure; often also a monitoring biomarker, may guide dosing or tx discontinuation; may be used as proof of mechanism
- **Safety:** Measures likelihood, presence, or extent of tox before or after tx or exposure
- **Surrogate endpoint:** A substitute outcome measure correlated w/ a direct measure of clinical benefit; for U.S. regulatory purposes, distinguished as validated, reasonably likely, or candidate; allows for rapid drug development

Types of Biomarkers and Examples

Types of Biomarker	Examples
Susceptibility/risk	*BRCA*1/2 mt & ↑ risk of breast CA
Prognostic	Gleason score in prostate CA & risk of progression
Diagnostic	Gene expression profiling for cell-of-origin subtype of DLBCL
Monitoring	PSA in prostate CA; M-spike in MGUS
Predictive	ER status in breast CA & response to endocrine tx
PD/response	FDG-PET (imaging biomarker) in DLBCL restaging
Safety	TPMT mt & metabolism of 6-MP
Surrogate end point	Durable major molecular response in CML

Steps in biomarker development

- **Identify marker of clinical utility:** Evaluate metabolic, biochemical, genetic, & molecular targets or pathways in animal models & preclinical studies
- **Evaluate analytical validity of assay:** Accuracy, precision, & reproducibility; appropriate specimen collection & handling & technical issues; if used to make individual pt decisions, must be done in a **CLIA environment** (http://www.cdc.gov/clia/regulatory/)
- **Clinical validity & utility assessment:** Phase I, II, & III clinical trials; internal validation & external validation; assess reproducibility of the result; provide a statistical design to assess clinical correlations
  - **Discovery** (may be done in small sample size to discover potential markers)
  - **Training** (test previously identified markers in a small independent cohort)
  - **Validation** (test marker in larger pop independent from training set to provide supportive evidence for clinical use)

Biomarkers in the precision medicine era (*Nat Rev Cancer* 2016;16:525)

- **Precision medicine:** Combining clinical data w/ molecular biomarkers to refine dz risk, dx, prog, & tx approach
- **Genomic & epigenomic** alterations, eg, *EGFR* mts in lung CA, *MLH1* promoter methylation after abnl MLH1 IHC in colon CA, (*Nat Rev Gastroenterol Hepatol* 2020;17:111), **RNA & protein** expression (eg, PD-L1 status) all in clinical use; preliminary: Metabolite & microbiomic biomarkers
- **Single molecule** vs. **panel biomarkers** (eg, Oncotype DX in BC, prognostic & predictive); **tissue-based** vs. **blood-based** ("liquid biopsy"; eg, Guardant360 CDx & FoundationOne Liquid CDx)
- To accelerate biomarker discovery, national cohorts established as data resource, incl. NIH's All of US Research Program (*NEJM* 2019;381:668)

BIOSTATISTICS

Descriptive statistics

- Describe or summarize a set of data
- **Continuous data:** Generally, prefer median & quartiles. Mean & standard deviations are useful for decision making; can be used descriptively if the distribution is symmetric
- **Categorical data:** Can be described by frequencies & percentages. Most commonly given as a prevalence = (# of total persons affected)/(total pop at risk). In some settings, (for a given time interval), use incidence = (# of new cases)/(pop at risk)
- **Time-to-event data:** Can be characterized by number of events, median follow-up for participants w/o an event, median survival, probability of event at a given follow-up time (eg, 65% probability of death by 5 y). Do not use rates (eg, number of deaths/sample size)

Measurement of comparisons & associations

- **Correlation (r):** Linear relationship b/w 2 continuous measures, ranging from −1 to +1. Generally avoided outside of methodologic studies
- **RR (relative risk):** Ratio of prevalence in "exposed" to prevalence in "nonexposed." RR = (proportion when exposed)/(proportion when not exposed)
- **Absolute risk difference:** Difference in risk. RD = risk when not exposed – risk when exposed
- **Odds:** Calculated as (# affected)/(# not affected)
- **OR (odds ratio):** A ratio of odds in "exposed" pop to odds in "nonexposed" pop. Less useful than absolute or RR differences but required for case-control studies & logistic regression

Confidence intervals

- **Variability of estimate:** Examples of estimates include means, proportions, or measures of association such as RR. Interpreted as a plausible range of values. Commonly 95% (often comparable to *p*-value cutoff of 0.05) but other values can be specified depending on situation & study question

Hypothesis testing

- A statistical test to determine the strength of evidence against a specific null hypothesis (H_0)
- **Choose 1-sided or 2-sided test:** 2-sided test is almost always used except under unusual circumstances; H_0 is rejected if the observation is statistically significantly different (< or >). Specify level of significance w/ α-value (commonly 0.05 but chosen depending on study question); α may be referred as type I error or FP rate
- **Calculate *p*-value:** If the *p*-value $< \alpha$, H_0 is rejected. If *p*-value $\geq \alpha$, H_0 is not rejected
- ***p*-Value** → probability of a result as extreme or more extreme than the one observed if null hypothesis true

Figure 2-1

	H_0 is true	H_0 is false
Fail to reject H_0	Correct	Type II error (β)
Reject H_0	Type I error (α)	Correct power = 1 – β

Estimation vs. inference

- Inference: Is something there? Assessed by *p*-value. Incorporates size of estimate & variability (often influenced by sample size)
- Estimation: How big is it? A central estimate (eg, mean or proportion) & 95% CI

Multiple hypothesis testing

- Testing multiple hypotheses increases risk of FPs. Informally assess evidence in light of multiple testing or make formal statistical correction used for multiple tests. Can control familywise error rates (probability of making at least 1 type I error) or first-degree relatives (FDRs) (proportion of type I errors)

Sample size calculation

- Info commonly needed: Study type, question, or end points (eg, survival, RR), hypothesis (ie, expected size or difference of effects), α, $1 - \beta$, test statistics, 1-sided vs. 2-sided test; for survival data → length of accrual & follow-up, median survival times & probabilities for H_0 & alternate hypothesis; specific statistical assumptions need to be satisfied (eg, no significant competing causes). Requires complex calculations involving considerable statistical judgment

Evaluating diagnostic procedures

- A test evaluated against a gold standard (a surrogate for true dz status) w/ observations classified as TP, TN, FP, & FN

Figure 2-2

	Dz	No Dz
Test +	TP	FP
Test –	FN	TN

Se = TP/(TP + FN)

Sp = TN/(TN + FP)

PPV = TP/(TP + FP)

PPN = TN/(TN + FN)

LR+ = Se/(1 – Sp)

LR– = (1 – Se)/Sp

- **ROC curve:** A graphical display of TP (Se) vs. FP (1 – Sp) for different cutoff points of a test. Evaluate the trade-off b/w Sn & Sp
- **Decision curve:** A graphical display of clinical net benefit against a threshold probability. A test w/ the highest net benefit leads to the best clinical outcome

Analysis of time-to-event data

- **Unique issues:** Not all pts enter study at the same time; some may withdraw or be lost to follow-up; not all pts have an event w/in the study period; observations can be censored. General approach: Analyze in terms of event probabilities
- **Methods:** Actuarial or life-table analysis for survival times; Kaplan–Meier (KM) product-limited estimates (KM survival curve) → graphical curve for cum. probabilities of survival; logrank test → compare KM curves
- **Competing risk:** Calculate incidence separately for event of interest (eg, CA recurrence) & competing event (eg, death from other causes)

Modeling and analysis of multiple variables

- **Modeling methods** → allow for analysis of multiple predictor variables for a given outcome w/ specific assumptions that model needs to satisfy
- **Methods:** Linear regression, Cox regression (for censored observations, eg, survival, uses assumption of proportional hazards), logistic regression (binary outcome). Use for prediction modeling, adjusting for confounders in observational studies

Guidelines for reporting statistics, figures, and tables in clinical research

- The following offer resources for reporting statistics in clinical research: *Eur Urol* 2020;78:97; *Eur Urol* 2019;75:358

Meta-analysis

- Summarize a set of studies w/ a specific study question; a summary effect measure w/ CI; forest plot → used to summarize studies; examine heterogeneity among the studies (use Cochran's Q, avoid I^2)
- Funnel plot → assesses possible publication bias; more useful if number of trials is large
- Sensitivity analysis → evaluate effect of incl./excluding certain studies

General principles

- **Good clinical practice (GCP)** guideline developed by the ICH (https://www.fda.gov/regulatory-information/search-fda-guidance-documents/e6r2-good-clinical-practice-integrated-addendum-ich-e6r1)
- **Health Insurance Portability and Accountability Act (HIPAA)** defines research as a systematic investigation incl. research development, testing, & evaluation, designed to develop or contribute to generalizable knowledge; covers both living & deceased individuals
- **Protected health information (PHI):** Unique pt identifiers such as name, medical record number, address, social security number, health/insurance plan, employers/family members, all elements of date except y, etc.

Key individuals/components

Principal investigator (PI): Detailed in GCP; oversees conduct of trial

Major Responsibilities of Principal Investigators
Maintain credentials (appropriate education & training)
Delegate responsibilities appropriately & supervise staff
Communicate w/ IRB (obtain approvals, reporting)
Ensure adequate resources (recruitment, time, environment)
Manage study-related documents (records, reports)
Manage data collection & data accuracy
Account for study drug (handling, storage, dispensing)
Confirm eligibility
Confirm informed consent
Assure compliance w/ the protocol (monitor & report deviations)
Compile progress reports & final report if needed
Ensure adequate care & safety of study pts (monitor AEs)
Evaluate study for early termination if needed & inform others

- **Sponsor:** Individual or organization pharmaceutical or nonpharmaceutical → assumes legal responsibility, ensures investigator appropriateness, ethics review, data quality assurance, AE reporting
- **Sponsor-investigator:** Individual initiates & conducts a clinical investigation & under whose immediate direction the investigational drug is being administered or dispensed. For administrative reasons, only **1** individual/organization. If a pharmaceutical company will be supplying the drug, but will not itself be submitting the IND, the company is not the sponsor
- **IND application:** For therapeutic trials, filed w/ the FDA; required to conduct clinical studies w/ an investigational drug involving interstate commerce for drugs as well as biologics (eg, vaccines); describes formulation, toxicology, & other drug-related info such as nonclinical efficacy; submitted by the study sponsor; FDA has 30 d to review initial submission. Certain protocols may be **IND-exempt** (https://www.fda.gov/media/79386/download)
- **Trial registration:** Section 801 of the FDAAA 801 requires responsible parties to register & submit summary results of clinical trials w/ ClinicalTrials.gov
- **Types of trials/funding:** Investigator-initiated trials (IITs), industry-sponsored trials (ISTs), cooperative group trials, trials conducted w/ the NCI/CTEP

Important documents

- **Protocol:** Includes aims/objectives, background, protocol schema, statistical consideration, tox/AEs, plan for dose modification for DLT, criteria for subject inclusion/exclusion, endpoints/outcome assessment, randomization procedure, data management plan, protection of human subjects, informed consent procedures, references
- **Informed consent:** Document detailing purpose of research, description of research procedures, drugs, possible risks/AEs, benefits, alternatives, financial costs, right to withdraw or refuse, termination, & confidentiality & privacy
- **Research authorization:** Obtains approval from the pt that PHI can be disclosed for research purposes, describes in detail how info is shared
- **Investigator's brochure:** Summary document of study drug info on physical, chemical, pharmaceutical properties, PK data, & prev studies (nonclinical & clinical)
- **Contract:** Details responsibilities, intellectual property, payment schedule, publication rights

- **Budget:** Details study-specific expenditures, includes items which are not billable to the pt or insurance

Protocol review process

- **Institutional review board (IRB):** Under FDA regulations, an IRB is an appropriately constituted group that has been formally designated to review & monitor biomedical research involving human subjects; can be local, central, or commercial; minimum of 5 members (incl. 1 scientist, 1 nonscientist, & 1 person not affiliated w/ institution) → ensures that risks are reasonable given potential benefits, risks are minimized, participant selection is equitable, informed consent is obtained properly, rights & welfare of participants are maintained as appropriate; may approve, disapprove, modification requirement, terminate/suspend
- **Institution-specific committees:** Conduct review in addition to IRB, often w/ a different focus (eg, to determine if protocols align w/ departmental or institutional interests)
- Certain research may be **exempt** from requirement for informed consent (eg, retrospective studies), but requests require IRB or privacy board review & **waiver of HIPAA authorization** & **informed consent.** The following criteria must be fulfilled: (1) Research could not be practically conducted w/o a waiver, (2) research could not be conducted w/o PHI, (3) use & disclosure is no more than minimum risk to participants' privacy

During and after the conduct of clinical trials

- **Ongoing review:** Modification, AEs, study reports, annual reports, audits; conducted by the institution (IRB), sponsor, & FDA
- **Data safety monitoring board (DSMB):** A group of experts that independently reviews trial data on a regular basis & gives advice to sponsor regarding safety, scientific validity, & merit of the trial for continuation or discontinuation; not required for all the trials but recommended for trials w/ assc. risk for significant morbidity or mortality, large trials, multicenter trials
  - May be preset & precalculated interim evaluation boundaries → helps determine threshold to stop or continue trial
  - FDA guidance on DSMB (https://www.fda.gov/media/75398/download)
  - Safety monitoring required for all, but not all require formal committee; may be external to the trial organizers, sponsors, & investigators
- **Meeting w/ FDA:** May be requested to ensure adequacy of trials for NDA & registration; often after phase I or phase II
- **New drug application (NDA):** Submitted by sponsor → includes preclinical data, clinical studies, info on safety & efficacy, proposed labeling & manufacturing detail. FDA approval for specific use evaluated in clinical trials; effectiveness of drug → OS or surrogate outcome; approved can be fast track for accelerated approval.
- **Postmarket studies/surveillance:** May be required as a condition for approval

Figure 2-3 Drug development overview.

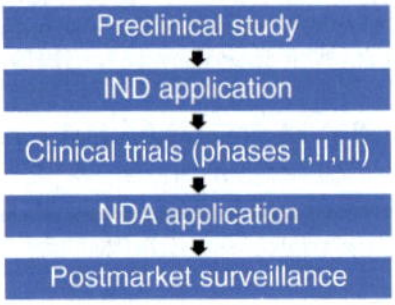

Special pathways for FDA approval

- **Fast track:** Expedites development/approval of drugs for unmet needs; must be requested by pharmaceutical company
- **Breakthrough therapy:** Expedites approval of drugs once the drug has shown preliminary evidence of improving clinically significant endpoints over available drugs
- **Accelerated approval:** Allows for drugs that treat serious conditions w/ unmet medical needs to be approved based on surrogate endpoints; phase IV confirmatory trials to confirm clinical benefit required
- **Priority review:** Designation that indicates the FDA will aim to take action on an application w/in 6 mos

BASIC RADIATION BIOLOGY AND PHYSICS

Definitions of photons and elementary particles in modern radiotherapy

- **Ionizing radiation (IR):** Photons that have adequate energy to eject orbital electrons
- **X-rays:** Energized photons, as produced from electrical current in linear accelerators
- **Gamma (γ) rays:** Energized photons that are emitted from the decay of radioactive nuclei (isotopes) or via electron–positron annihilation in PET imaging
- **Protons:** Positively charged particles w/ favorable dose distribution
- **Carbon ions:** Positively charged particles that are characterized by a dose distribution benefit related to the Bragg peak as well as a potential advantage a/w their high linear energy
- **Electrons:** Negatively charged particles that are for tx of shallow anatomical structures

Photon interactions with biologic material

- **Direct effects (minor for x-rays):** DNA molecules themselves are the direct targets of ionization, which ultimately trigger a chemical or biologic change
- **Indirect effects (major for x-rays):** Radiation ionizes other molecules in the cell (most frequently water) to produce **free radicals** that diffuse to & cause **damage to DNA**
- **Double stranded breaks (DSBs)** in DNA are thought to be the critical cellular lesion whose induction results in biologic effects, incl. cell killing, although many other types of molecular damage are also induced

Cellular response to IR

- **Mitotic death:** Cell death d/t chromosome missegregation during mitosis
- **Apoptosis:** A form of programmed cell death involving the action of caspases
- Alternative mechanisms of IR-induced lethality include necroptosis & autophagy. In addition, cells may go into senescence in which the cells remain viable but are incapable of further replication
- Cells that undergo **apoptotic death** in response to IR (eg, lymphoid cells, acinar cells of the salivary glands) are typically **more radiosensitive**

Repair of DNA DSBs

- A correlation exists between the probability of cell death & the induction of putative "lethal" chromosomal aberrations (eg, **dicentrics, rings,** etc.)
- Repair of DSBs occurs predominantly through either nonhomologous end-joining **(NHEJ)** or homologous recombination **(HR)**. Defects in these pathways promote radiosensitivity

Radiosensitivity and cell cycle

- Cells vary in radiosensitivity across the cell cycle: Generally, **more sensitive in M & G2** phases & **most resistant in late S phase**

Synergy of oxygen with radiotherapy

- **Oxygen enhances DNA damage** induced by free radicals, facilitating the **indirect action of IR**
- The oxygen enhancement ratio, dose of radiation required to produce a biologic effect under hypoxic conditions (often present in solid tumors resulting in radioresistance) divided by the dose under aerated conditions, generally in the range of 2–3 for x-rays

Understanding radiation response: The 4 Rs of radiobiology

- **Repair** of sublethal damage
- **Reassortment** of cells w/in the cell cycle
- **Repopulation** of cells during course of radiotherapy
- **Reoxygenation** of hypoxic cells

Basis for conventional dose fractionation

- Spares nl tissues by allowing for **repair of sublethal damage** (primarily DSBs) & **cellular repopulation** between fractions
- Augments tumor control by allowing for **reoxygenation** of hypoxic regions w/in the tumor & **reassortment** of cells into more radiosensitive portions of the cell cycle

Potential benefits of hypofractionated radiotherapy

- Hypofractionation is the use of dose fraction sizes greater than a standard 1.8–2.0 Gy
- **Radioresistant tumor histologies** (eg, melanoma, RCC) may respond more effectively to tx w/ large dose fraction sizes
- **Image-guided IMRT & SBRT/SABR** have enabled the use of large fraction sizes d/t improved anatomical targeting of radiotherapy & relative sparing of nearby nl tissues
- Large radiation doses (ie, >8 Gy) may be a/w additional mechanisms of CA cell death, incl. effects on the **tumor-associated stroma** (eg, endothelial cells)

- **Late effects on nl tissues,** which are radiation toxicities that manifest generally 3 mos to several years following RT, remain a concern a/w the use of higher radiation dose fractions

Chemical modifiers of radiation response

- **Radioprotectors** represent drugs that prevent or reduce the toxic effects of radiation against nl tissues. These are often **scavengers of IR-induced free radicals**. Radioprotectors are not in routine clinical use. The most well studied is amifostine for prevention of mucositis & xerostomia in head & neck cancer (*PLOS* 2014;9(5);e95968)
- **Radiosensitizers** are actively being developed & optimally enhance the effects of radiation against tumors while not increasing toxicity to nl tissues & organs
- **Hypoxic cell radiosensitizers & cytotoxins** are drugs that enhance the effects of radiation on radioresistant hypoxic tumor tissue or preferentially kill hypoxic tumor

Chemotherapy and radiotherapy

- Classical drugs used in cancer chemotherapy are frequently used sequentially or concurrently w/ radiotherapy to maximize therapeutic benefit. This has improved pt outcomes although also a/w ↑ overall tox
- **Drugs that show significant synergy w/ RT:** Dacarbazine, cisplatin, bleomycin, dactinomycin, doxorubicin, mitomycin C, 5-FU, capecitabine, gemcitabine
- Mechanisms for synergy vary widely: Include cell cycle effects, DNA damage response

Molecularly targeted therapy and radiotherapy

- Integration of molecularly targeted agents w/ chemoRT may provide therapeutic benefit by exploiting biologic & genetic differences between CA & nl tissue while minimizing additional tox, such as bevacizumab, cetuximab, & olaparib
- Studies are underway investigating targeted agents, incl. inhibitors of cell cycle checkpoints (CHK1/2, WEE1), the PI3K/AKT/mTOR pathway, androgen signaling, & immune checkpoints (CTLA-4, PD-L1, & PD-1)

Acute normal tissue effects

- Due to **cell killing of nl tissues** (eg, dermatitis, esophagitis, diarrhea) usually a/w early toxicities that are manifested during the course of RT or by **radiation-induced inflammatory cytokines** (eg, nausea, vomiting, fatigue) resulting generally in late adverse effects
- **Testes:** 0.1–0.15 Gy leads to temporary sterility. Doses of 6–8 Gy can lead to permanent sterility. Such doses have minimal effect on testosterone production
- **Ovaries:** Very sensitive to IR. Doses of 6–12 Gy result in sterilization of 50% of pts. There is age dependence, w/ lower doses needed to induce sterility in older pts. Sterility is a/w ovarian hormonal failure, resulting in premature menopause

Late normal tissue effects

- **Occur after a delay of mos to y** & can result from a combination of vascular damage &/or loss of parenchymal cells in the affected organ
- **Specific dose–volume relationships** have been linked to the risk of late organ tox. Some of these data are summarized below, derived from the QUANTEC project (*Int J Radiat Oncol Biol Phys* 2010;76:S1)

Site-Specific Tissue Effects

Organ	Outcome	Fraction Size (Gy)	Dose (Gy)	Likelihood or Risk
Brain[a]	Radionecrosis	<2.5	120	5%
Spinal cord[b]	Myelopathy	1.8–2	54 61	<1% <10%
Kidney[c]	Nephrotoxicity	1–2	10 (whole kidney)	5%
Heart[d]	Ischemic heart dz	1.8–2	30	RR ~ 1.5–3.3

[a]*Int J Radiat Oncol Biol Phys* 2010;76(3 Suppl):S20.
[b]*Int J Radiat Oncol Biol Phys* 2010;76(3 Suppl):S42.
[c]*Int J Radiat Oncol Biol Phys* 2010;76(3 Suppl):S108.
[d]*Int J Radiat Oncol Biol Phys* 2010;76(3 Suppl):S77.

Subsequent malignancy

- **Dose, volume, underlying genetics, & age of the pt** at the time of RT are critical determinants of the risk for a subsequent malignancy
- The likelihood of a subsequent CA is correlated w/ dose, but **there is no threshold dose** below which there is no additional risk of a subsequent malignancy
- **Latent period** for radiation-induced solid tumors is generally between **10 & 60 y**

EXTERNAL BEAM RADIATION THERAPY

What is EBRT?

- EBRT = a form of teletherapy (Greek for "distant") where therapeutic RT delivered by a machine outside the body to treat malignancies & some benign conditions in neoadjuvant, definitive, adjuvant, &/or palliative settings
- EBRT is a **local** therapy (exceptions: TBI = total body irradiation, TSEB = total skin electron beam)
- Contrast w/ brachytherapy (Greek for "short"): RT delivered internally by a source inside/near the tumor

Types of Radiation Used for EBRT		
IR	Electrons	**Used for superficial CAs,** such as skin & SC tissues
	Photons	**Most used in EBRT** High-energy x-rays created by a LINAC
	Protons	Deposits almost all energy in the Bragg peak → minimizes **radiation "exit dose"** beyond the target tissue Expensive & in limited supply around the country Indications: **Pediatrics**, re-RT, specific histologies
	Heavy ions (eg, carbon)	↑ relative biologic effectiveness (RBE) > photons/protons Extremely limited availability worldwide. High cost
	Neutrons	↑ RBE, greater than other forms of radiation Largely decreasing worldwide & current role is limited

Adapted with permission from *Leibel and Phillips Textbook of Radiation Oncology*. 3rd ed. Saunders: 2010.

How does a patient proceed from consultation to starting EBRT?

- Consultation visit: Radiation oncologist evaluates need for RT, schedules simulation scan
- **Simulation:** Pt undergoes planning scan, usually CT but occasionally MRI, in the tx position. May be coupled by fusion w/ a PET or MRI in the tx position to aid in target volume delineation
  1. Pt immobilized using variety of devices depending on the tx site
  2. Tx **"isocenter"** (point RT beam interaction) placed on the planning scan
  3. Isocenter & alignment tattoos placed on the pt
  4. Images fused (if applicable) & transferred to tx-planning software
- Draw volumes: Medical doctor (MD) contours target volumes & nl structures on the planning scan; if simple 2D tx, MD also places desired RT beams on the CT & selects beam angles
- Write Rx: MD prescribes a specific dose & fractionation of RT
- Tx planning:
  1. If 2D, physics staff verifies beams, calculates dose, & EBRT can begin immediately
  2. If 3D or more complex tx, physics staff generates custom plan for each tumor can take 1–2 wks for tx planning & QA review
- Tx plan reviewed by MD for approval. At least one other MD should also review plan for quality assurance
- Pt setup on tx machine: A "dry-run" session to double-check all tx & machine parameters
- EBRT begins either immediately after or 1 d after setup session

Terminology of EBRT: Delivery types

- **Conventional:** 2D RT w/ 2 beams such as AP-PA or opposed laterals; used for simple EBRT txs w/ lower total doses (eg, whole-brain RT, palliation for bone mets)
- 3D conformal RT (3DCRT): 3D tx plan using > 2 beams to treat a target region conformally (eg, pelvis for rectal CA; avoiding kidney dose in upper abdominal CA)
- **IMRT:** A computer-generated RT plan covers the planning target volume using **multiple beam angles or arcs** (volumetric modulated arc therapy **[VMAT]**); optimizes tx of target tissue while sparing high dose to critical nl tissues (eg, head & neck CAs, prostate CA). Requires contouring/delineation of both tx volumes & nl tissue organs at risk (OAR)
- Image-guided RT (IGRT): Daily or weekly 2D or 3D imaging to improve tx precision; used w/ IMRT, SRS, & SBRT to allow **smaller margins on tx volumes**
- 4DCT: Used to **account for internal motion** from breathing w/ contoured tumor in all phases of respiratory cycle, thus, ensuring that tumor volume is w/in beams during tx (eg, lung CA, upper abdominal CAs)
- Deep inspiration breath hold (DIBH): Pt holds breath for simulation & tx to account for internal motion from breathing but allows smaller margins than 4DCT or to expand lungs & push heart away from tx field (eg, left-sided breast CAs)

- Respiratory gating: Technique used to deliver RT only when a pt's breathing falls w/in certain phases of respiratory cycle (eg, upper abdominal CAs)
- SRS/SBRT: Discussed in "Stereotactic Radiotherapy" chapter

Dose and fractionation

- Units of RT dose = **Gy** = 1 J/kg; 1 Gy = 100 cGy
- Fractions = Number of sessions over which the total RT dose is delivered
- Dose & fractionation are determined according to multiple factors: Intrinsic tumor radiosensitivity, proximity of tumor to critical nl tissues, data from randomized trials, use of sequential or concurrent chemotherapy, pt convenience, pt tolerance
- Typically, RT is delivered in daily fractions M-F over wks, but can be given bid (eg, limited-stage SCLC w/ chemotherapy), & tid (eg, full-dose TBI prior to SCT)
- Fractionation terminology:
  - **Hypofractionation** = using higher RT dose per fraction, over fewer fractions: Moderate hypofractionation (eg, 2–3 Gy), ultrahypofractionation using 1–5 fractions (eg, **SBRT, radioresistant** tumors such as melanoma)
  - **Hyperfractionation** = using smaller RT dose per fraction, over more fractions

Common EBRT Doses and Fractionation

Site	Total Dose (Gy)	# Fractions
Breast	50–60 *(if hypofractionated 42.5)*	25–30 *(if hypofractionated 16)*
Prostate	78–86 *(if hypofractionated 40)*	43–48 *(if hypofractionated 5)*
Primary brain tumor	60	30
H&N definitive tx	70	33
Early-stage lung	48–60	3–4
Hodgkin lymphoma	20–36	13–20
Rectal preoperative	50.4	28
Postop tumor beds	50–66	25–33
Whole brain RT (palliative)	30	10

Leibel and Phillips Textbook of Radiation Oncology. 3rd ed. Saunders: 2010.

Side effects of EBRT

- During RT, pts seen in clinic at least once a wk by attending MD. Acute s/e actively managed during these visits
- **Acute s/e (<90 d):** Site-specific, listed in table below
  Fatigue & mild skin erythema are most common acute s/e
- **Late s/e (>90 d):** Site-specific & age-specific
- **Secondary malignancies:** Overall absolute risk of 2° RT-induced malignancy in adults is <1%. Risk ↓ w/ ↑ age

Children have ↑ risk of 2° malignancy. Latency after RT: >7 y for solid tumors, >2 y for liquid tumors (*Lancet Oncol* 2011;12:353–360)

Potential Side Effects Following EBRT

Site	Acute (<90 d)	Late (>90 d)
Breast	Skin erythema, skin desquamation, mild breast edema	Breast fibrosis, implant contracture, heart dz
Prostate	Urinary frequency & urgency, ↑ frequency BMs	Erectile dysfunction, painless rectal bleeding
Brain	Nausea, fatigue, hair loss	Subtle cognitive changes, radiation necrosis
H&N	Mucositis, xerostomia, dysgeusia, skin erythema, odynophagia	Xerostomia, skin fibrosis, dysgeusia, dental caries
GI	Diarrhea, rectal pain, nausea	Change in bowel habits
Lung	Cough, esophagitis	Pulm fibrosis, pneumonitis
Bone mets	Marrow suppression if very large field treated, esp. pelvis	Fracture risk
All pts	Fatigue, mild skin erythema	Radiation recall after certain chemotherapies

Follow-up after EBRT

- First post-tx visit occurs 4–8 wks after EBRT, depending on tx site & type of tx
- Imaging is a regular part of follow-up, incl. CT, PET, MRI
- Laboratories as indicated (eg, TSH after H&N RT, ESR/LDH for lymphomas)
- Pt is seen every 2–6 mos, alternating w/ other treating physicians

STEREOTACTIC RADIOTHERAPY

Definitions

- **SRS:** Stereotactic radiosurgery; used for brain parenchymal lesions in 1–5 fractions
- **SBRT:** Stereotactic body radiotherapy; used for extracranial lesions in 1–15 fractions
- Historically SBRT/SRS delivered w/ frame-based stereotactic pt setup for accurate delivery of highly conformal RT. Modern SBRT/SRS utilizes image guidance rather than frame-based stereotactic setup to deliver a high dose per fraction. The term "stereotactic" does not describe current techniques

Mechanism

- Uses **high dose per fraction to deliver a more biologically effective tumoricidal dose.** Conventional RT = ~2 Gy/fx. Stereotactic RT = ~5–24 Gy/fx
- Multiple nonparallel radiation beams converge on the tx target. Full dose is limited to region of overlap, nontarget areas receive smaller doses from limited beams

Delivery machines

- Often use image guidance to aid in tx accuracy incl. x-rays & cone beam CT scans
  - **LINAC:** Most common device, generates photons by a mechanism similar to an x-ray tube; typical tx consists of ~5–12 beams from different angles to converge on target or delivered over a 360° arc using VMAT
  - **MR LINAC:** MR-guided LINAC combines MR imaging w/ a LINAC, daily pre-tx MRIs & adaptive planning to account for day-to-day shift in target tissue & organs at risk (ORS)

Advantages

- Allows for delivery of higher dose per fraction, which increases BED delivered to tumor, thereby increasing efficacy of tx
- Allows for RT in fewer sessions, thereby decreasing overall length of tx. Increases pt convenience, allowing for prompt initiation of other therapies

Disadvantages

- More resource-intensive: Advanced pt positioning/immobilization, pt setup verification w/ onboard imaging, sophisticated tx planning software & physics teams
- Planning process takes longer given complexity of tx, making SBRT/SRS less feasible for urgent clinical needs
- Higher risk of radiation toxicity: Delivery of higher dose per tx sessions poses incr. risk of nl tissue injury d/t errors in pt setup/immobilization, internal organ motion during a single tx session (infrafractional motion), or between tx sessions (interfraction motion)
- Higher doses per fraction may require a dose reduction compared to what could be delivered w/ more fractions if the tumor is w/in or near a sensitive organ sites

Uses of SRS

Application	Results	Common Use
Brain metastases	No difference in OS & ↓ cognitive deterioration at 3 mo w/ SRS alone vs. SRS + WBRT for 1–3 brain mets (*JAMA* 2016;316(4):401)	1–5 brain mets; can consider up to 10 in select clinical circumstances
Meningioma	WHO Grade I: 5-y control >90%; lower for WHO Grade II & III (*Neurosurgery* 2020;87(50):879)	Small tumors in sites where complete excision is difficult; adjuvant RT for malignant meningiomas & subtotally resected dz
Pituitary adenoma	Local control >90% in functioning & nonfunctioning adenomas, risk of hypopituitarism in 80% of pts at 10 y (*Neuro-Oncology* 2020;22(3):318)	Tumors <3 cm in diameter & 3–5 mm or more from optic pathway

Uses of SBRT for Primary Disease		
Primary Disease	**Results**	**Common Use**
Early-stage NSCLC	92% 5-y LC; 5-y OS 40% (*RTOG 0236; JAMA Onc* 2018;4(9):1287)	Early-stage T1–2 NSCLC among pts who are poor surgical candidates; inoperable early-stage NSCLC
Primary liver	94% 2-y LC w/ proton SBRT for hepatocellular carcinoma & intrahepatic cholangiocarcinoma (*JCO* 2016;34(5):460)	Inoperable primary for hepatocellular carcinoma & intrahepatic cholangiocarcinoma
Prostate	85% failure-free survival at 5 y; similar to conventional RT (*Lancet* 2019;394(10196):385)	Rationale is for convenience & unique radiobiology of prostate CA, but data not yet sufficient to be standard of care
Pancreas	2-y local progression 32%, 2-y OS of 38% (*JAMA Onc* 2021; 7(5):735)	Inoperable pancreatic adenocarcinoma

Uses of SBRT for Metastatic Disease		
Application	**Results**	**Common Use**
Nonspinal bone metastases	SBRT a/w improved pain response at 2 wks, 3 mos, & 9 mos (*JAMA Oncol* 2019;5(6):872)	Painful, nonspinal bone mets in pts w/ life expectancy >2 y
Spine metastases	1-y LC ~85% (histology dependent (*J Nsg Spine* 2007;7:151). SBRT may improve pain control compared to conventional RT (*Radiother Oncol* 2018;128(2): 274)	Radioresistant histologies (melanoma, sarcoma, renal cell carcinoma); re-irradiation after conventional RT; postop following spine stabilization for pts w/ spinal instability d/t epidural spinal cord compression
Lung metastases	2-y LC 96%. Low toxicity (*JCO* 2009;27(10):1579)	1–3 lung mets
Oligometastatic lung cancer	Addition of local consolidative therapy (surgery or SBRT) improves OS in select pts w/ oligometastatic lung cancer (*JCO* 2019;37(18):1558)	Select pts w/ de novo oligometastatic lung cancer w/o progression on 1st line systemic therapy
Liver metastases	1–3 hepatic mets <6 cm, 2-y LC of 92%. Low tox (*JCO* 2009;27(10):1572)	Alternative to surgery

BRACHYTHERAPY

Definition

- Derived from "brachy" meaning "short," refers to tx of targets using radiation sources in short distance or close proximity to a target; this allows tx of a target, while minimizing radiation dose to nl tissues that would otherwise be traversed by an external beam
  - **Interstitial:** Inserted w/in a target tissue (eg, prostate LDR)
  - **Intracavitary:** Brachy source w/in a natural or applicator cavity (eg, HDR cervix, IVRT)
  - **Contact:** Placed close to a target (eg, contact applicator for skin CAs)
  - The high degree of dose localization depends on the **inverse-square law,** where the dose rate ↓ w/ square of the distance from the source ($1/\text{distance}^2$)

Figure 3-1 Permanent low–dose-rate prostate seed implant under TRUS guidance; U/S cradle and template shown with needles placed through the perineum into the prostate gland.

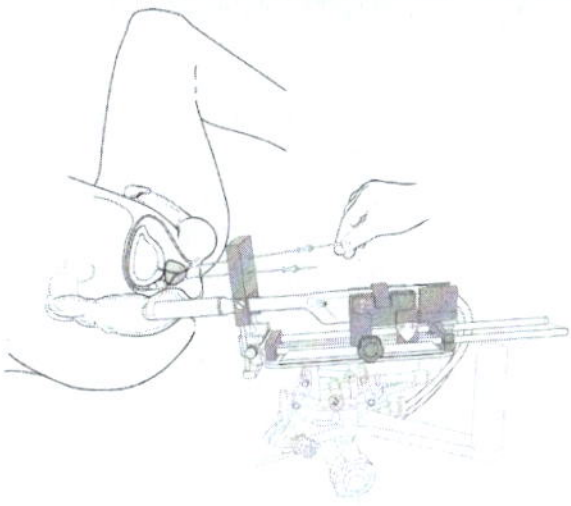

Figure 3-2 Intracavitary brachytherapy for cervical cancer using ring-and-tandem high–dose-rate applicator; applicator is shown in place in the vagina with tandem inserted into the uterus.

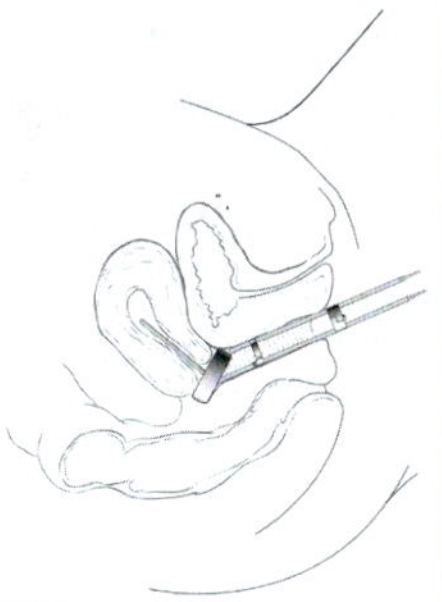

Sources used

- LDR txs (<12 Gy/h) typically use palladium-103 (Pd-103, $T_{½}$ = 17 d) or iodine-125 (I-125, $T_{½}$ = 59.4 d)
  - Generally used for permanent implants (eg, prostate CA)
- High–dose-rate (HDR) txs (>12 Gy/h) use sources such as iridium-192 (Ir-192, $T_{½}$ = 74 d)
  - Uses a remote afterloader & preplaced catheters to guide a physically small, high-activity source to the target rather than direct handling
  - Used for temporary implants (eg, cervical CA, intravaginal RT, & prostate cancer—especially when used in a combined modality regimen to treat locally advanced dz)
- Many other sources exist, incl. cesium-137, ruthenium-106, radium-226, & cobalt-60

Intraoperative radiation therapy

- Tx, generally of a single margin or entire surgical cavity, to sterilize at-risk margins
  - Can be performed w/ a multichannel HDR applicator (Ir-192, $T_{½}$ = 74 d) & a remote afterloader or can use solid applicators loaded w/ high-activity isotopes such as phosphorus-32 (P-32, $T_{½}$ = 14.3 d) or yttrium-90 (Y-90, $T_{½}$ = 64 h)
  - Low-energy photon & electron generators have been designed & also have been used, particularly in breast CA

Toxicities

- Nl tissues adjacent to the brachytherapy source can receive high radiation doses; however, there is a steep dose fall-off
- Interstitial & intracavitary tx often require anesthesia & carry risk of bleeding & infxn
  - **Breast:** Cosmetic changes to breast tissue, fat necrosis
  - **Prostate:** Acute urinary retention (3%), urethral irritation, chronic stricture (2–4%), proctitis (2%), erectile dysfunction (30%)
  - **Esophagus:** Esophagitis/dysphagia, tracheoesophageal fistula (up to 12%)
  - **Anorectal:** Proctitis, mucosal ulceration
  - **Bronchial:** Fistula (5–10%), hemoptysis (7–22%), stenosis, tracheomalacia
  - **Endometrial:** Vaginal shortening/stenosis, dyspareunia
  - **Cervical:** Cystitis, fistula, proctitis, vaginal shortening/stenosis

Brachytherapy: Primary Uses		
Site	**Clinical Results**	**Common Use**
Prostate	Excellent biologic control (10-y & 15-y b-PFS 85% & 80%) (ASCENDE-RT, *IJROBP* 2020;108(3):S62)	**Monotherapy** in low-risk pts & as a **boost to external beam** ± hormone Rx in intermediate & high-risk pts; also in **salvage** setting for isolated LR
Cervical cancer	Definitive: 5-y LC overall 92% (no difference by stage) w/ CRT (weekly cisplatin + EBRT), followed by MRI-based IGABT (EMBRACE-I, *Lancet Oncol* 2021;22(4):538)	Temporary LDR/HDR "ring-and-tandem"/"tandem and ovoids" applicator for intact cervix
Endometrial cancer	Postoperative: I–IIA intermediate- to high-risk 5-y LR RFS 95%, vaginal RFS 98% (PORTEC-2, *Lancet* 2010; 375(9717):816) Definitive: Overall 5-y LC 60–86%, I–II: 75–86%	Vaginal cylinder applicator following hysterectomy to treat cuff, salvage brachytherapy, or definitive combination Rx (incl. uterus) if surgery contraindicated
Vaginal cancer	Overall 5-y LC I: 77–86%; II: 50–84%, (*Brachytherapy* 2012;11(1):58)	Either intracavitary applicator w/ vaginal cylinder or interstitial implant if bulky dz
Esophageal cancer	Boost: 74% have complete response, w/ 71% subsequent locoregional control (RTOG 9207; *Cancer* 2000;88(5):988) Palliation: Obstructive sx relief in 67% No prior radiation: 18-m LRFS 75%	Previously used as both a boost to external beam, monotherapy for superficial lesions, & as salvage Rx for recurrence; use in non-palliative setting is investigational
Anorectal cancer	Anal (interstitial boost): 5-y LC 80–90% Rectal (intracavitary boost): 5-y LC 72–80% for limited dz	Previously used as both a boost to external beam, monotherapy for superficial lesions, & as salvage Rx for recurrence.
Head & neck	Lip: 5-y LC 90–95% Oral tongue: 5-y LC T1: 88%, T2: 83%, T3: 62% Floor of mouth: 5-y LC 75–90% Buccal mucosa: 5-y LC 81% Oropharynx (salvage): 5-y LC 57–69% Nasopharynx: 5-y LC (boost) T1: 2 82%, T3: 74% (salvage) 52%	**Usually salvage tx or boost** following definitive RT. Mostly interstitial implants, w/ the exception of nasopharynx, which is done w/ an intracavitary implant.
Breast	Boost: Women <40 y, reduction in LR from 19.5 to 10.2% (*NEJM* 2001;345(19):1378); 5-y LC 88–98% Intracavitary tx: 5-y LC 95–97% (*IJROBP* 2012;84(3):S186); 10-y IBTR 4.6% (B39; *Lancet* 2019;394(10215):14)	**Partial breast irradiation,** serves as a boost to the tumor bed after surgical resection; can be interstitial implant or intracavitary tx
Sarcoma	Post-op, 5-y LC 82% (*JCO* 1996;14(3):859) Salvage: LC 60%	IORT to treat at-risk margins w/ HDR applicator, or interstitial implant-based; salvage
Ocular melanoma	5-y LC: 85% COMS medium: 12-y OS enucleation 59% vs. brachy 57% (*Arch Ophthalmol* 2001;119(7):969)	Uses a temporary applicator "plaque" loaded w/ I-125 seeds that is sewn onto the eye & delivers radiation to the lesion over several days
Lung	Bronchial dz: LC 59–95% Interstitial brachytherapy in inoperable NSCLC: 1-y LC 86% Sublobar resection & implant: 5-y LC stage I: 94% (*IJROBP* 2011;79(4):1112)	Parenchymal: Either permanent seed implant sewn onto surgical bed or temporary HDR intraoperative txs using afterloader techniques. Bronchial: Endoluminal applicator
Pediatric	IORT 2-y LC 56%, 12% late toxicity Retinoblastoma: 4-y 60% eye preservation (*Ped Blood Cancer* 2004;43(2):134)	IORT can be used to sterilize surgical margins (neuroblastoma, sarcoma) & reduce RT exposure; eye plaque for retinoblastoma
Spine	Spine met: 6-m LRFS 83% (*Neurosurgery* 2012;71(5):1003)	Temporary P-32 plaque placed directly on dura after laminectomy

Other sites for which brachytherapy has been studied: bile duct, bladder, brain, coronary arteries, & penis/urethra.

TBI AND TSEB

Total Body Irradiation (TBI)

Definition and background

- TBI is a technique used in preparation & conditioning for pts w/ acute myeloid leukemia (AML), acute lymphoid leukemia (ALL) & occasionally for Hodgkin/Non-Hodgkin lymphomas prior to allogeneic HSCT (*IJROBP* 2018;101(3):P521)

Goals of TBI

1. **Immunosuppression through lymphocyte & aberrant cell eradication.** This is important to prevent rejection of donor hematopoietic cells among pts receiving HSCT
2. **Cytoreduction & eradication of residual leukemia & lymphoma cells.** Delivery of radiation via TBI does not depend on blood supply, drug absorption, or biodistribution. As a result, radiation delivered via TBI can reach sanctuary sites such as the testes & CNS less effectively treated via systemic therapy. Clones resistant to systemic therapy can still be radiosensitive

- Dose & fractionation vary across institutions
- Male pts w/ ALL at incr. risk of testicular relapse since the testicles are a sanctuary site w/ suboptimal penetration of chemotherapy; testicular boosts + TBI w/ 400 cGy in a single fraction delivered using electrons (*IJROBP* 2018;101(3):P521)

Low-dose TBI

- Low-dose TBI (200–400 cGy) given to pts receiving reduced intensity conditioning regimens (eg, cord blood transplant programs, older pts) at MSKCC
- Low-dose TBI generally well tolerated (*JCO* 2006;24(3):444); the most common acute toxicities include nausea & parotitis; severe toxicity rare

Full-dose TBI

- Full-dose TBI given in multiple fractions often 2–3 times per day to total doses of 1375 cGy in adults & 1500 cGy in children after high-dose chemotherapy at MSKCC
- Modern full-dose TBI is delivered in multiple fractions which significantly reduces toxicity compared to historical practices which delivered full-dose TBI in a single fraction (*IJROBP* 2018;101(3):P521)

Full-dose TBI: Acute and subacute toxicity

- **Nausea & emesis:** Effectively prevented w/ antiemetics (eg, ondansetron)
- **Dermatologic:** Erythema & alopecia commonly seen w/in the 1st wk
- **Parotitis:** Generally presents on tx 2nd d d/t damage to salivary serous cells → apoptosis & elevated amylase. Effect is dose dependent w/ spontaneous resolution of soreness in 5–6 d. Tylenol or icing can be helpful supportive care interventions
- **Pneumonitis:**
  - Clinical diagnosis presenting 1–2 mo after full-dose TBI completion
  - Most common sxs = dry cough, new/worsening dyspnea on exertion, low-grade fever
  - Modern TBI delivered w/ external lung shielding to reduce risk of pneumonitis by >50% (*Bio Blood Marrow Transplant* 2007;43:573)
- Rate of pneumonitis difficult to estimate d/t institutional variability in dose, fractionation, variability in lung shielding practices & possible contribution from high-dose chemotherapy (*IJROBP* 2018;101(3):P521)
  - Tx = prednisone (1 mg/kg) for 2–3 wks w/ slow taper over 1–4 mos

Full-dose TBI: Late toxicity

- **Pulmonary toxicity:** Etiology likely multifactorial. Presents as new or worsening dyspnea on exertion w/ reduced diffusion capacity on pulmonary function testing. Reduced lung dose is a/w reduced pulmonary toxicity & improved survival among children receiving TBI for allogeneic HSCT (*IJROBP* 2019;105(1):S189)
- **Cardiovascular toxicity:** Long-term survivors who as children received TBI & allogeneic HSCT may have elevated likelihood of developing cardiovascular risk factors such as high triglycerides & low high-density lipoprotein levels. Pts should undergo screening for cardiovascular risk factors (*Bio Blood Marrow Transplant* 2017;23(3):475)
- **Cataracts:** 10-y rate of cataracts ~40% w/ incidence increasing over time. Presents as opacification of lens on exam & can be permanently corrected w/ surgery (*British J of Haem* 2014;168(4):518)
- **Infertility:** Common in all male pts & in females >10 yo treated w/ TBI. However, pts undergoing allogeneic HSCT w/o TBI also at high risk for long-term endocrine dysfunction (*Cancer* 2002;95(5):1076)

- **Hypothyroidism:** Most common endocrinopathy seen after TBI (~25%). Pts require annual screening for hypothyroidism & possible early initiation of thyroid hormone replacement therapy
- **Impaired growth:** Pertinent to prepubescent pediatric pts treated w/ TBI. Etiology likely multifactorial (*Bone Marrow Transplantation* 2016;51:351)
- **Secondary malignancies:** Rates of leukemia, posttransplant lymphoproliferative disorders, & other secondary malignancies are elevated especially in children (*Bone Marrow Transplantation* 2016;51:351)

Total Skin Electron Beam (TSEB) Therapy

Definition and background

- TSEB uses electrons directed at the entire surface of the body. Electrons deliver therapeutic radiation dose to the pt's skin w/o penetration to deeper internal organs, minimizing tx toxicity (*Clin Transl Radiat Oncol* 2019;15:26)
- Recognized & efficacious tx for cutaneous T-cell lymphomas (CTCLs). Mycosis fungoides (MF) accounts for 50–70% of all CTCLs & is the most common application of TSEB (*Clin Transl Radiat Oncol* 2019;15:26)
- Pts w/ localized skin dz only are eligible for focal electron therapy w/ radiation field targeted to involved areas of dz only rather than TSEB. This approach frequently utilized for indolent & aggressive B-cell skin lymphomas
- TSEB & focal electron RT may be delivered in conjunction w/ systemic therapy &/or topical agents
- **Goals of TSEB & focal electron RT:**
  1. Inducing remission in definitive tx of newly diagnosed, nonlocalized CTCL
  2. Palliation of sxs incl. pruritis, erythroderma, & pain
- **Effective palliation for MF:** Historically TSEB delivered w/ dose of 30–36 Gy w/ >95% ORR. Modern approaches use 12 Gy in 8 fractions over 2 wks & achieve 87% ORR (*IJROBP* 2017;99(3):2017). At 12 Gy dose, tx can be repeated if needed

Technique

- Significant variation by institution
- Target of radiation includes skin varying from <0.5 mm (eyelid) to >5 mm (back), subcutaneous infiltration (>1.5 cm), blood present in the skin during irradiation & superficial involved lymph nodes (up to 2–3 cm depth)
- Modern techniques use a photon beam passed through a Lucite screen in front of the pt to generate the electron beam. This electron field then used to treat the pt in multiple standing positions (MSKCC: 6 positions, twice weekly) for dose homogeneity. Dz response is typically rapid. Other institutions treat only a few positions per tx session, thus total duration of tx is longer
- Supplemental electron boost dose is often given to areas w/ more limited exposure to TSEB (eg, top & soles of feet, scalp, perineum, axilla, & occasionally inframammary folds). Supplemental boost can also be given to areas of severe dz
- Shielding of the eyes & digits of the hands/feet used to reduce local reaction from field overlap. Scalp shielding appropriate in certain pts to prevent alopecia, incl. pts w/o evidence of direct scalp involvement

Toxicity

- At >10 Gy, mild erythema w/ dry desquamation & brisk changes at lesions. Overall, tx is well tolerated w/o significant toxicity at 12-Gy dose (*Clin Transl Radiat Oncol* 2019;15:26, *IJROBP* 2017;99(3):2017)
- At >25 Gy, transient edema of the hands & ankles w/ blisters requiring local shielding or tx breaks can occur
- Temporary nail loss & alopecia (100% by end of tx >25 Gy) w/ 4–6 mos' time to regenerate
- Long-term sequelae are rare at <10 Gy & very mild, even at typical doses to 25–30 Gy. The most common chronic cutaneous changes include wrinkling, telangiectasias, uneven pigmentation

RADIATION ONCOLOGY EMERGENCIES

Definition

- Acute oncologic emergencies that potentially require urgent tx w/ RT, eg, malignant spinal cord compression, brain mets, SVC syndrome, airway obstruction, & uncontrolled tumor hemorrhage (eg, abdominal, bronchial, gynecologic)

Malignant spinal cord compression

- **Definition:** Compression of dural sac & contents (spinal cord &/or cauda equina) by extradural tumor mass. Minimum radiographic evidence is indentation of thecal sac at level corresponding to clinical features (*JCO* 2005;12(15):3366)
  - Radiographic cord compression varies in severity & urgency for tx (see **ESCC** below)
  - **Myelopathy** consists of neurologic sxs attributable to clinical cord compression & is always an emergency

ESCC (Epidural Spinal Cord Compression) Scale	
Grade 0	Bone only dz (no visible tumor w/in spinal canal)
Grade 1a	Epidural impingement, w/o deformation of thecal sac
Grade 1b	Epidural impingement w/ deformation of thecal sac
Grade 1c	Epidural impingement w/ deformation of thecal sac & spinal cord abutment but w/o cord compression
Grade 2	Spinal cord compression, but w/ CSF visible around cord
Grade 3	Spinal cord compression, no CSF visible around cord

J Neurosurg Spine 2010;13(3):324.

  - **ESCC Grade 2–3** is **high-grade cord compression** & frequently causes myelopathy. Even asx radiographic-only dz should be considered an emergency
  - **ESCC Grade 1a–c** is **low-grade compression** & is more likely asx. Generally, radiation is warranted on an outpt basis
- **Workup:** H&P, MRI Total Spine (Se 93%, Sp 97%, accuracy 95%); neurosurgical eval. Important to assess for sx of **myelopathy** incl. weakness, numbness, gait ataxia, hyperreflexia, loss of proprioception, urinary retention, & bowel/bladder incontinence. Also evaluate for potential spinal instability, consisting of movement-related mechanical pain such as pain exacerbated by sitting or standing or lying flat (see **SINS** below)

SINS (Spine Instability Neoplastic Score) Criteria	
SINS Component	**Score**
Location	
Junctional (occiput–C2, C7–T2, T11–L1, L5–S1)	3
Mobile Spine (C3–C6, L2–L4)	2
Semi-rigid (T3–T10)	1
Rigid (S2–S5)	0
Pain relief with recumbence (lying down) or pain with movement/loading of spine	
Yes	3
Occasional pain but not mechanical	1
Pain-free lesion	0
Bone lesion quality	
Lytic	2
Mixed (lytic/blastic)	1
Blastic	0
Radiographic spinal alignment	
Subluxation/translation present	4
De novo deformity (kyphosis/scoliosis)	2
Nl alignment	0
Vertebral body collapse	
>50% collapse	3
<50% collapse	2
No collapse w/ >50% body involved	1
None of the above	0

Posterolateral involvement of spinal elements (ie, facet, pedicle, costovertebral joint fracture, or replacement w/ tumor)	
Bilateral	3
Unilateral	1
None of the above	0
Interpretation of the SINS Score	
0–6	Stable
7–12	Indeterminate (?impending instability)
13–18	Instability

J Clin Oncol 2011:29(22):3072.

Clinical Scenario	Treatment Options
High-grade ESCC, Clinical myelopathy	Start steroids (Dexamethasone 10 mg IV loading dose, followed by 4–6 mg q6–8h). Start PPI & consider PCP ppx. Generally, decompression followed by postoperative RT
High-grade ESCC, No clinical mylopathy	Tx varies according to the ***radiosensitivity*** of the histology: Conventional EBRT alone for **radiosensitive** histologies (ie, lymphoma, myeloma, breast prostate, small cell, seminoma, ovarian); decompression followed by postoperative SBRT for **radioresistant** histologies (ie, everything else)
Low-grade ESCC, No clinical myelopathy	Conventional EBRT for radiosensitive histologies & SBRT for radioresistant histologies
Mechanical instability (SINS 7–18)	Consider surgical stabilization vs. kyphoplasty followed by radiation

- **Radiation dosing schedules:**
  - Conventional EBRT → 3 Gy × 10 fractions, 4 Gy × 5 (most common), 8 Gy × 1
  - SBRT → 6 Gy × 5, 8–10 Gy × 3, or 18–24 Gy × 1
- **Prognosis:** Most important prognostic factor is ambulatory status. Other predictive factors are time to development of motor deficits (better functional outcome a/w slower development of motor deficits before RT) & favorable histology (*JCO* 2005;12(15):3366)

Brain metastases

- **Definition:** "Solitary" = 1 brain met, only site of dz; "Single" = 1 brain met, other sites of metastatic dz
- **Workup:** H&P, MRI brain w/ contrast
- **Prognostic factors:** Older RPA based on RTOG trials (*IJROBP* 2000;47(4):1001) now replaced by **GPA** → Developed for 6 common primary histologies (ie, NSCLC/Small cell, Melanoma, Breast, RCC, GI) & accounts for primary diagnosis, age, KPS, presence of extracranial mets (ECM), number of brain mets, total volume of mets, & hormone-receptor subtype in breast (ie, basal, luminal A, luminal B, or HER2+) (*JCO* 2012;30(4):419)
- **Treatment:**
  - Steroids (Dexamethasone 4 mg q6h, only if neurologic sx present)
  - Consider radiation &/or surgery based on clinical sxs, size & number of brain mets, performance status, prog, surgical candidacy, history of prior RT, & presence of leptomeningeal disease (LMD), availability of CNS-penetrant systemic tx
  - If neurologically asx, outpt tx is appropriate

Clinical Scenario	Treatment Options
Acutely sx w/ impending neurologic devastation	Surgery + Adjuvant SRS (if limited dz) or WBRT (if diffuse dz ± LMD); WBRT w/ clinical setup (if nonsurgical candidate)
Single large (>3 cm) met	Hypofractionated SRS alone; Surgery + Adjuvant SRS
Single small met, good prog	Single-fraction SRS alone; Surgery + Adjuvant SRS/SBRT
Limited mets (1–10 lesions), good prog	SRS alone + observation; Reserve WBRT or add'l SRS for salvage
Diffuse mets, good prog	WBRT alone
Reirradiation	SRS alone (if limited dz); Consider repeat WBRT (if diffuse dz) in select cases (ie, good KPS, limited ECM, prolonged DFS)

Poor prog/KPS	Best supportive care or WBRT alone
LMD	WBRT ± focal RT to bulky dz in brain or spine; Intrathecal chemotherapy; shunting if CSF obstruction suspected

Handbook of Evidence-Based Radiation Oncology. 3rd ed. Springer: 2018.

- **Radiation dose schedule:**
  - For WBRT: 3 Gy × 10 (most common); 4 Gy × 5
  - For SRS: 18–24 Gy × 1 (most common); 9 Gy × 3; 6 Gy × 5

SVC syndrome

- **Etiology:** NSCLC (50%), SCLC (22%), Lymphoma (12%), Met (9%), Other (7%)
- **Presentation:** Dyspnea, ↑ Venous pressure, ↓ Venous return; sx develop over wks to mos
- **Proposed grading system**

Grade	Category	Incidence (%)	Definition
0	Asymptomatic	10	Radiographic SVC obstruction w/o sx
1	Mild	25	Head/neck edema, cyanosis, plethora
2	Moderate	50	Head/neck edema w/ functional impairment (eg, mild dysphagia, cough, impairment of head, jaw or eyelid movements, visual disturbances)
3	Severe	10	Mild/moderate cerebral edema (HA, dizziness); mild/moderate laryngeal edema; or diminished cardiac reserve (syncope after bending)
4	Life-threatening	5	Significant cerebral edema (confusion, obtundation); significant laryngeal edema (stridor); or significant hemodynamic compromise (syncope w/o precipitating factors, HoTN, renal insufficiency)
5	Fatal	<1	

J Thorac Oncol 2008;3(8):811.

- **Workup:** CXR, CT scan
- **Treatment:** (*NEJM* 2007;356(18):1862)
  - Medical management: (1) Elevate head of bed; (2) Remove indwelling catheters (risk of thrombosis causing SVC syndrome); (3) Consider steroids &/or diuresis
  - Radiation tx: If treating palliatively, use 3 Gy × 10, 4 Gy × 5. If treating w/ curative intent, use dose & fraction schedule appropriate to the histology
  - Consider endovascular stent prior to RT for rapid symptomatic relief
  - Consider chemotherapy if SVC syndrome is d/t SCLC, NHL, or germ cell tumors

Airway obstruction

- **Workup:** CT, bronchoscopy
- **Treatment:**
  - Endobronchial debulking & stent placement for rapid sx relief & is followed by radiotherapy
  - External beam radiotherapy: Dose schedules: 3 Gy × 10, 4 Gy × 5, 2.5 Gy × 15

Uncontrolled tumor hemorrhage

- **Etiology:** Gynecologic, GI, Pulm, or other malignancies causing tumor erosion of vessels
- **Workup:** CT, endoscopy/colonoscopy/ERCP (if GI source), bronchoscopy (if pulm source), basic blood tests (CBC, chemistries)
- **Treatment:**
  - Medical management: (1) Transfuse RBCs; (2) Vaginal packing (if gynecologic etiology); (3) Endoluminal cauterization; (4) IR embolization (can provide rapid relief in some cases)
  - Radiation tx: Consider 3 Gy × 10, 4 Gy × 5, or 2.5 Gy × 15, or quad shot (ie, 3.7 Gy BID × 2 d, repeat q2wk × 2 PRN)

Indications for Surgery		
Indication	**Goal**	**Examples**
Curative resection	Resection of all macroscopic tumor at local, regional, or oligometastatic sites w/ curative potential	Right hemicolectomy & resection of limited liver mets for colon CA
Staging/ prognosis	Tumor excision to complete staging & provide prognostic information	Sentinel LN bx for breast CA/melanoma
Disease control	Resection of incurable dz by removing some cancer to decrease tumor burden, improve sxs, & prolong survival	Cytoreductive surgery for peritoneal mets
Palliation	Improve pain, obstruction, or infection caused by tumor	Intestinal bypass for malignant bowel obstruction
Diagnosis	Provide tissue for pathologic dx or molecular workup when other less-invasive methods are nondiagnostic or discordant	Excision of LN for suspected lymphoma

Relative Contraindications for Surgery		
Contraindication	**Reason**	**Examples**
Patient factors	Pt will not tolerate physiologic stress of surgery, is unlikely to have meaningful functional recovery, or prefers nonsurgical tx	Poor functional status, severe cardiopulmonary dz/ end-organ dysfunction, pt preference
Anatomic factors	Tumor removal requires resection of vital nonreconstructible structures, or would result in organ failure	Locally advanced pancreatic adenoCA encasing long segment of SMA; resection of large liver tumor would result in liver failure due to small liver remnant
Disease factors	Incurable, biologically aggressive dz w/ short expected survival & no potential impact from surgery	Gastric adenoCA w/ peritoneal mets

Alternatives to Surgery	
Treatment modality	**Techniques**
Radiation	Conventional, IMRT, SBRT, ablative radiation
Endoscopy	EMR/ESD, colonic stenting, biliary stenting
Interventional radiology	Percutaneous ablation, TAE

Principles of Neoadjuvant, Adjuvant, and Downstaging Therapy		
	Goals	**Examples**
Neoadjuvant	Improve survival in resectable dz by optimizing delivery of perioperative therapy. Select pts best suited for surgery by ruling out early progression while on tx; shrink tumor to make surgery less extensive or lower risk	Pancreaticoduodenectomy for resectable pancreatic adenoCA; neoadjuvant therapy for breast CA to facilitate breast-conserving therapy
Adjuvant	Treat microscopic residual local/ distant dz postresection to improve survival	Colon adenoCA w/ LN mets
Downstaging	Convert unresectable dz to potentially resectable	Locally advanced pancreatic adenoCA

Principles of palliative surgery

- Appropriate pt selection is crucial; balance risks of surgical intervention w/ benefit of relieving sxs & improving QoL
- Use the palliative triangle: Shared decision-making between pt, family, & surgeon (*Arch Surg* 2011;146(5):517)
- Multidisciplinary discussion to evaluate other tx modalities
- >50% of pts w/ incurable CA evaluated for surgical tx undergo palliative surgery; 90% achieve sx relief w/ surgery (*Arch Surg* 2011;146(5):517)

SURGICAL EMERGENCIES

Initial evaluation and management of surgical emergencies

- These potentially lifesaving steps should be taken as soon as possible by the physician requesting surgical consultation:
- **Evaluate need for immediate resuscitation:** If vital signs abnormal, secure airway, establish IV access, give supplemental oxygen, transfer to monitored setting. Transfer to ICU if needed
- **Start initial treatment based on suspected disease process:**
  - **Sepsis:** Start broad-spectrum abx, begin fluid resuscitation, add vasopressors if needed (*JAMA* 2017;317:847–848)
  - **Hemorrhage:** Immediate consultation for bleeding control (surgery, IR, GI), establish large-bore (14 or 16 gauge) peripheral IV access, minimize crystalloids, balanced resuscitation w/ blood products (1:1:1 ratio of pRBC:FFP:platelets), permissive hypotension (SBP 70–110 mmHg), correction of acidosis/hypothermia (*Surg Clin North Am* 2017;97:999)
- **Localize suspected disease process:** Obtain imaging studies if pt stable
- **Prepare patient for surgery:** NPO, stop AC, identify significant cardiopulmonary comorbidities, send type/screen & coagulation studies, place Foley catheter &/or NGT if needed
- **Assess prognosis & goals of care:** Discuss prognosis, goals of care, & whether additional CA-directed treatments are available to pt if they recover. **An emergency surgical intervention is not the appropriate treatment for many pts**
- Specific tx plans for common surgical emergencies described below

Malignant obstruction

- **History:** Abdominal pain, nausea, vomiting, obstipation
- **Exam:** Distended, tympanitic, mild tenderness. Immediate surgical consultation if unstable vital signs or significant tenderness
- **Labs:** AKI & electrolytes abnormalities common. Leukocytosis raises concern for bowel ischemia
- **Imaging:** CT abdomen/pelvis w/ water-soluble oral contrast & IV contrast to evaluate location & extent of obstruction, & assess for evidence of compromised bowel. Insert NGT if pt unable to tolerate oral contrast
- **Initial treatment:** Discuss prognosis, goals of care, & cancer-directed tx options w/ primary oncologist. Rarely, pts present w/ bowel ischemia or perforation. Emergency surgery may be appropriate if consistent w/ goals of care & overall prognosis. For clinically stable pts, start w/ nonoperative management: Insert NG & connect to LCWS for decompression. Make NPO, start fluid resuscitation, correction of electrolyte abnormalities. Further tx determined by location of obstruction. 79–90% can achieve sx resolution w/ surgical/endoscopic management (*Ann Surg* 2004;240:719–726)
  - **Gastric outlet obstruction:** Surgical bypass vs. endoscopic stenting after decompression & resuscitation complete
  - **Small bowel obstruction:** May resolve w/ nonoperative management. Consider diet modification & expectant management, especially if 1st episode of obstruction & systemic tx options available. Surgical management should be considered for recurrent obstruction, chronic sxs, failure of nonoperative management, or lack of effective tx options. Surgical management determined by nature of obstruction:
    - *Single point of obstruction:* Small bowel resection or bypass
    - *Multiple points of obstruction:* Palliative gastrostomy tube for decompression. May consider highly selective use of surgical management
  - **Large bowel obstruction:** Surgical emergency due to high-risk of perforation from closed loop obstruction (if pt has competent ileocecal valve). Selected pts w/o signs of impending perforation can undergo endoscopic stenting. Otherwise, pts require resection or diverting colostomy, if consistent w/ their GOC

Cholecystitis

- **History:** RUQ/epigastric pain, fevers. Often minimal sxs from immunosuppression
- **Exam:** RUQ/epigastric tenderness. Immediate surgical consultation if unstable vital signs or diffuse tenderness
- **Labs:** Leukocytosis, elevated AST/ALT common. Elevated Tbili raises suspicion for choledocholithiasis or cholangitis
- **Imaging:** RUQ u/s shows cholelithiasis or sludge, gallbladder wall thickening, pericholecystic fluid, positive sonographic Murphy sign. Biliary dilation raises suspicion for choledocholithiasis, cholangitis

- **Initial treatment:** If pt has unstable vital signs, immediate consultation w/ surgery & IR for percutaneous cholecystostomy tube for source control. If clinically stable, start w/ IV abx, NPO, IV fluids. Discuss prognosis, GOC, & need for further cancer-directed tx w/ primary oncologist. Further management determined by surgical risk (*N Engl J Med* 2015;373:357)
  - Low-risk surgical candidate: Cholecystectomy during admission
  - High-risk surgical candidate: Consult IR for percutaneous cholecystectomy. Interval cholecystectomy in several wks if risk factors can be addressed
- **If clinical signs of choledocholithiasis, cholangitis:** Consult gastroenterology to evaluate for ERCP vs. MRCP. Cholecystectomy after choledocholithiasis/cholangitis has resolved

Perianal abscess

- **History:** Perianal pain, fevers. Often minimal sxs due to immunosuppression
- **Exam:** Perianal tenderness, induration. Often lack fluctuance/purulence due to neutropenia
- **Labs:** Neutropenia common. Evaluate degree of thrombocytopenia for possible surgical intervention
- **Imaging:** Pelvic MRI if presentation & exam equivocal
- **Treatment:** IV abx, wait 2–3 d for neutropenia to resolve, transfuse platelets to correct thrombocytopenia, then OR for EUA, I&D of abscess, & Seton placement (*Oncology* 2015;29:581)

Diverticulitis

- **History:** Lower abdominal pain, fevers. Often minimal sxs from immunosuppression
- **Exam:** Lower abdominal tenderness. Immediate surgical consultation if unstable vital signs or diffuse tenderness
- **Labs:** Leukocytosis common. Evaluate degree of neutropenia, anemia, thrombocytopenia to assess surgical risk
- **Imaging:** CT abdomen/pelvis w/ IV contrast to evaluate for perforation, abscess, or phlegmon
- **Initial treatment:** Emergency surgery if pt has unstable vital signs, diffuse tenderness, or imaging shows diffuse free air. If clinically stable, start w/ nonoperative management: IV abx, NPO, IV fluids, IR consult for percutaneous drainage of abscess. Discuss prognosis, GOC, & need for further cancer-directed tx w/ primary oncologist. Further management dictated by response to initial tx. Immunocompromised pts at higher risk of developing recurrent diverticulitis w/ perforation, so are more likely to benefit from surgical intervention (*JAMA* 2014;311:287)
  - **Sxs resolve:** Advance diet & transition to oral abx. Discuss role for elective sigmoid colectomy in several wks if further systemic tx required (may avoid need for ileostomy/colostomy).
  - **Persistent sxs:** Repeat CT to evaluate for abscess/perforation. Discuss role for sigmoid colectomy during this admission (will require end colostomy)

Medically refractory immunotherapy-induced colitis

- **History:** Diarrhea, abdominal pain, distention, hematochezia, mucus in stools
- **Exam:** Lower abdominal tenderness. Immediate surgical consultation if unstable vital signs or diffuse tenderness
- **Labs:** Elevated CRP, C. diff, & CMV PCR negative
- **Imaging:** CT abdomen/pelvis w/ IV contrast ± oral contrast to evaluate severity & identify free air
- **Treatment:** Emergency surgery if pt has unstable vital signs, diffuse tenderness, or imaging shows diffuse free air. If clinically stable, start w/ nonoperative management: NPO, IV abx, IV fluids, serial abdominal exams. Multidisciplinary discussion w/ surgery, medical oncology, & gastroenterology to determine next steps. Surgery considered as last resort for refractory colitis after infectious workup has been repeated & other immunosuppressants have been considered. 4% of pts fail to respond to medical therapy & require colectomy (*J Immunother Cancer* 2020;8:e001488)

INTERVENTIONAL PULMONOLOGY

Introduction

Scope of practice: Interventional pulmonologists perform minimally invasive procedures to diagnose & stage lung CA & tumors that metastasize to the thorax; provide sx relief by debulking tumors obstructing central airways & manage pleural diseases, which include pleural effusions, pneumothoraxes, & their complications

When to consult

- Bx of lung nodules, mediastinal lymph nodes, & pleural lesions for dx, staging, & tissue acquisition
- Dx of diffuse lung diseases, drug-induced pneumonitis, opportunistic infections that warrant a lung bx
- Intervention for dyspnea from airway obstruction due to thoracic tumors, foreign bodies
- Management of hemoptysis, pleural effusions (diagnostic & therapeutic), & pneumothoraces
- Direct CA tx: Recent advances include bronchoscopic intratumoral injection of chemo & bronchoscopic ablation therapy of lung nodules

Diagnostic bronchoscopy

- Can provide cytologic & histopathologic tissue for dx of malignancy & complications of CA therapy (eg, pneumonitis, opportunistic infections); can also assist in evaluating extent of endobronchial tumor
- Multiple modalities have varying yields & risks
  - **Bronchial brushing & washings:** Brush bronchial mucosa for cells & bacteria (*AJRCCM* 2016;193(10):68)
  - **BAL:** Instillation of normal saline aliquots into isolated lung subsegment w/ lavage collection for cultures, cell counts, & cytology (*Thorax* 2013;68(suppl 1):i1)
  - **Transbronchial biopsy (TBBx):** Uses bx forceps to obtain alveolar tissue
  - **Cryobiopsy:** Specialized cryoprobe used to obtain frozen samples of lung parenchyma. Samples are larger, well-preserved, & have less crush artifact compared to TBBx assisting in molecular analysis (*Chest* 2020;157(4):1030)
  - **EBUS:**
    - **Radial EBUS** generates a 360° u/s image of lung parenchyma to allow peripheral lung nodule bx or placement of fiducial markers
      - **Linear EBUS** provides view of mediastinal lesions around the central airway parallel to the bronchoscope shaft; allows real-time sampling of mediastinal lesions for transbronchial nodule aspiration (TBNA). Cytologic specimens obtained can be used for molecular testing (*Chest* 2013;143(5 suppl):e191S)
- **Navigational bronchoscopy:** Employs sensors to link w/ 3D virtual airway map to guide bx of peripheral lung nodules
- **Robotic bronchoscopy:** Allows operator to navigate smaller airways into the lung periphery under direct visualization using electromagnetic or shape-sensing guidance to find target airways, & provide stability during sampling of target lesion (*J Thor Dis* 2020;12(6):3279)

Procedures	Diagnostic Yield	Complications
Bronchial brushing & washing	5% or 47% w/ visible endobronchial lesion	Pneumothorax
BAL	19%	Transient hypoxia
TBBx	34% for lesion <2 cm 63% for lesion >2 cm	Pneumothorax 1–4% (compared to 20% w/ CT-guided bx)
Cryobiopsy	95%	Bleeding 4–20% Pneumothorax 1–7%
EBUS	67–95%	Bleeding 1%
Navigational bronchoscopy	60–80% dependent on size & location of nodule	Pneumothorax 5%
Robotic bronchoscopy	85–95%	Pneumothorax 1–2%

Therapeutic bronchoscopy (TB)

- Used for airway obstruction, defined as >50% narrowing of the airway from endobronchial tumor, extrinsic compression or mixed
- TB w/ a rigid &/or flexible bronchoscope can be used along w/ other modalities to restore airway patency & provide symptomatic relief

- Choice of modalities depends primarily on type of obstruction, pt/tumor characteristics, operator preference, & availability of tools
- While TB provides immediate symptomatic relief, concomitant tx w/ RT &/or chemo-immunotherapy can provide more definitive & long-term benefit
- The following modalities can be used (*Chest* 2020;157(2):446):
  - **Endobronchial tumor:** Tumor debulking w/ electrocautery, laser, argon plasma coagulation, cryotherapy; mechanical debulking w/ large forceps, rigid bronchoscope, & PDT
  - **Extrinsic compression:** Balloon dilation & airway stents are primary modalities for resolving stenoses. Airway stents can be metallic or silicone. Metallic stents preferred for malignant airway obstruction w/ central airways as preferred targets. Lobar stents can be considered but have ↑ risk of complications
  - **Mixed obstruction:** Requires a combination of the above modalities & is guided by anatomy & operator preference
- **Complications:** Overall complication rate ~4–13%. Specific complications include bleeding (0.5–1%), refractory hypoxia (2%), & unexpected escalation of care (4.4%). Less common complications include airway trauma/laceration, stent migration, pneumothorax, injury to oropharyngeal & laryngeal structure, & death (0.5%) (*AJRCCM* 2016;193(1):68)
- **Outcomes:** >50% luminal patency is achieved in >90% of cases. Improvement in dyspnea (50–80%), HRQOL scores, quality adjusted survival, & median survival time reported (*Thorax* 2019;74(2):141)

Figure 4-1 Left panel: Metastatic colon cancer with complete mixed obstruction of the bronchus intermedius. **Middle panel:** Post debulking with persistent >50% obstruction. **Right panel:** Normal airway patency after placement of metallic stent in the bronchus intermedius.

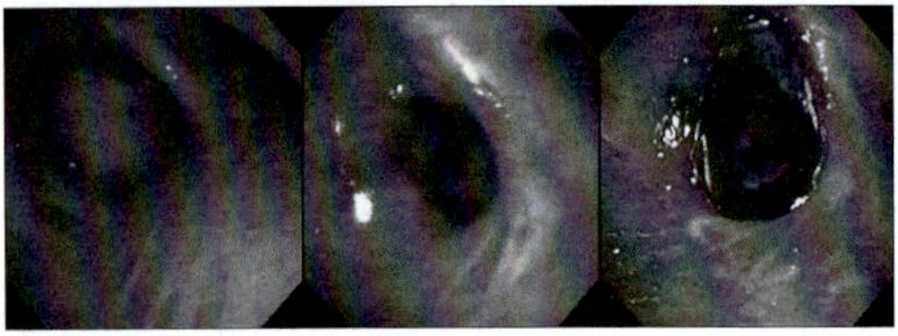

Whole lung lavage (WLL)

- Hematologic malignancies can cause acquired pulmonary alveolar proteinosis → common sxs are dyspnea, cough, & fevers
- For pts w/ moderate–severe hypoxemia, WLL is the most widely accepted form of tx
- Technique includes single lung lavage w/ double-lumen ETT & 15–20 L of normal saline in 0.8–1.5 L aliquots. Lavage fluid initially thick/milky → final lavage appears clear. Contralateral lung lavage performed 1–2 wks later
- WLL can improve sxs of exertional dyspnea & oxygenation despite only small changes in pulmonary function. 30–50% of pts require 1 lavage, while others require repeat lung lavages at intervals of 6–12 mos (*ERS* 2004;23(4):526)

Pleural diseases

Diagnostic procedures:

- **Thoracentesis**
  - **Indication:** To diagnose etiology of pleural effusion & provide dyspnea relief in symptomatic pts
  - **MPE:** Therapeutic thoracentesis can alleviate dyspnea in symptomatic pts & identify nonexpandable lung (30% of MPE). Pleural fluid cytology is diagnostic in 60% of MPE; however, diagnostic yield from sending >2 specimens is low & should be avoided (*Thorax* 2010;65(8):667)
    - **Pleuroscopy w/ pleural biopsy:** Involves use of a rigid pleuroscope to explore pleural space & obtain pleural biopsies for diagnostic purposes +/– concurrent placement of IPC. Diagnostic yield ~90–100%
      - **Indication:** Undx'd exudative effusions w/ a high suspicion of malignancy & to obtain additional tissue for molecular testing
      - **Complications:** Bleeding, infxn, pneumothorax (*J Thor Dis* 2020;12(5):2803)

Figure 4-2 Left panel: Metastatic breast cancer studding the pleura as noted on pleuroscopy. **Right panel:** Biopsy of the pleura with forceps during pleuroscopy.

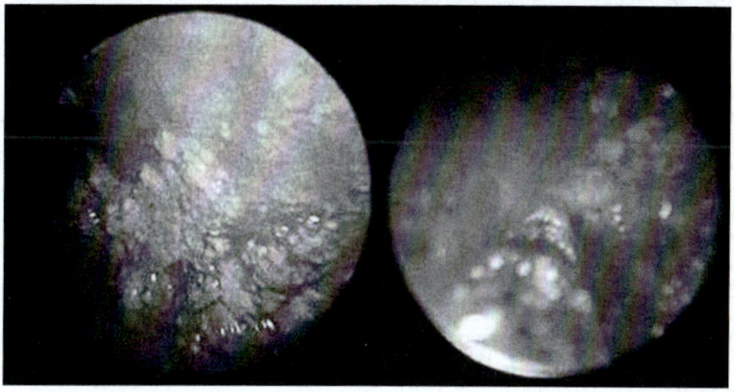

Therapeutic procedures:

- **IPC:**
  - **Indication:** Management of recurrent symptomatic MPE in pts w/ both expandable & nonexpandable lung. IPC placement is usually outpt but when performed as an inpt, decreases hospital stay. Typically remain in place for 2–6 wks, but can remain in place longer
  - **Patient selection:**
    - Pts w/ dyspnea improvement after thoracentesis +/– total lung reexpansion
    - Social support to assist in drainage at home is preferred
    - IPC best suited for pts requiring a short-term intervention while waiting for systemic therapy to take effect, those who prefer outpt management & a minimally invasive intervention, as well as those w/ expected shorter survival (eg, <2 mos) in need of palliative intervention
    - Spontaneous pleurodesis by IPC alone is achieved in ~40% of cases
- **Complications:** (1) Cellulitis & pleural space infxn → tx w/ oral or IV abx; catheter removal indicated if the infection fails to improve; (2) catheter blockage, may require intrapleural alteplase instillation or replacement of the IPC (rare) (*AJRCCM* 2018;198(7):839)
- **Pleurodesis:** Obliteration of the pleural space by induction of pleural inflammation & fibrosis using a sclerosant. This can be achieved using a pleuroscope (poudrage) or through an IPC or chest tube (slurry). Talc most common agent used as a sclerosant. Doxycycline & iodine are alternatives
  - Recent data suggests no difference in talc slurry vs. talc poudrage in success of pleurodesis (~80–90% success)
  - Lung & breast ca have better response to pleurodesis compared to other malignancies (*JAMA* 2020;323(1):60)
- **Indication:** Pts w/ rapidly recurrent MPE (<1 mo) who do not want a prolonged IPC or have failed spontaneous pleurodesis w/ IPC alone
- **Patient selection:**
  - Fit pts (ECOG 0–2) w/ an expandable lung, preference for a more definitive procedure, & expected >2–6 mos survival
  - Involves inpt stay postprocedure, inflammation can result in pain
- **Complications:** Infection including empyema, bleeding, rarely ARDS (*J Thor Dis* 2020;12(5):2803)

Image guidance

- The cornerstone of interventional radiologic therapies is advanced image guidance
- **Fluoroscopy:** Real-time x-ray imaging, utilizing lower dose than diagnostic radiography. Extensively used in vascular interventions (arterial & venous) & nonvascular interventions (eg, GI, GU, biliary interventions)
- **Digital subtraction angiography:** Fluoroscopic technique where precontrast image is "subtracted" from postcontrast images, providing accurate imaging of blood vessels
- **Contrast:** Iodinated contrast agents are commonly used for vascular imaging & interventions. Relative contraindications to contrast include renal insufficiency & hypersensitivity. Carbon dioxide can be an alterative contrast agent
- **Ultrasound:** Real-time imaging using sound waves. Advantages include lack of IR, multiplanar imaging capability, real-time visualization of needle & portability. Used in biopsies, drainages, vascular, nephrostomy, biliary access, musculoskeletal interventions including nerve blocks
- **CT:** Cross-sectional imaging modality using multiple x-rays, used for guidance in biopsies, drainages & ablations

Principles of embolization

- **Embolization:** Minimally invasive method of blocking normal or abnormal blood vessels using 1 or more embolic agents
- **Embolic agent:** A physical agent which is used to achieve desired embolic effect
- **Nontarget embolization:** When the embolic agent blocks blood flow w/in arteries supplying normal surrounding tissue
- Choice of embolic agent depends on the level of occlusion (capillary, arteriolar, or arterial), desired permanent or temporary embolic effect, risk of nontarget embolization, & the catheter delivery system being used
- Temporary embolic agents are used when there is high risk of end-organ damage & the desired embolic effect is temporary. Eg, acutely bleeding tumors, adjunct to other embolic agents, trauma. Most commonly used temporary embolic is Gelfoam
- Permanent embolic agents are used when total ischemia of the tumor is desired (HCC) or when a larger vessel can be safely sacrificed (eg, in acute bleeding). Permanent embolics include coils, particles, plugs, & glue
- Embolic agents are delivered using a combination of interventional catheters & wires in the desired arterial bed

Figure 4-3 Illustration depicting transarterial embolization using particles.

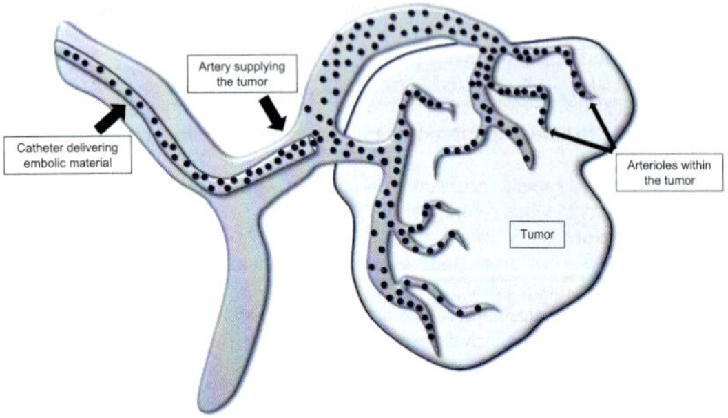

Principles of percutaneous ablation

- **Ablation:** Minimally invasive technique to treat tumors using needles or ablation probes
- Utilizes cytotoxic properties of thermal energy, electric field strength, or chemicals to cause tumor cell death
- **Thermal ablation technologies:** Cryoablation, microwave ablation, radiofrequency ablation, magnetic resonance guided focused u/s (MRgFUS)
- **Irreversible electroporation:** Nonthermal, electric current–based modality
- **Chemical Ablation:** Using cytotoxic chemicals (acetic acid & ethanol) to cause cell death
- **Image guidance:** Ablation procedures can be performed using u/s, CT, or MRI, w/ CT being the most common

TRANSARTERIAL THERAPIES

Transarterial embolization

- Transarterial "bland" embolization refers to delivery of embolic material w/o chemotherapeutic agents to the arteries supplying the tumor
- Mechanism: Occlusion of the terminal tumor arterioles by embolic material, leading to ischemic necrosis & cell death

Transarterial chemoembolization (TACE)

- Delivery of chemo agent directly into the artery feeding the tumor (*Lancet* 2002;359(9319):1734). Techniques include conventional TACE (cTACE) & drug-eluting bead TACE (DEB-TACE)
- **cTACE:** Delivery of chemotherapeutic agents (most commonly doxorubicin, cisplatin, &/or mitomycin C +/− lipiodol) followed by administration of an embolic agent (eg, gelfoam or particles)
  - Lipiodol (iodinated poppy seed oil) has selective uptake in target tumors → slows the washout of cytotxic drugs. In the liver, lipiodol passes through the hepatic sinosoids into the portal venules → dual embolization effect (*Cardiovasc Intervent Radiol* 2016;39(3):334)
- **DEB-TACE:** Refers to transarterial delivery of beads loaded w/ doxorubicin
  - Evolved to improve the PK of TACE & lower the systemic absorption of chemotherapeutic agent
  - The beads lodge in tumor microcirculation & release the drug over time (*Future Oncol* 2018;14(28):2969)

Figure 4-4 Transarterial chemoembolization. CT abdomen with contrast **A:** Shows large hypervascular metastatic lesion in segment 4A. Diagnostic angiography **B:** Shows enhancement of the metastatic lesion supplied by segment 4A branch, subsequently embolized using an emulsion of lipiodol and doxorubicin. **C:** Postembolization angiography shows stasis of flow within the feeding vessel. **D:** Follow-up CT 1 year later shows decreased size of the lesion with hyperdense lipiodol staining without recurrent disease.

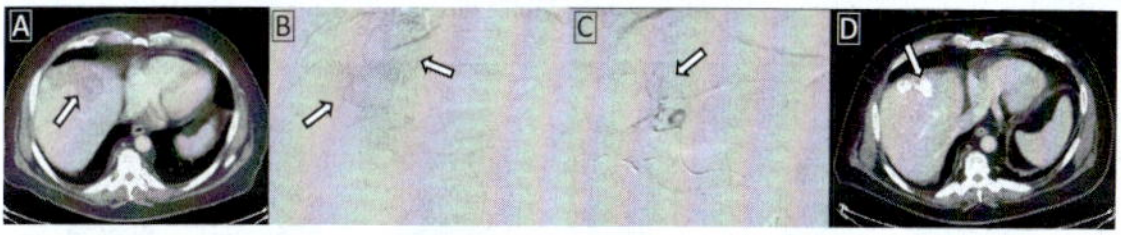

Selective internal radiation therapy (SIRT)

- Also known as transarterial radioembolization, SIRT refers to delivery of radioembolic beads loaded w/ radioactive compound into an artery feeding the tumor of interest (*Gastroenterology* 2016;151(6):1155)
- **Ytrium-90 (Y90):** Pure β-emitter w/ half-life of 64.2 h, decays to stable Zirconium-90 (Z90). Maximal electron penetration is 10 mm, making pt isolation unnecessary & minimizing off-target effects
- 2 Radioembolic beads are commercially available:
  - **SIR spheres** (Sirtex Medical, Lake Forest, IL): Resin-based, lower activity per particle. Larger number of microspheres needed to achieve desired dose
  - **TheraSpheres** (Boston Scientific, Marlborough, MA): Glass-based, higher activity per particle, lower number of microspheres needed to achieve desired dose
- **Radiation segmentectomy:** Administration of Y90 to single hepatic segment w/ the intention of segmental tissue ablation (*Radiology* 2018;287(3):1050)
- **Radiation lobectomy:** Administration of Y90 to entire hepatic lobe

Figure 4-5 Transarterial radioembolization. **A:** Hepatocellular carcinoma (HCC) lesion shown in segment 8. **B:** Subselective hepatic angiography shows tumor enhancement with predominant supply from the segment 8 artery. Radiation segmentectomy performed using Y90 delivered to segment 8. **C:** Follow-up CT 4 months later shows necrosis within the lesion without residual disease.

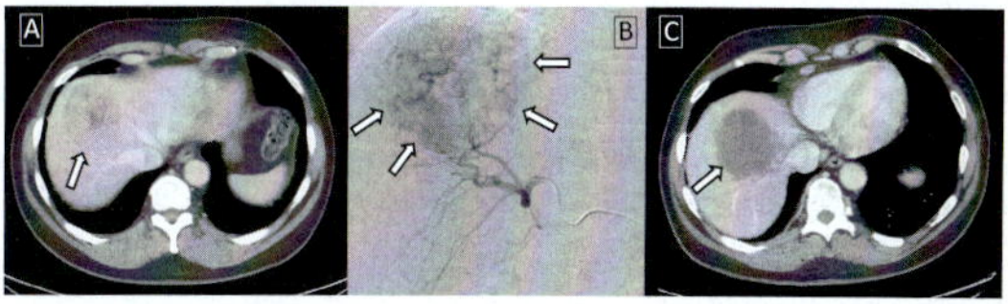

IMAGE-GUIDED PERCUTANEOUS ABLATION

Radiofrequency ablation (RFA)

- Conducted using interstitial electrodes inserted into the lesion & dispersive electrodes ("grounding pads") placed on skin surface
- Grounding pad closes the circuit, dispersing energy over large body surface area & decreasing probability of skin injury
- **RF waves:** Electromagnetic waves w/ frequencies ranging from 350–500 kHz
- **Mechanism:**
  - Dipolar molecules (like water) close to active interstitial electrode move in response to an alternating current produced by RF generator
  - Molecules constantly realign w/ electric poles w/ continuously alternating current; this motion causes friction & results in heat production, resulting in coagulation necrosis
  - Cell death occurs w/in few seconds at 55°C
- **Clinical application:** Used in liver, kidney, lung, & prostate cancers (*Eur Radiol* 2007;17(3): 725–733)

Microwave ablation

- Microwaves are higher-frequency electromagnetic waves (MHz to GHz)
- **Mechanism:**
  - Oscillating electrical field is transmitted from the antenna of microwave probe
  - Water molecules are polarized & carry electrical charge; rapid molecular agitation causes friction, leading to rise in water temperature, & heat
- Microwave creates higher temperatures & larger ablation zones, compared to RFA
- **Clinical application:** Hepatic, pulmonary, & renal malignancies/mets (*Lancet Gastroenterol Hepatol* 2018;3(5):317)

Figure 4-6 Lung microwave ablation. **A:** CT showed lung nodule in right upper lobe suspicious for metastatic disease. **B:** Intraprocedural axial CT with patient in prone position shows microwave ablation probe within the nodule. **C:** Follow-up CT 1 month later shows post-ablation changes around the nodule.

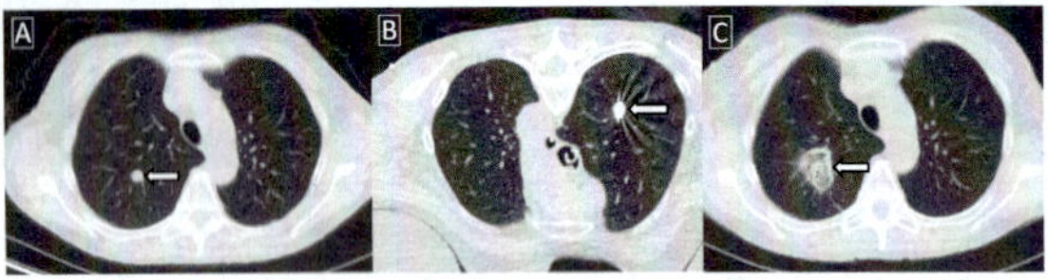

Cryoablation

- In contrast to RFA & microwave, cryoablation reduces the temperature of target lesion to below freezing (–20–-40°C)
- Cycling between cooling & thawing results in cell membrane disruption, dehydration, protein denaturation, intra- & extracellular ice formation, & vascular stasis → cell death
- The low thermal energy is transferred from tissue to tissue via conduction
- "Iceball" created by cryoablation probe can be seen w/ CT or u/s, allowing real-time monitoring during the procedure (*Abdom Radiol (NY)* 2016;41(4):754)

Irreversible electroporation (IRE)

- Nonthermal ablation technology that relies on pulses of high electrical current to disrupt cell membranes; thermal damage to surrounding structures is reduced; no "heat-sink"
- Electrical voltages may lead to muscular contractions; a muscle relaxant during the procedure is typically administered by anesthesiology
- Advantages over thermal ablation modalities:
  - Safer ablation of tumors near large blood vessels
  - Shorter ablation duration
- Clinical application: IRE has shown promise in liver, prostate, & pancreatic tumors (*Tech Vasc Interv Radiol* 2020;23(2):100675)

Chemical ablation

- Intratumoral instillation of acetic acid or alcohol, using percutaneously inserted needles under image guidance
- Destroys cells by protein denaturation & coagulation necrosis, in addition to entering vascular circulation, causing endothelial necrosis, platelet aggregation, thrombosis, & ischemic necrosis
- Clinical application: Primarily used in hepatocellular carcinoma in pts w/ cirrhosis (*World J Gastroenterol* 2014;20(43):15943)

Vertebral augmentation

- **Vertebroplasty:** Percutaneous injection of viscous bone cement (polymethyl methacrylate [PMMA]) for vertebral stabilization
- **Kyphoplasty:** Similar to vertebroplasty, w/ addition of vertebral height restoration by elevating the vertebral endplates using a balloon & facilitation cement injection under low resistance to minimize leakage. Performed under fluoroscopic image guidance & requires minimal sedation
- **Indications:** Osteoporotic compression fracture, vertebral mets ("pathologic fracture"), aggressive hemangioma, vertebral myeloproliferative dz
- In addition to clinical sxs of back pain & point tenderness, preprocedural MRI w/ or w/o contrast is essential for pt selection (*Lancet Oncol* 2011;12(3):225)

Figure 4-7 Kyphoplasty technique. Guiding cannula is passed through the pedicle and into the pathologic vertebral body. Once positioning is confirmed using multiple fluoroscopic views, a cavity may be created using a balloon (kyphoplasty) and bone cement is injected. Cannula is removed after cement injection.

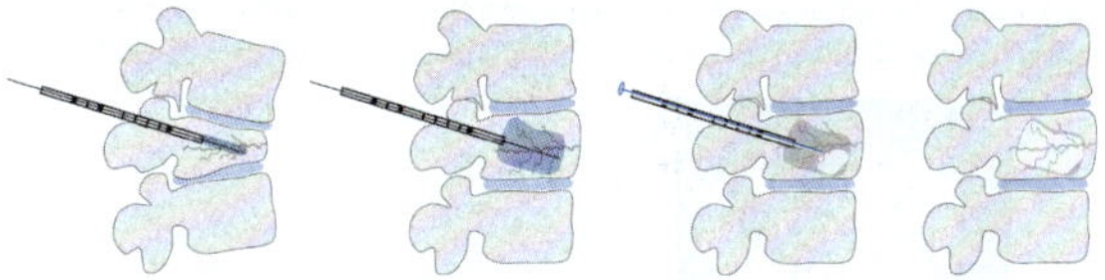

Figure 4-8 Kyphoplasty of an L5 metastasis. **A:** Sagittal STIR MRI image shows the metastatic lesion involving L5 vertebral body with collapse and mild posterior retropulsion. **B:** Lateral fluoroscopic image shows kyphoplasty cannulas inserted via the pedicles into the vertebral body and kyphoplasty balloons inflated within the vertebral body to create a cavity. **C:** Cement injection performed under fluoroscopic guidance.

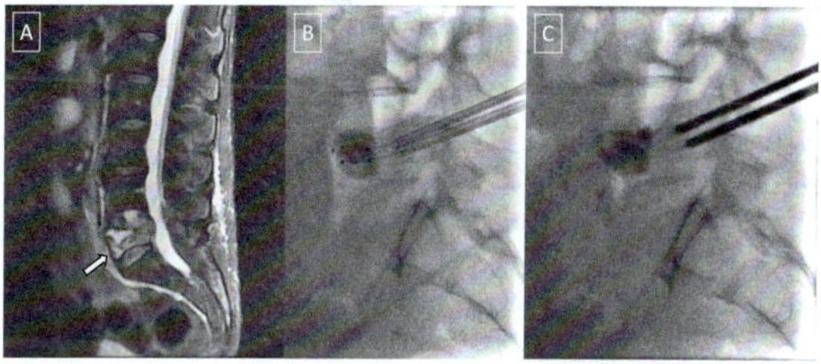

Cementoplasty and percutaneous screw fixation

- Cementoplasty refers to percutaneous injection of bone cement into the skeletal system. In the spine, the terms vertebroplasty/kyphoplasty are used. Outside the spine, the terms used include sacroplasty (sacrum), acetabuloplasty (acetabulum), & osteoplasty
- **Indications:** Painful pathologic fractures refractory to medical management &/or RT (met dz, myeloma), aggressive hemangioma
- Cementoplasty can be combined w/ percutaneous screw fixation to provide mechanical stabilization in certain areas of the skeleton under shear/torsional stress (*Diagn Interv Imaging* 2019;100(12):743)

Percutaneous cryoneurolysis

- The application of cold temperatures to a peripheral nerve, resulting in long term (but reversible) ablation of the nerve
- The procedure is technically similar to cryoablation of tumors & uses the same ablation probes
- **Indications:** Chronic postoperative pain, pain 2/2 metastatic disease (*AJR Am J Roentgenol* 2018;210(2):454)

Acute GI hemorrhage

- Majority of acute GI hemorrhages respond to medical or endoscopic management; some pts may require emergent tx by interventional radiologist. Successful intervention may avoid emergency surgery (*Medicine (Baltimore)* 2017;96(52):e9437)
- Diagnostic modality of choice includes **multi-phase CT angiography (CTA);** alternative modality is **nuclear medicine Tc 99m–labeled red blood cell scan** (↑ sensitivity)
- Catheter angiography of the artery supplying most likely site of bleeding is performed to evaluate for active extravasation or pseudoaneurysm
- If source of bleeding is identified, transcatheter embolization performed using embolic materials (temporary or permanent) to control hemorrhage
- In pts w/ portal hypertension presenting w/ acute variceal bleeding refractory to endoscopic management, emergent transjugular intrahepatic portosystemic shunt (TIPS) can decrease portal pressure; variceal embolization & splenic artery embolization can be used in select variceal bleeds (*N Engl J Med* 2010;362(25):2370)

Figure 4-9 Pseudoaneurysm embolization. **A:** CT abdomen with contrast shows large pseudoaneurysm arising from the gastroduodenal artery (GDA). **B:** Transradial angiography of replaced hepatic artery showed pseudoaneurysm arising from the GDA with outflow inferior pancreaticoduodenal arteries. **C:** Successful coil embolization performed of the outflow vessels and inflow GD.

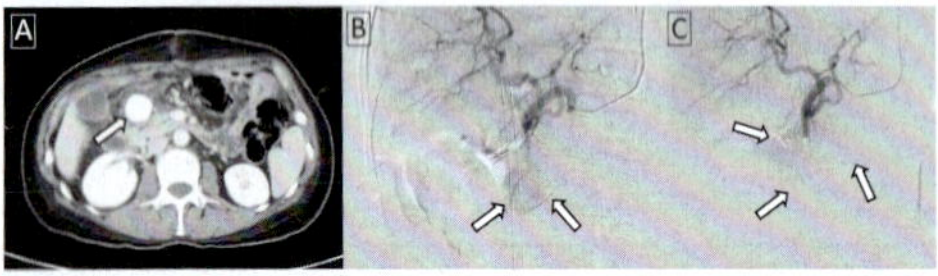

Venous thromboembolism

- VTE comprises deep vein thrombosis (DVT) & pulmonary embolism (PE); risk of VTE in CA pts ↑ compared to general pop
- Primary tx of VTE is AC; endovascular tx can be considered for sx control & prevention of clot-related sequelae
- Endovascular tx options for VTE include catheter-directed mechanical thrombectomy & thrombolysis using tPA to dissolve clot
  - Candidates for endovascular DVT therapy include pts w/ iliofemoral DVT to prevent postthrombotic syndrome (PTS) (*Lancet.* 2012;379(9810):31)
  - Candidates for endovascular PE therapy include pts w/ massive PE (sustained hypotension) & high-risk submassive PE (stable, right heart strain, elevated troponin) (*JACC Cardiovasc Interv* 2018;11(14):1401)
- In pts w/ contraindication to tPA (hemorrhagic brain mets), purely mechanical thrombectomy options can be used
- IVC filters: Percutaneously placed devices to prevent PE (*Circulation* 2005;112(3):416)
- Accepted indications for IVC filters:
  - Known DVT w/ contraindication to AC
  - Recurrent PE on therapeutic AC

Figure 4-10 **A:** CT venogram shows acute thrombus within left femoral vein. **B:** Initial fluoroscopic contrast injection from left popliteal vein access shows no contrast opacification of femoral vein and multiple collateral channels. **C:** After mechanical thrombectomy, venographic image shows recanalization of the femoral vein & minimal residual thrombus. **D:** Removed thrombus showed evidence of acute-on-chronic thrombosis (*darker*—acute clot, *lighter*—chronic clot).

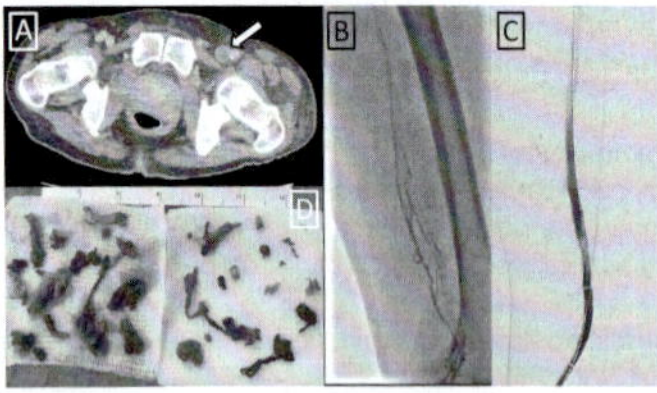

Acute urinary obstruction

- Obstructive uropathy w/ urosepsis represents a surgical emergency that requires urgent intervention to decompress the urinary collecting system
- Percutaneous nephrostomy placement by the interventional radiologist achieves rapid decompression of the collecting system
- Access to the renal collecting system is obtained using u/s guidance into the most dilated posterior lower pole calyx
- Once the calyx is punctured, contrast is injected under fluoroscopy to confirm positioning in collecting system (*Tech Vasc Interv Radiol* 2009;12(2):154)

Figure 4-11 Percutaneous nephrostomy placement. **A:** Contrast-enhanced CT shows moderate left hydronephrosis with delayed nephrograms. **B:** Illustration showing ideal access to the kidney in posterior calyx, in the so-called "avascular plane of Brodel." **C:** Ultrasound-guided access obtained to a posterior calyx of lower pole (*arrow* at needle tip). **D:** Final fluoroscopic image shows nephrostomy catheter in renal collecting system (*arrow*).

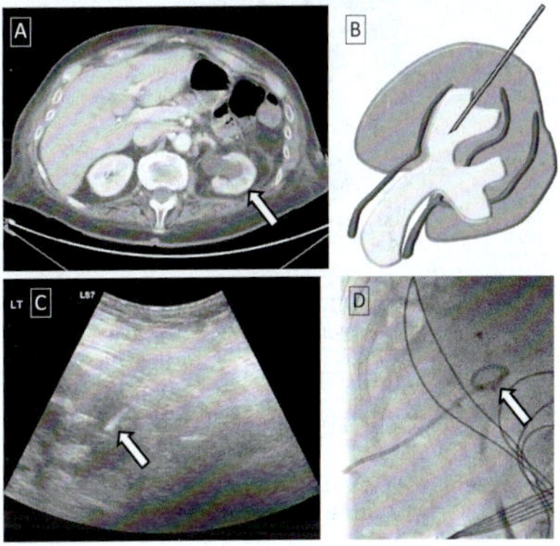

Biliary interventions

- Biliary obstruction may be 2/2 either benign or malignant etiologies; requires multidisciplinary discussions between GI endoscopists, interventional radiologists, & hepatobiliary surgeons
- Percutaneous biliary interventions include percutaneous transhepatic cholangiography (PTC), internal/external biliary catheter placement, & biliary stent placements
- Commonly accepted indications for percutaneous biliary intervention:
  - Pts w/ obstructive jaundice w/ or w/o cholangitis
  - Endoscopic techniques are not possible (hilar obstruction or surgically altered anatomy)
  - Endoscopic retrograde cholangiopancreatography is technically unsuccessful
- Contraindications: Coagulopathy (high risk of hemorrhage), allergy to contrast (*Gastroenterol Clin North Am* 2018;47(3):621)

Figure 4-12 Biliary catheter and stent placement. **A:** Coronal T2-weighted MRI image shows dilatation of left-sided biliary ducts with soft tissue filling defect near the hilum (*arrow*), suspicious for recurrent tumor. **B:** Cholangiogram via segment 3 duct access shows severe long segment stenosis of proximal 2/3rds of the common bile duct. **C:** Biliary catheter was placed beyond the stenosis and above the papilla. **D:** After resolution of acute symptoms of sepsis, patient was brought back for biliary stent placement (*long arrow*). The covering external catheter (*small arrow*) was removed after 1 week.

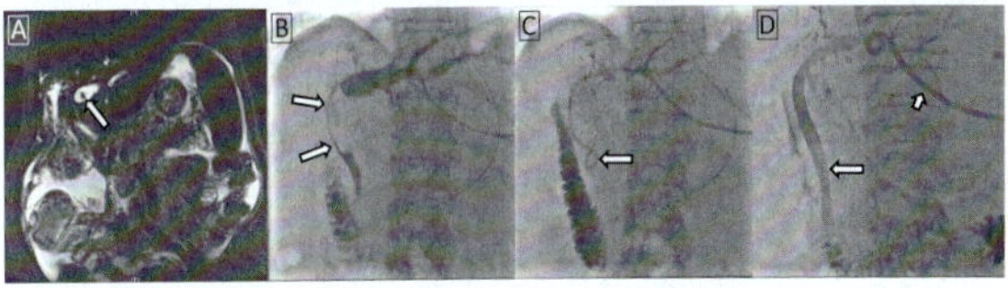

Hallmarks of cancer

Figure 5-1 Cancers share a set of common distinctive and complementary capabilities that enable tumor growth and metastatic dissemination. (Adapted with permission from *Cell* 2011;144:646.)

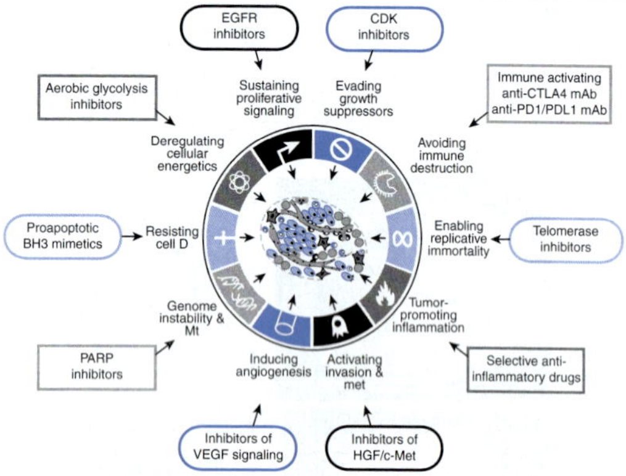

Emerging hallmarks: Phenotypic plasticity; biophysical properties

Cancer stem cells (CSCs)

The CSC hypothesis posits that CAs contain **relatively rare subpopulations of cells that are particularly capable of tumor regeneration** (*Nat Rev Drug Discov* 2014;13:497)

- Evidence for CSCs in a variety of CAs including AML, CRC, melanoma, gliomas, medulloblastoma, skin, head, & neck SCC
- CSCs can be slow-cycling & immune-evasive & thus **resistant to chemo, radiotherapy, & IO**
- Can be a dynamic cell state acquired by **phenotypically plastic & heterogeneous** tumor cells
- Characterized by **dedifferentiation,** activation of programs such as EMT & by epigenetic reprogramming
- Microenvironment plays a critical role in the resistance of CSCs to tx
- CSC-targeting txs aimed at stem-like programs & dedifferentiated states are being explored as a therapeutic strategy

Approaches for Targeting CSCs

Approach	Examples
Targeting CSC-dependent signaling pathways	Inhibitors of Wnt, TGF-β, Notch, Hedgehog, & YAP pathways
Targeting the tumor microenvironment	Inhibitors of stemness-inducing cytokines & chemokines & vasculature (eg, PGE2, CSF-1, CCL2, CXCL12, VEGF)
Differentiation therapy to force exit from the stem-like state	ATRA for APL, epigenetic modulators (eg, HDAC inhibitors, DOT1L inhibitors, IDH1/2 inhibitors)
CSC-targeted IO	Antibodies & CAR-T cells against CSC-specific cell-surface markers (eg, CD47, CD133)

MECHANISMS OF ONCOGENESIS

- Carcinogenesis proceeds in a stepwise fashion which can involve the activation of oncogenes as well as the inactivation of tumor suppressor genes

Mutations

- Alterations in DNA sequence or structure secondary to replication errors or carcinogens. Mut may impact prot fxn eg, loss of fxn, gain of fxn neomorphic (eg, *IDH1/2* or dominant neg eg, *TP53, ATM* T7271G, *H3.3* K27M, *H3.3* K36M)

Type of Mutation	Examples
Substitution transition G↔ A, C↔T transversion A/G ↔ C/T Can be silent (no change in AA), nonsense (early stop codon), **missense** (change in AA)	***JAK2* V617F** in PV, ET ***BRAF* V600E** in melanoma, HCL ***KRAS* G12D** in CRC, NSCLC ***EGFR* L858R** in NSCLC Note: 1st letter: Original AA, number: AA position, 2nd letter: Substituted AA
Deletion: Loss of 1 or more bases or larger DNA region	***EGFR* exon 19 del** in NSCLC **5q-**syndrome in MDS
Insertion: Insertion of 1 or more bases	***EGFR* exon 20 ins** in NSCLC

*__Amino Acid Nomenclature:__ Arg (R), His (H), Lys (K), Asp (D), Glu (E), Ser (S), Thr (T), Asn (N), Gln (Q), Cys (C), Gly (G), Pro (P), Ala (A), Val (V), Ile (I), Leu (L), Met (M), Phe (F), Tyr (Y), Trp (W)

Copy number alterations

- Deletion or duplication of genomic fragments (a few kb up to entire chromosomes)
- Clinically relevant egs:
  ***ERBB2 (HER2)* Amp:** Breast CA (avg of >6 gene copies/nucleus or *HER2/CEP17* ratio >2.2 via FISH), gastric CA. Predictive of response to trastuzumab
  ***MET* Amp:** Mechanism of acquired resistance to EGFR TKIs in NSCLC

Chromosomal rearrangements

- Can create gene fusions
- These rearrangements constitutively activate proto-oncogenes in an aberrant fashion; alternatively, dysregulate prot expression (ie, constitutively activate a TK)

Type	Examples
Translocation: Rearrangement of material btw nonhomologous chromosomes 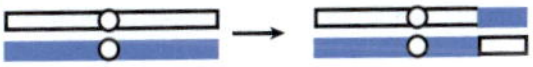 Reciprocal: Even exchange of material Robertsonian: 2 acrocentric chromosomes fuse near centromere w/ short arm loss	***BCR-ABL1* t(9;22)** in CML/Ph+ ALL ***PML-RARA* t(15;17)** in APL ***NPM1-ALK* t(2;5)** in ALCL ***RUNX1-RUNX1T1* t(8;21)** in AML M2 ***EWSR1-FLI1* t(11;22)** in Ewing sarcoma ***MYC-IGH t(8;14)*** in Burkitt lymphoma
Inversion: Chromosomal segment is reversed end-to-end (pericentric—includes centromere vs. paracentric—exclude centromere) 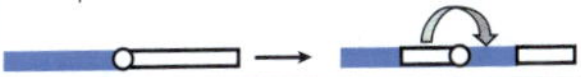	***EML4-ALK* t(2;2)** in NSCLC ***CBFB-MYH11* inv(16)** in AML M4 w/ eosinophilia
Deletion: Genetic material lost w/in a chromosome (interstitial) 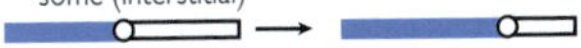	***TMPRSS2-ERG* del(21)** in prostate CA ***FIP1L1-PDGFRA*** in hypereosinophilic syndrome

Infections

- Play important roles as carcinogens in several dzs (see Cancer Epidemiology chapter for more extensive list). Carcinogenesis occurs through a variety of mechanisms (eg, chronic inflammation, specific actions of viral/bacterial prots, insertional mutagenesis)
  - **Viruses:** HPV (cervical & oropharyngeal CA; viral prots E6 & E7 inhibit TP53 & RB1), EBV (lymphoma), KSHV, HTLV1 (ATLL), HBV, & HCV (HCC)
  - **Bacteria:** *H. pylori* (gastric CA), bacterial CagA prot → activates tyrosine phosphatase SHP2 affecting various pathways involved in cell migration, adhesion, & apoptosis

Hormone receptors

- Breast & prostate CA are often driven by aberrant ER or AR signaling, respectively, & targeting these receptors represent standard-of-care tx for these CAs

GROWTH FACTOR SIGNALING

- **Growth factors (GFs)** are soluble prots whose binding to **growth factor receptors (GFRs)** activates downstream pathways (such as Ras/MAPK & PI3K/Akt/mTOR) that promote cellular growth, proliferation, inflammation, & cytoskeletal reorganization
- Most GFRs are transmembrane prots w/ intrinsic TK activity & are therefore known as RTKs
- Several RTKs can be targeted by **mAbs** (eg, trastuzumab for ERBB2, cetuximab for EGFR, see Monoclonal Antibodies chapter) or **small molecules** (eg, TKIs)
- **Growth-factor signaling** is regulated by positive & neg feedback loops, which convey specificity, & allow restoration of cellular homeostasis after the stimulus has ceased. Reactivation of RTK signaling after inhibition of overactive downstream components is a/w resistance & dictates the need for combination therapies (ie, simultaneous BRAF, MEK, & EGFR inhibition in *BRAF*^{V600E} CRC)

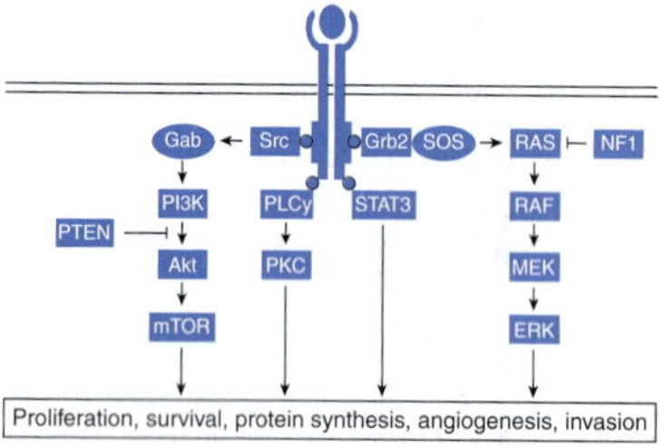

Figure 5-2 EGFR signaling: Ligand binding induces receptor dimerization and phosphorylation of intracellular TK domains (TKDs). Phosphorylated TKDs act as docking units for several proteins involved in signal propagation via different pathways. This series of signal transduction events culminates in a change in the cellular transcriptional program.

Growth Factor Receptor	Role in Carcinogenesis/Examples
ERBB family: Structurally related receptors, capable of forming homo or heterodimers, contain TK domains (except for ERBB3 [HER3]) (*Nat Rev Cancer* 2005;5:341)	
EGFR (ERBB1)	*EGFR* mts in lung CA, EGFR overexpressed in lung adenoCA, GMB, HNSCC
ERBB2 (HER2)	*ERBB2 (HER2)* amp & ERBB2 (HER2) overexpression: Breast CA & gastric CA
ERBB3 (HER3) & **ERBB4** (HER4)	Dimerize w/ other family members, overexpressed in multiple malignancies
FGFRs: FGFR1, FGFR2, FGFR3, FGFR4 (*Nat Rev Drug Discov* 2009;8:235)	*FGFR1* mts in GMBs & amps in squamous NSCLC *FGFR3* mts & overexpression in bladder CA
MET (HGFR)	*MET* mts in sporadic/hereditary papillary RCCs
KIT	*KIT* mts in GIST, melanoma, mast cell leukemia
PDGFRA	*PDGFRA* mts in GIST, role in angiogenesis
VEGFR	Angiogenesis, overexpressed in multiple CAs
IGF1R	Insulin signaling, potential predisposition to several CAs
RET	Mts & fusions in lung & thyroid CA
NTRKs: TRKA, TRKB, TRKC	Fusions in several CAs (*Nat Rev Clin Onc* 2018;15:731)
ALK	Fusions in NSCLC, mts in NB
MAPK Pathway	
NF1	*NF1* is a tumor suppressor gene, w/ mts a/w **neurofibromatosis type I,** juvenile myelomonocytic leukemia, melanoma
RAS	***KRAS*** most commonly mutated oncogene in CA: 90% pancreatic CA, 35% CRC, 25% NSCLC, 20% serous ovarian CA, 15% thyroid CA, etc. *NRAS* mutated in melanoma, HCC, thyroid CA (*Nat Rev Cancer* 2011;11:761)
RAF	***BRAF*** mts (& rare fusions) in melanoma, CRC, thyroid CA, glioma
MEK	Rare *MAP2K1 (MEK)* mts in several malignancies
ERK	Alterations in *MAPK1 (ERK)* rarely demonstrated in human CAs

PI3K-AKT-mTOR Pathway	
PI3K	PIK3CA mts in endometrial CA, breast CA, cervical CA, anal CA, CRC, can coexist w/ other driver mts (*JAMA Oncol* 2016;2:1565)
PTEN	***PTEN*** is a tumor suppressor gene, mts a/w **Cowden syndrome,** gliomas, endometrial CA, breast CA, ovarian CA
AKT	Rare ***AKT1*** mts in several malignancies
mTOR	Serine/threonine kinase, integrates several upstream pathways, plays role in angiogenesis, CRTC1 (TORC1) inhibited by mTOR inhibitors
TSC	*TSC1* or *TSC2* mts in **tuberous sclerosis,** lymphangioleiomyomatosis
STK11	*STK11 (LKB1)* mts in **Peutz–Jeghers syndrome** (hamartomatous GI polyps w/ ↓ malignant potential, hyperpigmented macules/patches on lips, & oral mucosa)

Cell cycle control

- **Cell cycle phases: G1** (growth phase, DNA replication prots formed, G1 checkpoint: Cycle arrest if DNA damage, metabolite depletion, growth factor withdrawal) → **S** (DNA synthesis, cell doubles DNA) → **G2** (2nd growth period, G2 checkpoint: Arrest if DNA damaged/improperly replicated) → **M** (mitosis, spindle assembly checkpoint: Arrest if sister chromatids misaligned) (*Nat Rev Cancer* 2009;9:153)
- **CDKs: Phosphotransfer enzymes** at the heart of cell cycle control
- **Cyclins:** Prots that bind to & positively regulate CDKs activity; CCND1 is overexpressed in **MCL** via t(11:14)
- **RB1:** Plays major role in **inhibiting G1-S phase progression,** hypophosphorylated RB1 sequesters E2F/DP thus repressing transcription → in the presence of growth factors, Cyclin D-CDK4/6 & Cyclin E-CDK2 sequentially phosphorylate RB1 → results in transcription of E2F target genes → cell cycle progression
- **Endogenous CDK inhibitors:** (Eg, CIP/KIP family which inhibit CDK2, INK family (CDKN2A) which inhibit CDK4 & CDK6). Inactivating germline *CDKN2A (P16INK4A)* mts in **FAMMM** (genetic predisposition to multiple moles, melanomas, & pancreatic CA)
- Alterations in the cyclin D- CDK4/5-Rb pathway in CAs: Association w/ breast CA, GMBs (*CDK4* amp), MCL (cyclin D2 overexpression via t(11:14)
- **CDK inhibitors as cancer treatment:** CDK4/6 inhibitors for ER+ breast CA (*NEJM* 2016;375:1925)

Figure 5-3 Cell cycle progression: Cyclin–CDK complexes regulate progression through different phases of the cell cycle; CDK inhibitors (members of the INK and CIP/KIP families) interact with specific cyclin–CDK complexes to block kinase activity. Anaphase promoting complex (APC) is activated upon chromosome alignment and leads CDK1 inhibition and exit from mitosis.

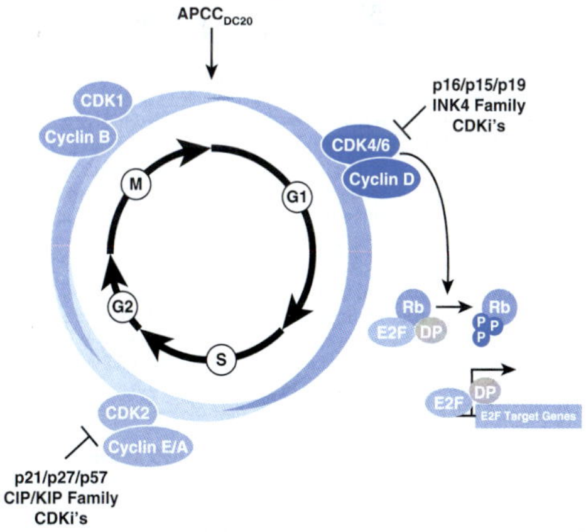

TRANSCRIPTION, APOPTOSIS, AND TP53

Transcriptional regulation

- Gene expression is modulated by transcription factors that bind gene promoters & enhancers. TFs are frequently genetically or epigenetically altered in CA
- 1 important class of TFs are nuclear receptors (ie, **ER** & **PR** in breast CA, RAR in APL, see Figure 5-4). Upon binding their cognate hormone, they translocate to nucleus → bind to response elements on the genome → affect target gene expression
- Transcription also regulated by various epigenetic mechanisms (histone modification, DNA-methylation, nucleosome remodeling, chromatin compaction, & looping)

Transcription Factor	Example
MYC family (Figure 5-4)	*MYCN (N-MYC)* & *MYCL1 (L-MYC)* amps in **neuroblastomas**. *MYC (C-MYC)* t(8;14) translocations in **Burkitt lymphoma**
ETS family	Gene fusions in prostate CA & Ewing sarcoma
WT1	*WT1* Mt in **Wilms tumor** & Denys–Drash syndrome

Figure 5-4 In cancer, upstream pathways (eg, Wnt, Shh, EGF) and dysregulation of MYC transcription itself by translocation/amplification, lead to constitutive c-myc expression that ↑ proliferation. The retinoic acid receptor (RAR) binds RA, allowing it to shuttle to the nucleus and regulate transcription.

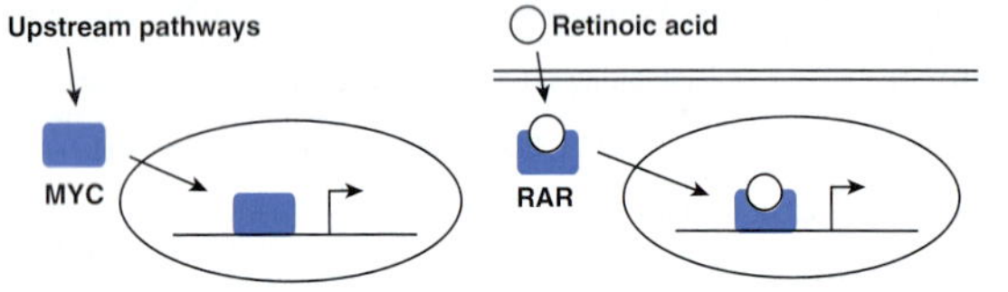

Apoptosis

- Physiologic process of programmed cell death, orchestrated via 2 major mechanisms:
  - **Extrinsic pathway:** An external "death signal" (ie, TNFα, FasL) binds to transmembrane receptors (TNFR1 & FAS) → death domains (TRADD & FADD) exposed → caspase activation → proteolysis of target prots in cell
  - **Intrinsic pathway:** Cell stress or DNA damage such as in the face of radiation or chemo → mitochondrial membrane perm via BAX/BAK, cytochrome C release → forms apoptosome w/ APAF-1/procaspase-9 → caspases activation.
- **BCL-2 family:** Regulate mitochondrial outer memb perm. Pro- & antiapoptotic:

Proapoptotic	Antiapoptotic
BAX, BAK, & BH3-only subset: NOXA, PUMA, BAD, BID, BIM	MCL-1, BCL-XL, **BCL-2** (overexpressed due to t(14;18) in follicular lymphomas)

- BCL-2 blocks apoptosis by inhibiting BAX/BAK. **Venetoclax** is a BCL-2 inhibitor (BH3 mimetic) used in AML & CLL/SLL. Bcl-xL & Mcl-1 inhibitors in clinical trials
- **Senescence:** Process by which cells enter irreversible cell-cycle arrest in response to cellular stresses (DNA damage, telomere shortening, oncogenic signals). In the context of oncogene signaling (ie, RAS or BRAF), can act as a tumor suppressive mechanism
- **Telomeres:** Repetitive DNA sequences at chromosome ends that shorten w/ cell division. Telomere loss → replicative senescence. Tumors often upregulate hTERT to maintain telomere length (*J Biomed Sci* 2018;25:22)

TP53

- Most frequently mutated tumor suppressor in CA
- p53 is a sequence-specific DNA binding prot that regulates transcription, is activated by stress signals (DNA damage, replicative stress, oncogenes, etc.) & is predominantly posttranslationally regulated. p53 is ubiquitinated by E3 ligase MDM2 & continuously degraded (MDM2 inhibitors are under investigation)
- DNA damage → ATM/ATR/CHK1→ phosphorylate p53 → inhibits MDM2 → ↑ **p53 activity**
- Oncogenic stress → ARF/p14 → sequester MDM2 → ↑ **p53 activity**
- p53 activation → multiple tumor suppressive outputs: (1) Cell-cycle arrest (via p21), (2) apoptosis (via Puma), (3) senescence (via p21), (4) DNA repair (via XPC/DDB2)
- **Li–Fraumeni syndrome:** Germline *TP53* Mt, leads to ↑ predisposition to sarcomas, breast CA, leukemias, brain tumors, adrenocortical CA

DNA repair mechanisms

- DNA repair is the process by which the cell repairs DNA lesions; many DNA repair genes are tumor suppressors & are a/w inherited CA syndromes (*Nat Rev Cancer* 2012; 12:801)
- Multiple pathways cooperate to perform efficient repair of DNA damage in the cell. Loss of a single pathway (eg, by inactivating mt) is often compensated by others
- PARP inhibitor development: PARP naturally binds to DNA single-strand break; PARP inhibition sequesters inhibited PARP on DNA. This PARP-SSB lesion requires homologous recombination (HR) to repair; in HR-deficient cells, such as those w/ *BRCA1*/*BRCA2* mt, these lesions lead directly to cell death, while normal (HR-proficient) cells are spared
- HR deficiency-associated CAs now thought to include breast, ovary, prostate, & pancreas CAs. PARP inhibitors approved for pts harboring *BRCA1* or *BRCA2* mt in various clinical & genomic contexts for these solid tumors

Mechanism	Examples
1-step repair: Direct reversal of DNA damage, MGMT removes alkyl group from O^6-guanine	GBM: Improved outcomes w/ alkylating agent temozolomide in tumors harboring *MGMT* **promoter methylation** or **loss**
NER: Endonuclease excises pyrimidine dimers (UVB-induced) & bulky adducts → DNA polymerase fills in gap using opposite strand as template	**Xeroderma pigmentosum:** Inherited defect in NER & ↑ skin CA risk ***POLE*** Mt: Ultramutated phenotype (CRC, endometrial CAs)
BER: Glycosylases, endonucleases, & DNA polymerases repair chemically altered bases (eg, oxidative damage)	***MUTYH*** (caretaker gene, encodes BER glycosylase) → germline mt in **HNPCC**
MMR: Corrects replication errors that escape polymerase editing in repetitive regions, involves MLH & MSH prots, a/w hypermutator phenotype	Germline mt in *MLH1*, *MSH2*, *MLH3*, *MSH6* → microsatellite instability (MSI-H), hallmark of **HNPCC (Lynch syndrome)**
Recombinational repair: DNA double-strand breaks mended by HR & NHEJ, involves various prots such as ATM, BRCA1, BRCA2	**Ataxia telangiectasia:** *ATM* mts, x-ray Sn, ↑ lymphoma risk ***BRCA* Mt:** Hereditary breast–ovarian CA syndrome

Angiogenesis

- Mediated by a number of growth factors & receptors including (1) HIF1α: In hypoxia, heterodimerizes w/ HIF1β in nucleus & leads to transcription of target genes, (2) **VEGF-VEGFR:** Initiate angiogenesis, (3) **ANG-TIE:** Helps maintain angiogenesis/vessel maturation → balanced by several inhibitors of angiogenesis (*NEJM* 2008;358:2039)

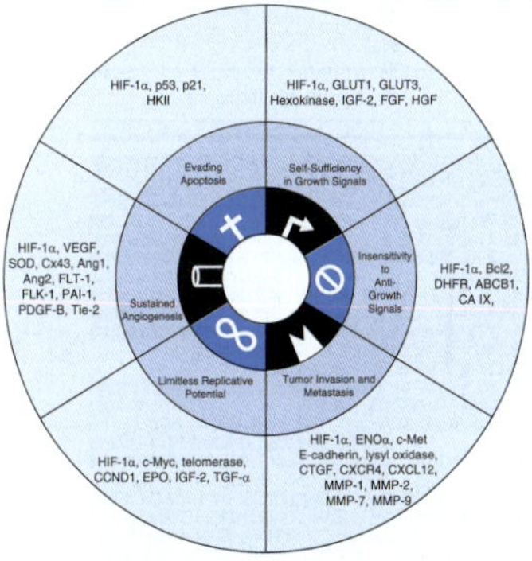

Figure 5-5 Effects of hypoxia on the hallmarks of cancer. Hypoxia and accumulation of HIF1 perturb the 6 hallmarks of cancer through a variety of signaling pathways. Of the hallmarks, the interaction between hypoxia and sustained angiogenesis has received the most attention. (Figure reproduced with permission from Betof AS, Dewhirst MW. Establishing the tumor microenvironment. In: Siemann DW, ed. Tumor Microenvironment. West Sussex, UK: John Wiley & Sons, Ltd.; 2011.)

- **VHL disease:** VHL ubiquitination mediates HIF1α response to hypoxia. Germline *VHL* mt a/w hemangioblastomas, RCCs, pheochromocytomas, PNETs; sporadic mts also occur in RCCs

Classic Sanger Sequencing	
Developed in 1977 by Frederick Sanger & colleagues	
Required reagents	DNA template (what you want to seq), DNA primer (known seq), dNTPs, ddNTPs, DNA polymerase
The principle	Mixing dNTPs & ddNTPs results in random chain termination yielding different sized DNA fragments → DNA fragments are separated by size → fragments are detected w/ radioactively or fluorescently labeled ddNTPs or DNA primers DNA polymerase CAN replicate & extend seq w/ dNTPs; DNA polymerase CANNOT extend seq w/ ddNTPs
Limitations	Poor seq quality in 1st 50 bp of seq Seq degradation after >700 bp Known DNA seq needed to design primers Cheap on a per-sample basis, expensive on a per-genome basis Impractical for large sequencing projects

Next Generation Sequencing	
The principle	Simultaneous sequencing of multiple short DNA (<250 bp) fragments Overlapping sequencing fragments can be reassembled
Depth of coverage	Measures number of times specific site has been sequenced ↑ Depth of coverage → ↑ quality of sequencing data 60× coverage does not mean whole genome sequencing 60×; it means 60× on avg Some sites >100× & some sites not sequenced
Allele depth	Measures number of times a specific mt was seen
Variant allele frequency (VAF)	VAF = Allele depth/Depth of coverage
Limitations	High initial equipment startup costs Quality of data depends on depth of coverage Sensitivity to identify rare mutants or tumor heterogeneity depends on depth of coverage

Figure 6-1 Example of a mutation using DNA sequencing by NGS method and visualized on IGV viewer.

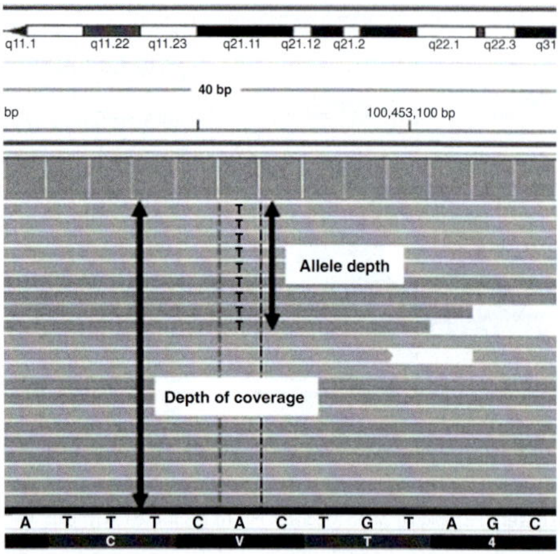

CYTOGENETICS

Cytogenetics

- **Definition:** The study of chr structure & its abnormalities
- Normal: 46 chrs, 22 pairs + XX vs. XY
  Each chr joined by centromere; short arm p, long arm q
- **Aneuploidy:** Additions/deletions of chrs

Karyotyping

- **Principle:**
  Cells are arrested in metaphase, while chrs are condensed
  Cells/chrs are stained w/ dyes; then images of the chrs are captured
  For hematologic malignancies, typically done on BM samples rather than on peripheral blood
- **Observed information:**
  Differences in numbers & size of chrs, centromere positions, position & number of satellite seq, degree, & distribution of heterochromatic regions
- **Limitations:**
  Small but important insertions & deletions may not be visible
- **Reciprocal (balanced) translocations:**
  Rearrangement of parts btw nonhomologous chrs: No net loss of genetic data, but fusion genes created vs. other genes rendered inactive
- **Unbalanced (robertsonian) translocation:**
  Fusion of 2 chrs near the centromere typically leading to loss of the p arms
  Often occurring w/ chrs 13, 14, 15, 21, 22
  Fusions of 13 & 14 do not lead to loss of genetic material

Common Nomenclature	
Symbol	**Meaning**
Formatting	Modal number, sex chrs, abnl abbreviation (1st chr; 2nd chr) (arm band number; arm band number) (eg, 46, XY, t(9;12)(p24;q13)
,	Separates chr modal number, sex chrs, & chr abnormalities
–	Loss of chr
()	Surrounds altered chrs & break points
+	Gain of chr
;	Separates rearranged chrs & breakpoints involving more than one chr
del	Deletion
der	Derivative chr (used when only one chr from a translocation is present)
dup	Duplication of portion of chr
ins	Insertion of portion of a chr
inv	Inversion
p	Short arm of chr
q	Long arm of chr
t	Translocation

Adapted from http://www.slh.wisc.edu/clinical/cytogenetics/basics/

Fluorescent in situ hybridizations (FISH)

- **Goal:** Detect presence/absence of a specific DNA seq (eg, fusion gene)
- **The principle:**
  - Fluorescent probes that are complementary to the genes/DNA seq of interest are allowed to hybridize to fixed & permeabilized cells/tissues
  - Fluorescence is detected as a marker for the gene(s) of interest
  - Yields quantitative detection of genes at the single cell level: 0, 1, 2, 3 or more copies of a given DNA seq
- **Applications:**
  - Gene amps, gene deletions, gene translocations
- **Benefits:**
  - Specific probes (different colors) can be designed to detect multiple targets simultaneously
  - Multiple cells can be assayed simultaneously
  - Spatial organization of the genes can be assayed: Allows assessing colocalization of 2 or more DNA seq pairs (eg, red + yellow probes colocalize → orange, suggesting 2 DNA seq of interest are in close proximity)
- **Limitations:**
  - Detection of targets depends on design & quality of the probes
  - Target identities must be known in advance to design probes

Selected Cytogenetic Aberrations in Oncology		
Disease	**Aberration**	**Significance**
Neuroblastoma	*MYCN* amp	Prog
Glioma/GMB	1p/19q codeletion	Phenotyping
Breast, Gastric Carcinomas	*ERBB2* (HER2) amp	Tx: Trastuzumab
Lung Adenoca	*ROS1, ALK, RET* rearrangements	Tx: TKI
Psa Adenoca	*TMPRSS2-ERG* t(21;21)	Dx
Alveolar Rhabdomyosarcoma	*PAX3-FOXO1* t(2;13)	Dx
Ewing Sarcoma	*EWSR1-FLI1* t(11;22)	Dx
Fibrosarcoma	*ETV6-NTRK3* t(12;15)	Dx
Inflammatory Myofibroblastic Tumor	*TPM3-ALK* t(2;5)	Tx: TKI
Solitary fibrous tumor	*NAB2-STAT6* inv(12)	Dx
Synovial sarcoma	*SS18-SSX1* t(X;18)	Dx
Follicular thyroid carcinoma	*PAX8-PPARγ* t(2;3)	Dx
Urothelial carcinoma	*FGFR3-TACC3*	Tx: FGFR inhibitors
CML	*BCR-ABL1* t(9;22) +8, +19, or i(17)(q10)	Dx; Dz Transformation
Myeloid/Lymphoid Neoplasms w/ Eosinophilia	Rearrangement of *PDGFRA* **or** *PDGFRB* **or** *FGFR1* **or** *PCM1-JAK2* t(8;9)	Dx
Follicular Lymphoma	*IGH-BCL2* t(14;18)	Dx
Mantle Cell Lymphoma	*CCND1-IGH* t(11;14)	Dx
Burkitt Lymphoma	*MYC-IGH* t(8;14) **or** *IGK-MYC* t(2;8) **or** *MYC-IGL* t(8;22)	Dx
EN MZL zone lymphoma, MALT type	t(11;18) t(14;18) t(3;14)	Pulmonary or gastric MALT Orbital or salivary gland MALT Thyroid or orbital or skin MALT
Lymphoplasmacytic Lymphoma	6q23 deletion	Dx
DLBCL	Translocation of BCL6 (3q27)	Dx
Acute Myeloid Leukemia	*RUNX1-RUNX1T1* t(8;21) **or** *CBFB-MYH11* inv(16)/t(16;16) *PML-RARA* t(15;17) **or** *RBM15-MKL1* t(1;22) *MLLT3-KMT2A* t(9;11) **or** Normal Karyotype *DEK-NUP214* t(6;9) **or** *RPN1-EVI1* inv(3)/ t(3;3) 11q23 rearrangement **or** *BCR-ABL1* t(9;22)	Good prog Good prog Int prog Bad prog Bad prog
MDS	del(11q) or -Y Normal, del(5q), del(12p), del(20q), double del(5q) del(7q), Monosomy 5, Trisomy 8, Trisomy 19, i(17)(q10) Monosomy 7, inv(3), t(3;3), del(3q) Complex Karyotype (≥3 abnormalities)	Very good prog Good prog Int prog Poor prog Very poor prog
CLL	del(13) Trisomy 12 **or** del(6q) 17p13 deletion or del(11)	Good prog Int prog Poor prog
B-ALL	Hyperdiploid (X, 4, 14, 21) **or** *ETV6-RUNX1* t(12;21) *IL3-IGH* (5;14) *BCR-ABL1* t(9;22) **or** t(v;11q23) **or** Hypodiploid Near haploid **or** low hypodiploid **or** Intrachromosomal amp of chr 21	Good prog Int prog Poor prog Worse prog

RNA sequencing

- **Definition:** Laboratory technologies used to determine the ribonucleotide seq of mRNA which are used to infer changes in the transcript seq including gene fusions & expression levels
- **Steps:** RNA extraction → mRNA enrichment (rRNA depletion—optional) → cDNA synthesis → Target enrichment (optional) → Adaptor ligation → Sequencing → Analysis
- **Techniques:**
  - **Targeted enrichment:** Adapted by laboratories interested in custom panels where a smaller number of genes are targeted as opposed to the whole transcriptome; can be accomplished via hybridization capture based or PCR enrichment methods. Most panels allow gene fusion detection & limited expression analysis. Pros: Simple to implement, 5–10 d TAT, low-input RNA, compatible w/ FFPE tissue. Cons: Not comprehensive approach, can miss events not targetable by the panel
  - **Whole transcriptome sequencing:** Allows the profiling of the full transcriptome including mRNA transcripts & noncoding RNA. MRNA targeted sequencing possible via enrichment of polyadenylate transcripts which comprise only 1–2% of the whole transcriptome. These methods enable:
    1) Assessment of expression levels of all detected transcripts at a given time & the identification of gene expression signatures related to dz or drug response
    2) Identification of transcript variants & gene fusions
  - **Direct sequencing:** Generate reads by directly sequencing full length RNA w/o modification or reverse transcription; experimental & used for discovery
- **Clinical utilities:**
  - Analysis of differential gene expression: Quantitative difference in genes expression levels btw individuals
  - Complement the limitations of purely genetic information leading to adv understanding of dz pathophysiology (alternate tumors driver alterations, resistance mechanisms to some drugs, etc.)
  - Identification of biomarkers for targeted therapy (eg, crizotinib for *ALK* fusion-positive lung carcinoma & *ROS1* fusion-positive lung carcinoma; trametinib for *BRAF* fusion-positive melanoma; entrectinib for *NTRK1* fusion-positive malignancies)

Selected Gene Fusions detected by RNA Sequencing

Gene	Encodes	Common Partners
ALK	RTK	*EML4, FN1, KIF5B, STRN, TPM1/3/4*
RET	RTK	*KIF5B, CCDC6, NCOA4*
ROS1	RTK	*CD74, SDC4, SLC34A2, GOPC, TPM3*
TFE3	Transcription factor	*ASPSCR1, RBM10, NONO*
FGFR3	RTK	*TACC3*
FGFR2	RTK	*TACC2, BICC1*
BRAF	Serine threonine kinase	*AGK, KIAA1549, MKRN1, TRIM24*
ERG	Erythroblast transformation specific transcriptions factors	*TMPRSS2, SLC45A3, FUS, EWSR1*
NTRK1	NTRK-1	*TPM3, LMNA, TPR*
NTRK3	NTRK-3	*ETV6, SQSTM1, EML4*

Cancer immunology basics

- The immune system plays an important role in CA surveillance; Rx's that modulate & amplify the immune system are referred to as **immunotherapies**
- **Innate immunity:** 1st line of defense, include Mϕ, DC, & NK cells, complement system. Pattern recognition receptors (eg, Toll-like receptors) recognize conserved molecular patterns on microbes; recognition via these receptors leads to cytokine production, recruitment & activation of additional immune cells, resulting in killing of pathogens; microbial & cellular fragments are then produced & taken up by Ag-presenting cells (Mϕ, B-cells, & DC), ultimately activating the adaptive immune system
- **Adaptive immunity:** Generates lifelong immune "memory" → consists of T- & B-cells, which lead to cellular & humoral immunity, respectively; their activation occurs via TCR & BCR that are highly diverse & specific

T-cells

- Thymus-derived lymphocytes, recognize Ag-complexed w/ MHC

Cell	Activated by	Effect	Cytokines Produced
CD4+ (eg, helper T-cells)	MHC class II (HLA-DR) on APC (DC, **Mϕ**)	Differentiate into either Th1, Th2, Th17, or Treg	Th1: IFN-γ, IL-2 Th2: IL-4, IL-5, IL-10 Th17: IL-17, IL-23 Treg: IL-10, TGF-β
CD8+ (eg, CTL)	MHC class I (HLA-A, B, C) on all cell types	Once active can directly kill cells	IFN-γ, IL-2, granzyme, perforin

- **CD4+ cells:** Regulate the immune response; activate Th1, Th2, Th17, or Treg responses depending on cytokine milieu when they see Ag on class II MHC; can also activate Mϕ & NK cells, which mediate effector functions of T-cell subsets → IL-2 regulates their proliferation & activation role in tumor immunology; both preclinical models & pts w/ ↓ CD4 function (eg, HIV pts) show ↑ rates of malignancies
- **Th1 cells: (Cellular immune response),** activate CTL & Mϕ
  Cytokines—activated by IFN-γ, inhibited by IL-10 & IL-4
  CTLs play an important role in detecting virus-infected cells & recognition of tumor cells (tumors frequently express MHC class I, however tumors can also downregulate MHC class I expression & evade CTLs)
- **Th2 cells: (Humoral immune response)** leads to B-cell activation, Ab class switching & Ab production, & activation of eosinophils
  Cytokines—activated by IL-4 & IL-10. Inhibited by IFN-γ
- **Th17 cells:** Activated by IL-1, TGF-β, & IL-6, produce IL-17; found in a variety of malignancies & a/w both pro- & antitumor effects (*Am J Pathol* 2013;182:1)
- **Treg:** Maintain self-tolerance by suppressing expansion of cells directed against self-Ag; may also inhibit tumor-reactive cells (*JCO* 2006;24:5373). Tregs are activated in the same milieu as effector cells & specific subsets develop to suppress specific arms of immunity based on environmental cues (*Science* 2009;326:986)
  Type 1 Tregs are activated by IL-10, then produce further IL-10 & TGF-β (*CCR* 2008;14:3706)

Natural killer (NK) cells

- Part of innate immune response. NK cells express inhibitory & activating KIRs that mediate NK function & play an important role in preventing relapse after allogeneic transplantation in AML (*NEJM* 2012;367:805); NK cells express Fc receptors & play a role in mediating ADCC
- Cytokines: Produce IFN-γ, activated by IL-2

B-cells

- Part of adaptive immune system, produce Ab & serve as APCs
- Role of Ab: (1) Activate C'-mediated cytotoxicity via Fc portion of Ab, (2) ADCC, (3) interact w/ cell surface receptors that regulate cell growth

Dendritic cells

- Stimulated by microbes via pattern recognition receptors, cytokines, &/or T-cell signals → they then differentiate & migrate to different tissues & become active APCs

- Very effective APC, critical for development of Ag-specific effector CD8+ T-cells
- 2 main types (though others exist)
  - **CD11c⁺ myeloid DC:** Respond to GM-CSF & are the most efficient APCs, especially for activation of naïve T-cells; play a role in activating tumor-specific CTLs via IL-12
  - **CD11c⁻ plasmacytoid DC:** Express IL-3 receptor, circulate in the peripheral blood & help mediate innate immune responses, particularly against viruses
- Augmentation of DC function as APC may serve as platform for CA immunotherapy approaches such as tumor vaccines for DC presentation of tumor Ag to T-cells

Macrophages (Mϕ)

- Derived from monocytes, specialized phagocytes, function as APCs, recognize cell surface receptors for C′ & Fc receptors for immunoglobulin, thus can mediate Ab-dependent cellular uptake
- 2 main activation states, M1 & M2
  - **M1:** Produce nitric oxide (NO) synthase, IL-12 & TNF; kill tumor via NO & TNF, a/w improved outcomes in oncology pts (*Eur Respir J* 2009;33:118)
  - **M2:** Produce arginase, IL-10, TGF-β, prostaglandin E2; promote angiogenesis, limit the Th1 response & help tumor growth

Immune surveillance and immunoediting

- **Immunodeficiency** is a/w malignancy, as seen in organ transplant recipients, HIV pts, pts w/ rheumatic dzs & pts on immunosuppression Rx; this supports the role of the immune system in CA prevention
- **The 3 E's of CA immunoediting:** Explanation for the immune system's role in CA elimination & growth (Review: *Nat Immunol* 2002;3:991)
  - ***Elimination***—The innate immune system (NK & Mϕ) is activated by inflammatory cytokines (produced by tumors); innate system activation leads to ↑ secretion of inflammatory cytokines (IL-2 & INF-γ), activating DCs & Mϕ resulting in Ag presentation, T-cell activation (both CD4+ & CD8+) & production of CTLs leading to cell death & eradication of developing tumors
  - ***Equilibrium***—Elimination of tumor cells leads to selection of less immunogenic cells; this period of selection & elimination can lead to transient control of tumor growth
  - ***Escape***—Tumors escape the immune system via loss of molecules on tumor cells important for immune activation (eg, MHC loss w/ β2M mts); tumors can secrete immunosuppressing cytokines (IL-10 & TGF-β) & downregulate IFN-γ; in addition, tumors often express nonmutated self-Ag, which the immune system will, by definition, not react against; tumors can express molecules that inhibit T-cell function (eg, PD-L1/B7-H1, which bind an inhibitory receptor on T-cells [PD-1] & lead to their inhibition) (*Immunology* 2007;450:903). Ubiquitous CD47 ("Don't eat me" signal) w/ ↑ expression on tumor cells mediates escape from phagocytosis
- **TME**—Immune cells are found in tumors, the exact composition of these cells has been a/w pt outcomes; eg, high concentration of TILs (CD8+ cells) are a/w better outcomes & ↑ response to chemotherapy, Tregs & myeloid-derived suppressor cells are a/w worse outcomes, the exact role of Th17 in tumors is still being elucidated; the milieu of cytokines & chemokines also plays a role in outcome; some cytokines (VEGF, IL-1, IL-8) lead to endothelial cell proliferation, migration, & activation; tumor-associated Mϕ help promote tumor cell invasion & mets (*Nat Rev Cancer* 2012;12:298; *Immunology* 2011;121(1):1). Expression of PD-L1 in tumor microenvironment can be indicator of improved likelihood of response to immune checkpoint blockade
- **Tumor-associated antigens (Ag)**—Antitumor effect of immune system dependent upon recognition of tumor-associated Ag, either known shared Ag (eg, CA testis Ag, NY-ESO-1, WT1) or pt specific. Pt-specific tumor-associated Ag are derived from somatic mts unique to each tumor that produce altered peptides (eg, neoantigens) which can break "tolerance to self" & may be recognized by immune system
- **Tumor mutational load** correlates w/ incr. response to immunotherapy (*NEJM*; 2014;371:2189). Pembrolizumab approved in 2020 for metastatic/unresectable dz w/ TMB >10 mut/Mb based on KEYNOTE-158 (*Lancet Oncol* 2020;21(10):1353). Clonal neoantigen burden correlates w/ response to PD-1/CTLA-4 blockade (*Science* 2016;351:1463)

Background

- Activation of naive T-cells requires 3 **signals:**
  - **Signal 1:** Antigenic peptide recognition presented by MHC molecules to TCR
  - **Signal 2:** Interaction of add'l receptors & ligands to provide costimulatory or coinhibitory (checkpoint) signals, regulating T-cell activation/fate
  - **Signal 3:** Cytokines support differentiation into specific subsets
- **Role in CA**
  - CA cells can dysregulate coinhibitory/stimulatory signals to evade the immune system
  - Therapies targeting costimulatory pathways are a major class of CA immunotherapy: mAb/ligands that enhance costimulatory signals (Fig. 7-1, left) or block coinhibitory (checkpoint) receptors (Fig. 7-1, right) can lead to effective antitumor immunity

Figure 7-1 T-cell activation is regulated by activating (*light blue*) and inhibitory (*blue*) signals.

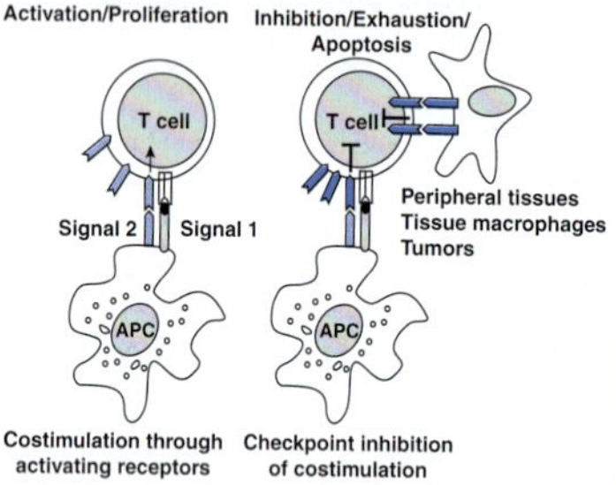

Activating Receptors/Ligands and Targeting Agents			
Receptor	**Ligand**	**Drugs**	**Development**
CD28	B7-1,2	TGN1412	Phase 1 terminated* (*NEJM* 2006;355:1018)
ICOS	B7-H2	Vopratelimab	Phase 1/2
CD137 (4-1BB)	4-1BBL	Utimolumab Urelumab AGEN2373 ADG106	Phase 1 (*JCO* 2008;26:3007) Phase 1/2 Phase 1 Phase 1
OX40	OX40L	MEDI6469 PF-04518600 MOXR0916	Phase 1/2 (*Nature Comm* 2021;12;1047) Phase 1/2 Phase 1
CD40	CD40L	Several mAbs	Phase I (*JCO* 2009;27:4371; *JCO* 2007;25:876)
CD27	CD70	Varilumab	Phase 1 (*Blood Adv* 2020;12:1917)
GITR	GITRL	TRX518 MK-4166/1248 BMS-986156	all Phase I

*Trial stopped after development of cytokine release syndrome with SIRS/MOF in the first six treated patient.

Inhibitory Receptors/Ligands and Targeting Agents			
Receptor	**Ligand**	**Drugs**	**Development**
PD-1	PD-L1/2	**Anti-PD-1:** Pembrolizumab, Nivolumab, Cemiplimab **Anti-PD-L1:** Atezolizumab, Avelumab, Durvalumab	**Approved** in melanoma, lung (NSCLC & SCLC), Hodgkin lymphoma, HNSCC, cutaneous squamous cell ca, urothelial cell CA & RCC (*JAMA* 2017;318:1647; *NEJM* 2012;366:2443; *NEJM* 2012;366:2455) Phase 1 (>500) in multiple CAs
CTLA-4	B7-1/2	Ipilimumab Tremelimumab	Approved: **Ipilimumab** melanoma, renal cell CA, NSCLC, mesothelioma (*NEJM* 2010;363:711; *NEJM* 2018;378:1277; *NEJM* 2019;381:2020) Phase 2,3 for various CAs
VISTA-R	VISTA	JNJ-61610588, CI-8993	Phase 1
Unclear	B7-H3	Enoblituzumab	Phase 1/2
TIM3	GAL9	TSR022, MBG453, Sym023	Phase I
LAG3	MHC	Eftilagimod alpha LAG525 Sym022 BMS-986016	Phase 1/2a Phase 1 Phase 1/2 Phase 1/2
TIGIT	PVR	Tiragolumab	NSCLC: FDA Breakthrough Therapy designation in combo w/ atezolizumab (*JCO* 2020;38(15):9503); phase 1/2 in multiple other CAs

Checkpoint inhibitors

- CPI enhance antitumor immunity by blocking negative regulators of T-cell function
  - **Anti-cytotoxic T-lymphocyte antigen 4 (CTLA-4):** Ipilimumab
  - **Anti-programmed death 1 (PD-1):** Nivolumab, pembrolizumab, cemiplimab, dostarlimab
  - **Anti-programmed death-ligand1 (PD-L1):** Atezolizumab, avelumab, durvalumab

Immune-related adverse events (irAE)

- Inflammatory adverse events (distinct from chemotherapy s/e) arising from CPIs, often very similar to autoimmmune/autoinflammatory conditions
- Incidence varies & may occur in up to 60% of pts treated w/ combined CPIs (*Nat Rev Clin Oncol* 2019;16:563; *JAMA Oncol* 2019;5:1008): Wide range of severity, from mild to potentially life-threatening
- Greater incidence in setting of combination therapy (CTLA4 + PD-(L)1)
- Incidence is a/w increasing doses of CTLA4 (ipilimumab), while there is no dose-dependent association w/ PD-(L)1 therapies
- Highly variable time of onset (may be in 1st few wks after starting tx or after cessation of therapy)
- Overall, the types of irAEs do not seem to be specific to underlying CA type
- Most common irAEs: Rash, colitis, & endocrinopathies
- Unclear which pts will develop irAEs, though there is incr. concern in pts w/ a history of autoimmune dz (area of ongoing study; *J Immunother Cancer* 2021;9:e002121)
- Some may be antibody driven, others T-cell mediated (under investigation) (*PNAS* 2016; 113(42):11919–11924; *Ann Oncol* 2017;28(3):583–589; *Nature Medicine* 2019;25:1243–1250)
- Potential association between clinical response & irAE but data remain conflicting (*JCO* 2015;33(28):3193; *JCO* 2019;37(30):2730)

irAEs may affect nearly any tissue/system (*NEJM* 2018;378:158–168)

- HEENT: Uveitis, retinitis, scleritis mucositis, dry mouth
- Skin: Rash, vitiligo, psoriasis, pruritus, Stevens–Johnson syndrome, bullous pemphigoid
- Cardiac: Myocarditis (*NEJM* 2016;375:1749), pericarditis
- Pulmonary: Pneumonitis, pleuritis
- Liver: Hepatitis
- Renal: Acute interstitial nephritis, glomerulonephritis
- Pancreatic: Pancreatitis
- GI tract: Gastritis, enteritis, colitis
- Neurologic: Neuropathy, encephalitis, meningitis, Guillain–Barré Syndrome
- Endocrinopathies: Autoimmune diabetes, adrenal insufficiency, hyperthyroidism, hypothyroidism, hypophysitis, central diabetes insipidus, hypoparathyroidism
- Hematologic: Thrombocytopenia, aplastic anemia, neutropenia, hemolytic anemia
- Vascular/rheumatologic: Vasculitis, arthralgia, dermatomyositis, myositis

  **This list is not comprehensive.

Principles of management of irAEs

- Always r/o other etiologies (ie, inflammation, infection, progression)
- Graded in severity from 1 to 5 (G1–G5) according to the CTCAE
- Pts receiving CPI must be monitored closely for irAEs; tx of irAEs should be started promptly once recognized to prevent morbidity & mortality
- The majority of irAEs can be managed as an outpt but hospitalization should be considered for grade ≥3 or severe grade 2 irAEs
- Corticosteroids are the backbone of tx for most irAEs combined with pausing/stopping CPI
- For pts who require high-dose corticosteroids for management of irAEs, current evidence suggest that efficacy of CPI not impacted, except possibly for hypophysitis (*Cancer* 2018;124(18):3706). However, pts being treated w/ high-dose steroids for other reasons & before initiation of CPI may have lower response to CPI (*Cancer* 2020; 12(3):546)

Cutaneous irAE

- Most common irAE, >1/3 to 1/2 of pts receiving CPI. Usually low grade in severity, w/ grade 3–4 events <5% (highest rate w/ nivolumab+ipilimumab) (*Oncologist* 2016;21(10):1230)
- Most common manifestation is erythematous, reticular, & maculopapular rash, but a wide range of dermatologic manifestations can occur; vitiligo, psoriasis, lichenoid dermatitis, bullous pemphigoid, among others (*JCO* 2019;37;2746–2758)

Management: CTCAE Grading Based on BSA, Morbidity, and Duration	
Grade	**Management**
1–2 (<30% BSA)	Supportive, topical emollients, topical steroids, oral antihistamines for pruritus. Continue CPI
3 (>30% BSA)	+ Steroids (prednisone 1 mg/kg daily PO) 1–2 wks. CPI should be delayed until baseline or G1. Consider dermatology & skin biopsy
G4 (>30% BSA + systemic sxs)	IV methylprednisolone 1–2 mg/kg. Dermatology consultation, consider other immunosuppressants (infliximab, MMF, cyclophosphamide). Discontinue CPI

Diarrhea and colitis

- Most commonly seen in pts treated w/ CTLA-4 ab (10–20%) (*Front Immmunol* 2017;8;1547); highest incidence in CTLA4 + PD-(L1) combo; median time to onset is 6–8 wks after initiation of therapy, rapid onset, large volume, can be bloody
- Always r/o other etiologies & look for other associated irAEs
- Imaging is not sensitive for diagnosis. Gold standard is colonoscopy, which can predict severity (including additional #BMs/day) & guide management

Management: CTCAE Grading Based on #BMs, Morbidity, and Duration	
Grade	**Management**
1 (<4 BMs) 2 (4–6 BMs)	Workup for blood, stool, screening labs (HIV, Hep, TB) in case infliximab is needed. Sx management & loperamide, consider budesonide, consider steroids in G2 (prednisone 1 mg/kg daily PO) Continue CPI only if G1
3 (>7 BMs) 4 (>7 BM + systemic sxs)	Hospitalization, steroids (prednisone 1–2 mg/kg daily). Colonoscopy to evaluate severity. Discontinue CPI IV methylprednisolone 1–2 mg/kg, if no improvement in 72 h consider infliximab 5 mg/kg, MMF 0.5–1 g, or tacrolimus

Endocrinopathies

- Presentation nonspecific, includes fatigue, nausea, headache, &/or depression
- Unlike other irAE, endocrinopathies are usually permanent & require indefinite hormone replacement. Syndromes include:
  - Hypophysitis: 3% CTLA4, <0.5% PD-(L)1, 6% in combination therapy (*JAMA Oncol* 2018;4(2):173–182). Diagnosis is challenging. 8 AM ACTH w/ cortisol. Systemic steroids can affect ACTH & cortisol results. Consult endocrinology for diagnosis & management
  - Hyper- & hypothyroidism: 2.9% & 6.6%, respectively (*JAMA Oncol* 2019;5(7):1008–1019). The former is often transient & may precede hypothyroidism. Routine monitoring of thyroid function test (TSH, free T4) is required before every cycle or at least once a mo. Treat hyperthyroidism only if symptomatic (β-blockers or NSAIDs), do not use methimazole, steroids rarely used. Tx for hypothyroidism is hormone replacement (levothyroxine) which is usually long lasting
  - Adrenal insufficiency: The most severe of endocrinopathies, can present as adrenal crisis. In this case hospitalization for stress-dose steroids & support for sx management (dehydration/hypotension, electrolyte abnormalities) is required
  - Diabetes mellitus: Very rare (<1%) (*JAMA Oncol* 2018;4(2):173–182), more common w/ PD-(L)-1 or combination therapy, check glucose levels w/ regular labs. Steroids are not effective, tx is insulin

Adoptive cell therapy

- **Mechanism:** Direct or indirect killing of tumor or infected cells by antigen-specific lymphocytes
- **DLI:** HLA-matched lymphocytes, used for tx of relapse after allogeneic SCT for CML & AML, & to lesser degree ALL. EBV-specific lymphocytes used for EBV-associated PTLD refractory to rituximab. Viral-specific lymphocytes used for opportunistic viral infections post SCT, including CMV, BK, & JC virus
- **TIL:** Lymphocytes isolated from tumors, cultured & expanded in vitro & infused back into pt, typically preceded by lymphodepletion (*NEJM* 1988;319:1676; *JCO* 2016;34:2389)
- **Genetically modified lymphocytes**
  - **CAR:** Autologous or allogeneic lymphocytes engineered to express non–MHC-restricted Ag receptor using Ag-specific monoclonal Ab variable regions fused w/ TCR & costimulatory receptor domains (eg, CD28) in 1 molecule (*PNAS* 1993;90:720)
  - **Engineered TCR:** Autologous lymphocytes engineered to express MHC-restricted tumor-specific TCR (*Science* 2006;314:126)

Engineered TCRs Recently in Clinical Trials

Tumor Antigen	HLA-Restriction	Cancer Type
gp100	HLA-A*02	Melanoma
MART-1	HLA-A*02	Melanoma
MAGE-A3	HLA-A*02	Melanoma, synovial sarcoma, esophageal CA
MAGE-A3	HLA-A*01	Melanoma, multiple myeloma
MAGE-A3/A6	HLA-DBP1*04	Pan-CA
MAGE-A4	HLA-A*24	Esophageal CA
MAGE-A4	HLA-A*02	Synovial sarcoma
NY-ESO-1	HLA-A*02	Melanoma, synovial sarcoma, multiple myeloma
HPV E7	HLA-A*02	HPV-associated CAs
CEA	HLA-A*02	Colon CA
WT1	HLA-A*02	AML
WT1	HLA-A*24	MDS, AML

Vaccines

- **Mechanism:** Enlarge the pool of tumor-specific T-cells from naive repertoire or reactivate existing T-cells that may be in an anergic state. Should also focus on stimulating memory T-cell reactivity, which has superior proliferative capacity & persistence
- **Challenge:** Ensure the proper homing of these T-cells to tumor & curtail the plethora of mechanisms by which tumors evade immunity. CA vaccines have been more successfully used in settings w/ less immune suppression (premalignant lesions or adjuvant therapy after resection) (eg, HPV16 vaccination in pts w/ high-grade VIN (*NEJM* 2009;361:1838); autologous tumor cell–BCG vaccine for resected stage II/III colon CA w/ ↑RFS (*Lancet* 1999;353:345))
- **Targets:** Overexpressed tumor Ag (eg, MUC-1, HER2, hTERT), carcinoembryonic Ag (eg, CEA, AFP), recurrent mutated Ag (eg, *KRAS*), CA testis Ag (eg, MAGE, NY-ESO-1), viral Ag (eg, HPV, HCV), microenvironment factors (eg, VEGF)
- **Adjuvants:** Enhance the immunogenicity of an Ag (eg, cytokines, microbes, mineral salts, oil emulsions or surfactants, particulates, viral vectors)

Vaccine Platforms
Protein: Full-length proteins, not restricted to specific HLA types. Use of CA testis Ag is a popular choice due to its lack of expression on normal adult tissues
Peptide: Easier preparation than whole protein, but typically HLA-restricted. Peptides can be from CA testis Ag or tumor-specific Ag (eg, viral, mutated proteins)
DNA/RNA: Vector encoding an Ag of interest is used. Supporting factors can be added into the sequence (eg, cytokines, immune checkpoint inhibitor)
Tumor cells: Autologous (eg, OncoVAX®) or allogenic tumor cells (eg, GVAX)
Dendritic cell (DC): Typically involve generating DC ex vivo, most commonly from monocytes by culture w/ cytokine cocktails for DC maturation. DCs are then loaded w/ autologous/allogeneic tumor-cell lysates or specific Ag & are infused back into the pt
Vectored: Ag of interest are introduced w/ a recombinant viral vector (eg, vaccinia, adenovirus, fowlpox, *Listeria monocytogenes*)

- **Sipuleucel T:** 1st **FDA-approved** therapeutic vaccine. Autologous PBMC activated ex vivo w/ a recombinant fusion protein (PA2024) which consists of PAP fused to GM-CSF. PBMC cell mixture contains DC precursors, T-cells, B-cells, & Mϕ in variable proportions. ↑ OS in metastatic CRPC (*NEJM* 2010;363:411)

Bispecific antibodies (BsAbs) (*Nat Rev Clin Oncol* 2020;17:418)

- **Mechanism:** Binds tumor Ag leading to immune-mediated tumor cell elimination either by AICD or functioning as a T-cell engager (eg, bridges polyclonal cytotoxic T-cells & target on malignant cells). Unimpaired by the immunosuppressive tumor microenvironment, bypasses need for prior immunization, HLA Sp, or costimulatory molecules. In addition, BsAbs can greatly enhance the therapeutic index in radioimmunotherapy of solid tumors
- **Targeting strategies:** BiTE®, CrossMab (allows for 1:2 valency), TriKE, DART, SMITE, ImmTAC

Bispecific Antibodies Recently in Clinical Trials

Antibody	Targets	Cancer Type
Blinatumomab	CD19 & CD3	CD19+ B-cell malignancies **(FDA approved)**
Amivantamab-vmjw	EGFR & MET	NSCLC w/ *EGFR* exon 20 insertions **(FDA approved)**
Multiple	BCMA & CD3	R/R multiple myeloma
Multiple	CD20 & CD2	R/R NHL
Flotetuzumab	CD123 & CD3	CD123+ hematologic malignancies
Solitumab	EpCAM & CD3	EpCAM+ solid tumors
Catumaxomab	EpCAM, CD3, & FcγR	Malignant ascites in pts w/ EpCAM+ carcinomas
Pasotuxizumab	PSMA & CD3	Prostate CA
Cibisatamab	CEA & CD3	CEA+ solid tumors
Vanucizumab	Ang2 & VEGF	Colorectal CA
Duligotuzumab	EGFR & HER2	HNSCC
PRS-343	HER2 & CD137	HER2+ solid tumors
Tebentafusp	Gp100/HLA-A2 & CD3	Uveal melanoma (*NEJM* 2021;385(13):1196)

Oncolytic viruses (OV)

- **T-VEC:** Modified HSV-1 designed to replicate in & lyse tumor cells while promoting regional & systemic antitumor immunity. Insertion & expression of the gene encoding GM-CSF results in recruitment & activation of APCs. **FDA-approved** based on ↑ durable response rate in RCT of pts w/ unresectable or metastatic melanoma randomized to intralesional T-VEC vs. scGM-CSF (16.3% vs. 2.1% $p < 0.001$) (*JCO* 2015;33:2780)

Immune modulatory strategies—non–T-cell checkpoint*

- **CD47 ("Don't eat me signal"):** Serves as a ligand of signal regulatory protein-1 (SIRP-1). CD47 is overexpressed in AML, NHL, HNSCC, bladder CA, & breast CA. SIRP-1 is expressed on **Mϕ**, granulocytes, dendritic cells, neurons, & endothelial cells
  Targeting strategies: Anti-CD47 can disrupt the interaction between CD47 & SIRPa which enables phagocytosis of tumor cells (*NEJM* 2018;379:1711)
- **CSF1R:** CSF1 signaling a/w anti-inflammatory M2/**TAMs** phenotype & myeloid-derived suppressor cells
  Targeting strategies: Anti-CSF1R Ab emactuzumab (*Lancet Oncol* 2015;8:949); small molecule inhibitor of CSF1R (PLX3397) (*NEJM* 2015;373:428)
- **Adenosine:** Serves as a danger signal & in immune regulation. Produced during inflammatory processes through CD73 & CD39. Several tumors can express these ectonucleotidases. Adenosine through $A_{2A}R$ can ↓ Ag presentation from DC, ↓ IFNγ, ↑ M2-like phenotype, ↑ T_{reg}, ↓ T_H1
  Targeting strategies: Adenosine 2A receptor antagonist
- **NK cells:** Anti-KIR binds to inactivating KIRs, which prevents KIR-mediated inhibition of NK cells & permit NK cell–mediated antitumor cytotoxicity (*Blood* 2014;123:678). Phase I/II trials for advanced solid tumors

*T-cell agonists/checkpoint inhibitors: discussed elsewhere.

Principles of CAR T-cell therapy

- CAR: Ab-derived extracellular scFv linked to intracellular T-cell signaling domains of the TCR
- Pt or allogeneic T-cells modified to express tumor Ag-specific CAR then reinfused → **cytotoxic activity redirected to tumor cells** in an **HLA-independent** manner
- CAR generations: 1st: target-specific scFv + TCR signaling domain (eg, CD3z); **2nd (currently approved products):** adds cytoplasmic signaling domains of T-cell costim receptors (eg, CD28, 4-1BB) to provide "**signal 2**"; 3rd: experimental, adds >1 costim domain; 4th: experimental, adds "armored" domain w/modifications to enhance CAR function (eg, express costimulatory ligands, secrete cytokines, etc.)
- **Costim domain affects CAR T-cell persistence** & **toxicity profile**: CD28 costim associated w/ faster onset of T-cell activity, more cytokine-related toxicity, & earlier CAR T-cell exhaustion compared to 4-1BB costim. 4-1BB a/w longer persistence
- Pts receive **conditioning** ("lymphodepletion") prior to CAR T-cell infusion (may ↓ Tregs, ↓ immune cells competing for cytokines, ↑ APC activation); most common is Flu/Cy

CAR T-cell manufacturing

- Autologous T-cells collected; activated; transduced w/ γ-retrovirus, lentivirus, or nonviral method (eg, *Sleeping Beauty* system); expanded; cryopreserved under GMP conditions; usually takes 10–14 d
- Strategies may vary by center (eg, bead-based vs. cell-based expansion, separate CD4+/CD8+ expansions, product w/ fixed CD4:CD8 ratio)

Current clinical applications (*Cytotherapy* 2016;18:1393; *NEJM* 2019;380:1726)

- Requires expertise of specialized center
- **R/R B-ALL:** Rates of MRD-CR ~70% following CD19-targeted CAR T-cell therapy in children & adults (*NEJM* 2018;378(5):449)
- **R/R CLL & B-NHL:** ↓ rates of CR to CD19-targeted CAR T-cell therapy vs. B-ALL; responses observed across range of histologies (DLBCL, T/FL, MCL, FL, etc.)
- Responses also seen in pts w/ relapsed B-cell malignancies following allogeneic HCT
- Bispecific CAR T-cells under active investigation (eg, CD19/CD22 & CD19/CD20)
- **R/R MM:** BCMA target w/ 4-1BB costim; ORR 73% (33% CR) (*NEJM* 2021;284(8):705)
  → Bivalent BCMA-targeting CAR T-cell demonstrated efficacy in recent Phase 2 trial
- AML, solid tumors: CAR T-cell therapy under active investigation against wide range of tumor-specific targets (CD33, MUC16, mesothelin, EGFR, HER-2, etc.)
- Association between greater CAR T-cell expansion & greater antitumor response observed in most (but not all) series

Major toxicities and management (*Blood* 2016;127:3321, *Nat Rev Clin Oncol* 2020;17:147)

- **CRS:** SIRS h–d after CAR T-cell infusion, w/ fevers, myalgias, malaise; more severe cases w/ **capillary leak syndrome** a/w hypoxia, HoTN, multiorgan dysfunction, coagulopathy
  → Characterized by ↑ inflammatory cytokines (esp IL-6) & T-cell activation & expansion
  → Association between ↑ dz burden, ↑ CAR T-cell dose, & more severe CRS; several centers use risk-adapted CAR T-cell dosing (↓ T-cell dose if ↑ dz)
  → May be fatal. Requires expert consultation. Pts may require intensive supportive care including ICU admission, intubation/mechanical ventilation & vasopressors
  → Treat severe CRS w/ **tocilizumab** (mAb to IL-6R) ± corticosteroids
- **ICANS:** Range of largely reversible neurologic sx (delirium, confusion, aphasia, obtundation, seizures, headache); can occur w/ or w/o CRS; related to disruption of BBB & ↑ **cytokines in CSF;** treat w/ **corticosteroids** &/or **anti–IL-6 therapy** if CRS also present
- **On-target/off-tumor effects:** depend on CAR T-cell target & its expression in normal tissues (eg, B-cell aplasia in pts receiving CD19-targeted CAR T-cells → pts may require IVIG for hypogammaglobulinemia)

Special concerns

- Ag escape: CD19-targeted CAR tx → **CD19$^-$ relapse** BCMA-targeted CAR tx → **BCMA loss**
- Role of allogeneic HCT in pts w/ B-ALL & MRD CR to CAR T-cell therapy remains unclear; favored in adults w/o prior HCT, though some have extended remission w/o HCT
- Pts receiving CAR T-cells produced by viral transduction methods presently require ongoing testing for replication-competent retrovirus/lentivirus (theoretical risk; not seen to date in transduced pt cells or during pt monitoring)

Adoptive cell therapy (ACT) using TILs

- Involves infusion of autologous TILs, which are isolated from resected tumor specimens & expanded ex vivo
- Unlike antitumor TCRs or CAR therapies, conventional TIL therapy uses naturally occurring T cells from the tumor microenvironment that are not genetically engineered

Steps Involved During TIL Therapy

Step	Details	Rationale
Tissue harvest	1 or more tumor samples are obtained from a surgical resection. Sections are digested into single-cell suspension & expanded in vitro	Isolate pure cultures of TIL clones capable of recognizing tumor antigens
Lymphodepletion	Cyclophosphamide (60 mg/kg × 2 d) + Fludarabine (25 mg/m^2 × 5 d). TBI has also been given in some protocols	Depletes immunosuppressive cell populations (ie, MDSCs, Treg cells) (*Science* 2002;298(5594):850). Promotes cytokines that promote T-cell proliferation/survival (*J Exp Med* 2005;202(7):907). Reduces cytokine sinks
Infusion of TILs	Administration of TILs expanded ex vivo	Infuses TILs that show tumor reactivity, capable to expand after administration.
IL-2 infusion	600,000–720,000 IU/kg IV. q8–12h × 6–12 doses	Supports TILs' expansion & effector function (*Curr Oncol Rep* 2012;14(5):468)

Toxicities related to TIL therapy

- Majority of toxicity is a/w lymphodepletion & IL-2
- Lymphodepletion: Commonly see thrombocytopenia, anemia, & neutropenia for 1–2 wks. Neutropenia can be managed w/ colony-stimulating factor
- IL-2: Can cause fever, rigors, & in some cases capillary leak syndrome, manifested as peripheral edema, effusions, reduced urine output, acute kidney injury w/in h of infusion. Sxs are usually transient & subside w/ supportive measures (*JITC* 2014;2(1):26); *J immunother* 2001;24(4):287)
- TILs: Transient infusion–related reactions are most common. Due to the use of naturally occurring polyclonal T-cells w/ native TCRs, the risk of serious or severe cytokine-associated toxicities such as CRS significantly reduced compared to other cellular therapies. Persistent autoimmune toxicity has rarely been reported (*Opthalmol* 2009;116(5):981; *JCO* 2005;23(10):2346)

Current evidence of TILs

- **Melanoma:** Most of the proof of clinical benefit to date has been in melanoma. Pooled analysis & meta-analysis in pts w/ advanced melanoma showed ORR between 41% & 50%, w/ CRs in up to 22%. Recent pivotal phase II trial for pts who previously received PD-(L)1 blockade showed ORR of 36% w/ median DOR not reached at 18.7 mos. Safety profile consistent w/ known lymphodepletion & IL-2 toxicities (*JCO* 2021;39(24):2656; *JCO* 2021;39(suppl 15):1004; *Annals Oncol*, 2019;30(12):1902; *CCR* 2011;17(13):4550)
- **HPV-associated carcinomas:** A phase II trial showed ORR of 28% & 18% in the cervical & noncervical CA cohort, respectively, w/ HPV-reactive T-cells correlating w/ response (*CCR* 2019;25(5):1486). An additional phase II study resulted in 44% ORR in previously treated cervical CA pts (*JCO* 2019;37(suppl 15):2538)
- **NSCLC:** A phase I trial evaluated the safety & efficacy of TILs in NSCLC pts after tx w/ nivolumab, ORR 25% including tumors negative for PD-L1 expression & harboring *EGFR* mutations (*Cancer Res* 2020;80(16):suppl)
- **HNSCC:** An ongoing phase II clinical trial evaluating TILs combined w/ pembrolizumab in CPI-naive pts w/ HNSCC showed an ORR 44% w/ a median DOR not reached at 8.6 mos. AE profile was consistent w/ known AE profiles of pembrolizumab, lymphodepletion, & IL-2 regimens (*JITC* 2020;8(3):suppl)

PRINCIPLES OF HEREDITARY CANCER SYNDROMES AND HEREDITARY BREAST AND OVARIAN CANCERS

- Causes of CA: 80% sporadic, **15–20% familial, 5–10% hereditary**
- Inherited CAs **arise from highly penetrant germline mts;** "familial" CAs may be caused by interaction of low-penetrance genes, gene-environment interactions, or both
- Over 200 hereditary CA susceptibility syndromes
- Traditionally, pts should have **genetic counseling (GC) before genetic testing (GT)** to determine eligibility, discuss benefits, risks & potential unanticipated findings, guide interpretation & reproductive considerations; however, this is shifting as eligibility expands & because GT is often needed before surgical/therapeutic decision-making
- Family members: Refer at-risk relatives of index pts for GC/GT
- Reproductive options: Preimplantation GT
- Offer referral to psychosocial support services given burden of dz & impact on family

Genetic Testing Outcome and Clinical Significance/Screening Recommendation	
Positive: Pathogenic mt	Pt is at higher-than-population risk of CA; gene/syndrome-specific screening recommendations
Variant of uncertain significance (VUS)	Pt may be at higher-than-population risk of CA; offer research & individualized recommendations based on personal/FHx
Negative for known mt in family	True Negative. Pt is at or near population risk of CA; screen as per general population guidelines
Negative: No known mt in family	Uninformative Negative. Pt is at unclear risk; offer research & individualized recommendations based on personal/FHx

Biology of hereditary breast and ovarian cancers

- **Germline mts in: *BRCA1* (ch 17q), *BRCA2* (ch 13q);** see table for addn'l genes
- Ashkenazi Jewish (AJ) founder mts: *BRCA1* 187delAG & 5385insC, *BRCA2* 6174delT
- **Gene function:** Double-stranded DNA damage repair by homologous recombination
- **Inheritance:** Autosomal dominant

Epidemiology and cancer risk

- **Incidence:** ~5% of all breast CA, 10–15% of all ovarian CA, ~6% metastatic prostate CA, ~5–10% pancreatic CA attributable to *BRCA;* higher prevalence of *BRCA* mts in AJ individuals (1:40 unselected population)
- **Penetrance:** 50–85% risk of breast CA by age 70; *BRCA1* confers 30–50% risk of ovarian CA, 10–30% for *BRCA2* carriers
- **Lifetime CA risks:** Breast (50–85%), ovarian (10–50%), prostate, second primary breast, male breast, pancreas
- **Prognosis:** *BRCA1/2* does not impact overall survival in breast CA (*Templeton PLoS* 2016;5:11)

Pathology

- **Breast CA:**
  - *BRCA1:* ~15% medullary carcinomas; basal-like molecular subtype, higher grade; ~80% TNBC
  - *BRCA2:* More varied pathology spectrum, similar to sporadic CA; more HR+ (luminal molecular subtype)
- **Ovarian CA:** High-grade serous carcinoma
- **Prostate CA:** Higher Gleason score, nodal involvement, de novo metastatic

Risk assessment

- **Genetic testing if:** Breast CA ≤ age 45; breast CA ≤ age 50 w/ 2nd 1° breast CA or ≥1 relative w/ breast, ovarian, pancreas, or prostate CA; TNBC ≤ age 60; metastatic breast or prostate CA, pancreas CA, or ovarian CA at any age; AJ. Refer to GC for additional GT criteria
- **Risk assessment models:**
  - Empirical: Estimate probability that testing will detect a *BRCA1/2* mt (NCI, Myriad, University of Pennsylvania models, Manchester scoring system)
  - Genetic risk: Estimate mt carrier probabilities & CA risks (BRCAPro, Tyrer–Cuzick, BOADICEA)

Genetic testing

- Comprehensive **full sequencing & large rearrangement analysis of** *BRCA1/2*
- *BRCA1/2* testing often performed in context of multi-gene panel w/ other moderate-risk breast &/or ovarian CA genes (*see table below*)

- If AJ & known familial mt, 1st test for known familial mt & all AJ founder mts
- If AJ & no known familial mt, 1st test for AJ founder mts; further testing if negative

Management

- **Breast CA:** SBE beginning age 18. CBE q6–12mo beginning age 25. Annual breast MRI beginning age 25 or younger based on earliest onset in affected family member. After age 30, screen w/ **annual MRI & mammogram**. Risk-reducing bilateral mastectomy (rrBLM)↓ breast CA risk by ≥90%; discuss w/ all known *BRCA* mt carriers
- **Male breast CA:** SBE beginning age 35. CBE q12mo beginning age 35. Consider mammogram beginning age 40
- **Ovarian CA:** rrBSO ↓ ovarian CA risk by 85–90% & possibly breast CA risk by approximately 50% if performed premenopausally; a/w lower all-cause, breast CA-specific, & ovarian CA-specific mortality (*JAMA* 2010;304:967); rrBSO after completion of child-bearing, ideally between ages 35–40 for pts w/ *BRCA1*. Reasonable to delay to age 40–45 in pts w/ *BRCA2*, assuming they have maximized breast CA prevention (ie, s/p rrBLM)
- **Prostate:** Digital rectal exam & PSA beginning age 40
- **Pancreas:** No definitive evidence supporting screening; consider investigational imaging & screening studies
- **Chemoprevention:** Consider tamoxifen or raloxifene but limited evidence
- **Lifestyle measures:** Limit EtOH consumption, weight loss; OCPs may reduce risk of ovarian CA

Treatment

- Surgery: **Same as for non-mt carriers,** though more strongly **consider bilateral** (risk-reducing) mastectomy during surgical tx
- Chemotherapy: Same as for non-mt carriers; anthracycline/taxane combination w/ benefit in *BRCA1* mt; ***BRCA*-associated breast CA may be particularly platinum-sensitive** (*Breast Cancer Res Treat* 2014;147:401)
- **PARP inhibitors:** Approved for breast, ovarian, pancreas, & prostate CAs w/ germline *BRCA* mts (*JCO* 2015;33:244); longer PFS w/ maintenance olaparib vs. placebo in pancreas (*NEJM* 2019;381:317), olaparib vs SOC in metastatic HER2 (–) breast (*NEJM* 2017; 377:1700), adjuvant olaparib in high-risk HER2 (–) early breast (*NEJM* 2021;384:2394), & maintenance olaparib in newly diagnosed advanced ovarian (*NEJM* 2018;379:2495)
- Endocrine: Same as for non-mt carriers
- Her2-targeted: Same as for non-mt carriers

Reproductive considerations

- Biallelic *BRCA* mts: Fanconi anemia (AR childhood d/o; discuss GT for partner to determine reproductive risk. IVF w/ preimplant GT (PGT) available if positive)

Additional breast/ovary risk genes

Genes	Associated Cancers
PALB2	Breast, pancreas, ovarian
ATM	Breast, pancreas, prostate, ovarian[a]
CHEK2	Breast, colon
RAD51C/RAD51D	Ovarian, breast[a]
BARD1	Breast[a]
BRIP1	Ovarian

[a]For these cancers, the link between the gene and cancer is uncertain.

LYNCH SYNDROME

Biology, epidemiology, clinical presentation, and pathology

- **Germline mt in DNA MMR** gene (*MLH1, MSH2, MSH6, PMS2*) or 3′ del in *EPCAM/TACSTD1* gene (leads to *MSH2* silencing)
- **Gene function:** Correct mispaired bases as a result of replication error
- **Phenotypic hallmark: MSI** (accumulation of errors during DNA replication, especially in repetitive sequences known as microsatellites) in the tumor
- **Inheritance:** Autosomal dominant
- **Incidence:** ~3% of all CRC (mean age 43); 2–5% of endometrial CA
- **Lifetime CA risks:** Colon (10–60%), endometrial (10–60%), others (<10%; gastric, ovarian, pancreatic, urethral, renal pelvis, GBM, small intestine)
- **Muir–Torre syndrome:** LS variant w/sebaceous neoplasms, often in *MSH2* mt carriers
- **Prognosis:** MSI-H CRC & endometrial CA have better prognosis than if MSS
- Colon CA: MSI-H, poorly differentiated w/medullary features, mucinous histology, TILs; predilection for proximal colon; more rapid progression from adenoma to carcinoma than in sporadic CRC
- Endometrial CA: MSI-H, mixed histologies **(majority endometrioid, poorly differentiated)**

Risk assessment models and genetic testing

- **Amsterdam II criteria (1999): Specific** (50% pts meeting criteria have MMR gene mt) but **not sensitive** (stringent criteria miss up to 68% pts MMR gene mt)
- **Revised Bethesda Guidelines (2002):** Broader criteria than Amsterdam model, cost-effective, but difficult to apply in practice

Types of Testing	
IHC for MMR protein expression	Sn ~83%, Sp 89%; perform IHC on all 4 MMR proteins to pinpoint appropriate gene(s) for mt analysis; absence of 1 or more protein(s) in tumor suggestive of LS except if MLH1 absent–reflex test tumor for *BRAF* V600E mt &/or MLH1 promoter hypermethylation which would suggest a sporadic etiology
MSI analysis	Sn 77–89%, Sp 90%; MSI-H if ≥2/5 markers positive; use when FHx is not strongly suggestive to determine who should undergo germline mt testing; helpful if IHC inconclusive or normal but clinical suspicion high

- **Test tumor tissue 1st:** If positive tumor tissue testing (MSI-H or IHC abnormal) refer for GC & germline GT
- **Universal screening for LS:** All CRCs & endometrial CA regardless of age
- **If no tumor tissue available but strong FHx:** Refer for GC/GT
- If tumor MSI-H or IHC-abnormal further work-up for LS is indicated, irrespective of tumor type

Management

- **CRC:** Colonoscopy beginning age 20–25 or 2–5 y younger than youngest affected relative (whichever 1st), repeat q1–2y; discussion of subtotal colectomy in CRC-affected LS pt; in pts w/ PMS2/MSH6, CRC risk is lower & recommendations re: age to start are controversial
- **Endometrial/Ovarian:** Discuss TAH/BSO upon completion of childbearing; controversial in PMS2 where OC risk limited
- **Other:** Consider upper EGD & noninvasive capsule endoscopy q2–3y beginning age 30–35; consider annual U/A age 30–35; site-specific eval. & heightened attention to sxs
- **Chemoprevention:** ASA reduces CA risks in hereditary CRC carriers (*Lancet* 2011;378:2081)

Treatment

- **MSI-H tumors may be more resistant to fluorouracil**-based chemotherapy (*JCO* 2010;28:3219) w/ implications for stage II CRCs
- Increased tumor immunogenicity suggests high likelihood of response to IO across MSI-H tumors
- **MMRd predicts response to ICI in CRC** (*NEJM* 2015;372:2509); MSI can be used as a biomarker for PD-1/PD-L1 blockade

Reproductive considerations

- Biallelic *MMR* mts cause CMMRD, rare AR childhood disorder; discuss testing partner for *MMR* status to determine reproductive risk; IVF w/ PGT available if positive

FAMILIAL ADENOMATOUS POLYPOSIS (FAP)

Biology

- ***APC* gene mts** (ch5q21)
- **Gene function:** Regulation of β-catenin–mediated gene transcription
- 2 variants: **Classical** & **attenuated (AFAP);** phenotypic variability dependent on location of particular *APC* mt (penetrance for classical FAP ~100%)
- **Inheritance:** Autosomal dominant; ~25% of mts occur de novo

Epidemiology

- **Incidence/prevalence:** FAP + AFAP account for <1% of all CRC

Clinical presentation

- **FAP:** >100 (100–1,000s) polyps by age teens-30s; lifetime risk of CRC approaches 100% by age 50
- **AFAP** typically <100 polyps; later onset (incidence rises after age 40, approaches 70% by age 80)
- **Location of dz:** FAP: L-sided CRC more common; AFAP: R-sided CRC
- **Associated nonmalignant findings (more common w/ FAP):** Desmoid tumors (distal *APC* mt), congenital hypertrophy of retinal pigment epithelium (CHRPE, central *APC* mt), mandibular osteomas, supernumerary teeth, epidermal cysts, adrenal cortical adenomas
- **Associated malignant conditions:** Thyroid tumors, gastric small intestinal polyps w/ 5–10% risk of duodenal or ampullary adenocarcinoma, Turcot syndrome (colonic polyposis + brain tumors), possibly pancreatic CA

Genetic testing

- Sn to identify *APC* gene mt currently 70–90%
- Comprehensive **full sequencing** & **large rearrangement analysis of** *APC*
- *APC* testing often performed in context of multi-gene panel w/ other polyposis risk genes (*MUTYH, GREM1, POLE, POLD1, NTHL1, MSH3, BMPR1A, SMAD4, PTEN, STK11*, etc.)

Screening and risk reduction

- **Personal history of FAP:** Flexible sigmoidoscopy or colonoscopy q12mo beginning age 10–15; review surgical options (colectomy or proctocolectomy) once adenomas develop; prophylactic proctocolectomy usually indicated in the 2nd decade for classical FAP
- **Personal or FHx of AFAP:** Colonoscopy & polypectomy q2–3y beginning late teens; consider prophylactic surgery if polypectomy no longer feasible
- **At-risk, no testing (preference or access):** Annual flexible sigmoidoscopy or colonoscopy age 10–15 until age 24; if negative, less frequent intervals; if using flexible sigmoidoscopy, consider colonoscopy q5y beginning age 20 in case pt has AFAP
- Consider **chemoprevention** w/ NSAIDs (*NEJM* 2006;355:885; *Lancet* 2020;395:1855)

Additional surveillance

- Bowel surveillance following surgery: If retained rectum, endoscopic exam q6–12mo of remaining tract & ileal pouch/ileostomy
- Annual thyroid exam ± U/S
- Consider abdominal CT or MRI if FHx of symptomatic desmoid tumor

LI–FRAUMENI SYNDROME

Biology

- **Germline mt in** *TP53*
- Brazilian founder mt: p.Arg337His, Ashkenazi Jewish founder mt: p.Gly334Arg
- **Gene function:** Tumor suppression
- **Inheritance:** Autosomal dominant; ~20% mts occur de novo

Epidemiology and clinical presentation

- **Incidence:** Up to 8% female breast CA in pts <30 yrs, 6–50% pediatric adrenocortical carcinoma (ACC); Brazilian founder mt prevalence (1:375)
- **Lifetime CA risks:** Overall >70% for males, >90% for females. Breast (54%; avg dx age 33), CNS (19%), osteo or soft tissue sarcoma (5–22%), ACC (13%), others: leukemia/lymphoma, colon, head/neck, melanoma. Up to 50% risk to develop multiple primary CAs
- **Prognosis:** Improved OS w/ surveillance (5y OS: 88.8% w/ vs. 59.6% w/o, *Lancet Oncol* 2016;17:1295). Certain mts pose lower lifetime CA risks d/t differing genotype/phenotype correlations

Pathology

- **Breast:** Propensity for Her2+, malignant phyllodes tumors
- **ACC:** LFS-associated ACC more typical before age 12 but no difference btw LFS-associated & sporadic in sex or tumor stage
- **ALL:** ~50% w/ hypodiploid ALL will have LFS

Risk assessment criteria

- **Classic criteria:** Sarcoma < age 45 + 1st-degree relative w/ cancer <45 & 1st or 2nd-degree relative w/ cancer <45 or sarcoma at any age
- **Chompret criteria:** Revision of Classic criteria to account for pts w/ core LFS CAs, regardless of FHx
- **LFS-like criteria:** More inclusive of FHx <60, consider LFS screening

Genetic testing

- Comprehensive **full sequencing & large rearrangement analysis of** *TP53*
- Consider *TP53* testing w/ other CA risk genes in multi-gene panel depending on personal/FHx
- Clonal hematopoiesis &/or germline mosaicism can yield *TP53*+ germline mt at lower allele frequency

Management

- WBMRI detection rate for new, localized primary cancers 7% (*JAMA Oncol* 2017;3:1634)
- **Children:** Abdominal/pelvic U/S q3–4mo, U/A q3–4mo, bloodwork q4mo, annual brain MRI, WBMRI
- **Adults**: SBE beginning age 18, CBE beginning age 20–25, annual MMG & breast MRI beginning age 20–25 (or earlier if FHx); consider rrBLMRM, annual brain MRI & WBMRI, colonoscopy q2–5y beginning age 40 (or 10y prior to earliest CRC CA in family), annual dermatology exam, labwork q3–4mo, annual abdominal U/S
- **Minimize exposure to radiation when possible**

Reproductive considerations

- Consider preimplantation GT (**PGT**)

OTHER GENETIC SYNDROMES

VHL disease

- **Genetics:** *VHL* gene mt; AD; very high penetrance
- **Clinical presentation: CNS hemangioblastoma;** retinal angiomas, ccRCC (low risk in type 2A, high risk in type 2B), pheochromocytomas (low risk in type 1, high risk in type 2A/B), pancreas serous cystadenomas & neuroendocrine tumors, epididymal cystadenomas
- **Testing criteria:** FHx of VHL w/ hemangioblastoma, pheochromocytoma, or RCC. If no FHx, ≥2 hemangioblastomas & a visceral tumor. GT for *VHL* can detect almost all cases of VHL dz
- **Management of carriers:** Annual retinal exam beginning age 1 w/ close monitoring for neurologic disturbance; annual metanephrine testing beginning age 5–15; annual abd U/S beginning age 8; MRI of brain & cervical spine q2y & auditory testing beginning age 16

Hereditary diffuse gastric cancer

- **Genetics:** *CDH1* (*E-cadherin*) & *CTNNA1* gene mt; AD; incomplete penetrance
- **Clinical presentation:** 40–80% lifetime risk of diffuse gastric CA (DGC, median age 38); 43–55% risk of **lobular breast CA**
- **Testing criteria:** Family criteria ≥1 of following: 2 gastric CA w/ at least 1 DGC; 1 DGC at any age + 1 lobular breast CA <age 70; 2 lobular breast CA <age 50. Individual criteria: DGC <age 50; DGC any age if Māori ethnicity; DGC any age w/ cleft lip/palate; DGC + lobular breast CA both <age 70; b/l lobular breast CA <age 70; gastric in situ signet ring cells or pagetoid spread of signet ring cells <age 50
- **Management of carriers:** Prophylactic total gastrectomy (gastric CA rare <age 20), EGD surveillance (efficacy unknown); breast: Annual MMG/MRI beginning age 30 (or earlier if FHx), consider rrBLM

Cowden syndrome

- **Genetics:** *PTEN* gene mt; Autosomal dominant (AD); very high penetrance
- **Clinical presentation: Hamartomatous tumors** in multiple organs (skin, mucosa, GI tract); breast CA (lifetime risk 25–50%), endometrial CA, thyroid CA, macrocephaly; **trichilemmomas** (skin-colored warty papules) **& papillomatous papules** are pathognomonic
- **Testing criteria:** Pathognomonic: Lhermitte–Duclose dz, mucocutaneous lesions (*J Med Genet* 2000;37:828)
- **Management of carriers:** Annual skin & pelvic exams, thyroid U/S, high-risk breast CA screening, discussion of rrBLM & hysterectomy, early colonoscopy

Other hereditary cancer predisposition syndromes

Syndrome	Genes	Associated Tumors/Features
BAP1 cancer	*BAP1*	Uveal melanoma, mesothelioma, RCC
Birt–Hogg–Dubé	*FLCN*	Chromophobe renal CA, fibrofolliculoma, a/w spontaneous PTX
Carney	*PRKAR1A*	Adrenal CA, thyroid CA, GCT, schwannoma, pituitary adenoma
DICER1	*DICER1*	Pleuropulmonary blastoma, pulomary cysts, thyroid neoplasia, ovarian tumors
Familial Atypical Multiple Melanoma & Mole	*CDKN2A* (encodes p16)	Early-onset melanoma, ↑ risk of pancreatic in some families
Familial MTC	*RET*	MTC, no pheo or parathyroid involvement
Hereditary GIST	*KIT, PDGFR*	Multicentric/large GIST; hyperpigmented elbow, knee, perineum w/ mastocytosis (urticarial pigmentosa)
Hereditary paraganglioma & pheochromocytoma	*SDHA, SDHAF2, SDHB, SDHC, SDHD, TMEM127, MAX*	Paraganglioma, pheochromocytoma, RCC
Hereditary papillary renal cell carcinoma	*MET*	Multiple bilateral papillary renal tumors

Hereditary leiomyomatosis & renal cell cancer	*FH* (fumarate hydratase)	Skin nodules (leiomyomata), uterine fibroids (leiomyomas & leiomyosarcomas), type II papillary RCC
Juvenile polyposis	*SMAD4/DPC4, BMPR1A*	Colon hamartomas in children a/w ↑ risk of colon CA
Multiple endocrine neoplasia, Type 1	*MEN1* (ch11)	Anterior pituitary, parathyroid, adrenal cortex, pancreatic islet tumors
Multiple endocrine neoplasia, Type 2	*RET*	Medullary thyroid carcinoma (MTC risk 95% recommend ppx thyroidectomy), pheo, hyperparathyroid (HPT). MEN 2b: Earlier onset & more aggressive; a/w mucosal neuromas, marfanoid phenotype, ganglioneuroma, megacolon
Neurofibromatosis, Type 1	*NF1* (ch17q11.2)	Neurofibrosarcomas, pheo, optic gliomas, meningiomas
Neurofibromatosis, Type 2	*NF2* (ch22)	Bilateral vestibular schwannomas
Nevoid basal cell carcinoma syndrome (Gorlin syndrome)	*PTCH1, SUFU*	Medulloblastoma, basal cell carcinoma
Peutz–Jeghers	*STK11*	Pigmented mucocutaneous macules, GI hamartomas (benign); ↑ risk of colon CA, breast CA, ovarian CA, small bowel CA & pancreas CA
Rhabdoid predisposition	*SMARCB1, SMARCA4*	Rhabdoid tumors, choroid plexus CA, central PNET
Telomere biology disorder	*TERT*	Dysplastic nails, pigmentation of chest/neck, oral leukoplakia, BMF
Tuberous sclerosis I & II	*TSC1/TSC2*	RCC, SEGA (astrocytoma), hamartoma, cardiac rhabdomyoma
Werner	*WRN/RECQL2*	Thyroid CA, melanoma, sarcoma; a/w bilateral cataracts, DM, osteoporosis, CAD, infertility

PHARMACOGENETICS AND PHARMACOGENOMICS

Introduction

- **Pharmacogenetics:** Effect of heritable genes on response to drugs. Study of single genes & interindividual differences in drug-metabolizing enzymes
- **Pharmacogenomics:** Effect of inherited & acquired genetic variation on drug response. Study of the functions & interactions of all genes in the genome & how the overall variability of drug response may be used to predict right tx for individual pts & contribute to the design new drugs
- **Polymorphisms:** Common variations in a DNA sequence that may lead to ↓ or ↑ activity of the encoded gene (SNP, micro- & minisatellites)
- **SNPs:** Single-nucleotide polymorphisms that may cause an amino acid exchange in the encoded protein, account for >90% of genetic variation in the human genome

Phase I drug-metabolizing enzymes

- Genetic polymorphisms reported for *CYP450* isoforms 2C8, 2C9, 2C19, 2D6, & 3A4

CYP3A4/5

- CYP3A isoenzymes account for ~50% of the metabolic activity of all CYP450 enzymes
- Substrates include etoposide, paclitaxel, & vincristine
- SNP frequencies of *CYP3A4* relatively low in most populations (14% in Caucasians & 10% in Japanese individuals) making it difficult to link genotype to PK or PD of CYP3A4 substrates
- Study conducted by the National Children's CA Group Pediatric ALL trial set out to correlate the association between relapse & tox of 1,204 pts w/ CYP3A4*1B, CYP3A5*3, & CYP3A5*6 SNPs. Trial results were neg; however, 1st 2 variants had a statistically significant ↑ risk of peripheral neuropathy

CYP2C8

- Involved in metabolism of paclitaxel to inactive metabolite, 6α-hydroxy paclitaxel
- 6 Allele variants have been identified; CYP2C8*3 occurs most frequently in Caucasians, while CYP2C8*2 occurs most frequently in African Americans. Both variants result in reduced enzymatic activity & ↑ exposure to paclitaxel

CYP2C19

- Involved in activation of thalidomide through 5-hydroxylation
- CYP2C19*2 homozygotes have shown poor metabolizing phenotype, may respond poorly to thalidomide tx

CYP2D6

- Involved in the conversion of tamoxifen to 4-hydroxytamoxifen which is subsequently converted to endoxifen (both more potent antiestrogens than tamoxifen)
- CYP2D6 homozygous variant or heterozygous genotype individuals have ↓ plasma endoxifen conc. compared to homozygous wild-type subjects after 4 mos of therapy

Non-P450 phase I metabolizing enzymes

Dihydropyrimidine dehydrogenase (DPD): The 1st & rate-limiting step in catabolism of pyrimidine bases, uracil & thymidine

- 5-FU & capecitabine (prodrug for 5-FU) metabolized by DPD to inactive metabolites in liver
- DPD deficiency leads to increased exposure & prolonged $T_{1/2}$ of 5-FU → sev. myelosuppression, GI & neurologic tox
- 39 polymorphisms & mts of the DPD gene are known; DPD*2A the most common polymorphism → inactive enzyme in 0.9% of Caucasian pts

Phase II drug-metabolizing enzymes

Thiopurine methyltransferase (TPMT): Involved in the metabolism of thiopurines (6-MP, AZA) through S-methylation to inactive metabolites

- TPMT*2, TPMT*3A, & TPMT*3C account for 95% of pts w/ TPMT deficiency
- Pts who carry TPMT polymorphisms are at risk of sev. hematologic tox; pts homozygous for TPMT allele variation have 4x increased risk of tox
- Appropriate 6-MP dose reductions for TPMT-deficient pts have allowed for similar tox & survival outcomes when compared to pts w/ normal levels
- Tests for TPMT genotype & phenotype are commercially available

Uridine diphosphate glucuronosyltransferase 1A1 (UGT1A1)

- Microsatellite mt results in UGT1A1*28 polymorphism leading to ↓ UGT1A1 expression & activity
- UGT1A1*28 polymorphism typically found in pts w/ Gilbert syndrome; frequency 12–27% in Africans, 5–15% in Caucasians, 1.2–5% in Asians (*BJP* 2006;62(1):35)
- Important role in the metabolism of etoposide, epirubicin, & most importantly irinotecan
- **Irinotecan:** Prodrug activated to ethyl-10-hydroxycamptothecin (SN-38) via carboxyl esterase. SN-38 undergoes UGT1A1-catalyzed glucuronidation to form inactive SN-38 glucuronide (SN-38G). Reduced UGT1A1 activity leads to ↑ exposure to SN-38 ↑ tox **(diarrhea, myelosuppression)** limiting optimal clinical use

Drug transporters

P-gp (MDR-1)

- P-gp & its encoding gene MDR-1 (ABCB1) expressed in high levels in brain vessels, adrenal glands, kidney, liver, & GI tract
- P-gp is involved in the transport of hydrophobic drugs including doxorubicin, paclitaxel, irinotecan, hormones, & carcinogens
- Multidrug resistance proteins act as drug efflux pumps rendering cells resistant to cytostatic drugs
- Three most common SNPs are P-gp*6 (22–56% in Caucasians), P-gp*7, & P-gp*8

Drug targets

5,10-Methylenetetrahydrofolate reductase (MTHFR)

- Involved in metabolism of 5,10-methylenetetrahydrofolate to 5-methylenetetrahydrofolate, methyl donor for the methylation of DNA, homocysteine, & DNA synthesis
- Reduced MTHFR activity affects intracellular folate pools → ↑ tox in pts treated w/ antifolates

Thymidylate synthase (TS)

- Essential enzyme in de novo synthesis of thymidylate, precursor of thymidine triphosphate, essential for DNA synthesis & repair
- TS gene promoter is polymorphic & has 2 (TSER*2) or 3 (TSER*3) 28-bp tandem repeat sequences
- In vitro studies show TS promoters w/ the TSER*3 sequence generate 3× higher mRNA than those w/ the TSER*2 sequence
- Inhibition of TS by FdUMP is 1 of the 1° mechanisms of action of 5-FU
- TS expression levels inversely correlate w/ the sensitivity of tumors to 5-FU; therefore, TSER*2 homozygotes respond better to 5-FU than TSER*3 homozygotes or heterozygotes (*Devita, Hellman, and Rosenberg's Cancer: Principles & Practice of Oncology*. 10th ed. 2014; *Annu Rev Med*. 2015;66:65; *Br J Haematol* 2003;122(2):240)

ANTIBODY DRUG CONJUGATES

Agent	Epitope	Conjugated Drug
Ado-trastuzumab emtansine	HER2	Mertansine
Enfortumab vedotin-ejfv	Nectin 4	Monomethyl auristatin E (MMAE)
Fam-trastuzumab deruxtecan-nxki	HER2	DX-8951 derivative, DXd
Moxetumomab pasudotox-tdfk	CD22	Pseudomonas exotoxin PE38
Polatuzumab vedotin-piiq	CD79b	MMAE
Sacituzumab govitecan-hziy	Trop-2	Irinotecan derivative SN-38
Tagraxofusp-erzs	CD123	Diphtheria toxin

Ado-trastuzumab emtansine (Kadcyla)

- **Mechanism:** HER2-targeted antibody–drug conjugated to the antimicrotubular maytansinoid agent, mertansine (DM1)
- **Dosing:** 3.6 mg/kg every 3 wks, no renal or hepatic adjustments
- **PK/PD:** $T_{1/2}$ ~4 d
- **AEs: Hepatotoxicity, ↓ LVEF,** pancytopenia, GI tox, neuropathy, ↓ K
- **DDI:** CYP3A4 substrate

Enfortumab vedotin-ejfv (Padcev)

- **Mechanism:** Anti-Nectin 4 human IgG1; after binding, internalized ADC releases antimicrotubule agent MMAE, producing cell cycle arrest/apoptosis
- **Approved indication:** Urothelial cancer
- **Dosing:** 1.25 mg/kg (max 125 mg) IV d 1, 8, & 15 of 28-d cycles; avoid use in mod./sev. hepatic impairment; no adjustment for renal impairment; manufacturer-recommended dose reductions available for toxicity
- **PK/PD:** $T_{1/2}$ 3.4 d for ADC, 2.4 d for MMAE; MMAE metabolized hepatically (CYP3A4)
- **Adverse effects (AEs):** Skin rxns (mostly maculopapular rash/pruritus, some sev. rxns), hyperglycemia, peripheral neuropathy, ocular disorders (mostly corneal), alopecia, diarrhea, dysgeusia, low vomiting risk, myelosuppression
- **DDI:** Strong CYP3A4 inhibitors/inducers likely increase/decrease MMAE exposure; no specific dose adjustments recommended; MMAE is a P-glycoprotein substrate
- **Clinical pearls:** Prophylactic artificial tears suggested; median 3.8 mos to grade ≥2 neuropathy, 1.9 mos to ocular disorders

Fam-trastuzumab deruxtecan-nxki (Enhertu)

- **Mechanism:** HER2-targeted antibody–drug conjugated to a topoisomerase I inhibitor (DXd, an exatecan derivative)
- **Approved indications:** Breast cancer, gastric cancer
- **Dosing:** Breast cancer (unresectable/metastatic): 5.4 mg/kg q3wks; gastric cancer (locally advanced/metastatic): 6.4 mg/kg q3wks; adjust for neutropenia, neutropenic fever, thrombocytopenia, cardiotoxicity, infusion rxns, pulmonary toxicity; 1st-dose reduction breast 4.4 mg/kg, gastric 5.4 mg/kg, 2nd-dose reduction breast 3.2 mg/kg, gastric 4.4 mg/kg
- **PK/PD:** $T_{1/2}$ ~5–6 d
- **AEs:** Hepatotoxicity, ↓ LVEF, pancytopenia, GI tox, ILD, ↓ K, alopecia, ↑ LFT, ↑ Tbili, fatigue, headache
- **DDI:** Minor CYP3A4 substrate, P-gp substrate

Moxetumomab pasudotox-tdfk (Lumoxiti)

- **Mechanism:** CD22-directed antibody–drug fused to Pseudomonas exotoxin (PE38) which is internalized & causes inhibition of protein synthesis & apoptotic cell death
- **Approved indication:** Hairy cell leukemia
- **Dosing:** 0.04 mg/kg on d 1, 3, 5 of 28-d cycle administered w/ 1 L isotonic IV before & after + H1 & H2 antagonists before + oral corticosteroid after infusion; consider low-dose aspirin on d 1–8 of each cycle; delay infusion for ≥grade 2–3 SCr; grade 2 capillary leak syndrome delay tx, grade 3–4 discontinue; discontinue for hemolytic uremic syndrome
- **PK/PD:** $T_{1/2}$ 1.4 h
- **AEs:** Capillary leak syndrome, infusion rxns, hemolytic uremic syndrome, ↓ albumin, ↓ Ca, ↓ Phos, ↑ LFTs
- **DDI:** N/A

Polatuzumab vedotin-piiq (Polivy)

- **Mechanism:** Anti-CD79b humanized IgG1; after binding, releases antimicrotubule agent MMAE, producing cell cycle arrest & apoptosis
- **Approved indication:** Diffuse large B-cell lymphoma
- **Dosing:** 1.8 mg/kg IV every 21 d; avoid use in mod./sev. hepatic impairment; no adjustment for mild/mod. renal impairment; manufacturer-recommended dose reductions available for hematologic toxicity, neuropathy
- **PK/PD:** $T_{1/2}$ 12 d for ADC, 4 d for MMAE; MMAE metabolized hepatically (CYP3A4)
- **AEs:** Myelosuppression, neuropathy, diarrhea, low emetogenicity, infusion rxns, infxns
- **DDI:** Strong CYP3A4 inhibitors/inducers likely increase/decrease MMAE exposure; no specific dose adjustments recommended; MMAE is a P-glycoprotein substrate
- **Clinical pearls:** HSV/VZV & PJP prophylaxis required, consider 1° GCSF prophylaxis

Sacituzumab govitecan (Trodelvy)

- **Mechanism:** Antitrophoblast cell-surface antigen 2 (Trop-2) antibody coupled to topoisomerase 1 inhibitor SN-38; binds to Trop-2 & is internalized so SN-38 can cause DNA damage, apoptosis, & cell death
- **Approved indications:** Breast cancer, urothelial cancer
- **Dosing:** 10 mg/kg d 1 & 8 of 21-d cycle; slow infusion if infusion rxn occurs; reduce dose for neutropenia & neutropenic fever; hold dose for grade 3–4 diarrhea, reduce dose for grade 3–4 nausea/vomiting
- **PK/PD:** $T_{1/2}$ 15.3 h; free SN-38 $T_{1/2}$ 19.7 h
- **AEs:** Diarrhea, nausea/vomiting, cytopenia, ↓ Ca, ↓ Na, ↑ LFTs, fatigue
- **DDI:** UGT1A1 substrate

Tagraxofusp-erzs (Elzonris)

- **Mechanism:** Recombinant IL-3-diphtheria toxin fusion protein; internalization releases truncated diphtheria toxin, producing protein synthesis inhibition & cell death
- **Approved indication:** Blastic plasmacytoid dendritic cell neoplasm
- **Dosing:** 12 mcg/kg IV d 1–5 of 21-d cycles; do not dose after cycle d 10 if doses delayed for toxicity; hold if AST &/or AST >5× ULN, &/or if creatinine >1.8 mg/dL or creatinine clearance <60 mL/min; additional hold criteria in package insert
- **PK/PD:** $T_{1/2}$ 0.7 h
- **AEs:** Capillary leak syndrome (BBW), hypersensitivity rxns, transaminitis, myelosuppression (20% febrile neutropenia), hyperglycemia, low vomiting risk
- **DDI:** No DDI studies conducted
- **Clinical pearls:** Manufacturer-recommended monitoring & management of capillary leak, including predose parameters for administration, available; first cycle must be inpt; premedicate each dose w/ H1RA, H2RA, acetaminophen, & corticosteroid

MONOCLONAL ANTIBODIES

Source Infixes Used for Naming Monoclonal Antibodies	
-o-	Mouse
-xi-	Chimeric
-zu-	Humanized
-u-	Human

Devita, Hellman, and Rosenberg's Cancer: Principles and Practice of Oncology. 9th ed. 2011.

Dosing Note: Most monoclonal antibodies do not require renal or hepatic dose adjustments; this is therefore not stated for each individual drug.

Alemtuzumab (Campath)
- **Mechanism:** Binds to CD52
- **Dosing:** Given IV or SQ, ↑ from 3 to 10 mg IV daily or 3 to 10 mg SQ 3×/wk; if tolerated, may ↑ to 30 mg IV/SQ 3× weekly
- **PK/PD:** Clearance ↓ w/ repeated dosing (due to ↓ of CD52 receptors), $T_{1/2}$ ~11 h after 1st 30-mg dose
- **AEs: Pancytopenia (DLT, time to nadir ~30 d),** GI upset, pneumonitis, HoTN, HTN, HSR
- **Clinical pearls:** Premedicate before every dose, ppx for PCP & HSV, risk of CMV infxn during & at least 2 mos after last dose. Avoid live virus vaccines

Amivantamab (Rybrevant)
- **Mechanism:** Binds to EGFR & MET
- **Dosing:** <80 kg = 1,050 mg IV & ≥80 kg = 1,400 mg IV. Wk 1: 350 mg on D1, remaining dose D2; wks 2–4: full infusion D1; wk 5 onward: full infusion every 2 wks
- **PK/PD:** $T_{1/2}$ ~11 d
- **AEs:** Rash, infusion rxns, musculoskeletal pain, paronychia, nausea, fatigue, stomatitis, constipation, ILD/pneumonitis
- **Clinical pearls:** For adv/met *EGFR* ex20ins+ NSCLC; premedicate w/ antihistamines, antipyretics, & glucocorticoids

Atezolizumab (Tecentriq)
- **Mechanism:** Binds to PD-L1
- **Dosing:** 840 mg every 2 wks, 1,200 mg IV every 3 wks, or 1,680 mg every 4 wks; hold for hepatic tox, ↑ Scr, & immune-mediated AEs
- **PK/PD:** $T_{1/2}$ ~27 d
- **AEs:** Immune-mediated tox, lymphocytopenia, GI tox, rash, infusion rxn, metabolic abnormalities, pneumonitis, ↑ liver enzymes, endocrinopathies
- **DDI:** No known pathways of metabolism
- **Clinical pearls:** Tx immune–related tox w/ steroids (prednisone 1–2 mg/kg/d), can increase complications post allogeneic HSCT

Avelumab (Bavencio)
- **Mechanism:** Binds to PD-L1
- **Dosing:** 800 mg or 10 mg/kg every 2 wks; consider holding tx if renal or hepatic toxicity develop
- **PK/PD:** $T_{1/2}$ ~6.1 d; 1° elimination is proteolytic degradation
- **AEs:** Immune-mediated tox, diarrhea, hepatitis B reactivation, infusion rxn, skin rash, fatigue, leukopenia, ↑ liver enzymes, arthralgia
- **DDI:** No known pathways of metabolism; Avoid corticosteroids since it may diminish the therapeutic effect of immune checkpoint inhibitors
- **Clinical pearls:** Tx immune–related tox w/ steroids (prednisone 1–2 mg/kg/d)

Bevacizumab (Avastin)
- **Mechanism:** Binds to VEGF
- **Dosing:** 5–15 mg/kg IV every 14–21 d, temporarily hold for proteinuria
- **PK/PD:** $T_{1/2}$ ~20 d
- **AEs:** HTN, thrombosis, GIB, thrombocytopenia, proteinuria
- **DDI:** No known pathways of metabolism
- **Clinical pearls:** Pts w/ SBP >150 mmHg or DBP >100 mmHg, recent hemoptysis, surgery/bx, or new onset of thrombosis require further evaluation before initiating tx

Blinatumomab (Blincyto)

- **Mechanism:** Binds CD19 on malignant B-cells & CD3 on T-cells
- **Dosing:** Cycle 1:9-mcg continuous infusion daily (d 1–7), followed by 28-mcg continuous infusion daily (d 8–28); cycle 2–5: 28-mcg continuous infusion daily (1–28) every 6 wks;. Cycles for MRD: 28-mcg continuous infusion
- **PK/PD:** $T_{1/2}$ ~2 h
- **AEs:** CRS, neurologic tox, fever, peripheral edema, diarrhea, ↑ liver enzymes
- **DDI:** No known pathways of metabolism, avoid live, & inactivated vaccines
- **Clinical pearls:** Admission required for initiation & for subsequent cycles for varying duration dependent on disease burden

Brentuximab vedotin (Adcetris)

- **Mechanism:** Binds CD30
- **Dosing:** 1.8 mg/kg every 3 wks, adjust dose for tx-related tox
- **PK/PD:** $T_{1/2}$ ~5 d
- **AEs: Peripheral neuropathy (DLT),** pancytopenia, URI
- **DDI:** CYP3A4 inhibitors/inducers (↑/↓ conc. of brentuximab)

Cemiplimab-rwlc (Libtayo)

- **Mechanism:** Binds to PD-1
- **Dosing:** 3 mg/kg intravenously over 90 min every 3 wks (total of 4 doses)
- **PK/PD:** $T_{1/2}$ = 20.3 d
- **AEs:** Musculoskeletal pain, fatigue, rash, diarrhea, lymphopenia, hyponatremia, hypophosphatemia, ↑ AST, anemia, & hyperkalemia. Possible immune-mediated adverse rxns, infusion rxns, complications of HSCT, embryo-fetal toxicity
- **DDI:** No known pathways of metabolism
- **Clinical pearls:** Tx immune–related tox w/ steroids (prednisone 1–2 mg/kg/d)

Cetuximab (Erbitux)

- **Mechanism:** Binds EGFR
- **Dosing:** 400 mg/m^2 IV loading dose, 250 mg/m^2 IV weekly
- **PK/PD:** $T_{1/2}$ ~112 h
- **AEs:** Acneiform rash (w/ in 1st 2 wks), pruritus, ↓ Mg, GI upset, anemia, HSR
- **DDI:** No known pathways of metabolism
- **Clinical pearls:** Not used in pts w/ mutated *KRAS*

Daratumumab (Darzalex)

- **Mechanism:** Binds to CD38
- **Dosing:** 16 mg/kg IV, dosing interval varies from once weekly to every 4 wks
- **PK/PD:** $T_{1/2}$ ~18 d
- **AEs:** Fatigue, lymphocytopenia, neutropenia, thrombocytopenia, infusion rxn, fever, upper respiratory sxs, herpes zoster
- **DDI:** No known pathways of metabolism
- **Clinical pearls:** Requires premedications before & after the infusion, antiviral ppx should be started w/in 1 wk of tx & continued for 3 mos post tx, interferes w/ RBC antibody screening & cross-matching

Dinutuximab (Unituxin)

- **Mechanism:** Binds to GD2
- **Dosing:** 17.5 mg/m^2/d IV for 4 consecutive d, given in combination w/ GMCSF, IL-2, & isotretinoin
- **PK/PD:** $T_{1/2}$ ~10 d
- **AEs:** HoTN, capillary leak syndrome, urticaria, thrombocytopenia, lymphocytopenia, anemia, fever, fluid retention
- **DDI:** No known pathways of metabolism, avoid live & inactivated vaccines, monitor use w/ antihypertensive agents
- **Clinical pearls:** Requires premedications

Durvalumab (Imfinzi)

- **Mechanism:** Binds to PDL-1
- **Dosing:** 10 mg/kg every 2 wks
- **PK/PD:** $T_{1/2}$ ~18 d
- **AEs:** Immune-mediated tox, infusion rxn, skin rash, metabolic abnormalities, hypothyroidism, diarrhea, lymphocytopenia, ↑ liver enzymes, fatigue, cough
- **DDI:** No known pathways of metabolism, avoid corticosteroids since it may diminish the therapeutic effect of immune checkpoint inhibitors
- **Clinical pearls:** Tx immune–related tox w/ steroids (prednisone 1–2 mg/kg/d)

Elotuzumab (Empliciti)

- **Mechanism:** Binds to the signaling lymphocytic activation molecule family member 7 (SLAMF7)
- **Dosing:** Cycle 1–2 given in combination w/ lenalidomide & dexamethasone or pomalidomide & dexamethasone: 10 mg/kg IV once weekly on a 28-d cycle; cycle 3 & more given in combination w/ lenalidomide & dexamethasone: 10 mg/kg IV every 2 wks of a 28-d cycle; cycle 3 & more given in combination w/ pomalidomide & dexamethasone: 20 mg/kg IV every 4 wks of a 28-d cycle. Withhold or discontinue tx for toxicity (hepatic & infusion rxns)
- **PK/PD:** $T_{1/2}$ ~82 d
- **AEs:** Fatigue, high blood pressure, diarrhea, ↓ Ca, leukopenia, thrombocytopenia, ↑ alk phos, hepatotoxicity, ↑ blood glucose, infxn, infusion rxns, 2° malignancy
- **DDI:** No known pathways of metabolism, avoid live & inactivated vaccines
- **Clinical pearls:** Antiviral ppx should be started prior to tx, requires premedication, can interfere w/ assays for M-protein monitoring

Gemtuzumab (Mylotarg)

- **Mechanism:** Binds CD33, once internalized calicheamicin derivative is released
- **Dosing:** AML: 9 mg/m^2 for 2 doses, APL: 6 mg/m^2 for 2 doses
- **PK/PD:** Initial $T_{1/2}$ ~45 h
- **AEs:** SOS, myelosuppression, HSR, metabolic abnormalities
- **DDI:** No known pathways of metabolism, avoid live & inactivated vaccines
- **Clinical pearls:** Requires premedications, monitor for signs of SOS

Ibritumomab (Zevalin)

- **Mechanism:** CD20-directed radioimmunoconjugate (bound to yttrium-90)
- **Dosing: Step (1)** rituximab IV; **step (2)** rituximab IV then ibritumomab IV, dose (0.3–0.4 mCi/kg) dependent on plt count (do not administer if plts <100,000 K/mcL)
- **PK/PD:** Distributes to all lymphoid cells, yttrium-90 $T_{1/2}$ ~64 h
- **AEs:** Prolonged pancytopenia (B-cell recovery starts in ~12 wks)
- **DDI:** Anticoagulants (↑ risk of bleeding)

Ipilimumab (Yervoy)

- **Mechanism:** Binds to CTLA-4
- **Dosing:** 3 mg/kg IV every 3 wks (up to 4 doses); tx can be held due to ↑ liver enzymes
- **PK/PD:** $T_{1/2}$ ~15 d
- **AEs:** Musculoskeletal pain, fatigue, rash, diarrhea, & immune-mediated AEs (BBW, commonly includes dermatitis, endocrine disorders, enterocolitis, hepatitis)
- **DDI:** No significant drug interactions
- **Clinical pearls:** Tx immune–related tox w/ steroids (prednisone 1–2 mg/kg/d)

Isatuximab (Sarclisa)

- **Mechanism:** CD38-directed cytolytic antibody
- **Dosing:** 10 mg/kg IV C1D1, 8, 15, 22; C2 onward 10 mg/kg IV on D1 & 15 every 28 d
- **PK/PD:** Total-body clearance decreases w/ increasing/multiple doses, near elimination from plasma ~2 mos after last dose
- **AEs:** Infusion-related rxns, neutropenia, upper respiratory infxn, hypertension, diarrhea, second primary malignancies
- **DDI:** Interferes w/ serologic testing (indirect Coombs test) & serum protein electrophoresis & immunofixation tests
- **Clinical pearls:** Requires premedication w/ dexamethasone (dose varies on regimen) APAP, H2 antagonists, & diphenhydramine

Margetuximab (Margenza)

- **Mechanism:** Binds to extracellular domain of HER2
- **Dosing:** 15 mg/kg IV every 21 d until POD/toxicity; hold tx for LVEF reductions
- **PK/PD:** Time to steady state is 2 mos, $T_{1/2}$ 19.2 d
- **AEs:** BBW for LVEF dysfunction, infusion-related rxns, fatigue, nausea, diarrhea, palmar-plantar erythrodysesthesia, ↑ liver enzymes, ↑ SCr, ↑ aPTT/INR
- **DDI:** Avoid anthracycline-based therapy for up to 4 mos after stopping margetuximab due to increased risk of cardiac dysfunction
- **Clinical pearls:** ECHO/MUGA w/in 4 wks prior to initiation of therapy & every 3 mos during & upon completion of therapy

Mogamulizumab (Poteligeo)

- **Mechanism:** Binds to CCR4
- **Dosing:** 1 mg/kg IV C1D1, 8, 15, 22; then 1 mg/kg IV C2+D1, 15 every 28 d until POD/toxicity; hold tx for rash ≥grade 2
- **PK/PD:** $T_{1/2}$ 17 d
- **AEs:** Infusion-related rxns, rash, fatigue, diarrhea, musculoskeletal pain, upper respiratory tract infxns, autoimmune complications reported
- **DDI:** No known pathways of metabolism
- **Clinical pearls:** Premedicate w/ APAP & acetaminophen, increased risks of sev. GVHD & transplant-related death in pts receiving pretransplant mogamulizmab

Naxitamab (Danyelza)

- **Mechanism:** Binds to GD2
- **Dosing:** 3 mg/kg/d (max 150 mg) on d 1, 3, 5 given every 4 wks until partial or complete response, followed by 5 cycles administered every 4 wks, further cycles can be given every 8 wks; requires dose interruption/discontinuation for toxicity
- **PK/PD:** Metabolized by catabolic pathways into small peptides, $T_{1/2}$ 8.2 d
- **AEs:** Infusion-related rxns, neurotoxicity, bone marrow suppression, hypersensitivity, hypertension, nausea (mod. emetic potential), urinary retention
- **DDI:** No known pathways of metabolism
- **Clinical pearls:** Requires premedications & tx w/ GM-CSF prior to & during each tx cycle

Necitumumab (Portrazza)

- **Mechanism:** Binds to EGFR
- **Dosing:** 800 mg IV on D 1 & 8 of a 21-d cycle, in combination w/ gemcitabine & cisplatin
- **PK/PD:** $T_{1/2}$ ~14 d
- **AEs:** Rash, ↓ electrolytes, vomiting, diarrhea, infusion-related rxns
- **DDI:** No known pathways of metabolism
- **Clinical pearls:** Serum electrolytes should be monitored prior to each dose & at least 8 wks after completion

Nivolumab (Opdivo)

- **Mechanism:** Binds to PD-1
- **Dosing:** Dosing dependent on dz, 240 mg every 2 wks or 480 mg every 4 wks; 1 mg/kg, 3 mg/kg or 360 mg in combination w/ ipilimumab at varying intervals, tx can be held due to ↑ liver enzymes or Scr & immune-mediated AEs
- **PK/PD:** $T_{1/2}$ ~25 d
- **AEs:** Pancytopenia, metabolic abnormalities, GI tox, pneumonitis, hypophysitis, ↑ liver enzymes, ↑ Scr, rash, infusion rxns
- **DDI:** No known pathways of metabolism
- **Clinical pearls:** Tx immune–related tox w/ steroids (prednisone 1–2 mg/kg/d), can increase complications post allogeneic HSCT

Obinutuzumab (Gazyva)

- **Mechanism:** Binds CD20 causing cell death
- **Dosing:** Dosing dependent on dz, CLL starts at 100 mg IV, FL starts at 1,000 mg IV weekly
- **PK/PD:** $T_{1/2}$ ~26–37 d
- **AEs:** Neutropenia, lymphocytopenia, ↑ liver enzymes, ↑ Scr, ↓ electrolytes, infusion rxns
- **DDI:** No known pathways of metabolism, avoid live & inactivated vaccines, monitor antihypertensive therapy
- **Clinical pearls:** Premedications required, screen for HBV prior to tx

Ofatumumab (Arzerra)

- **Mechanism:** Binds CD20
- **Dosing:** 300 mg IV × 1, then 2,000 mg IV weekly × 7 doses, then 2,000 mg every 4 wks × 4
- **PK/PD:** $T_{1/2}$ ~18 d
- **AEs:** Neutropenia (may be >2 wks), URI
- **DDI:** No known pathways of metabolism, avoid live & inactivated vaccines
- **Clinical pearls:** Premedicate for HSR

Olaratumab (Lartruvo)

- **Mechanism:** Binds PDGFR-α
- **Dosing:** 15 mg/kg on d 1 & 8 every 3 wks in combination w/ doxorubicin for 8 cycles, then continue as monotherapy
- **PK/PD:** $T_{1/2}$ ~11 d

- **AEs:** Fatigue, neuropathy, ↓ electrolytes, pancytopenia
- **DDI:** No known pathways of metabolism

Panitumumab (Vectibix)

- **Mechanism:** Binds EGFR
- **Dosing:** 6 mg/kg IV every 14 d. Adjust dose for tox (HSR, dermatologic)
- **PK/PD:** $T_{1/2}$ ~7.5 d
- **AEs: Acneiform rash,** ↓ Mg, ↓ Ca, eyelash growth, HSR
- **DDI:** No known significant interactions
- **Clinical pearls:** No therapeutic benefit in pts w/ mutated *KRAS*

Pembrolizumab (Keytruda)

- **Mechanism:** Binds to PD-1
- **Dosing:** 2 mg/kg IV every 3 wks, tx can be held due to ↑ liver enzymes
- **PK/PD:** $T_{1/2}$ ~27 d
- **AEs:** Immune-mediated tox, fatigue, rash, metabolic abnormalities, lymphocytopenia
- **DDI:** No known pathways of metabolism
- **Clinical pearls:** Tx immune–related tox w/ steroids (prednisone 1–2 mg/kg/d)

Pertuzumab (Perjeta)

- **Mechanism:** Binds to HER2 (binds to a different HER2 epitope than trastuzumab)
- **Dosing:** 840 mg IV × 1, then 420 mg every 3 wks
- **PK/PD:** $T_{1/2}$ ~18 d
- **AEs:** Cardiotoxicity, HSR, diarrhea, leukopenia, neutropenia
- **DDI:** No known pathways of metabolism

Ramucirumab (Cyramza)

- **Mechanism:** Binds to VEGFR2
- **Dosing:** Dosing dependent on dz; colorectal/gastric: 8 mg/kg IV every 2 wks as part of combination therapy; NSCLC 10 mg/kg every 21 d w/ docetaxel
- **PK/PD:** $T_{1/2}$ ~14 d
- **AEs:** HTN, diarrhea, proteinuria, neutropenia, anemia, infusion-related rxns
- **DDI:** No known pathways of metabolism
- **Clinical pearls:** Premedications required; pts w/ HTN should be controlled prior to administration & BPs monitored closely

Rituximab (Rituxan)

- **Mechanism:** Binds CD20
- **Dosing:** 375 mg/m^2 IV, frequency dependent on regimen
- **PK/PD:** Detectable in serum for 3–6 mos after completion
- **AEs:** Lymphopenia (B-cell recovery after ~6 mos), viral reactivation
- **DDI:** Live vaccines
- **Clinical pearls:** Split dose over 2 d for ALC ≥20,000/mcL or high tumor burden, screen for HBV prior to tx

Tafasitamab (Monjuvi)

- **Mechanism:** Binds CD19
- **Dosing:** 12 mg/kg IV C1D1, 4, 8, 15, & 22, then C2 & C3D1, 8, 15, 22, then C4+D1, 15 of 28-d cycle until POD/toxicity; hold therapy if plts ≤50,000/mcL or ANC ≤1,000/mcL × 7 d
- **PK/PD:** $T_{1/2}$ 17 d
- **AEs:** Infusion-related rxns, myelosuppression, fatigue, diarrhea, peripheral edema, cough, pyrexia, respiratory tract infxn
- **DDI:** No known pathways of metabolism
- **Clinical pearls:** Premedicate w/ APAP, H2 antagonist, diphenhydramine, &/or glucocorticosteroid, synergy w/ lenalidomide, check for CD19 expression before CAR-T

Trastuzumab (Herceptin)

- **Mechanism:** Binds to HER2
- **Dosing:** Loading dose 4–8 mg/kg IV, followed by 2–6 mg/kg maintenance dose IV weekly or every 21 d
- **PK/PD:** $T_{1/2}$ ~6–16 d
- **AEs: CMP (DLT),** GI upset, rash, fever, pain
- **DDI:** Anthracyclines (potential ↑ in cardiac tox)

Information based on publicly available drug inserts from Genzyme, Genentech, Seattle Genetics, Eli Lilly, Teva, GlaxoSmithKline, Janssen, United Therapeutics Corp, Bristol-Myers Squibb, Wyeth, Amgen, Incyte, Kyowa Kirin, Macrogenics, Sanofi Genzyme.

Class	Drugs	Mechanism
Cytidine analogs	Cytarabine Gemcitabine	Inhibition of DNA polymerase, incorporated into DNA & terminates chain elongation; gemcitabine also inhibits RNA reductase
Hypomethylating agents	Azacytidine Decitabine	Inhibition of DNA methylation via incorporation into DNA & RNA
Folate antagonists	Methotrexate Pemetrexed Pralatrexate	Inhibition of DHFR & thymidylate synthase (TS) results in inhibition of reduced folates & purine synthesis. S-phase specific.
Purine analogs	Cladribine Clofarabine Fludarabine Nelarabine Pentostatin	Incorporation of metabolites into DNA causing DNA strand breaks, decreased DNA synthesis & repair via inhibition of DNA polymerase & RNA reductase
Pyrimidine analogs	Capecitabine Fluorouracil	Metabolized to F-UMP & FdUMP to interfere w/ RNA & DNA synthesis. F-UMP is falsely incorporated into RNA to replace uracil, leading to inhibition of cell growth. FdUMP inhibits TS, depleting thymidine triphosphate, a necessary component of DNA synthesis
Thiopurines	Mercaptopurine Thioguanine	False metabolite incorporated into DNA/RNA, inhibiting their synthesis
Miscellaneous	Hydroxyurea	Inhibition of ribonucleoside diphosphate reductase, halting cell cycle at G1/S phase I

Devita, Hellman, and Rosenberg's Cancer: Principles & Practice of Oncology. 10th ed. 2014; *Cancer Chemotherapy and Biotherapy: Principles and Practice*. 5th ed. 2010.

Cytarabine (ara-C, Cytosar-U)

- **Dosing:** Can be administered IV, SC, or IT
- **Standard dose:** 100–200 mg/m^2/d 24-h continuous IV infusion × 5–7 d
- **High dose:** 1,000–3,000 mg/m^2 IV q12h × 3 d. No hepatic or renal dose adjustments recommended by PI
- **PK/PD:** Wide & rapid distribution, crosses BBB (conc. 40–50% plasma), hepatic metabolism, eliminated via deamination in liver, plasma, & peripheral tissue, $T_{1/2}$ 1–3 h
- **AEs: Myelosuppression** (DLT, BBW, nadir biphasic 7–9 d/15–24 d), N/V (low-to-mod. emetogenic potential depending on dose), diarrhea, mucositis, stomatitis, GI ulceration, hepatotoxicity, neurotoxicity (cerebellar dysfunction, reversible, high dose), rash, conjunctivitis (high dose)
- **DDIs:** Cyclophosphamide (case reports), MTX (↑ formation of ara-CTP), fludarabine (↑ formation of ara-CTP), gentamicin (potential ↓ efficacy of gentamicin), digoxin (↓ absorption of digoxin)
- **Clinical pearls:** Conjunctivitis prophylaxis w/ corticosteroid eyedrops w /high dose (start at least 6 h prior), monitor for s/s of neurotoxicity w/ high dose

Gemcitabine (Gemzar)

- **Dosing:** 800–1,250 mg/m^2 IV, cycles & d of administration vary based on indication. Adjustments: No renal or hepatic dose adjustments recommended
- **PK/PD:** Intracellular metabolism by nucleoside kinases, renal excretion (92–98%), $T_{1/2}$ of metabolite 1.7–19.4 h
- **AEs: Myelosuppression (DLT, ↑ w/ infusional),** edema, dyspnea, flu-like syndrome, ↑ LFTs, ↑ Tbili, infusion rxn, proteinuria, N/V (low emetogenic potential), pneumonitis (rare), TTP/HUS (rare)
- **DDI:** Cisplatin (↓ clearance of gemcitabine)
- **Clinical pearls:** Irritant, radiation sensitizer (caution w/ thoracic RT), can cause radiation recall

Azacytidine (5-Azacytidine, Vidaza, Onureg)

- **Dosing:** 75–100 mg/m²/d SC/IV × 7 d every 4 wks. Oral: 300 mg daily D1–14 of 28D cycle. Caution in pts w/ renal & hepatic dysfunction
- **PK/PD:** Does not cross BBB, hepatic metabolism via hydrolysis, bioavailability of SC ~89%, renal excretion (50–85%), ~0.5-4 h
- **AEs:** Myelosuppression, N/V (mod. emetogenic potential), injection site rxn (SQ), pyrexia, headache, ↑ LFTs, nephrotoxicity, rigors, arthralgia
- **DDI:** No significant drug interactions
- **Clinical pearls:** Unexplained reductions in serum bicarbonate levels <20 mEq/L, consider 50% dose adjustment

Decitabine (Dacogen)

- **Dosing:** 20 mg/m² daily × 5 d every 28 d
- **PK/PD:** Metabolism via deamination, $T_{1/2}$ ~30–35 min
- **AEs:** Myelosuppression (up to 90%, recovery 28–50 d), nausea (minimal), diarrhea, pyrexia, insomnia, fatigue, petechiae, hyperglycemia, hypokalemia, hypomagnesemia, ↑ Tbili
- **DDI:** No significant drug interactions

Methotrexate (MTX, Trexall)

- **Dosing:** Can be administered IV, PO, IT
- Dosing dependent on malignancy, range 30–40 mg/m²/wk to 100–12,000 mg/m² IV once. CrCl 10–50 mL/min: 50% of dose; CrCl <10 mL/min: avoid; HD: 50% of dose. Tbili 3.1–5 mg/dL or LFTs >3× ULN: 75% of dose; Tbili >5 mg/dL: avoid
- **PK/PD:** Extensive distribution into 3rd-space fluids (effusions, ascites, ↑ $T_{1/2}$), renal excretion (80–90% as unchanged drug)
- **AEs:** Myelosuppression, mucositis, N/V (mod. emetic potential w/ doses ≥250 mg/m²), photosensitivity, nephrotoxicity (intratubular precipitation, direct tubular toxin), ↑ LFTs, ↑ Tbili, neurotoxicity, pneumonitis
- **DDI:** Probenecid, PCNs, ASA, NSAIDs, PPIs, phenytoin, sulfonamides (↓ excretion of MTX), leucovorin (↓ MTX activity)
- **Clinical pearls:** Vigorous hydration & urinary alkalinization for high doses (↓ incidence of renal failure), doses >500 mg/m² require leucovorin rescue. Consider glucarpidase for MTX overdose or toxic plasma levels in pts w/ delayed clearance due to renal tox. Ensure no pleural effusions or ascites prior to IV dosing

Cladribine (Leustatin)

- **Dosing:** 0.09 mg/kg/d IV continuous infusion × 7 d. Doses can vary based on indication & route of administration. Renal: CrCl 10–50 mL/min: 75% of dose; CrCl <10 mL/min: 50% of dose; CAPD: 50% of dose. Caution in pts w/ hepatic dysfunction
- **PK/PD:** Penetrates CSF (conc. ~25% plasma); renal excretion, $T_{1/2}$ 5.4 h (adults), ~19.7 h (children)
- **AEs: Myelosuppression** (**BBW,** dose-dependent, prolonged), **neurotoxicity** (**BBW,** dose-related, doses above FDA labeling, including paraparesis & quadriparesis), **renal tox** (**BBW,** dose-related, doses above FDA labeling), headache, rash, dizziness, fever, fatigue, prolonged lymphopenia, infxn
- **DDI:** No major DDI

Clofarabine (Clolar)

- **Dosing: ALL (≤21 y):** 52 mg/m²/d IV × 5 d every 2–6 wks; **AML (induction):** 30 mg/m²/d × 5 d; **AML (consolidation):** 20 mg/m²/d × 5 d. CrCl 30–60 mL/min: Reduce dose by 50%, use w/ caution in hepatic impairment
- **PK/PD:** Intracellular metabolism to active metabolite; renal excretion; $T_{1/2}$ 7 h (adults). 5 h (children), ↑ in elderly/renal impairment
- **AEs: Myelosuppression (DLT),** N/V, diarrhea, **SIRS/capillary leak,** ↑ opportunistic infxns, renal tox, ↑ LFTs/Tbili (w/in 10 d, duration ≤15 d), cardiac tox
- **DDI:** Warfarin (↑/↓ warfarin effects), nephrotoxins (cumulative nephrotoxicity)
- **Clinical pearls:** Consider corticosteroid prophylaxis (hydrocortisone 100 mg/m² d 1–3 for prevention of capillary leak/SIRS)

Pemetrexed (Alimta)

- **Dosing:** 500 mg/m² d 1 every 21 d. Renal: CrCl <45 mL/min: Avoid **concomitant NSAID use.** CrCl 45–79 mL/min & NSAID w/ short $T_{1/2}$ (ibuprofen, indomethacin, ketoprofen, ketorolac): Avoid NSAID 2 d before, d of, & 2 d following tx. Any CrCl & NSAID w/ long $T_{1/2}$ (nabumetone, naproxen, oxaprozin, piroxicam): Avoid NSAID 5 d before, d of, & 2 d following tx
- **PK/PD:** Renal excretion, $T_{1/2}$ 3.5 h

- **AEs: Myelosuppression (DLT),** mucositis, **fatigue (DLT),** hand–foot syndrome, anorexia, GI tox, ↑ LFTs
- **DDI:** NSAIDs (↓ renal excretion)
- **Clinical pearls:** Folic acid 400–1,000 µg daily (initiate 7 d prior, continue during tx, & for 21 d after last dose) to reduce GI & heme tox, cyanocobalamin 1,000 µg IM (initiate 7 d prior to tx, then administer every 3 cycles) to prevent GI & heme tox. Dexamethasone 4 mg PO twice daily × 3 d (initiate 1 d prior to tx) to prevent cutaneous rxns

Pralatrexate (Folotyn)

- **Dosing:** 30 mg/m² IV weekly × 6 wks, 1 wk rest. Use caution in renal impairment. Tbili >1.5 mg/dL or AST/ALT >2.5 × ULN: Omitted in trials, use w/ caution. Grade 3 hepatotoxicity (on tx): Hold, ↓ to 20 mg/m²; grade 4 hepatotoxicity (on tx): D/C. Adjust dose for tox (hematologic, mucositis)
- **PK/PD:** 67% protein bound, renal excretion (35%), $T_{1/2}$ 12–18 h
- **AEs: Mucositis (DLT), myelosuppression (DLT),** ↑ LFTs, anorexia, fatigue, edema, rash, hypokalemia, nausea, cough, epistaxis, night sweats
- **DDI:** Probenecid, PCN, cephalosporins, aspirin, NSAIDs (↓ renal excretion)
- **Clinical pearls:** Folic acid 1–1.25 mg/d (initiate 10 d prior, continue during tx, & for 30 d after last dose) to reduce GI & heme tox & cyanocobalamin 1,000 µg IM (initiate w/in 10 wks prior to initial dose, then every 8–10 wks) to reduce GI & heme tox

Fludarabine (Fludara)

- **Dosing:** 20–30 mg/m² IV × 3–5 d every 28 d (dosing varies based on malignancy). CrCl 50–79 mL/min: ↓ dose to 20 mg/m² IV; CrCl 30–49 mL/min: ↓ dose to 15 mg/m² IV; CrCl <30 mL/min: avoid use. No hepatic dose adjustments recommended
- **PK/PD:** Intracellular metabolism to active metabolite; $T_{1/2}$ ~20 h (adults), 12.4–19 h (children), renal excretion (60%)
- **AEs: Myelosuppression (DLT, BBW,** nadir 10–14 d, recovery 5–7 wks), immunosuppression, N/V (low emetogenic potential), fever (60–69%), fatigue, diarrhea, weakness, cough (10–44%), PNA, infxn (33–44%), AIHA, autoimmune effects, **neurotoxicity (BBW;** rare; seen at high doses; agitation, coma, confusion, seizures)
- **DDI: Pentostatin (fatal pulmonary tox, BBW),** imatinib (↓ fludarabine effects), live vaccines (vaccinial infxn may occur)
- **Clinical pearls:** Recommend antiviral & antipneumocystis prophylaxis

Nelarabine (Arranon)

- **Dosing:** 1,500 mg/m²/dose IV d 1, 3, 5 every 21 d. Use caution in CrCl <50 mL/min (↓ ARA-G clearance). Closely monitor w/ mod.-to-sev. hepatic impairment (Tbili >3× ULN)
- **PK/PD:** Hepatic metabolism to ARA-G (active metabolite); $T_{1/2}$ (ARA-G): 2 h (adults), 3 h (children)
- **AEs:** Myelosuppression, **neurotoxicity (DLT, BBW,** somnolence, headache, seizures, fatigue, hypoesthesia, D/C if ≥grade 2), ↑ LFTs, ↑ Tbili, hyperkalemia, myalgia, arthralgia, cough, dyspnea, blurred vision
- **DDI:** Pentostatin (↓ conc. of nelarabine), live vaccines (vaccinial infxn may occur)

Pentostatin (Nipent)

- **Dosing:** 4 mg/m² IV every 2 wks. Use w/ caution in pts w/ CrCl <60 mL/min
- **PK/PD:** Renal excretion (~50–96%), $T_{1/2}$ ~6 h (↑ 18 h w/ CrCl <50 mL/min)
- **AEs:** Myelosuppression (nadir 7 d), **CNS tox, hepatotoxicity, nephrotoxicity (BBWs** occurred when used at higher than recommended doses), fever, fatigue, headache, rash, ↑ LFTs, myalgia, cough, infxn
- **DDI: Fludarabine (fatal pulmonary tox, BBW),** carmustine, etoposide, high-dose cyclophosphamide (fatal pulmonary edema & HoTN)

Trifluridine and tipiracil (Lonsurf)

- **Dosing:** 35 mg/m² (based on trifluridine component) PO BID on d 1–5 & d 8–12 of 28-d cycle, round dose to nearest 5 mg. Max per dose: 80 mg (trifluridine). CrCl >30 mL/min: No dose reduction; CrCl 15–29 mL/min: 20 mg/m² (based on trifluridine component)
- **PK/PD:** Eliminated via thymidine phosphorylase to form inactive metabolite. Trifluridine $T_{1/2}$ 2.1 h (at steady state); tipiracil $T_{1/2}$ 2.4 h (at steady state)
- **AEs:** Myelosuppression, fatigue, N/V (mod. emetogenic potential), decreased appetite, diarrhea, abdominal pain, weakness, fever
- **DDI:** No significant drug interactions
- **Clinical pearls:** Administered orally twice daily w/ in 1 h of morning/evening meals; available in 2 tablet strengths (trifluridine 15 mg/tipiracil 6.14 mg & trifluridine

20 mg/tipiracil 8.19 mg); dose is rounded to nearest 5 mg of trifluridine; blood counts should be checked prior to d 1 & d 15 of each cycle

Capecitabine (Xeloda)

- **Dosing:** 1,000–1,250 mg/m^2 PO twice daily × 2 wks every 21 d. Renal: CrCl 30–50 mL/min: 75% of dose; CrCl <30 mL/min: use contraindicated
- **PK/PD:** Oral prodrug of 5-FU, converted via 3-step activation process. Bioavailability ~80%, protein binding <60%, hepatic & tissue metabolism (active metabolite: 5-FU), renal excretion (96%), $T_{1/2}$ 0.5–1 h
- **AEs:** Diarrhea, hand–foot syndrome, myelosuppression, mucositis, neurologic tox, coronary vasospasm
- **DDI:** Inhibits CYP2C9 weakly, warfarin (BBW), oral anticoagulants (↑ levels of anticoagulants), phenytoin (↑ levels of phenytoin), leucovorin (↑ tox of capecitabine)
- **Clinical pearls:** Increased risk of fatal/sev. AEs w/ DPD deficiency. Available as 150-mg & 500-mg tablets, take w/in 30 min after a meal, radiation sensitizer, uridine triacetate used as antidote in cases of overdose, accidental ingestion, & possible DPD deficiency

Fluorouracil (5-FU, Adrucil)

- **Dosing:** Dose, schedule, & administration (IVB vs. IV continuous infusion) are based on malignancy. Common ranges, IVB: 400–600 mg/m^2/dose; IV continuous infusion 200–1,500 mg/m^2/d. No renal or hepatic dose adjustments recommended; use w/ caution
- **PK/PD:** Extensive tissue distribution; saturable catabolism; excretion via metabolism, lung, & urine; $T_{1/2}$ 8–20 min after IVB
- **AEs:** Dependent on dose & administration (IV bolus vs. IV continuous infusion), **diarrhea (DLT), mucositis (DLT),** N/V (low emetogenic potential), myelosuppression (bolus > continuous infusion), neurotoxicity, coronary artery vasospasm, conjunctivitis, hand–foot syndrome (continuous infusion > bolus), alopecia, nail changes
- **DDI:** CYP2C9 substrates (↓ substrate levels), cimetidine (↓ clearance of 5-FU), oral anticoagulants (↑ levels of anticoagulants), leucovorin (↑ tox of 5-FU)
- **Clinical pearls:** AEs w/ DPD deficiency (prolonged clearance, ↑ tox), radiosensitizer; leucovorin is given w/ bolus administration to ↑ intracellular half-life of 5-FU (↑ cytotoxicity). Uridine triacetate used as antidote in cases of overdose or DPD deficiency

Mercaptopurine (6-MP, Purinethol)

- **Dosing:** 1.5–2.5 mg/kg/d oral daily (duration dependent on malignancy). CrCl <50 mL/min: Every 48 h. No hepatic dose adjustments recommended
- **PK/PD:** Erratic PO absorption, poor CNS penetration, metabolized hepatically via **xanthine oxidase** & methylation via TPMT
- **AEs:** Myelosuppression, GI tox (N/V, anorexia, diarrhea, stomatitis), cholestatic jaundice, ↑ risk of infxn
- **DDI: Allopurinol, Febuxostat (↑ mercaptopurine tox, reduce dose by 50–75%),** azathioprine
- **Clinical pearls:** TPMT deficiency (may require up to 90% dose reduction)

Thioguanine (6-TG, Tabloid)

- **Dosing:** 60 mg/m^2/d × 14 d; 2 mg/kg/d orally. No renal dose adjustments recommended.
- **PK/PD:** Erratic PO absorption, hepatic metabolism via TPMT, $T_{1/2}$ 5–9 h
- **AEs:** Myelosuppression, GI tox (N/V, anorexia, diarrhea, stomatitis), cholestatic jaundice, ↑ risk of infxn, hyperuricemia, photosensitivity, 2° malignancy
- **DDI:** No significant drug interactions
- **Clinical pearls:** TPMT deficiency (may require up to 90% dose reduction)

Hydroxyurea (Droxia, Hydrea)

- **Dosing:** 20–30 mg/kg oral daily; titrate dosing for WBC & plt count. CrCl <60 mL/min: 50% of dose. No hepatic dose adjustments recommended
- **PK/PD:** Readily absorbed, widely distributed including CSF, 75–80% protein bound, metabolism via hepatic & GI tract, renal excretion, $T_{1/2}$ ~2–4 h
- **AEs: Myelosuppression (DLT, primarily granulocytopenia w/in 2–5 d),** GI ulceration (including mucositis), skin pigmentation, rash, squamous carcinoma (skin)
- **DDI:** Didanosine, stavudine (↑/↓ conc. of hydroxyurea, fatal pancreatitis), radiation (↑ tissue sensitivity to radiation)
- **Clinical pearls:** Consider BID–QID dosing for rapid WBC reduction

Info based on publicly available drug inserts from Allos, Bedford, Berlex, Bristol Myers—Squibb, Celgene, Centocor Ortho Biotech, Eisai, Genzyme, GlaxoSmithKline, Hoffman-LaRoche, Hospira, Lilly, & Teva.

ALKYLATING AGENTS

Drug Class	Agents	Mechanism
Alkyl sulfonates	Busulfan	Bifunctional agent, cytotoxicity via DNA alkylation & cross-linking
Aziridines	Thiotepa	Aziridinium analog of nitrogen mustard metabolite; bifunctional agent, cytotoxicity via DNA alkylation & cross-linking
Nitrogen mustards	Bendamustine, chlorambucil, cyclophosphamide, ifosfamide, mechlorethamine, melphalan	Bifunctional agent activated to yield 2 aziridinium ring moieties; cytotoxicity via DNA alkylation & cross-linking
Nitrosoureas	Carmustine (BCNU), lomustine (CCNU)	Bifunctional agent w/ reactive intermediates, cytotoxicity via DNA alkylation & cross-linking; inhibits nucleic acid synthesis enzymes
Platinum compounds	Carboplatin, cisplatin, oxaliplatin	Bifunctional agent w/ reactive intermediates; cytotoxicity via DNA platination & cross-linking
Triazenes/methylating agents	Dacarbazine, procarbazine, Temozolomide	Monofunctional agent activated to cause DNA methylation; do not cross-link; procarbazine also metabolized to free radical species
Marine-derived tetrahydroisoquinoline alkaloid	Trabectedin Lurbinectedin	Blocks the cell cycle at the G2/M phase by binding to the minor DNA groove, altering DNA transcription

Devita, Hellman, and Rosenberg's Cancer: Principles & Practice of Oncology. 10th ed. 2014; *Cancer Chemotherapy and Biotherapy: Principles and Practice*. 5th ed. 2010.

Busulfan (Busulfex [IV], Myleran [PO])

- **Dosing:** 1.8 mg/m^2/d PO (adjust for goal leukocyte counts ≥15,000/mm^3) OR 120 mg/m^2/d IV divided every 6–24 h over 3–4 d OR 0.8–1 mg/kg/dose IV every 6 h over 3–4 d; dose per IBW or ABW (lower value) or adjusted BW (obesity); adjust dose per PK & target AUC (~1,200 mM × min [900–1,500 mM × min])
- **PK/PD:** PO bioavailability ~80% (variable/age dependent), penetrates BBB, hepatic metabolism, $T_{1/2}$ 2.5 h
- **AEs: Myelosuppression (DLT),** hepatic VOD (↑ risk w/ AUC >1,500 μM × min), mucositis, seizure, pulm fibrosis (rare)
- **DDI:** Glutathione-depleting substrates (APAP, MNZ; ↑ busulfan conc.), azole antifungals (↑ busulfan conc.), phenytoin (↓ busulfan conc.)
- **Clinical pearls:** Administer w/ ppx anticonvulsant (levetiracetam, phenytoin). Monitor signs of hepatic VOD (wt gain, ascites, ↑ Tbili, hepatomegaly)

Thiotepa

- **Dosing:** 0.3–0.4 mg/kg IV every 1–4 wks OR 150–250 mg/m^2/dose IV divided 1–2 daily × 3 d before HSCT OR 60 mg instilled via intravesical administration weekly × 4 wks OR 10 mg IT 1–2 weekly or monthly. Consider dose reduction for renal or hepatic impairment or hematologic tox
- **PK/PD:** Hepatically metabolized via CYP2B6 & 2C11 to 1° metabolite TEPA; both thiotepa & TEPA therapeutically active & renally eliminated, $T_{1/2}$ 1.2–2 h; TEPA 3–21 h
- **AEs: Myelosuppression (nadir: 2–3 wks),** CNS dysfunction, amenorrhea, spermatogenesis inhibition, dermatitis, alopecia, 2° malignancies
- **DDI:** Potent CYP2B6 inhibitor
- **Clinical pearls:** Tight dressings & ointments should be avoided as thiotepa is excreted in sweat. Pt should shower often to reduce risk of skin irritation

Bendamustine (Bendeka, Treanda)

- **Dosing:** 70–120 mg/m²/d IV × 2 d every 21–35 d. Renal: CrCl <40 mL/min: Not recommended. Hepatic: Mild impairment: use w/ caution; AST or ALT ≥2.5 times ULN or Tbili ≥1.5 times ULN: not recommended. Tox ≥ grade 3: Reduce dose.
- **PK/PD:** 94–96% protein bound; hepatic metabolism via hydrolysis, CYP1A2; fecal excretion; $T_{1/2}$ = ~40 min; metabolites 30 min–3 h
- **AEs: Myelosuppression (DLT; nadir: ~3 wks),** N/V (mod. emetogenic risk), fever, ↑ bili, peripheral edema, rash, diarrhea, HSR
- **DDI:** CYP1A2 inhibitors (amiodarone, ciprofloxacin, fluvoxamine; ↑ bendamustine), CYP1A2 inducers (carbamazepine, phenytoin, phenobarbital, rifampin; ↓ bendamustine)
- **Clinical pearls:** Allopurinol may ↑ skin tox risk. Premedicate w/ prior HSR ≤ grade 2 (antihistamines, antipyretics, corticosteroids). Only Bendeka formulation can be infused over 10 min

Chlorambucil (Leukeran)

- **Dosing:** Induction 0.1–0.2 mg/kg/d PO × 3–6 wks, maintenance 2–4 mg/d PO OR 0.4 mg/kg PO intermittently, biweekly, or monthly. Consider dose reduction w/ renal impairment or hematologic tox. No hepatic dose adjustments recommended. Discontinue if generalized skin rash develops
- **PK/PD:** Rapid, complete absorption, highly protein bound (99%), hepatic metabolism to active compound & renal excretion, $T_{1/2}$ 1.5 h
- **AEs: Myelosuppression (nadir: 3 wks),** hepatotoxicity, skin rxns, pulm tox, CNS disturbances, 2° malignancies
- **DDI:** No significant drug interactions

Cyclophosphamide (Cytoxan, Neosar)

- **Dosing:** 1–5 mg/kg/d PO OR 75–100 mg/m²/d PO × 14 d every 4 wks OR 250–1,800 mg/m²/dose IV × 1–4 d every 3–4 wks OR 40–50 mg/kg IV divided over 2–5 d OR 50–60 mg/kg/d IV × 2–4 doses prior to HSCT. Consider dose adjustment w/ renal & hepatic impairments
- **PK/PD:** PO bioavailability >75%; prodrug hepatically activated via CYP2B6, 3A4, & 2C9 (metabolites reduce glutathione); renal excretion, $T_{1/2}$ 3–12 h
- **AEs: Myelosuppression (DLT; recovery: 7–10 d),** hemorrhagic cystitis, nephrotoxicity, SIADH, N/V (high [>1,500 mg/m²], mod. [≤1,500 mg/m² or PO] emetogenic risk), cardiotoxicity, alopecia, sterility, 2° malignancies
- **DDI:** CYP3A4 inducers (phenobarbital, phenytoin, carbamazepine; ↑ cyclophosphamide metabolism to active metabolites), CYP3A4 inhibitors (aprepitant, azole antifungals; ↓ cyclophosphamide metabolism)
- **Clinical pearls:** Properly hydrate pt pre/post-tx. Hemorrhagic cystitis due to accumulation of acrolein in the bladder, can be prevented w/ MESNA (cumulative dose 60–100% of cyclophosphamide dose)

Ifosfamide (Ifex)

- **Dosing:** 1,200–3,000 mg/m²/d IV × 3–5 d every 2–3 wks OR 5,000 mg/m² IV every 2 wks. Consider dose reduction w/ renal or hepatic impairment
- **PK/PD:** Prodrug hepatically activated via CYP3A4 & 2A6, renal excretion, $T_{1/2}$ 3–15 h
- **AEs: Myelosuppression (DLT; nadir 8–14 d),** hemorrhagic cystitis, nephrotoxicity (proximal tubular damage), SIADH, reversible neurotoxicity (somnolence, disorientation, lethargy), N/V (high [≥2 g/m²], mod. [<2 g/m²] emetogenic risk), alopecia
- **DDI:** CYP3A4 inducers/inhibitors (↑/↓ metabolism to active metabolites)
- **Clinical pearls:** Properly hydrate pt pre/post-tx. Hemorrhagic cystitis due to accumulation of acrolein in the bladder, can be prevented w/ MESNA (cum. dose 60–100% of ifosfamide dose). Neurotoxicity due to an accumulation of chloroacetaldehyde, can be treated w/ methylene blue or thiamine

Mechlorethamine (Mustargen)

- **Dosing:** 0.1–0.4 mg/kg/d IV × 1–4 d OR 6 mg/m² IV on d 1, 8 in a 28-d cycle. No renal or hepatic dose adjustments recommended
- **PK/PD:** Rapid spontaneous hydrolysis w/in plasma & limited hepatic metabolism, renal excretion, $T_{1/2}$ 15–20 min
- **AEs:** Myelosuppression, N/V (high emetogenic risk), anticholinergic effects (diaphoresis, lacrimation, diarrhea), encephalopathy (high-dose tx), gonadal atrophy, alopecia, 2° malignancies
- **DDI:** No significant drug interactions

- **Clinical pearls:** Causes irritation to skin/mucous membranes if contact occurs. Limited stability in solution & must be administered w/in 30 min of preparation. **Vesicant** (treat w/ sodium thiosulfate)

Melphalan (Alkeran, Evomela, Pepaxto)

- **Dosing:** 2–10 mg PO daily OR <0.05–0.15 mg/kg PO daily OR 0.2–0.25 mg/kg/d PO × 4–5 d every 4–6 wks OR 4–9 mg/m^2/d PO × 4–7 d every 4–6 wks OR 16 mg/m^2 IV every 2–4 wks OR 30 mg/m^2 IV × 1 dose (mini-BEAM) OR 140–200 mg/m^2 once 2–5 d prior to HSCT OR 100 mg/m^2/d × 2 doses prior to HSCT (Evomela only), 40 mg IV × 1 dose every 28 d (Pepaxto). Renal: Mod./sev. renal impairment: Reduce PO dose; BUN >30 mg/dL: reduce IV dose by up to 50% (Alkeran, Evomela). Consider reduction w/ cell count tox
- **PK/PD:** Variable bioavailability (25–90%) & protein binding (53–92%), spontaneous hydrolysis or alkylation in plasma or tissues, renal excretion (20–30%), $T_{1/2}$ 1–2 h
- **AEs: Delayed myelosuppression (nadir: 4 wks),** mucositis, esophagitis, diarrhea, pulm fibrosis (chronic use), 2° malignancies
- **DDI:** Carmustine (↑ risk of lung tox)
- **Clinical pearls:** Limited stability in solution & must be administered w/in an h of preparation when at room temperature. Improved bioavailability when taken on an empty stomach. Cryotherapy during infusion can ↓ mucositis. Do not substitute melphalan flufenamide (Pepaxto) for or w/ melphalan hydrochloride (Evomela, Alkeran). Melphalan flufenamide is the pro-drug of melphalan

Carmustine, BCNU (BiCNU, Gliadel [implantable wafer])

- **Dosing:** 150–200 mg/m^2 IV every 6–8 wks OR 75–100 mg/m^2/d IV × 2–3 d every 6–8 wks OR 300 mg/m^2 IV once (BEAM regimen) OR 600 mg/m^2 IV once (CBV regimen). Consider reduced dose for renal impairment & hematologic tox
- **PK/PD:** ~80% protein bound, penetrates BBB, hepatic metabolism, renal excretion, $T_{1/2}$ <30 min; active metabolite 67 h
- **AEs: Delayed myelosuppression (DLT; nadir: 4–6 wks),** N/V (high [>250 mg/m^2], mod. [≤250 mg/m^2] emetogenic risk), HoTN, ↑ LFTs. Cum. doses >1,500 mg/m^2—renal failure, pulm fibrosis
- **DDI:** Melphalan (sensitize pts to lung tox)
- **Clinical pearls:** Evaluate renal function when cum. doses >1,000 mg/m^2. Chronic marrow hypoplasia may result after repeated dosing. A/w 2° malignancies

Lomustine, CCNU (CeeNU)

- **Dosing:** 100–130 mg/m^2 PO every 6 wks. Consider dose reduction for renal impairment or prior cell count nadir
- **PK/PD:** Complete absorption, penetrates BBB, hepatic metabolism to active metabolites, renal excretion, $T_{1/2}$ active metabolite 16–48 h
- **AEs: Delayed myelosuppression (DLT; nadir: 4–6 wks),** N/V (mod. emetogenic risk), ↑ LFTs, 2° malignancies, cum. doses >1,500 mg/m^2 a/w renal failure, pulm fibrosis less frequent than w/ carmustine
- **DDI:** No significant drug interactions
- **Clinical pearls:** Evaluate renal function when cum. doses >1,000 mg/m^2. Chronic marrow hypoplasia may result after repeated dosing. Take w/o food to ↓ N/V

Carboplatin (Paraplatin)

- **Dosing:** 300–400 mg/m^2 IV every 4 wks. Often dosed per **Calvert formula:** Total dose = target AUC × (GFR + 25). Common target AUC 3–7.5 every 3–4 wks or AUC 2 for 3–5 d per mo. Renal (nonCalvert dosing): CrCl 41–59: 250 mg/m^2; CrCl 16–40: 200 mg/m^2. Thrombocytopenia/neutropenia: 75% of dose
- **PK/PD:** Renal excretion, $T_{1/2}$ ~2–6 h (platinum ≥5 d)
- **AEs: Delayed myelosuppression (DLT; nadir: ~3–4 wks),** HSR, nephrotoxicity, ototoxicity, peripheral neuropathy, N/V (mod. emetogenic risk), electrolyte imbalance, ↑ LFTs
- **DDI:** Sorafenib (↑ carboplatin tox), topotecan (↑ topotecan tox)
- **Clinical pearls:** Cap GFR at 125 mL/min in Calvert formula

Cisplatin (Platinol)

- **Dosing:** 20–100 mg/m^2/d IV × 1–5 d every 3–4 wks. SCr >1.5 mg/dL or BUN >25 mg/dL: Do not use. Consider dose reduction for renal impairment
- **PK/PD:** Highly protein bound (>90%), nonenzymatic metabolism, renal excretion (>90%), $T_{1/2}$ <1 h; protein-bound platinum 1–5 d

- **AEs:** Nephrotoxicity, **N/V acute/delayed 2–5 d post dose (DLT; high emetogenic risk),** peripheral neuropathy (cum. dose 300–600 mg/m^2; reversible), ototoxicity & hearing loss (cum. dose >400 mg/m^2; irreversible), electrolyte disturbance, Raynaud phenomenon, HSR, ↑ LFTs
- **DDI:** AG (↑ nephrotoxicity), loop diuretics (↑ nephrotoxicity & ototoxicity), phenytoin (↓ phenytoin conc.), topotecan (↑ topotecan tox), vinorelbine (granulocytopenia)
- **Clinical pearls:** Properly hydrate pt pre/post-tx. Mannitol can be used to ↑ UOP. Antiemetic Rx must cover delayed N/V period. Monitor renal function, electrolytes, & signs of hearing loss & neuropathy frequently. **Vesicant** (at conc. >0.4 mg/mL)

Oxaliplatin (Eloxatin)

- **Dosing:** 85–130 mg/m^2 IV every 2–3 wks. Renal: CrCl <30 mL/min: reduce dose to 65 mg/m^2. Reduce dose for prolonged neuropathy & grade 3–4 GI & cell count tox
- **PK/PD:** Highly protein bound (>90%), hydrolyzed to reactive metabolites, renal excretion, $T_{1/2}$ 391 h (platinum metabolites)
- **AEs: Neurotoxicity (DLT),** myelosuppression, pharyngolaryngeal dysesthesia, peripheral neuropathy, ↑ LFTs, ↑ SCr, fever
- **DDI:** No significant drug interactions
- **Clinical pearls:** Cold temperatures can worsen peripheral neuropathy

Dacarbazine (DTIC-Dome)

- **Dosing:** 250 mg/m^2/d IV × 4–5 d every 3 wks OR 375 mg/m^2/dose IV on d 1, 15 every 4 wks (ABVD regimen) OR 800–850 mg/m^2 IV every 3–4 wks. Consider dose adjustment w/ renal impairment
- **PK/PD:** Prodrug hepatically activated via CYP1A2, minimally bound to protein (~5%), renal excretion, $T_{1/2}$ 19 min; active metabolite 5 h
- **AEs: Myelosuppression (DLT; nadir: 21–25 d), N/V (DLT but can become tolerant; high emetogenic risk),** flu-like sx, injection-site pain, photosensitivity
- **DDI:** CYP1A2 inducers/inhibitors (↑/↓ conversion to active metabolites)

Procarbazine (Matulane)

- **Dosing:** 1–6 mg/kg/d PO OR 100 mg/m^2/d PO × 7 d every 21 d (BEACOPP regimen) OR 60–70 mg/m^2/d PO × 14 d every 6 wks. Consider dose reduction for hepatic impairment
- **PK/PD:** Rapid & complete absorption, prodrug hepatically activated, penetrates BBB, renal excretion of metabolites, $T_{1/2}$ 1 h
- **AEs: Delayed myelosuppression (DLT; nadir: 4 wks),** N/V (mod. emetogenic risk), paresthesias, somnolence, depression, agitation, azoospermia, ovarian failure, 2° malignancies
- **DDI:** Alpha/beta agonists (↑ BP), antidepressants, antipsychotics, carbamazepine, cyclobenzaprine, linezolid, methadone, & tramadol (serotonergic effect), hypoglycemic agents (hypoglycemic effect). Many medications interact w/ MAO inhibitors, review medication list before starting procarbazine
- **Clinical pearls:** As an MAO inhibitor, pts should avoid foods high in tyramine. EtOH should be avoided due to disulfiram rxn. Risk of hemolysis w/ G6PD deficiency

Temozolomide (Temodar)

- **Dosing:** 100–200 mg/m^2/d IV or PO × 5–7 d every 14–28 d OR 75 mg/m^2/d IV or PO × 6 wks. Consider dose reduction for renal impairment or nonhematologic tox ≥ grade 3
- **PK/PD:** Rapid & complete absorption, prodrug spontaneously hydrolyzed to active metabolite in plasma, penetrates BBB, renal excretion (~38%), $T_{1/2}$ ~2 h
- **AEs: Myelosuppression (DLT; nadir: 21 d),** N/V (mod. emetogenic risk), HA, fatigue, constipation, ↑ LFTs, peripheral edema, seizure, alopecia, muscle pain, vision changes
- **DDI:** Valproic acid (↓ clearance of temozolomide)
- **Clinical pearls:** PO form should be administered consistently on either an empty stomach or w/ food, as food will affect bioavailability. ↑ risk of PCP, consider ppx

Trabectedin (Yondelis)

- **Dosing:** Soft tissue sarcoma: 1.5 mg/m^2 CIV over 24 h; dose reductions for preexisting hepatic impairment. Prior to each tx cycle, ANC should be ≥1,500/mm^3; platelets ≥100,000/mm^3; Tbili ≤ULN; & Aϕ, ALT, AST, & CPK ≤2.5× ULN
- **PK/PD:** Hepatically metabolized by CYP3A4; $T_{1/2}$: ~175 h; excretion: feces (58%), urine (6%)
- **AEs:** Bone marrow suppression, cardiomyopathy, hepatotoxicity, hypersensitivity, rhabdomyolysis, thromboembolism

- **DDI:** Strong CYP3A4 inducers (avoid use, ↓ conc. of trabectedin), strong CYP3A4 & P-gp inhibitors (avoid use, ↑ conc. of trabectedin)
- **Clinical pearls:** Premedicate w/ dexamethasone 20 mg IV 30 min prior to starting. Trabectedin is a vesicant

Lurbinectedin (Zepzelca)

- **Dosing:** Small-cell lung cancer: 3.2 mg/m^2 IV once every 21 d; dose reductions for hepatotoxicity & heme toxicity during tx. Prior to each tx cycle, ANC should be ≥1,500/mm^3; platelets ≥100,000/mm^3
- **PK/PD:** Hepatically metabolized by CYP3A4; $T_{1/2}$ 51 h; excretion: feces (89%), urine (1%)
- **AEs:** Myelosuppression, hepatotoxicity, GI toxicity
- **DDI:** Strong CYP3A4 inducers (avoid use, ↓ conc. of lurbinectedin), strong CYP3A4 inhibitors (avoid use, ↑ conc. of lurbinectedin)
- **Clinical pearls:** Mod. emetic potential. Premedicate w/ dexamethasone & 5HT3 antagonist prior to eachtx

Info based on publicly available drug inserts from ESP Pharma, Inc.; GlaxoSmithKline LLC; Bedford Laboratories; Cephalon, Inc.; Baxter Healthcare Corporation; Lundbeck LLC; Apo-Pharma USA, Inc.; E.R. Squibb & Sons, L.L.C.; Teva Parenteral Medicines, Inc.; Sanofi-Aventis U.S. LLC; Sigma-Tau Pharmaceuticals, Inc.; Merck Sharp & Dohme Corp; Spectrum Pharmaceuticals, Inc.; Jazz Pharmaceutical, Inc.; Oncopeptides AB (publ); & Janssen & Sanofi-Aventis.

ANTIMICROTUBULAR AGENTS

Drug Classification	Agents	Mechanism
Epothilone B analog Macrolides isolated from mycobacteria	Ixabepilone	Induces mitotic arrest at G2/M phase by binding to β-tubulin subunit
Halichondrin B analog Isolated from marine sponge *Halichondria okadai*	Eribulin	Inhibits microtubule growth phase, leading to G2/M cell-cycle block
Taxanes Isolated from the bark of the pacific yew tree, produced by fungal endophyte *Taxomyces andreanae*	Cabazitaxel Docetaxel Paclitaxel Albumin-bound paclitaxel	Stabilize microtubules & inhibit disassembly by binding to the β subunit of tubulin & inducing cycle arrest. Cell cycle specific, late G2 mitotic phase
Vinca alkaloids Isolated from periwinkle plant (*Vinca rosea*)	Vinblastine Vincristine Vinorelbine	Inhibit microtubule formation & disrupt the formation of the mitotic spindle, arresting the cell at M/S phases

Devita, Hellman, and Rosenberg's Cancer: Principles & Practice of Oncology. 10th ed. 2014. Info based on publicly available drug inserts from Sanofi-Aventis, Bristol-Myers Squibb, Celgene, Bedford Laboratories, Teva Pharmaceuticals, GlaxoSmithKline, Eisai Inc.

Ixabepilone (Ixempra)

- **Dosing:** 40 mg/m^2 IV over 3 h every 3 wks, BSA capped at 2.2 m^2. No renal dose adjustments recommended. AST or ALT >10× ULN or Tbili >3× ULN: Avoid use. Adjust dose for tox (neutropenia, neuropathy).
- **PK/PD:** Hepatic metabolism via CYP3A4 to inactive metabolites
- **AEs:** Leukopenia, fatigue, alopecia, mucositis, myalgia, peripheral neuropathy, N/V (low emetogenic potential)
- **DDI:** CYP3A4 inducers/inhibitors (↓/↑ conc. of ixabepilone)
- **Clinical pearls:** Can overcome resistance to taxanes & vinca alkaloids. Contains Cremophor, a/w HSRs—premedicate w/ H1RA & H2RA

Eribulin (Halaven)

- **Dosing:** 1.4 mg/m^2 IV over 2–5 min on d 1, 8 of 21-d cycle. Renal—CrCl 30–50 mL/min: 1.1 mg/m^2. Hepatic—mild: 1.1 mg/m^2; mod.: 0.7 mg/m^2. Adjust dose for tox (neutropenia, thrombocytopenia)
- **PK/PD:** $T_{1/2}$ ~ 40 h
- **AEs:** Fatigue, neutropenia (nadir 13 d), alopecia, peripheral neuropathy, QTc changes, N/V (low emetogenic potential)
- **DDI:** No significant drug interactions
- **Clinical pearls:** Discontinue if tox occurs at 0.7-mg/m^2 dose

Cabazitaxel (Jevtana)

- **Dosing:** 25 mg/m^2 IV over 1 h every 3 wks. CrCl <30 mL/min: Use w/ caution. Hepatic—mild: 20 mg/m^2; mod.: 15 mg/m^2. Adjust dose for tox (myelosuppression, GI, & neuropathy)
- **PK/PD:** CNS distribution > other taxanes, hepatic metabolism via CYP3A4/5, $T_{1/2}$ 95 h
- **AEs: Myelosuppression (DLT, nadir 12 d),** GI, neuropathy, dyspnea, arthralgia, fatigue, N/V (low emetogenic potential)
- **DDI:** CYP3A4 inducers/inhibitors (↓/↑ conc. of cabazitaxel)
- **Clinical pearls:** Contains polysorbate 80, a/w HSRs—premedicate w/ corticosteroids, H1RA, & H2RA prior to administration. Administered w/ continuous prednisone throughout tx

Docetaxel (Taxotere)

- **Dosing:** 60–100 mg/m^2 IV over 1 h every 3 wks. No renal dose adjustments recommended. Hepatic dose adjustments recommended based on indication. Adjust dose for tox (neutropenia & GI)
- **PK/PD:** Extravascular distribution & tissue binding, metabolism via CYP3A4, $T_{1/2}$ 11 h
- **AEs: Myelosuppression (DLT, nadir 7 d),** edema (dose-dependent), cutaneous rxns, nail changes, alopecia, neuropathy, GI, N/V (low emetogenic potential)

- **DDI:** CYP3A4 inducers/inhibitors (↓/↑ conc. of docetaxel)
- **Clinical pearls:** Administer corticosteroids × 3 d starting **1** d prior to ↓ fluid retention, reduce severity of HSRs. **Irritant w/ vesicant potential** (elevate extremity & cold compresses)

Paclitaxel (Taxol)

- **Dosing:** 60–250 mg/m^2 IV over **1**–24 h weekly or every 3 wks. No renal dose adjustments recommended. Hepatic dose adjustments according to infusion times. Adjust dose for tox (sev. peripheral neuropathy or neutropenia: reduce by 20%)
- **PK/PD:** Distributed into body fluids & tissues, hepatic metabolism via CYP2C8 & CYP3A4, $T_{1/2}$ (3-h infusion): 13–20 h
- **AEs: Myelosuppression (DLT, nadir 11 d),** alopecia, neuropathy, myalgia, GI, N/V (low emetogenic potential)
- **DDI:** CYP2C8, CYP3A4 inducers/inhibitors (↓/↑ conc. of paclitaxel)
- **Clinical pearls:** Contains Cremophor, a/w HSRs—premedicate w/ corticosteroids, H1RA, & H2RA prior to administration. Peripheral neuropathy ↑ w/ shorter infusion, myelosuppression ↑ w/ longer infusion. **Irritant w/ vesicant potential** (elevate extremity & cold compresses)

Albumin-Bound Paclitaxel (Abraxane)

- **Dosing:** 260 mg/m^2 IV over 30 min every 3 wks *or* 100–125 mg/m^2 on d **1**, 8, 15 of 21–28 d cycle based on indication. No renal dose adjustments recommended. Hepatic dose adjustments based on AST/Tbili & indication. Adjust dose for tox (neutropenia, thrombocytopenia, neuropathy).
- **PK/PD:** Extravascular distribution & tissue binding, hepatic metabolism via CYP2C8 & CYP3A4, $T_{1/2}$ 27 h
- **AEs: Myelosuppression (DLT),** abnl ECG, alopecia, myalgia, neuropathy, N/V (low emetogenic potential)
- **DDI:** CYP2C8 inducers (rifampin)/inhibitors (gemfibrozil), CYP3A4 inducers/inhibitors (↓/↑ conc. of albumin-bound paclitaxel)
- **Clinical pearls:** ↓ HSR due to solvent-free formulation, routine premedications not required

Vinblastine (Velban)

- **Dosing:** 3–6 mg/m^2 IV every 7 d, varies depending on indication. No renal dose adjustments recommended. Tbili >3 mg/dL: 50% of dose
- **PK/PD:** Binds extensively to tissues (liver), does not penetrate CNS, hepatic metabolism via CYP3A4, $T_{1/2}$ 25 h
- **AEs: Myelosuppression (DLT, nadir 5–10 d),** constipation, alopecia, HTN, bone/jaw pain, neuropathy, N/V (min. emetogenic potential)
- **DDI:** CYP3A4 inducers/inhibitors (↓/↑ conc. of vinblastine)
- **Clinical pearls:** Implement bowel regimen pre/post dose. Fatal if given intrathecally. **Vesicant** (elevate extremity & warm compresses)

Vincristine (Oncovin)

- **Dosing:** 0.4–1.4 mg/m^2 IV (may cap dose at 2 mg) every 7 d, varies depending on indication. No renal dose adjustments recommended. Tbili >3 mg/dL: 50% of dose
- **PK/PD:** Poor CNS penetration, hepatic metabolism via CYP3A4, $T_{1/2}$ 85 h
- **AEs:** Peripheral neuropathy**,** constipation, alopecia, N/V (min. emetogenic potential)
- **DDI:** CYP3A4 inducers/inhibitors (↓/↑ conc. of vincristine)
- **Clinical pearls:** Implement bowel regimen pre/post dose. Fatal if given intrathecally. **Vesicant** (elevate extremity & warm compresses). NOT interchangeable w/ liposomal vincristine (Marqibo)

Vinorelbine (Navelbine)

- **Dosing:** 25–30 mg/m^2 IV every 7 d. No renal dose adjustments recommended. Tbili 2.1–3 mg/dL: 50% of dose; Tbili >3 mg/dL: 25% of dose. Adjust dose for toxicities (neutropenia, neurotoxicity).
- **PK/PD:** Binds to plts & lymphocytes, hepatic metabolism via CYP3A4 to active metabolite, $T_{1/2}$ 28–44 h
- **AEs: Myelosuppression (DLT, nadir 7–10 d),** GI, neuropathy, alopecia, N/V (min. emetogenic potential)
- **DDI:** CYP3A4 inducers/inhibitors (↓/↑ conc. of vinorelbine)
- **Clinical pearls:** Fatal if given intrathecally. **Vesicant** (elevate extremity & warm compresses)

ANTITUMOR ANTIBIOTICS

Drug Class	Agents	Mechanism
Anthracyclines/ Anthracenedione	Daunorubicin, doxorubicin, epirubicin, idarubicin/mitoxantrone	Inhibits topo II by intercalating DNA → DNA breaks & gen. of free radicals
Actinomycins	Dactinomycin	Intercalates into DNA between guanine–cytosine bases → inhibit topo II → DNA breaks
Others	Bleomycin, mitomycin	Gen. of oxygen-free radicals causing DNA breaks (G2 & M phase), intercalates into DNA → DNA breaks (nonspecific)

Devita, Hellman, and Rosenberg's Cancer: Principles & Practice of Oncology. 10th ed. 2014.

Daunorubicin (Cerubidine)

- **Dosing:** 30–90 mg/m^2/dose × 3 d. Max lifetime cumulative dose = 550 mg/m^2. Tbili 1.2–3 mg/dL: ↓ dose by 25%, SCr or Tbili >3 mg/dL: ↓ dose by 50%.
- **PK/PD:** Extensive extravascular distribution (including placenta) but no BBB penetration, hepatically metabolized to active metabolite via cytoplasmic reductases, substantial renal excretion, $T_{1/2}$ parent drug 14–20 h; metabolites 24–48 h
- **AEs: Myelosuppression (DLT, nadir 10–14 d),** mucositis, cardiac tox, N/V (mod. emetogenic potential), alopecia, transient LFT ↑, red/orange urine, "radiation recall," 2° malignancy
- **DDI:** P-gp inhibitors, taxanes, trastuzumab, & bevacizumab (↑ cardiotoxicity)
- **Clinical pearls:** Dexrazoxane (cardiac protection) w/ cumulative dose >435 mg/m^2—10:1 ratio for dose. ECHO or MUGA prior to Rx. Liposomal daunorubicin+cytarabine (CPX-351) should not be interchanged w/ conventional daunorubicin
- **Vesicant** (DMSO topical solution/dexrazoxane, elevate extremity, & cold compresses)

Doxorubicin (Adriamycin)/Liposomal doxorubicin (Doxil)

- **Dosing:** 20 mg/m^2 weekly or 40–60 mg/m^2 every 3 wks. Max lifetime cumulative dose = 550 mg/m^2 or < if >65 y, HTN, heart dz, mediastinal radiation or cyclophosphamide. Tbili 1.2–3 mg/dL: ↓ dose by 50%, Tbili 3.1–5 mg/dL: ↓ dose by 75%, & Tbili > 5 mg/dL: HOLD.
- **PK/PD:** Extensive extravascular distribution but no BBB penetration, hepatically metabolized to active metabolite, min. renal excretion; $T_{1/2}$ parent drug 1–3 h, metabolites 3–3.5 h
- **AEs: Myelosuppression (DLT, nadir 10–14 d),** mucositis, N/V (>60 mg/m^2/dose = high, ≤60 mg/m^2/dose = mod. emetogenic potential), cardiotoxicity, transient ↑ in LFTs, red/orange urine, alopecia, "radiation recall," 2° malignancy
- **DDI:** P-gp inhibitors, CYP3A4 inhibitors, taxanes, trastuzumab, & bevacizumab (↑ cardiotoxicity). Contraindicated w/ conivaptan
- **Clinical pearls:** Liposomal doxorubicin ↓ N/V & cardiac tox compared to doxorubicin, has mild myelosuppression but also has hand–foot syndrome & acute infusion rxn. Liposomal daunorubicin/cytarabine is NOT interchangable. Dexrazoxane (cardiac protection) w/ cumulative dose >300 mg/m^2—10:1 ratio for dose. ECHO or MUGA prior to Rx. **Vesicant** (DMSO topical solution or dexrazoxane, elevate extremity, & cold compresses)

Epirubicin (Ellence)

- **Dosing:** 100–120 mg/m^2 every 3–4 wks or 60 mg/m^2 d 1, 8 every 28 d. Max lifetime cumulative dose = 900 mg/m^2. SCr > 5 mg/dL: ↓ dose, no adjustments suggested. Tbili 1.2–3 mg/dL or AST 2–4× ULN: ↓ dose by 50%; Tbili >3 mg/dL or AST >4× ULN: ↓ dose by 75%.
- **PK/PD:** Extensive hepatic metabolism, renal/fecal excretion, $T_{1/2}$ = 33 h
- **AEs: Myelosuppression (DLT, nadir 10–14 d),** alopecia, hot sweats, diarrhea, N/V (>90 mg/m^2 = high emetogenic potential, ≤90 mg/m^2 = mod.), cardiotoxicity
- **DDI:** Taxanes, trastuzumab, & bevacizumab (↑ cardiotoxicity)
- **Clinical pearls:** Dexrazoxane (cardiac protection) w/ cumulative dose >540 mg/m^2—10:1 ratio for dose. ECHO or MUGA prior to Rx. **Vesicant** (DMSO topical solution/dexrazoxane, elevate extremity, & cold compresses)

Idarubicin (Idamycin PFS)

- **Dosing:** 12 mg/m^2/d × 3 d. Max lifetime cumulative dose = 180–225 mg/m^2. Tbili 2.6–5 mg/dL: ↓ dose by 50%, Tbili >5 mg/dL: HOLD. Dose reduction advised w/ renal impairment: no specific adjustments suggested
- **PK/PD:** Extensive tissue binding including CSF, hepatic metabolism to active metabolite, hepatic/renal excretion, $T_{1/2}$ 12–27 h
- **AEs: Myelosuppression (DLT, nadir 10–14 d),** mucositis, N/V (mod. emetogenic potential), cardiotoxicity, transient LFT ↑, red/orange urine, alopecia, radiation recall
- **DDI:** Taxanes, trastuzumab, & bevacizumab (↑ cardiotoxicity)
- **Clinical pearls:** Dexrazoxane (cardiac protection) w/ cumulative dose >110 mg/m^2—10:1 ratio for dose. ECHO or MUGA prior to Rx. **Vesicant** (DMSO topical solution/ dexrazoxane, elevate extremity, & cold compresses)

Dactinomycin (Cosmegen)

- **Dosing:** 12–15 μg/kg/d or 400–600 μg/m^2/d × 5 d. No renal or hepatic dose adjustments (may consider dose reduction in pt w/ hyperbilirubinemia)
- **PK/PD:** Extensive extravascular distribution but no BBB penetration, min. metabolism, renal excretion (30%), $T_{1/2}$ 36 h
- **AEs:** Myelosuppression (nadir 14–21 d), VOD, N/V (mod. emetogenic potential), alopecia, erythema, radiation recall
- **DDI:** Immunosuppressants (↑ immunosuppressant effects)
- **Clinical pearls:** The risk of fatal hepatic SOS is ↑ in children <4 y of age. **Vesicant** (elevate extremity & cold compresses)

Bleomycin (Blenoxane)

- **Dosing:** 5–15 units/m^2 weekly × 3 wks. CrCl <50 mL/min: Dose reductions required
- **PK/PD:** Poor oral bioavailability, SQ absorption similar to IV, intracavitary route is possible, no BBB penetration, renal excretion (60–70%), $T_{1/2}$ 3 h
- **AEs: Pulm tox/pneumonitis (DLT, 10%),** HSR (after dose 1–2), mucositis, cutaneous rxns (hyperpigmentation, erythema, skin peeling), HoTN
- **DDI:** Oxygen (↑ pulm tox), nephrotoxic drugs (↓ clearance)
- **Clinical pearls:** Risk of bleomycin-induced pneumonitis ↑ w/ cumulative dose >400 units, >70 y, underlying lung dz, prior irradiation to chest, high oxygen exposure–conc., ↑ use of G-CSF

Mitomycin (Mutamycin)

- **Dosing:** 10–15 mg/m^2 IV every 6–8 wks or 20–40 mg weekly intravesicular instillation. SCr >1.7 mg/dL: Avoid use
- **PK/PD:** Hepatic metabolism & renal excretion (10% unchanged), $T_{1/2}$ 17–78 min
- **AEs: Myelosuppression (DLT, nadir 4–6 wks),** TTP/HUS, fever, interstitial pneumonitis, N/V (low emetogenic potential), mucositis
- **DDI:** Tamoxifen (HUS), vinblastine (pulm edema)
- **Clinical pearls: Vesicant** (DMSO topical solution, elevate extremity, & cold compresses). Hematologic recovery ~8–10 wks

Mitoxantrone (Novantrone)

- **Dosing:** 12 mg/m^2/d × 3 d, 12–14 mg/m^2 every 3 wks
- **PK/PD:** Poor oral bioavailability, distributes extensively into tissues & RBCs, renal/fecal excretion, $T_{1/2}$ = 23–215 h (↑ w/ hepatic impairment)
- **AEs: Myelosuppression (DLT, nadir 10–14 d),** N/V (low emetogenic potential), alopecia, mucositis (<doxo), blue/green tears/urine, HA, dizziness, 2° malignancy
- **DDI:** Weak CYP3A4 inhibitor, ↑ effect of immunosuppressants
- **Clinical pearls:** Cardiotoxic risk ↑ w/ cumulative doses >140 mg/m^2. ECHO or MUGA prior to Rx. **Irritant w/ vesicant potential** (DMSO topical solution, elevate extremity & cold compresses)

Info based on publicly available drug inserts from Accord Healthcare, Bedford Laboratories, Pharmacia & Upjohn Company, Hospira, Janssen, Pfizer, Lundbeck, & Bristol-Myers Squibb.

TOPOISOMERASE INHIBITORS

Drug Class	Agents	Mechanism
Topoisomerase I inhibitors	Irinotecan (CPT-11), liposomal irinotecan, topotecan	Inhibition causes cleavable DNA complex stabilization & prevents religation of cleaved strand as well as causing single-strand DNA breaks (S phase specific)
Topoisomerase II inhibitors	Etoposide (VP-16), etoposide phosphate, teniposide, anthracyclines (see *Antitumor Antibiotics Chap.*)	Inhibition of enzyme w/c cuts both strands of the DNA helix simultaneously in order to manage DNA tangles & supercoils causing accumulation of cleaved DNA strand breaks

Devita, Hellman, and Rosenberg's Cancer: Principles & Practice of Oncology. 10th ed. 2014. *Cancer Chemotherapy and Biotherapy: Principles and Practice*. 5th ed. 2010.

Irinotecan, CPT-11 (Camptosar)

- **Dosing:** 125 mg/m^2 × 4 wks w/ 2 wks rest. Homozygous for UGT1A1*28 allele & hepatic impairment (Tbili > ULN): ↓ dose, no specific adjustments suggested
- **PK/PD:** Extensive extravascular distribution, active drug (SN-38) hepatically glucuronidated via UGT1A1, renal excretion (25%), remainder eliminated via hepatic metabolism & biliary excretion, $T_{1/2}$ 6–12 h (irinotecan), 10–20 h (SN-38)
- **AEs: Diarrhea (DLT, early & delayed),** myelosuppression (neutropenia), abdominal pain, N/V (mod. emetogenic potential), alopecia, fatigue, ↑ LFTs & Tbili, pulmonary tox (uncommon)
- **DDI:** CYP3A4 inducers/inhibitors (↓/↑ conc. of irinotecan)
- **Clinical pearls:** Diarrhea <24 h: Acute cholinergic effect produced by inhibition of acetylcholinesterase by prodrug, treat w/ atropine. Diarrhea >24 h: Mucosal cytotoxicity, treat w/ loperamide &/or octreotide. Liposomal irinotecan (Onivyde) for tx of metastatic pancreatic CA in combination w/ 5-FU refractory to gemcitabine

Topotecan (Hycamtin)

- **Dosing:** 0.75–1.5 mg/m^2 daily × 5 d w/ 2 wks rest or 2.3 mg/m^2/d PO × 5 d w/ 2 wks rest. Renal (IV): CrCl 20–39 mL/min: ↓ dose to 0.75 mg/m^2/dose; (PO): CrCl 30–49 mL/min: ↓ dose to 1.5 mg/m^2/dose; CrCl <30 mL/min: ↓ dose to 0.6 mg/m^2/dose
- **PK/PD:** Rapid oral absorption w/ 40% bioavailability, widely distributed w/ significant CSF penetration (CSF conc. ~30% of plasma), metabolism via rapid plasma hydrolysis to inactive metabolite, renal excretion, $T_{1/2}$ (IV) 2 – 3CS h, (PO) 3–6 h
- **AEs: Myelosuppression, predominately neutropenia (DLT/BBW, nadir 9–14 d),** N/V (low emetogenic potential), diarrhea, fatigue, alopecia, skin rash, transient ↑ LFTs, stomatitis, interstitial lung disease
- **DDI:** P-gp inhibitors ↑ conc. of topotecan
- **Clinical pearls:** Do NOT administer w/ neutrophils <1,500/mm^3 & plts <100,000/mm^3. Myelosuppression ↑ w/ extensive prior radiation or previous bone-marrow suppressive chemotherapy. Risk of thrombocytopenia ↑ w/ extensive prior carboplatin tx

Etoposide, VP-16 (Toposar, VePesid)

- **Dosing:** 50–120 mg/m^2/d IV × 3 d every 3–4 wks. Oral dosing 2:1 of IV dose (round to nearest 50-mg capsule). Tbili 1.5–3 mg/dL or AST >3× ULN: 50% of dose. CrCl <50 mL/min: 75% of dose
- **PK/PD:** Oral bioavailability 50%, poor BBB penetration, hepatically metabolized via CYP3A4/5, renal excretion (56%), $T_{1/2}$ 4–11 h
- **AEs: Myelosuppression, predominately neutropenia (DLT/BBW, nadir 7–14 d),** N/V (low-to-mod. emetogenic potential), HoTN during infusion, alopecia, HRS, fever, 2° malignancy
- **DDI:** CYP3A4 inducers/inhibitors (↓/↑ conc. of etoposide). P-gp inhibitors (↑ conc. of etoposide)
- **Clinical pearls:** Etoposide phosphate is water soluble & does not contain polyethylene glycol, polysorbate 80, or ethanol & can be given over 5 min w/o HoTN. Risk of 2° malignancy (AML via 11q23 translocation) usually occurs 2–3 y after administration of etoposide. Slow infusion to ↓ risk of HoTN

Teniposide, VM-26 (Vumon)

- **Dosing:** 165 mg/m^2/dose d 1, 4, 8, 11 of alternating consolidation cycles. No renal or hepatic dose adjustments recommended. Down syndrome (50% of dose)
- **PK/PD:** Good tissue distribution, limited BBB penetration, highly protein bound (99.4%), extensive hepatic metabolism via CYP3A4, renal excretion (44%), $T_{1/2}$ 5 h
- **AEs: Myelosuppression (DLT/BBW, nadir 7–10 d),** mucositis, diarrhea, N/V (mild-to-mod. emetogenic potential), HoTN during infusion, alopecia, rash, HSR
- **DDI:** CYP3A4 inducers/inhibitors (↓/↑ conc. of teniposide). P-gp inhibitors (↑ conc. of teniposide)
- **Clinical pearls:** Risk of 2° malignancies > etoposide. HRS including anaphylaxis-like rxns have been reported & have been linked to Cremophor in vials

Info based on publicly available drug inserts from Pfizer, GlaxoSmithKline, Bristol-Myers Squibb, & Merrimack Pharmaceuticals.

Figure 9-1 Cell cycle–specific drugs.

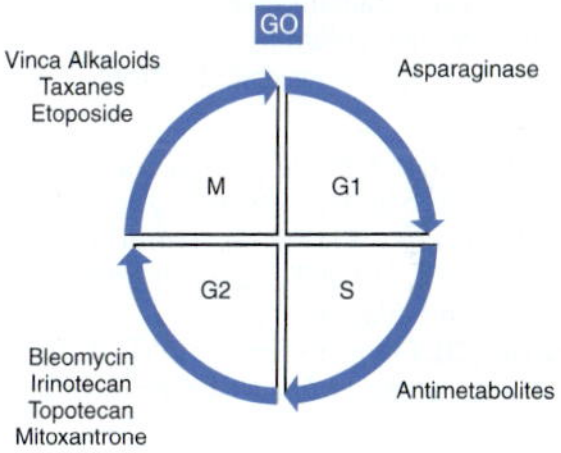

Figure 9-2 Mechanism of antimetabolites.

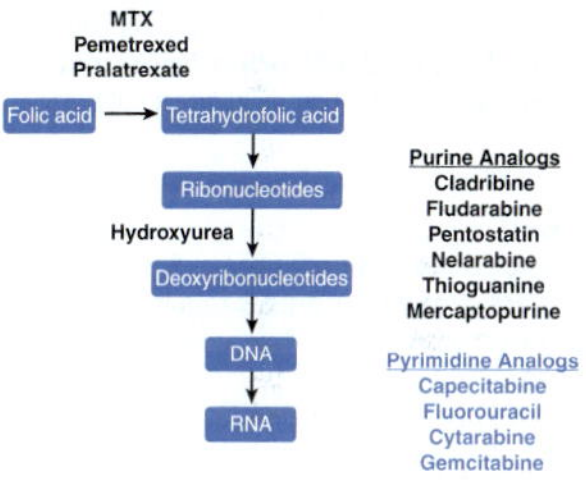

Drug Classification	
Immunomodulating agents/ immunotherapy	Decitabine and cedazuridine, interferon alpha-2b, interleukin-2, lenalidomide, pomalidomide, tazemetostat, thalidomide

Decitabine and cedazuridine (Inqovi)

- **Mechanism:** Decitabine (see antimetabolite chapter). Cedazuridine is a cytidine deaminase (CDA) inhibitor that prevents degradation of oral decitabine
- **Dosing:** Decitabine 35 mg/cedazuridine 100 mg for 5 d per 28-d cycle; delay next cycle if toxicity develops during tx (SCr ≥2 mg/dL; serum bilirubin ≥2× ULN; AST/ALT ≥ 2× ULN)
- **PK/PD:** Decitabine metabolized by CDA, cedazuridine converted to epimer by physiochemical degradation; $T_{1/2}$ 1.5 h (decitabine); $T_{1/2}$ 6.7 h (cedazuridine), excreted in urine & feces
- **AEs:** Anemia, neutropenia, thrombocytopenia, myalgia, arthralgia, mouth sores, nausea/vomiting, diarrhea, edema, rash, ↑ transaminases
- **DDI:** No known pathways of metabolism
- **Clinical pearls:** Take on an empty stomach (2 h before or after a meal)

Interferon alfa-2b (Intron A)

- **Mechanism:** ↑ activity of cellular & innate immune responses
- **Dosing:** 2–30 million units/m^2 typically 3× weekly, given IM/SQ/IV, dose adjustments for tox (hematologic, HSR, neuropsychiatric) & according to indication
- **PK/PD:** Bioavailability IM 83%, SQ 90%; does not penetrate CSF; primarily renal metabolism; $T_{1/2}$: IV ~2 h, IM/SQ ~2–3 h
- **AEs: Neuropsychiatric (DLT),** neutropenia, ↑ AST/ALT
- **DDI:** Inhibits CYP1A2 (weak), theophylline (↓ theophylline clearance), ribavirin (risk of worsening mental depression)

Interleukin-2 (Aldesleukin, Proleukin)

- **Mechanism:** ↑ lymphocyte mitogenesis & cytotoxicity
- **Dosing:** 600,000 units/kg IV every 8 h, repeat after 9 d (total 28 doses/course), SCr <1.5 mg/dL before starting Rx, hold for signs of hepatic failure, dose adjustments for tox (CV dz, CNS, dermatologic, GI, infxn, respiratory)
- **PK/PD:** Renally metabolized, $T_{1/2}$ IV initial ~10 min, renally excreted
- **AEs: Capillary leak syndrome (BBW, onset immediately after tx initiation), CNS tox (BBW), infxn (BBW),** GI bleeding/intestinal perforation, ↑ Tbili, renal insufficiency
- **DDI:** Live vaccines, steroids (counteract immunostimulant effects)

Lenalidomide (Revlimid)

- **Mechanism:** Immunomodulatory, antiangiogenic, & antineoplastic characteristics
- **Dosing:** 10–25 mg PO daily, renal adjustments required for CrCl <60mL/min, no hepatic dose adjustments recommended, dose adjustments for tox (thrombocytopenia, neutropenia, dermatologic)
- **PK/PD:** Rapid absorption, protein binding ~30%, $T_{1/2}$ 3–5 h (3-fold ↑ in mod.-to-sev. renal impairment), renally excreted, HD removes ~40% of a dose in a single session
- **AEs: BM suppression (BBW), thromboembolic events (BBW),** peripheral edema, peripheral neuropathy, GI upset, rash
- **DDI:** Digoxin (↑ digoxin conc. ~14%)
- **Clinical pearls: Must be registered w/ REMS program (RevAssist),** consider anticoagulation ppx when used w/ dexamethasone after assessment of RFs

Pomalidomide (Pomalyst)

- **Mechanism:** Displays immunomodulatory & antineoplastic characteristics
- **Dosing:** 4 mg PO daily, avoid if SCr >3 mg/dL or Tbili >2 mg/dL & AST/ALT >3× ULN. Adjust dose for tox (neutropenia, thrombocytopenia)
- **PK/PD:** Hepatically metabolized, $T_{1/2}$ ~8 h, excreted in urine & feces
- **AEs:** Neutropenia, anemia, thrombocytopenia, neuropathy, VTE
- **DDI:** CYP3A4/1A2 or P-gp inhibitors/inducers (↑/↓ conc. of pomalidomide)
- **Clinical pearls: Must be registered w/ REMS program (POMALYST REMS),** consider anticoagulation ppx after assessment of RFs

Tazemetostat (Tazverik)

- **Mechanism:** Inhibitor of histone methyltransferase EZH2 (enhancer of zeste homolog 2), EZH1, & some EZH2 gain-of-function mts
- **Dosing:** 800 mg PO twice daily, no renal or hepatic dose adjustments recommended, adjust dose for toxicity (neutropenia, thrombocytopenia, anemia)
- **PK/PD:** Bioavailability ~30%, protein binding 88%, hepatically metabolized, $T_{1/2}$ ~3 h, excreted in urine & feces
- **AEs:** Anemia, neutropenia, prolonged partial thromboplastic time, abdominal pain, musculoskeletal pain, electrolyte abnormalities, nausea, vomiting, ↑ triglycerides, ↑ transaminases, alopecia
- **DDI:** CYP3A4 or P-gp inhibitors/inducers (↑/↓ conc. of tazemetostat); inhibits CYP2C8; induces CYP3A4
- **Clinical pearls:** EZH1/2 mt is not required to be treated w/ tazemetostat

Thalidomide (Thalomid)

- **Mechanism:** Displays immunomodulatory & antiangiogenic characteristics
- **Dosing:** 50–800 mg PO daily; no renal or hepatic dose adjustments recommended; adjust dose for tox (ANC ≤750/mm^3, constipation, oversedation, peripheral neuropathy).
- **PK/PD:** Bioavailability ~90%, protein binding ~60%, metabolized by nonenzymatic hydrolysis in plasma, $T_{1/2}$ ~6 h, renally excreted
- **AEs: Thromboembolic events (BBW),** leukopenia, peripheral neuropathy, diarrhea, constipation, orthostatic HoTN, rash
- **DDI:** Dexamethasone (↑ thrombogenic effect of thalidomide)
- **Clinical pearls: Must be registered w/ REMS program (STEPS);** consider anticoagulation ppx after assessment of RFs

Drug Classification	
HDAC inhibitors	Belinostat, panobinostat, romidepsin, vorinostat

Belinostat (Beleodaq)

- **Mechanism:** Inhibits HDAC enzymes causing termination of cell growth & apoptosis
- **Dosing:** 1,000 mg/m^2 IV d 1–5 every 21 d, no renal or hepatic dose adjustments
- **PK/PD:** $T_{1/2}$ ~1 h; metabolism via UGT1A1, CYP2A6, CYP2C9, & CYP3A4
- **AEs:** Edema, ↑ QTc, fatigue, rash, anemia, thrombocytopenia, GI tox, ↑ liver enzymes
- **DDI:** Substrate of CYP2A6, CYP2C9, CYP3A4, P-glycoprotein, & UGT1A1; inhibits CYP2C8 & CYP2C9
- **Clinical pearls:** ↓ dose to 750 mg/m^2 for pts homozygous for UGT1A1*28 allele

Panobinostat (Farydak)

- **Mechanism:** Inhibits HDAC enzymes causing termination of cell growth & apoptosis
- **Dosing:** 20 mg PO QOD × 3 doses during wk 1 & 2 of a 21-d cycle for max of 8–16 cycles, given w/ bortezomib & dex; no renal adjustment; ↓ dose for hepatic impairment; adjust dose for heme/non heme tox; ↓ dose w/ strong CYP3A4 inhibitors; avoid concomitant use w/ strong CY3A4 inducers/CYP2D6 substrates; Prior to each tx cycle, ANC should be ≥1,500/mm^3; platelets ≥100,000/mm^3
- **PK/PD:** $T_{1/2}$ ~37 h, bioavailability ~21%, AUC ↓ when given w/ high–fat meal
- **AEs: CV events (BBW), diarrhea (BBW),** bone marrow suppression
- **DDI:** Substrate CYP2C19, CYP2D6, CYP3A4, P-glycoprotein; Inhibits CYP2D6; QTc-prolonging medications
- **Clinical pearls:** REMS program; Measure QTcF prior to initiation (must be <450 ms); mod. emetic potential

Romidepsin (Istodax)

- **Mechanism:** Inhibits HDAC enzymes causing termination of cell growth & apoptosis
- **Dosing:** 14 mg/m^2 IV d 1, 8, & 15 of 28-d cycle; no renal dose adjustments; use w/ caution in sev. hepatic impairment; adjust dose for tox
- **PK/PD:** Protein binding ~94%, $T_{1/2}$ ~3 h, metabolism via CYP3A4 or P-gp
- **AEs:** Pancytopenia, diarrhea, QTc prolongation, electrolyte wasting, hyperuricemia, hyperglycemia
- **DDI:** CYP3A4/P-gp inhibitors/inducers (↑/↓ conc. of romidepsin), QTc-prolonging medications (↑ QTc-prolonging effect)
- **Clinical pearls:** Monitor serum electrolytes (K & Mg) & ECG in pts w/ significant CV dz

Vorinostat (Zolinza)

- **Mechanism:** Inhibits HDAC enzymes causing termination of cell growth & apoptosis
- **Dosing:** 400 mg PO daily, no renal dose adjustments, mod. hepatic impairment (Tbili >1.5–3× ULN): 200 mg daily & contraindicated in sev. impairment (Tbili >3 mg/dL). Adjust dose for tox (↑ SCr, ↓ appetite, ↓ K, N/V, neutropenia, leukopenia, thrombocytopenia)
- **PK/PD:** Bioavailability fasting ~43%, protein binding ~71%, glucuronidated & hydrolyzed, $T_{1/2}$ ~2 h, renally excreted
- **AEs:** Thrombocytopenia, anemia, QTc prolongation, ↑ SCr, diarrhea, hyperglycemia, electrolyte wasting, proteinuria, thrombosis
- **DDI:** Oral anticoagulants (↑ risk of bleeding), valproic acid (risk of sev. thrombocytopenia & GI bleeding), QTc-prolonging medications (↑ QTc-prolonging effect)
- **Clinical pearls:** Encourage oral hydration as pts may develop diarrhea, monitor electrolytes (K & Mg), SCr, & glc

Information based on publicly available drug inserts from Merck, Novartis, Bristol-Myers Squibb, Spectrum, & Celgene.

Activity of Various Tyrosine Kinase Inhibitors (TKIs)

	JAK	ALK	MET	EGFR	HER2	FGFR	PDGFR	VEGFR	RET	FLT3	SRC	Bcr-abl	KIT	RAF	ROS1	MEK	TRK	CSF1
Afatinib				X	X													
Alectinib		X							X									
Avapritinib							X						X					
Axitinib								X										
Bosutinib											X	X						
Binimetinib																X		
Brigatinib		X								X					X			
Cabozantinib			X					X	X	X			X		X			
Capmatinib			X															
Ceritinib		X													X			
Cobimetinib																X		
Crizotinib		X	X												X			
Dacomitinib				X	X													
Dabrafenib														X				
Dasatinib							X				X	X	X					
Encorafenib														X				
Entrectinib		X															X	
Erdafitinib						X	X	X	X									
Erlotinib				X														
Gefitinib				X														
Gilteritinib										X								
Imatinib							X					X	X					
Larotrectinib																	X	
Lapatinib				X	X													
Lenvatinib						X	X	X	X				X					
Lorlatinib		X													X			
Midostaurin							X	X		X			X					
Nilotinib							X					X	X					
Neratinib			X	X														
Osimertinib				X	X													
Pazopanib						X	X	X					X					
Pexidartinib										X			X					X
Ponatinib						X	X	X	X	X	X	X	X					
Regorafenib						X	X	X	X				X	X				
Ripretinib							X											
Ruxolitinib	X																	
Selpercatinib								X	X									
Sorafenib							X	X	X	X		X	X					
Sunitinib							X	X	X	X		X						
Trametinib																X		
Tivozanib							X	X										
Vandetanib				X				X	X		X							
Vemurafenib														X				

Activity of Various Miscellaneous Pathway Inhibitors

	PI3Kδ	PI3Ka	BTK	PARP1/2/3	CDK4/6	Smo (Hh)	BCL-2	IDH2	IDH1	MET	XPO1
Alpelisib		X									
Copanlisib	X										
Duvelisib	X										
Idelalisib	X										
Umbralisib	X										
Ibrutinib			X								
Acalabrutinib			X								
Zanubrutinib			X								
Olaparib				X							
Palbociclib					X						
Ribociclib					X						
Rucaparib				X							
Niraparib				X							
Abemaciclib					X						
Sonidegib						X					
Glasdegib						X					
Venetoclax							X				
Vismodegib						X					
Enasidenib								X			
Ivosidenib									X		
Selinexor											X
Tepotinib										X	
Talazoparib				X							

Abemaciclib (Verzenio)

- **Dosing:** 150 mg PO BID + AI or fulvestrant, 200 mg PO BID as monotherapy. No renal adjustments. Withhold therapy & consider dose reduction for grade 3+ hepatotoxicity
- **PK/PD:** Metabolism via CYP3A4, $T_{1/2}$ = 18.3 h
- **AEs:** Diarrhea (86–90%), neutropenia, nausea, abdominal pain, infxns, fatigue, anemia, leukopenia, decreased appetite, vomiting, headache, thrombocytopenia, VTE (rare)
- **DDI:** Avoid strong CYP3A4 inducers. Consider dose reduction w/ mod.-strong CYP3A4 inhibitors
- **Clinical pearls:** Mod.-high emetic potential. Antiemetics may be necessary to prevent nausea & vomiting

Acalabrutinib (Calquence)

- **Dosing:** 100 mg PO BID; Dose reduce/interrupt therapy for hematologic toxicity (thrombocytopenia, neutropenia) per labeling
- **PK/PD:** Metabolism via CYP3A4 to active metabolite, $T_{1/2}$ = 3.5 h
- **AEs:** Fatigue, diarrhea, headaches, myalgias, cytopenias, HTN, atrial fibrillation
- **Clinical pearls:** Avoid PPIs/H2 blockers/antacids (can separate H2 blockers 2 h after dose & antacids 2 h before/after acalabrutinib), monitor for drug interactions

Afatinib (Gilotrif)

- **Dosing:** 40 mg PO once daily; 30 mg PO once daily in sev. renal impairment (eGFR 15–29 mL/min/1.73 m^2); *hold for:* ≥ grade 3 rxn; ≥ grade 2 diarrhea × 2 or more consecutive d; ≥ grade 2 cutaneous rxns for ≥7 d or intolerable; ≥ grade 2 renal impairment; reinstitute at 10 mg/d < dose at w/c rxn occurred; not studied in sev. (Child–Pugh C) hepatic impairment
- **PK/PD:** Minimal enzymatic metabolism, $T_{1/2}$ 37 h
- **AEs:** Diarrhea, stomatitis, rash/pruritus, paronychia, ↓ appetite, bullous/exfoliative skin disorders, ILD, keratitis, hepatic tox, left ventricular dysfunction
- **DDI:** P-gp inhibitors/inducers: Reduce/increase daily dose by 10 mg
- **Clinical pearls:** Take 1 h before or 2 h after a meal

Alectinib (Alecensa)

- **Dosing:** 600 mg PO BID; dose reduce by 150 mg BID & d/c in pts unable to tolerate 300 mg PO BID for ALT/AST ≥5× ULN w/ Tbili ≤2× ULN, Tbili >3× ULN, symptomatic bradycardia, CPK elevation >5× ULN; no adj. for renal/hepatic (not studied in sev. (CrCl <30 mL/min) renal impairment or mod.-to-sev. hepatic impairment)
- **PK/PD:** Metabolized by CYP3A4 to *M4*, *M4* is substrate of P-gp, concentrations in CSF similar to free concentrations in plasma; $T_{1/2}$ alectinib/M4 is 33 h/31 h
- **AEs:** Fatigue, constipation, edema, myalgia, hepatotoxicity, ILD/pneumonitis, bradycardia, sev. myalgia/↑CPK
- **DDI:** No clinically meaningful effects
- **Clinical pearls:** Take w/ food

Alpelisib (Piqray)

- **Dosing:** 300 mg PO QD w/ food; no renal or hepatic dose adjustments; dose reduce based upon toxicity, discontinue therapy if dose reduction below 200 mg daily is necessary
- **PK/PD:** Primarily metabolized by hydrolysis, lesser extent CYP3A4; $T_{1/2}$ 8–9 h
- **AEs:** Diarrhea, hyperglycemia, rash, fatigue, lymphocytosis, alopecia, weight loss, anorexia, stomatitis
- **DDI:** Avoid **strong** CYP3A4 inducers, avoid BCRP inhibitors
- **Clinical pearls:** Take w/ food; monitor for pancreatitis; minimal–low emetic risk; contraception needed during therapy & 1 wk after last dose

Avapritinib (Ayvakit)

- **Dosing:** 300 mg PO daily on empty stomach; no adjustment for mild/mod. hepatic/renal impairment (no data for sev. impairment); manufacturer-recommended 2° reductions available for toxicity
- **PK/PD:** $T_{1/2}$ 32–57 h; hepatic metabolism (major CYP3A4)
- **AEs:** Intracranial hemorrhage (incidence 1–3%), wide range of CNS adverse rxns, mod./high vomiting risk, edema, diarrhea, lacrimation, hair color changes
- **DDI:** Reduce starting dose for concomitant mod. CYP3A4 inhibitor (100 mg daily); avoid use w/ strong CYP3A4 inhibitors/inducers
- **Clinical pearls:** Premedicate w/ antiemetic; median time to CNS toxicity 6.1 wks

Axitinib (Inlyta)

- **Dosing:** Starting dose 5 mg PO every 12 h ↑/↓ based on tolerability. No renal dose adjustments recommended. Hepatic: Child–Pugh class B: 50% nl dose, ↑ as tolerated. Child–Pugh class C: Not studied
- **PK/PD:** Bound to albumin, hepatic metabolism via CYP3A4/5, $T_{1/2}$ 2.5–6 h
- **AEs:** HTN, fatigue, GI, hand–foot syndrome/rash, LFTs & electrolyte abnormalities, ↑ SCr (55%), proteinuria, hematologic
- **DDI:** CYP3A4 inhibitors/inducers (↑/↓ conc. of axitinib), warfarin
- **Clinical pearls:** Monitor: Hepatic, renal, & thyroid function; U/A (proteinuria); & BP. D/C 24 h prior to surgery (impaired wound healing)

Bosutinib (Bosulif)

- **Dosing:** 400 mg PO daily–500 mg PO daily (consider dose escalation to 600 mg PO daily for previously treated pts if no CHR by wk 8 or a CCyR by wk 12)
  - **Renal:** CrCl 30–50 mL/min: 300 mg (newly diagnosed)–400 mg PO daily; CrCl <30 mL/min: 200 (newly diagnosed)–300 mg PO daily
  - **Hepatic:** 200 mg PO daily
- Hematologic, hepatic toxicities, grade 3/4 diarrhea: Hold Rx & resume at ↓ dose
- **PK/PD:** Hepatic metabolism via CYP3A4, $T_{1/2}$ 22.5 h
- **AEs:** Edema, diarrhea (82%), ↓ Mg, rash (35%), ↑ LFTs, hematologic
- **DDI:** CYP3A4 inhibitors/inducers (↑/↓ conc. of bosutinib), PPI/H2 blocker/antacid (↓ bosutinib absorption), QTc-prolonging agents, warfarin
- **Clinical pearls:** Take w/ food. Diarrhea should resolve after a wk into Rx (tolerance) w/ antidiarrheal support. Monitor: CBCs, LFTS, EKG baseline & intermittently. Separate H2 blocker/antacid from bosutinib dose by more than 2 h **(avoid PPIs)**

Binimetinib (Mektovi)

- **Dosing:** 45 mg PO BID; Tbili 1.5–3 × ULN & any AST elevation or Tbili >3 × ULN & any AST elevation: decrease to 30 mg BID; grade 2 AST or ALT elevations if no improvement in 2 wks hold therapy until grade ≤1 then resume at same dose; grade 3 AST or ALT elevation 1st occurrence interrupt for up to 4 wks & if improves grade ≤1 then resume at reduced dose, if no improvement permanently discontinue & if recurrent grade 3 consider permanently discontinuing; grade 4 AST or ALT elevation 1st occurrence permanently discontinue or withhold for up to 4 wks & if improves grade ≤1 resume at reduced dose; for recurrent grade 4, permanently discontinue

- **PK/PD:** Metabolism primarily via UGT1A1, converted to active metabolite via CYP1A2, CYP2C19, $T_{1/2}$ = 3.5 h
- **AEs:** ↓ LVEF, ophthalmic changes, GI tox, rash, fatigue, ↑ LFTs, ↑ GGT, ↑ CPK, ↑ SCr, HTN, peripheral edema, skin rash, cytopenia
- **Clinical pearls:** Mod. or high emetic potential, monitor for signs of uveitis, rhabdomyolysis, VTE, & ILD

Brigatinib (Alunbrig)

- **Dosing:** 90 mg PO once daily × first 7 d; then increase to 180 mg PO once daily (if tolerated); sev. hepatic impairment (Child–Pugh C)—reduce dose by 40%; sev. renal impairment (CrCl 15–29 mL/min)—reduce dose by 50%
- **PK/PD:** Hepatic metabolism via CYP2C8 & 3A4; $T_{1/2}$ = 25 h
- **AEs:** ILD, HTN, bradycardia, visual disturbances, pancreatic enzymes ↑, hyperglycemia, CPK elevation
- **DDI:** CYP3A4 inhibitors/inducers (↑/↓ conc. of brigatinib)
- **Clinical pearls:** Take w/ or w/o food. Monitor—BP, heart rate, signs of ILD during lead-in dosing period, vision changes, CPK, blood glucose

Capmatinib (Tabrecta)

- **Dosing:** 400 mg orally twice daily; First-dose reduction: 300 mg orally twice daily; 2nd-dose reduction: 200 mg orally twice daily; Permanently stop in pts who are unable to tolerate 200 mg orally twice daily
- **PK/PD:** Primarily metabolized by CYP3A4 & aldehyde oxidase; $T_{1/2}$ = 6.5 h
- **AEs:** The most common adverse rxns (≥20%) are peripheral edema, nausea, fatigue, vomiting, dyspnea, & decreased appetite. Warnings for ILD/pneumonitis, hepatotoxicity, risk of photosensitivity, embryo-fetal toxicity
- **DDI:** Strong & mod. CYP3A Inducers: Avoid concomitant use
- **Clinical pearls:** Take w/ or w/o food; Swallow tablets whole

Cabozantinib (Cometriq and Cabometyx)

- **Dosing:** Renal: CrCl <30 mL/min: Use caution. Reduce dose for mild or mod. hepatic impairment (Cabometyx). Dose adjust for rx-induced tox
  - **Renal cell carcinoma (Cabometyx):** 60 mg PO once daily
  - **Metastatic medullary thyroid cancer (Cometriq):** 140 mg PO once daily
- **PK/PD:** ≥99.7% protein bound, hepatic metabolism via CYP3A4, fecal (54%) & urinary (27%) excretion, $T_{1/2}$ 55 h
- **AEs:** HTN (33%), fatigue, skin tox (hand–foot syndrome, alopecia, rash, hair color changes (34%), GI, ↑ LFTs, hematologic
- **DDI:** CYP3A4 inhibitors/inducers (↑/↓ conc. of cabozantinib)
- **Clinical pearls:** Take on an empty stomach. Monitor: Proteinuria, BP, renal & hepatic function, electrolytes (Ca, phos, K, Mg). Stop Cabometyx at least 28 d prior to surgery

Ceritinib (Zykadia)

- **Dosing:** 750 mg PO once daily; dose reduce by 150 mg/d for AST/ALT >5× ULN w/ Tbili ≤2× ULN, QTc >500 ms on ≥2 separate EKGs, sev./intolerable N/V or diarrhea despite optimal therapy, persistent hyperglycemia >250 mg/dL despite optimal therapy, symptomatic bradycardia, lipase/amylase >2× ULN; reduce dose by 1/3 for unavoidable concomitant CYP3A inhibitor
- **PK/PD:** Metabolized by CYP3A4 & substrate of P-gp, $T_{1/2}$ 41 h
- **AEs:** Diarrhea, nausea, elevated transaminases, vomiting, abdominal pain, fatigue, constipation, ↓ appetite, GI tox, hepatotoxicity, ILD/pneumonitis, QTc prolongation, hyperglycemia, bradycardia, pancreatitis
- **DDI:** ↑/↓ exposure w/ concurrent CYP3A4 inhibitors/inducers; may inhibit CYP3A/CYP2C9 & clinically affect fentanyl, cyclosporine, tacrolimus, sirolimus, phenytoin, warfarin
- **Clinical pearls:** Administer on empty stomach, supplied as 150-mg capsules

Cobimetinib (Cotellic)

- **Dosing:** 60 mg PO daily for 21 d out of a 28-d cycle. No renal or hepatic dose adjustments recommended. Adjust for CYP3A4 inhibitors. Adjust dose for tox
- **PK/PD:** Hepatic metabolism through CYP3A & UGT2B7 glucuronidation, $T_{1/2}$ 44 h
- **AEs:** Diarrhea, N/V, skin tox (photosensitivity, acneiform rash, cutaneous malignancies), ocular disorders (retinal detachment, uveitis), hemorrhage, cardiomyopathy, rhabdomyolysis, LFT elevations
- **DDI:** CYP3A inhibitors/inducers (↑/↓ conc. of cobimetinib)
- **Clinical pearls:** Monitor LFTs, CPK, SCr, LVEF, blood pressure, dermatologic exams, & ophthalmic exams

Copanlisib (Aliqopa)

- **Dosing:** 60 mg as a 1-h intravenous infusion on D1, D8, & D15 of a 28-d cycle; Renal: No dosage adjustments in labeling, CrCl ≥15 mL/min does not alter PK; Hepatic: Mild impairment–no adjustment, mod.—reduce dose to 45 mg, sev.—not studied
- **PK/PD:** Hepatic metabolism via CYP3A. $T_{1/2}$ 39 h
- **AEs:** Hypertension, bone marrow suppression, diarrhea, nausea, vomiting, hyperglycemia, hypertriglyceridemia, skin rash, infxn (PCP), pneumonitis
- **DDI:** Strong CYP3A4 inhibitors/inducers
- **Clinical pearls:** Monitor: Pneumonitis, blood pressure, blood glucose, consider PCP prophylaxis, minimal emetic potential

Crizotinib (Xalkori)

- **Dosing:** 250 mg PO BID. Renal: CrCl <30 mL/min: 250 mg PO once daily. Hepatic: Use w/ caution in impairment. Rx-related tox (heme, effusion/edema, rash): Hold & restart at ↓ dose
- **PK/PD:** Hepatic metabolism via CYP3A4, $T_{1/2}$ 42 h
- **AEs:** Edema, fatigue, dizziness, GI (↓ appetite, taste alteration), lymphopenia, ↑ ALT, neuropathy, vision disorders (onset <2 wks: visual impairment, diplopia, photopsia), hepatotoxicity, ILD/pneumonitis, QTc prolongation, bradycardia, sev. visual loss
- **DDI:** CYP3A4 inhibitors/inducers (↑/↓ conc. of crizotinib), QTc-prolonging agents
- **Clinical pearls:** Monitor: Pneumonitis, ECG, LFTs, ophthalmic evaluations

Erdafitinib (Balversa)

- **Dosing:** 8 mg PO QD, w/ a dose increase to 9 mg PO QD if serum phosphate level is <5.5 mg/dL & no ADR ≥ grade 2 at 14–21 d; no hepatic or renal dose adjustments; dose adjust based upon toxicity
- **PK/PD:** Primarily bound to alpha-1-acid glycoprotein; primarily CYP2C9 & CYP3A4 metabolized; $T_{1/2}$ 59 h
- **AEs:** Hyperphosphatemia, central serous retinopathy/retinal pigment epithelial detachment, ↑ SCr, hyponatremia, ↑ LFT, dry eye, stomatitis, diarrhea, dry mouth, decreased appetite, fatigue, onycholysis, dysgeusia, anemia, palmar-plantar erythrodysesthesia
- **DDI:** Avoid mod./strong CYP2C9 & CYP3A4 inhibitors/inducers, avoid coadministration of CYP3A4 substrates w/ narrow therapeutic windows, dose reduce/avoid OCT2 substrates, avoid serum phosphate altering agents until after initial dose determination (14–21 d)
- **Clinical pearls:** Take w/ or w/o food; minimal to low emetic risk; confirm *FGFR* mt

Erlotinib (Tarceva)

- **Dosing:** 100–150 mg PO daily. No renal dose adjustments recommended. Hepatic: Tbili >3× ULN &/or ↑ ALT/AST >5× ULN: ↓ dose
- **PK/PD:** Hepatic metabolism via CYP3A4, $T_{1/2}$ 36 h
- **AEs:** Rash (up to 75%—DLT), GI (nausea, vomiting, diarrhea), pyrexia, fatigue, cough, dyspnea, paronychia, ILD, renal failure, hepatotoxicity, GI perforation, bullous/exfoliative skin disorders, CVA, MAHA w/ thrombocytopenia, ocular disorders, hemorrhage in pts taking warfarin
- **DDI:** CYP3A4 inhibitors/inducers (↑/↓ conc. of erlotinib), PPI/H2 blocker/antacid (↓ erlotinib absorption), cigarette smoking/CYP1A2 inducers ↓ erlotinib plasma concentrations
- **Clinical pearls:** Take on empty stomach. Monitor: Skin tox (possible exfoliative rash)

Dabrafenib (Tafinlar)

- **Dosing:** 150 mg PO BID; dose reductions in increments of 50 mg PO BID, permanently discontinue if unable to tolerate 50 mg PO BID; mod.-to-sev. hepatic impairment may increase exposure (not studied); not studied in renal impairment
- **PK/PD:** Metabolized by CYP2C8/CYP3A4, substrate of P-gp & BCRP, inhibits OATP1B1 & OATP1B3, $T_{1/2}$ 8–22 h (including metabolites)
- **AEs:** Hyperkeratosis, headache, pyrexia, arthralgia, papilloma, alopecia, hand–foot syndrome (single-agent), pyrexia, rash, chills, headache, arthralgia, cough (in combo w/ trametinib), cutaneous/non-cutaneous malignancies, tumor promotion in *BRAF* WT melanoma, hemorrhage, cardiomyopathy, uveitis, sev. febrile rxns, skin tox, hyperglycemia, hemolytic anemia in G6PD-deficient pts
- **DDI:** Inhibitors/inducers of CYP2C8/CYP3A4; dabrafenib induces CYP3A4/CYP2C9
- **Clinical pearls:** Administer 1 h or 2 h after a meal, s/e profile differs between monotherapy/combination therapy w/ trametinib

Dacomitinib (Vizimpro)
- **Dosing:** 45 mg PO daily
- **PK/PD:** Hepatic metabolism via oxidation & glutathione conjugation, $T_{1/2}$ 70 h
- **AEs:** Diarrhea, nausea, hand–foot syndrome, rash, paronychia, chest pain, insomnia, ↑ glucose, LFTs, conjunctivitis, ↓ K/Na/Ca/Mg, anemia, musculoskeletal pain
- **DDI:** Substrate of CYP2D6 (minor) & strong CYP2D6 inhibitor. Avoid use of PPIs (↓ dacomitinib absorption)
- **Clinical pearls:** If using an H2 blocker or antacid, administer dacomitinib at least 6 h prior to or 10 h after the H2 blocker or antacid

Dasatinib (Sprycel)
- **Dosing:** 100 mg PO daily–140 mg PO daily. Adjust dose for Rx-related tox
- **PK/PD:** Hepatic metabolism via CYP3A4, $T_{1/2}$ 3–5 h
- **AEs:** Skin tox, edema (peripheral & pulmonary), hematologic, hepatotoxicity, pulmonary hypertension
- **DDI:** CYP3A4 inhibitors/inducers (↑/↓ conc. of dasatinib), PPI/H2 blocker/antacid (↓ dasatinib absorption), QTc-prolonging agents, warfarin (↑/↓ warfarin effects)
- **Clinical pearls:** Monitor: Pleural effusions (CXR if indicated). Antacid therapy at least 2 h prior to or after dasatinib dose; do not use with H2 antagonists or PPIs

Duvelisib (Copiktra)
- **Dosing:** 25 mg PO BID. **Renal:** No dose adjustments recommended. **Hepatic:** Hold for grade 3 ALT/AST elevation & resume once <3 × ULN
- **PK/PD:** Metabolism CYP3A4 & substrate of p-gp, $T_{1/2}$ 4.7 h
- **AEs:** Infxns (CMV, PCP), colitis/noninfectious diarrhea, pneumonitis, rash, hepatitis, neutropenia, thrombocytopenia
- **Clinical pearls:** Initiate PJP prophylaxis & continue until CD4+ >200, consider viral prophylaxis & CMV monitoring while on tx. Reduce to 15 mg BID w/ concomitant strong CYP3A4 inhibitors

Enasidenib (Idhifa)
- **Dosing:** 100 mg PO daily. **Renal:** No dose adjustments recommended. **Hepatic:** Bilirubin >3 × ULN for ≥14 d: reduce to 50 mg PO daily
- **PK/PD:** Metabolism CYP3A4 & substrate of p-gp, mean terminal $T_{1/2}$ 19–482 h (active metabolite)
- **AEs:** Hyperbilirubinemia (indirect), differentiation syndrome,
- **Clinical pearls:** May cause differentiation syndrome which may warrant hospitalization, dexamethasone, hydroxyurea, &/or supplemental oxygen. Use p-gp substrates w/ narrow therapeutic index w/ caution

Encorafenib (Braftovi)
- **Dosing:** Colorectal cancer (metastatic): 300 mg PO once daily, Melanoma (metastatic or unresectable): 450 mg PO once daily, Hepatic adjustments: hold for grade 3/4 AST/ALT elevations; colorectal 1st dose reduction 225 mg once daily, 2nd dose reduction 150 mg once daily, subsequent changes permanently discontinue; melanoma 1st reduction 300 mg once daily, 2nd dose reduction 225 mg once daily, subsequent changes permanently discontinue
- **PK/PD:** Metabolism primarily via CYP3A4 & CYP2C19, CYP2D6 to lesser extent, major CYP3A4 substrate, $T_{1/2}$ of 3.5 h
- **AEs:** Dermatologic, ocular toxicity, QTc prolongation, GI tox, arthralgias, cytopenias, hyperglycemia, ↑ GGT, ↑ LFTs, ↑ SCr
- **Clinical pearls:** Mod. emetic potential, QT prolongation, monitor for signs of uveitis, monitor for drug interactions

Entrectinib (Rozlytrek)
- **Dosing:** 600 mg orally once daily. Pediatric pts 12 y + BSA >1.50 m^2: 600 mg once daily; BSA 1.11–1.50 m^2: 500 mg once daily; BSA 0.91–1.10 m^2: 400 mg once daily
- **PK/PD:** Metabolized primarily by CYP3A4
- **AEs:** ≥20%: Fatigue, constipation, dysgeusia, edema, dizziness, diarrhea, nausea, dysesthesia, dyspnea, myalgia, cognitive impairment, increased weight, cough, vomiting, pyrexia, arthralgia, & vision disorders. Warnings for congestive heart failure, CNS effects, skeletal fractures, hepatotoxicity, hyperuricemia, QT interval prolongation, vision disorders, embryo-fetal toxicity

- **DDI:** Mod./strong CYP3A4 inhibitors: For pts 12 y & older & a BSA >1.50 m^2, reduce the dose of entrectinib if coadministration of mod./strong CYP3A inhibitors cannot be avoided. For pediatric pts 12 y & older w/ a BSA ≤1.50 m^2, avoid coadministration w/ entrectinib. Avoid coadministration w/ entrectinib & mod./strong CYP3A inducers
- **Clinical pearls:** May be taken w/ or w/o food; Swallow capsules whole

Gefitinib (Iressa)

- **Dosing:** 250 mg PO daily. No renal or hepatic dose adjustments recommended. Adjust dose for Rx-induced toxicities
- **PK/PD:** Hepatic metabolism via CYP3A4, $T_{1/2}$ 41 h
- **AEs:** Skin tox (rash, acne, dry skin), GI (nausea, vomiting, diarrhea), ILD, hepatotoxicity, GI perforation, diarrhea, ocular disorders/keratitis, bullous/exfoliative skin disorders
- **DDI:** CYP3A4 inhibitors/inducers (↑/↓ conc. of gefitinib), PPI/H2 blocker/antacid (↓ gefitinib absorption), warfarin
- **Clinical pearls:** Monitor: Skin tox, worsening pulm function & diarrhea; for pts w/ difficulty swallowing solids: immerse tablet in 4–8 oz of water & stir × 15 min, drink liquid or administer via NG tube, rinse container w/ 4–8 oz of water & drink/administer via NG tube

Gilteritinib (Xospata)

- **Dosing:** 120 mg PO daily. **Renal:** No dose adjustments recommended; data not available in sev. impairment. **Hepatic:** No dose adjustments recommended
- **PK/PD:** Metabolism CYP3A4 & substrate of p-gp, mean terminal $T_{1/2}$ 113 h (active metabolite)
- **AEs:** QT prolongation, differentiation syndrome, PRES, pancreatitis
- **Clinical pearls:** May cause differentiation syndrome which may warrant hospitalization, dexamethasone, hydroxyurea, &/or supplemental oxygen. Monitor QTc interval

Glasdegib (Daurismo)

- **Dosing:** 100 mg PO daily; No renal or hepatic dose adjustments recommended; adjust dose for Rx-induced toxicities
- **PK/PD:** Hepatically metabolized through CYP3A4; Time to peak ~2 h; $T_{1/2}$ ~14.4 h
- **AEs:** ↑ QTc; fatigue; skin rash; nausea; metabolic abnormalities; ↑ liver enzymes; anemia; thrombocytopenia; musculoskeletal pain; elevated Scr; dyspnea; fever
- **DDI:** CYP3A4 major substrate; QTc-prolonging agents
- **Clinical pearls:** Verify pregnancy status of females with 7 d of drug administration because of risk of sev. birth defects

Ibrutinib (Imbruvica)

- **Dosing:** 420–560 mg PO daily. **Renal:** No adjustments, no data in CrCl <25 mL/min **Hepatic:** Child–Pugh class A—140 mg daily, AVOID in Child–Pugh class B or C. Rx-related tox: Adjust dose per indication
- **PK/PD:** Metabolism via CYP3A4 (major), CYP2D6 (minor) to active metabolite; $T_{1/2}$ 4–6 h
- **AEs:** Bleeding/bruising, diarrhea, arthralgias, rash, cytopenia, infxn, tumor lysis syndrome, atrial fibrillation
- **DDI:** CYP3A4 inhibitors/inducers (↑/↓ conc. of ibrutinib), anticoagulants (↑ bleeding risk)
- **Clinical pearls:**. Hold 3–7 d pre- & postminor & major procedures (respectively). Inhibits BCRP (↑ conc. of sensitive substrates, eg, digoxin, MTX). Early lymphocytosis seen (onset d w/ median time to resolution: 8 wks). Avoid grapefruit juice/Seville oranges

Idelalisib (Zydelig)

- **Dosing:** 150 mg PO twice daily. **Renal:** No adjustments, no data in CrCl <15 mL/min **Hepatic:** ALT >5–20× ULN or bilirubin >3–10× ULN; hold until ≤1× ULN & resume at 100 mg BID. Discontinue if AST/ALT >20× ULN or bilirubin >10× ULN. Rx-related tox: Hold & adjust dose for indication (eg, diarrhea, cytopenias, CMV)
- **PK/PD:** Bioavailability unknown; metabolism via CYP3A4 (major), P-gp to inactive metabolite; $T_{1/2}$ 8.2 h
- **AEs:** Hepatotoxicity, diarrhea/colitis, pneumonitis, cutaneous skin rxns (SJS/TEN), cytopenias, fatigue, infxns, arthralgias
- **DDI:** CYP3A4 inhibitors/inducers (↑/↓ conc. of idelalisib), warfarin (↑ warfarin exposure)
- **Clinical pearls:** Strong inhibitor of CYP3A4 & UGT1A1, CYP2C9 (↑ conc. of sensitive substrates). Lymphocytosis seen (peak by wk 2 w/ postulated time to resolution of 12 wks). Opportunistic infxns (CMV & PCP) observed post marketing

Imatinib (Gleevec)

- **Dosing:** 400–800 mg PO daily. **Renal:** CrCl 40–59 mL/min: max 600 mg; 20–39 mL/min: max 400 mg; <20 mL/min: 100 mg daily. **Hepatic** (bili >3× ULN or AST/ALT >5× ULN): Consider ↓ dose 25%. Rx-related tox: Adjust dose per indication
- **PK/PD:** Metabolism via CYP3A4 (major), CYP1A2, 2D6, 2C9, 2C19 (minor); $T_{1/2}$ 18 h (adults), 14.8 (children)
- **AEs:** Nausea (mod. emetic potential), edema (periorbital edema, pulm, peripheral), fatigue, skin tox, hematologic, GI, ↑ LFTs
- **DDI:** CYP3A4 inhibitors/inducers (↑/↓ conc. of imatinib), warfarin (↑ warfarin effects)
- **Clinical pearls:** 800-mg doses should be split BID for tolerance. Inhibits CYP3A4 (↑ conc. of sensitive substrates)

Ivosidenib (Tibsovo)

- **Dosing:** 500 mg PO daily. No renal or hepatic dose adjustments recommended; effect of sev. hepatic impairment on PK unknown
- **PK/PD:** Metabolism CYP3A4, CYP2C9, CYP2B6, & substrate of p-gp, $T_{1/2}$ 93 h
- **AEs:** Hyperbilirubinemia (indirect), differentiation syndrome
- **Clinical pearls:** May cause differentiation syndrome which may warrant hospitalization, dexamethasone, hydroxyurea, &/or supplemental oxygen. Monitor QTc interval. Reduce dose to 250 mg daily w/ concomitant strong CYP3A4 inhibitors

Lapatinib (Tykerb)

- **Dosing:** 1,250 mg PO once daily (w/ capecitabine), 1,500 mg PO once daily (w/ letrozole). No renal dose adjustments recommended. Pre-existing hepatic impairment (Child–Pugh class C): ↓ 1,000 mg–750 mg w/ capecitabine & ↓ 1,500 mg–1,000 mg w/ letrozole
- **PK/PD:** Incomplete, variable absorption; highly protein bound; hepatic metabolism via CYP3A4; $T_{1/2}$ 25 h
- **AEs:** Diarrhea, nausea, hand–foot syndrome (w/ capecitabine), rash, fatigue; diarrhea, rash, nausea, fatigue (w/ letrozole); hepatotoxicity, LVEF dysfunction, diarrhea, ILD, prolonged QTc, sev. cutaneous rxns
- **DDI:** CYP3A4 inhibitors/inducers (↑/↓ conc. of lapatinib), inhibits CYP2C8 & P-gp, PPI/H2 blocker/antacid (↓ lapatinib absorption), QTc-prolonging agents, warfarin (↑/↓ warfarin effects)
- **Clinical pearls:** Take on empty stomach. Monitor: QTc, electrolytes, LVEF, baseline & periodic

Larorectinib (Vitrakvi)

- **Dosing:** 100 mg PO Q12h; no renal dose adjustments; mod.-to-sev. (Child–Pugh class B & C) hepatic impairment reduce dose by 50%
- **PK/PD:** Hepatically metabolized via CYP3A4; bioavailability ~34%; time to peak ~1 h; $T_{1/2}$ ~2.9 h
- **AEs:** Transaminase increase (onset 2 mos), neurotoxicity (onset 3 mos), hypoalbumenia, nausea, anemia, neutropenia, arthalgia, cough, fever
- **DDI:** CYP3A4 major substrate; P-gp minor substrate
- **Clinical pearls:** Avoid grapefruit

Lenvatinib (Lenvima)

- **Dosing:** 24 mg or 18 mg PO once daily. Decrease dose for sev. renal (CrCl <30 mL/min) or sev. hepatic dysfunction. Adjust dose for Rx-induced tox
  - **Differentiated thyroid cancer:** 24 mg PO once daily monotherapy
  - **Renal cell carcinoma:** 18 mg PO once daily (in combination w/ everolimus)
- **PK/PD:** Hepatic metabolism through CYP3A (minor substrate). $T_{1/2}$ ~28 h
- **AEs:** HTN, diarrhea, stomatitis, arthralgia/myalgia, skin tox (hand–foot syndrome, alopecia, rash), dysphonia, proteinuria, renal dysfunction, thyroid dysfunction, QTc prolongation, hypocalcemia, cardiac dysfunction, arterial thromboembolic events, hemorrhage
- **DDI:** No interactions
- **Clinical pearls:** Monitor BP, LFTs, UA, electrolytes, thyroid function

Lorlatinib (Lorbrena)

- **Dosing:** 100 mg PO once daily. For CrCl 15–29 mL/min, dose reduce to 75 mg PO once daily. No hepatic dose adjustments
- **PK/PD:** Hepatic metabolism primarily through CYP3A4, 48% urinary excretion (<1% unchanged drug), $T_{1/2}$ ~ 24 h
- **AEs:** Edema (57%), peripheral neuropathy (47%), ↑ cholesterol, ↑ triglycerides, ↑ glucose, weight gain, ↑ K, ↓ Mg/Phos, diarrhea, nausea, vomiting, arthralgia, myalgia, visual disturbance, dyspnea, cognitive effects, mood effects

- **DDI:** Avoid in combination w/ strong CYP3A4 inhibitors or inducers. Discontinue strong CYP3A4 inducers for at least 3 half-lives prior to initiation of lorlatinib
- **Clinical pearls:** Monitor serum cholesterol, triglycerides, blood pressure & serum fasting glucose at baseline & periodically thereafter. Initiate or increase dose of lipid-lowering agents as needed. Rare but serious s/e's: CNS toxicity (seizures, suicidal ideation), pneumonitis, & atrioventricular block

Midostaurin (Rydapt)

- **Dosing:** AML: 50 mg PO q12h on d 8–21 post induction & consolidation. Systemic Mastocytosis: 100 mg PO q12h. Renal or hepatic dose adjustments needed
- **PK/PD:** Metabolism CYP3A4, mean terminal $T_{1/2}$ 19–482 h (active metabolite)
- **AEs:** QTc prolongation, fatigue, rash, hepatotoxicity, nausea
- **Clinical pearls:** Administer w/ food, strongly consider antiemetic prophylaxis prior to each dose, monitor LFTs, supplied as 25-mg capsules

Neratinib (Nerlynx)

- **Dosing:** 240 mg once daily. **Renal:** No dose adjustment. **Hepatic:** Mild/mod. impairment—no adjustment. Sev. hepatic impairment: Reduce to 80 mg once daily
- **PK/PD:** Metabolism CYP3A4 P-gp inhibitor, $T_{1/2}$ 7–17 h
- **AEs:** Diarrhea/GI toxicity, skin rash, liver toxicity
- **Clinical pearls:** Administer w/ food; administer antidiarrheal prophylaxis during the first 56 d of therapy; monitor LFTs
- **DDI:** CYP3A4 inhibitors/inducers, PPIs, P-gp substrates

Nilotinib (Tasigna)

- **Dosing:** 300–400 mg PO every 12 h. **Renal:** No dose adjustments. **Hepatic:** (Child–Pugh A, B or C) start at 200–300 mg every 12 h, as tolerated. Dose adjust for Rx-induced tox (hepatic, hematologic, QTc, amylase/lipase)
- **PK/PD:** Metabolism via CYP3A4, $T_{1/2}$ = 17 h
- **AEs:** QTc prolongation, fatigue, rash, alopecia, hepatotoxicity, cardiac & vascular occlusive events, pancreatitis, fluid retention
- **DDI:** CYP3A4 inhibitors/inducers (↑/↓ conc. of nilotinib), PPI/H2 blocker/antacid (↓ nilotinib absorption), QTc-prolonging agents, warfarin (↑/↓ warfarin effects)
- **Clinical pearls:** Take on empty stomach. Inhibits CYP3A4 (↓ conc. of sensitive substrates). Monitor: QTc, liver enzymes, lipids, & glc at baseline & periodically. Antacid therapy at least 2 h prior to or after nilotinib dose (AVOID H2 blocker/PPI)

Niraparib (Zejula)

- **Dosing:** 200–300 mg PO daily; No renal dose adjustments recommended; Tbilli 1.5–3 × ULN & any AST: reduce dose to 200 mg daily; adjust dose for Rx-induced tox
- **PK/PD:** Metabolized by carboxylesterases; bioavailability ~73%; time to peak ~3 h; $T_{1/2}$ 6h
- **AEs:** Thrombocytopenia, anemia, neutropenia, hypertension, PRES, increased incidence of MDS/AML, skin rash, metabolic abnormalities, fatigue, ↑ liver enzymes, asthenia, musculoskeletal pain, increased SCr
- **DDI:** P-gp minor substrate
- **Clinical pearls:** Mod.-to-high emetic potential

Olaparib (Lynparza)

- **Dosing:** 300 mg PO BID. **Renal:** CrCl 31–50 mL/min: 200 mg BID; no data in CrCl <30 mL/min. **Hepatic:** No recommendations; no data for bilirubin >1.5× ULN & AST/ALT ≥2.5× ULN. Adjust dose for Rx-related tox
- **Concomitant CYP3A4 inhibitor: (strong)** 100 mg BID/**(mod.)** 150 mg BID
- **PK/PD:** Metabolism via CYP3A4; urinary excretion (44%), fecal excretion (42%); $T_{1/2}$ ~11.9 h
- **AEs:** Anemia, thrombocytopenia, neutropenia, nausea (low-emetic potential), fatigue, URI, myalgias, rash, increases in creatinine, 2° MDS/AML, pneumonitis
- **DDI:** CYP3A4 inhibitors/inducers (↑/↓ conc. of olaparib)

Osimertinib (Tagrisso)

- **Dosing:** 80 mg PO once daily; concurrent use w/ strong CYP3A4 inducer: Increase to 160 mg PO once daily; can reduce to 40 mg for tx-related tox
- **PK/PD:** Metabolized by CYP3A & dealkylation to 2 active metabolites
- **AEs:** Diarrhea, rash, dry skin, nail tox, ILD/pneumonitis, QTc prolongation, cardiomyopathy
- **DDI:** Strong CYP3A4 inducers ↓ exposure; inhibits BCRP (↑ exposure of rosuvastatin, sulfasalazine, topotecan)

Palbociclib (Ibrance)

- **Dosing:** 125 mg PO once a d × 21 d followed by 7 d off (28-d cycle). No hepatic or renal dose adjustment required. Dose adjusts for strong CYP3A inhibitors. Dose adjusts for Rx-induced tox
- **PK/PD:** Bioavailability 46%, food ↓ absorption, 85% protein bound, hepatically metabolized through CYP3A & SULT2A1, fecal (74.1%) & renal (17.5%) elimination, $T_{1/2}$ 29 h
- **AEs:** Neutropenia (75%), thrombocytopenia (17%), infxns, nausea, stomatitis, diarrhea, rash, alopecia, PE (1%)
- **DDI:** CYP3A inhibitors or inducers (↑/↓ conc. of palbociclib). Palbociclib is a weak CYP3A inhibitor
- **Clinical pearls:** Take w/ food. Monitor CBC on d 1 of each cycle & d 14 of the 1st 2 cycles. Available only through specialty pharmacies

Pazopanib (Votrient)

- **Dosing:** 800 mg PO daily. **Renal:** none. **Hepatic:** Tbili >1.5–3× ULN: 200 mg daily; Tbili >3× ULN: Use not recommended. Adjust dose for strong CYP3A4 inhibitors. Adjust dose for Rx-induced tox
- **PK/PD:** Bioavailability ↑ w/ food, hepatic metabolism via CYP3A4, $T_{1/2}$ 31 h
- **AEs:** HTN, diarrhea, edema, fatigue, hair color change, alopecia, hyperglycemia, hepatic, hematologic, GI, ILD/pneumonitis
- **DDI:** Statin (↑ hepatotoxicity of pazopanib), QTc-prolonging agents, CYP3A4 inhibitors/inducers (↑/↓ conc. of pazopanib), warfarin (↑/↓ warfarin effects), PPIs, P-gp, & BRCP inhibitors
- **Clinical pearls:** Take on empty stomach. Monitor: LFTs, LVEF, BP, thyroid, & ECG

Pexidartinib (Padcev)

- **Dosing:** 400 mg PO twice daily on empty stomach; reduce for mild-to-sev. renal dysfunction (200 mg in AM, 400 mg in PM); no adjustment for mild hepatic impairment (no data for mod./sev.), however avoid in active liver/biliary tract disease; manufacturer-recommended 2° reductions available for toxicity
- **PK/PD:** $T_{1/2}$ 26.6 h; hepatic metabolism (major CYP3A4); mixed fecal/renal excretion
- **AEs:** Hepatotoxicity (BBW, REMS program, 2 irreversible cases), hair color changes, elevated LDH, elevated cholesterol, myelosuppression, dysgeusia, minimal/low vomiting risk, eye edema
- **DDI:** Reduce starting dose for concomitant mod./strong CYP3A4 or UGT inhibitors; exposure reduced w/ concomitant acid-reducing agents; mod. CYP3A4 inducer
- **Clinical pearls:** Requires frequent LFT monitoring; may impair female & male fertility

Ponatinib (Iclusig)

- **Dosing:** 45 mg PO daily. **Renal:** No dose adjustments recommended. **Hepatic:** ALT/AST ≥3× ULN + bilirubin >2× ULN + alk phos <2× ULN: discontinue. AST/ALT >3× ULN, interrupt therapy until <3× ULN; restart at -1 dose level (45 > 30 > 15 mg). If tox occurs at 15 mg, DC therapy. Adjust dose for Rx-induced tox
  - **Concomitant strong CYP3A4 inhibitor:** 30 mg daily
- **PK/PD:** Hepatic metabolism via CYP3A4, $T_{1/2}$ 24 h
- **AEs:** Pancreatitis, ↑ LFTs, rash, cardiovascular events (HTN, HF, thromboembolism), fatigue, myelosuppression, GI, hyperglycemia, neuropathy, ocular tox, fluid retention
- **DDI:** CYP3A4 inhibitors/inducers (↑/↓ conc. of ponatinib)
- **Clinical pearls:** Active against *BCR-ABL* T315I mt. Monitor: Pancreatic enzymes, LFTs, CBC, s/sx VTE

Regorafenib (Stivarga)

- **Dosing:** 160 mg PO daily × 21 d of a 28-d cycle. No renal or hepatic dose adjustments recommended. Adjust dose for Rx-induced tox
- **PK/PD:** Metabolism via CYP3A4 & UGT1A9, $T_{1/2}$ 28 h
- **AEs:** HTN, palmar plantar erythrodysesthesia, diarrhea, mucositis, fatigue, electrolyte imbalances, hematologic, hepatic, GI, proteinuria, cardiac, wound healing impairment
- **DDI:** CYP3A4 inhibitors/inducers (↑/↓ conc. of regorafenib), warfarin (↑/↓ warfarin effects)
- **Clinical pearls:** Take w/ low-fat breakfast. Discontinue at least 2 wks prior to surgery (wound healing). Monitor: Blood pressure, rash, LFTs, electrolytes, CBC

Ribociclib (Kisqali)

- **Dosing:** 600 mg PO daily × 21 d of a 28-d cycle; CrCl 15–30 mL/min reduce dose to 200 mg daily; Mod.-to-sev. (Child–Pugh class B & C) reduce dose to 400 mg daily; Adjust dose for Rx-induced tox
- **PK/PD:** Hepatically metabolized through CYP3A4; 70% protein binding; time to peak 1–4 h; $T_{1/2}$ ~30–50 h

- **AEs:** Neutropenia, SJS/TENs, nausea, ↑ liver enzymes, ILD, QTc prolongation, alopecia, metabolic abnormalities, pruritis, gastroenteritis, infxns, arthralgia, increase Scr
- **DDI:** CYP3A4 major substrate; CYP3A4 mod. inhibitor
- **Clinical pearls:** Mod.-to-high emetic potential; LHRH agonist should be administered to pre/perimenopausal women receiving ribociclib in combination w/ an aromatase inhibitor or fulvestrant

Ripretinib (Qinlock)

- **Dosing:** 150 mg PO once daily; no adjustment for mild hepatic or mild/mod. renal impairment (no data for mod./sev. hepatic or sev. renal impairment); manufacturer-recommended 2° reductions available for toxicity
- **PK/PD:** $T_{1/2}$ ripretinib 14.8 h, equally active metabolite 17.8 h; hepatic metabolism (major CYP3A4 for ripretinib & active metabolite)
- **AEs:** Alopecia, fatigue, myalgia, diarrhea, increased aPTT, hand-foot syndrome, minimal/low vomiting risk, cardiac dysfunction (including heart failure), hypertension, new 1° skin cancers
- **DDI:** No guidance for dosing w/ CYP3A4 inhibitors; avoid use w/ strong CP3A4 **inducers;** P-gp inhibitor
- **Clinical pearls:** Assess baseline cardiac ejection fraction before initiation; hold for ≥1 wk pre-elective surgery & ≥2 wks post major surgery

Rucaparib (Rubraca)

- **Dosing:** 600 mg PO oral q12h; No renal or hepatic dose adjustments; adjust dose for Rx-induced tox
- **PK/PD:** Hepatically metabolized through CYP2D6; AUC increase & Tmax delayed followed by high-fat meal; 70% protein binding; bioavailability ~36%; Time to peak ~1.9 h; $T_{1/2}$ ~26 h
- **AEs:** Increase incidence of MDS/AML, skin rash, increase cholesterol, abdominal pain, constipation, anemia, ↑ liver enzymes, fatigue, asthenia, increase Scr, upper respiratory tract infxn
- **DDI:** Minor Substrate CYP1A2, CYP2D6, CYP3A4, P-gp; Inhibitor CYPA2 (mod.) & CYP3A4 (weak)
- **Clinical pearls:** Test for presence of *BRCA* mt; Mod.-to-high emetic potential

Ruxolitinib (Jakafi)

- **Dosing:** 5–25 mg PO every 12 h (doses based on plt count & disease indication). Dose adjustments based on response & tox
- **PK/PD:** Hepatic metabolism via CYP3A4, $T_{1/2}$ 3 h
- **AEs:** Edema, dizziness, headache, ↑ cholesterol, increased infxn risk (herpes zoster/HBV/TB reactivation)
- **DDI:** CYP3A4 inhibitors/inducers (↑/↓ conc. of ruxolitinib); avoid concomitant fluconazole >200 mg & strong CYP3A4 inhibitors
- **Clinical pearls:** Avoid abrupt discontinuation of therapy (disease flare in myeloproliferative neoplasm pts)
- **Monitor:** Dose adjust for hepatic & renal function, CBC every 2–4 wks until stable dose

Selinexor (Xpovio)

- **Dosing:** 60–80 mg twice weekly; 100 mg once weekly. No adjustments for mild-to-sev. renal dysfunction (no data for end-stage renal disease) or mild hepatic dysfunction (no data for mod./sev. hepatic impairment); manufacturer-recommended 2° reductions for toxicity available
- **PK/PD:** $T_{1/2}$ 6–8 h; hepatic metabolism (CYP3A4)
- **AEs:** Myelosuppression, diarrhea, mod./high vomiting risk, hyponatremia, pneumonia, ocular toxicity (new/worsening cataract)
- **DDI:** No significant interactions known (no pt-level data)
- **Clinical pearls:** Premedicate w/ antiemetic; trials indicate worse toxicity in elderly

Selpercatinib (Retevmo)

- **Dosing:** For adults & peds pts ≥12 y old: <50 kg: 120 mg orally twice daily; ≥50 kg: 160 mg orally twice daily; Reduce dose for sev. hepatic impairment (Tbili >3 –10× ULN)
- **PK/PD:** Metabolized predominantly by CYP3A4; $T_{1/2}$ = 32 h
- **AEs:** The most common adverse rxns, including laboratory abnormalities, (≥25%) ↑ LFTs, ↑ glucose, ↓ leukocytes, ↓ albumin, ↓ calcium, dry mouth, diarrhea, ↑ creatinine, hypertension, fatigue, edema, ↓ platelets, ↑ total cholesterol, rash, ↓ sodium, & constipation. Warnings of hepatotoxicity, hypertension, QT interval prolongation, hemorrhagic events, hypersensitivity, tumor lysis syndrome, risk of impaired wound healing, embryo-fetal toxicity

- **DDI:** Avoid concomitant use of acid reducing agents (PPIs, H2 receptor antagonists, & locally acting antacids) as they will ↓ selpercatinib plasma concentrations; avoid concomitant use of strong/mod. CYP3A inhibitors or inducers; if strong/mod. CYP3A inhibitors cannot be avoided, reduce the dose of selpercatinib & monitor QT interval more frequently; selpercatinib is mod. CYP2C8 inhibitor & a weak CYP3A inhibitor
- **Clinical pearls:** Take w/ or w/o food (unless administered w/ a PPI); Swallow capsules whole; withhold for ≥7 d prior to elective surgery & until wound healing has occurred

Sorafenib (Nexavar)

- **Dosing:** 400 mg PO every 12 h. No renal or hepatic dose adjustments required. Adjust dose for tox
- **PK/PD:** Hepatic metabolism via CYP3A4, $T_{1/2}$ 25–48 h
- **AEs:** Sensory neuropathy, HTN, rash, hepatic, hematologic, GI, alopecia, thyroid, cardiac (QTc prolongation)
- **DDI:** CYP3A4 inhibitors/inducers (↑/↓ conc. of sorafenib), warfarin (↑/↓ warfarin effects), carboplatin & paclitaxel (↑ AUC of sorafenib & paclitaxel), irinotecan (UGT1A1 substrates), docetaxel (↑ AUC), 5-FU (↑ AUC), CYP2B6 & CYP2C8 substrates (↑ exposure)
- **Clinical pearls:** Take on empty stomach. Monitor: Amylase/lipase, LFTs, BP

Sunitinib (Sutent)

- **Dosing:** 37.5–50 mg PO daily. Use caution in sev. renal or hepatic impairment. Adjust dose by 12.5 mg for tx-related tox
- **PK/PD:** Hepatic metabolism via CYP3A4, $T_{1/2}$ 40–60 h (parent) & 80–110 h (active metabolite)
- **AEs:** Diarrhea, nausea, mucositis/stomatitis, HTN, peripheral edema, rash, hand–foot syndrome, skin discoloration, hair color changes, altered taste, CV events (MI, myocardial ischemia, ↓ LVEF, CHF), ↑ QTc, TLS (RCC & GIST w/ ↑ tumor burden), thrombotic microangiopathy, proteinuria, sev. skin tox (SJS/TEN), thyroid dysfunction, hypoglycemia, ONJ, impaired wound healing
- **DDI:** CYP3A4 inhibitors/inducers (↑/↓ conc. of sunitinib), P-gp inhibitors (↑ conc. of sunitinib), QTc-prolonging agents, warfarin (↑/↓ warfarin effects)
- **Clinical pearls:** Monitor: LVEF, ECG, BP, oral exam prior to tx (ONJ risk)

Sonidegib (Odomzo)

- **Dosing:** 200 mg PO once daily. No hepatic dose adjustments, has not been studied in mod. or sev. hepatic impairment. No renal dose adjustments
- **PK/PD:** Hepatic metabolism through CYP3A, $T_{1/2}$ 28 d
- **AEs:** Muscle spasms, alopecia, myalgia, diarrhea, pruritus, headache, sev. birth defects, rhabdomyolysis
- **DDI:** CYP3A inhibitors/inducers (↑/↓ conc. of sonidegib)
- **Clinical pearls:** Take on an empty stomach. Pts should be counseled on embryo–fetal tox & to avoid blood donation. Monitor: CK, & SCr

Talazoparib (Talzenna)

- **Dosing:** 1 mg PO once daily. **Renal:** Reduce to 0.75 mg PO daily for CrCl 30–59 mL/min & 0.5 mg PO daily for CrCl 15–29 mL/min. CrCl <15 mL/min: Not studied. **Hepatic:** None
- **PK/PD:** Minimal hepatic metabolism, 69% excreted in urine (55% as unchanged drug), $T_{1/2}$ = 90 h
- **AEs:** Fatigue (62%), anemia (53%), nausea (49%), neutropenia, headache, thrombocytopenia, vomiting, diarrhea, decreased appetite, alopecia
- **DDI:** P-gp inhibitors or BCRP inhibitors (↑ talazoparib exposure). Consider dose reduction if used concomitantly
- **Clinical pearls:** Monitor CBC at baseline & monthly thereafter. 2° malignancy (MDS/AML) have been reported (rarely) in clinical trials

Tepotinib (Tepmetko)

- **Dosing:** 450 mg PO once daily; **Renal:** CrCl ≥30 mL/min—none (not studied <30 mL/min); **Hepatic:** Mild/mod. impairment—none (not studied in sev. impairment)
- **PK/PD:** Hepatic metabolism through CYP3A4 & 2C8; $T_{1/2}$ = 32 h
- **AEs:** ILD, hepatotoxicity, edema, fatigue
- **DDI:** CYP3A inhibitors/inducers (↑/↓ conc. of tepotinib), dual CYP3A + P-gp inhibitors, P-gp substrates w/ narrow therapeutic window
- **Clinical pearls:** Take w/ food. Monitor—LFTs, signs of ILD, signs of edema

Trametinib (Mekinist)

- **Dosing:** 2 mg PO once daily; dose reductions in increments of 0.5 mg PO daily, permanently discontinue if unable to tolerate 1 mg PO daily; not studied in mod.-to-sev. hepatic impairment or in renal impairment
- **PK/PD:** Metabolized by deacetylation or monooxygenation or in combination w/ glucuronidation; $T_{1/2}$ 4–5 d
- **AEs:** Rash, diarrhea, lymphedema (single-agent) pyrexia, nausea, rash, chills, diarrhea, vomiting, hypertension, peripheral edema (in combo w/ trametinib), cutaneous/non-cutaneous malignancies, hemorrhage, VTE, cardiomyopathy, ocular tox (RVO), ILD, serious febrile rxns, skin tox, hyperglycemia
- **DDI:** Not a substrate of CYP enzymes; inhibits CYP2C8, substrate of P-gp
- **Clinical pearls:** Administer 1 h before or 2 h after a meal; store in the refrigerator

Tivozanib (Fotivda)

- **Dosing:** 1.34 mg PO QD ×21 d then off ×7 d (28-d cycle); no renal dose adjustments; dose reduce to 0.89 mg in mod. hepatic impairment (tbili >1.5–3× ULN); dose reduce for toxicity
- **PK/PD:** Highly protein bound; metabolized predominantly by CYP3A4; $T_{1/2}$ 111 h
- **AEs:** Hypertension, cardiac failure, arterial thrombosis, hemorrhage, proteinuria, stomatitis, reverse posterior leukoencephalopathy syndrome, thyroid dysfunction, anorexia, rash
- **DDI:** Avoid Strong CYP3A4 inducers
- **Clinical pearls:** Take w/ or w/o food; mod.-to-high emetic risk (use antiemetics); hold tivozanib 24 h before surgery & wait to restart for 2 wks; monitor blood pressure 2 wks after initiating & monthly while on therapy; monitor TSH/T4 at initiation & at regular intervals during therapy; monitor for allergic rxns in pts w/ allergies to FD&C Yellow No.5 (tartrazine)

Umbralisib (Ukoniq)

- **Dosing:** 800 mg once daily; **renal:** CrCl ≥30 mL/min—no adjustment (not studied <30 mL/min); **hepatic:** Mild/mod. impairment—no adjustment (not studied in sev. impairment)
- **PK/PD:** Metabolism CYP2C9, CYP3A4, CYP1A2, $T_{1/2}$ 91 h
- **AEs:** Hematologic, diarrhea/colitis, infxns/opportunistic infxns, rash
- **Clinical pearls:** Administer w/ food; Administer PCP prophylaxis during tx; consider antiviral prophylaxis to prevent CMV infxn. Contains FD&C Yellow No. 5-caution w/ allergy

Vandetanib (Caprelsa)

- **Dosing:** 300 mg PO once daily. Renal: CrCl <50 mL/min: 200 mg daily. Mod.-to-sev. hepatic impairment: Use not recommended. Adjust dose for tox
- **PK/PD:** Hepatic metabolism via CYP3A4, $T_{1/2}$ 19 d
- **AEs:** HTN, ↑ QTc, skin tox, photosensitivity, insomnia (13%), fatigue, GI, hematologic, corneal abnormalities, hepatic, ↑ SCr, ILD, ischemic cerebrovascular events, HF
- **DDI:** CYP3A4 inhibitors/inducers (↑/↓ conc. of vandetanib), QTc-prolonging agents
- **Clinical pearls:** QTc >450 ms: Withhold Rx. Monitor: Electrolytes, TSH, ECG, renal & hepatic function, BP, s/s HF

Vemurafenib (Zelboraf)

- **Dosing:** 960 mg PO every 12 h. No renal or hepatic dosing. Adjust dose for tox
- **PK/PD:** Metabolism through CYP3A4, fecal excretion (94%), $T_{1/2}$ 57 h
- **AEs:** Edema, fatigue, arthralgia/myalgia, skin tox (photosensitivity, rash), GI, ↑ GGT, cough, NM, skeletal, hepatic, QTc prolongation, hepatic, radiation sensitization & radiation recall, kidney dysfunction
- **DDI:** CYP3A4 inhibitors/inducers (↑/↓ conc. of vemurafenib), P-gp inhibitors (↑ conc. of vemurafenib), QTc-prolonging agents, warfarin (↑/↓ warfarin effects), CY1A2 substrates (↑ conc.)
- **Clinical pearls:** Monitor: LFTs, EKG, electrolytes, SCr, skin tox, s/s of uveitis

Venetoclax (Venclexta)

- **Dosing:**
  - **CLL:** Wk 1: 20 mg daily, wk 2: 50 mg daily, wk 3: 100 mg daily, wk 4: 200 mg daily, wk 5+: 400 mg daily
  - **AML (unfit for induction):** Day 1: 100 mg, Day 2: 200 mg, Day 3+: 400 mg

- **Adjustments**
  - **Renal:** No adjustments (↑ TLS risk w/ impairment); **Hepatic:** None
  - **Strong CYP3A4 inhibitor**
    - Initiation & ramp up phase: Contraindicated
    - Maintenance: Avoid use or if necessary reduce venetoclax dose by 75%
  - **Mod. CYP3A4 inhibitor or P-gp inhibitor**
    - General: Avoid use or if necessary, reduce venetoclax dose by 50%
    - May resume original venetoclax dose inhibitor 2–3 d after inhibitor discontinuation
    - Rx-related tox: Adjust dose per indication
- **PK/PD:** Venetoclax is a substrate of CYP3A4/5 & P-glycoprotein (P-gp). Strong inhibitor of P-gp; $T_{1/2}$ 26 h
- **AEs:** TLS, diarrhea, nausea, myelosuppression
- **DDI:** CYP3A4 inhibitors/inducers (↑/↓ conc. of venetoclax), P-gp inhibitors (↑ conc. of venotoclax), p-gp substrates (↑ substrate)
- **Clinical pearls:** Take w/ low fat meal. Avoid grapefruit juice/Seville oranges & star fruit. All pts should be on allopurinol prior to initiation. Monitor: TLS labs, serum creatinine, CBC

Vismodegib (Erivedge)

- **Dosing:** 150 mg PO once daily. No renal or hepatic dose adjustments required
- **PK/PD:** Metabolism through oxidation, glucuronidation, & pyridine ring cleavage. $T_{1/2}$ ~4 d
- **AEs:** Muscle spasms, alopecia, weight loss, arthralgias, ageusia
- **DDI:** No known significant interactions
- **Clinical pearls:** Monitor pregnancy status. Pts should be counseled on embryo–fetal tox & to avoid blood donation

Zanubrutinib (Brukinsa)

- **Dosing:** 160 mg PO BID or 320 mg PO once daily; Sev. hepatic impairment (Child–Pugh C): 80 mg PO BID; grade 3 neutropenic fever, grade 4 neutropenia >10 d, grade 3 thrombocytopenia w/ bleeding, grade 4 thrombocytopenia (lasting >10 d), nonhematologic toxicity grade ≥3: 1st occurrence interrupt & resume at 160 mg BID or 320 mg once daily when grade ≤1, 2nd occurrence interrupt tx & resume at 80 mg BID or 160 mg once daily when grade ≤1, 3rd occurrence interrupt tx & resume at 80 mg once daily when grade ≤1, 4th occurrence discontinue therapy
- **PK/PD:** Metabolism 1° via CYP3A & major CYP3A4 substrate, $T_{1/2}$ ~2–4 h
- **AEs:** Cytopenias, rash, HTN, afib, ↑ LFTs, diarrhea, fatigue, skin rash, ↓ K, muscle pain
- **Clinical pearls:** Screen for hepatitis B prior to starting therapy, minimal or low emetic potential, hold 3–7 d prior to & after surgery

Info based on publicly available drug inserts from Janssen, Boehringer Ingelheim, Gilead, Pfizer, Exelixis, Genentech, Bristol-Myers Squibb, AstraZeneca, Eisai, Novartis, GlaxoSmithKline, Ariad, Bayer, & Incyte. Accessed April 2021.

Class	Drugs	Mechanism
Androgen receptor signaling inhibitor	Enzalutamide	No known agonist properties, inhibits DNA binding, nuclear translocation → cell apoptosis
CYP17 inhibitor	Abiraterone	Irreversible binding of CYP17 → ↓ production of androgen precursors dehydroepiandrosterone & androstenedione
Antiandrogen	Bicalutamide, flutamide, nilutamide apalutamide	Inhibition of androgen uptake via binding inhibition in target tissue
GnRH agonist	Goserelin, leuprolide	Agonist of LHRH → continuous stimulation leads to ↓ LH/FSH → suppression of steroidogenesis
GnRH antagonist	Degarelix	Binds to GnRH → ↓ LH/FSH production → suppression of steroidogenesis
Aromatase inhibitor	Anastrozole & letrozole (nonsteroidal), exemestane (steroidal)	Inhibition of aromatase → prevention of androstenedione to estrone & testosterone to estradiol conversion
ER antagonist/SERD	Fulvestrant	Competitive binding to ER in target tissue → ↓ regulation of ER
SERM	Raloxifene, tamoxifen	Competitive binding to ER in target tissue → ↓ DNA synthesis, accumulation of cells in G0 & G1 phase

Enzalutamide (Xtandi)

- **Dosing:** 160 mg oral daily (4–40-mg capsules). No renal or hepatic dose adjustments recommended. Concomitant strong CYP2C8 inhibitors: 80 mg oral daily. Adjust/withhold dose for grade ≥3 tox
- **PK/PD:** Rapid absorption, ~97–98% protein bound, hepatic metabolism via CYP2C8 & CYP3A4, renal excretion (~70%), $T_{1/2}$ 5.8 d
- **AEs:** Peripheral edema, fatigue, HA, hot flashes, diarrhea, back pain, arthralgia, dizziness, seizure (0.9%)
- **DDI:** Strong CYP3A4 inducer, mod. CYP2C9 & 2C19 inducer, avoid use w/ narrow therapeutic index agents metabolized via these enzymes, CYP3A4 inducers (↓ conc. of enzalutamide), strong CYP2C8 inhibitors (gemfibrozil, ↑ conc. of enzalutamide), CYP2C8 inducers (↓ conc. of enzalutamide), warfarin (↑ risk of bleeding)
- **Clinical pearls:** Can be taken w/ or w/o food. Potential ↑ in CV dz risk w/ androgen deprivation Rx

Abiraterone (Zytiga)

- **Dosing:** 1,000 mg oral daily (4–250-mg tablets). No renal dose adjustment recommended. Hepatic (prior): Child–Pugh class B: 250 mg oral daily, Child–Pugh class C: avoid; hepatic (during): AST/ALT >5× ULN or Tbili >3× ULN: withhold until AST/ALT <2.5× ULN & Tbili <1.5× ULN, resume at 750 mg oral daily, if recurrent, ↓ to 500 mg oral daily
- **PK/PD:** ↑ absorption w/ food (AUC ↑ 10-fold), >99% protein bound, extensive distribution, hydrolyzed to active metabolite, metabolism via CYP3A4/SULT2A1 to inactive metabolites, $T_{1/2}$ 14–16 h
- **AEs:** Mineralocorticoid excess (edema, HTN, ↓ K), fatigue, ↑ TG, hyperglycemia, ↑ LFTs, joint swelling, hot flashes, cough, insomnia
- **DDI:** Strong inhibitor of CYP1A2, CYP2D6, CYP2C8; mod. inhibitor of CYP2C9, CYP2C19, CYP2C8. Strong CYP3A4 inhibitors/inducers (↑/↓ effect of abiraterone), CYP2D6 substrates w/ narrow therapeutic index (eg, thioridazine, ↑ effect of substrate)
- **Clinical pearls:** Take on empty stomach (at least 1 h before or 2 h after food), administered in combination w/ prednisone 5 mg oral twice daily (suppression of ACTH drive). Monitor LFTs before starting, every 2 wks × 3 mos, then monthly while on Rx

Bicalutamide (Casodex)

- **Dosing:** 50 mg oral daily in combination w/ LHRH analog OR 150 mg oral daily as monotherapy. No renal dose adjustment recommended. Use caution in mod.-to-sev. hepatic impairment; ALT >2× ULN: D/C
- **PK/PD:** 96% protein bound, extensive hepatic metabolism, mod. renal excretion (~36%), $T_{1/2}$ ~6 d (↑ to 10 d in sev. liver dz)
- **AEs:** Peripheral edema, pain, hot flashes, breast pain, gynecomastia (38–39%), constipation/diarrhea, pelvic pain, weakness, bone pain, dizziness, dyspnea, ↓ glc tolerance
- **DDI:** CYP3A4 inhibitor, CYP3A4 substrates (↑ conc. of substrate), warfarin (↑ bleeding risk)
- **Clinical pearls:** Can be taken w/ or w/o food. Potential ↑ in CV dz risk w/ androgen deprivation Rx

Flutamide (Eulexin)

- **Dosing:** 250 mg oral every 8 h. No renal dose adjustment recommended. Use contraindicated in sev. hepatic impairment, ALT >2× ULN: Avoid use
- **PK/PD:** ~94% protein binding, extensive hepatic metabolism, renal excretion, $T_{1/2}$ 5–6 h
- **AEs: Hepatotoxicity (BBW),** gynecomastia, hot flashes, breast tenderness, impotence, ↓ libido, tumor flare, ↑ AST (transient), ↑ LDH (transient), N/V, diarrhea
- **DDI:** Abiraterone, mod.-to-strong CYP1A2 inhibitors, mod.-to-strong CYP3A4 inhibitors. Dasatinib (↑ levels of flutamide), CYP1A2 inducers, CYP3A4 inducers (↓ levels of flutamide), warfarin (↑ risk of bleeding)
- **Clinical pearls:** Supplied as 125-mg capsule. Can be taken w/ or w/o food. Potential ↑ in CV dz risk w/ androgen deprivation Rx. Measure LFTs before starting Rx

Nilutamide (Nilandron)

- **Dosing:** 300 mg oral daily × 1 mo, then 150 mg oral daily. No renal dose adjustments recommended. Sev. hepatic impairment: Contraindicated. ALT >2× ULN or jaundice (on Rx): D/C
- **PK/PD:** Rapid absorption, extensive hepatic metabolism, renal excretion (62%), $T_{1/2}$ 38–59 h, 59–126 h (metabolites)
- **AEs: Interstitial pneumonitis (BBW),** HA, hot flashes, insomnia, breast tenderness, impotence, ↓ libido, tumor flare, ↑ AST/ALT, N/V, constipation, **impaired dark adaptation (up to 57%)**
- **DDI:** CYP2C19 inhibitors/inducers (↑/↓ conc. of nilutamide), ethanol (intolerance)
- **Clinical pearls:** Supplied as 150-mg tablet. Can be taken w/ or w/o food

Apalutamide (Erleada)

- **Dosing:** 240 mg oral daily. No renal & hepatic dose adjustments recommended.
- **PK/PD:** Bioavailability is 100%, extensive hepatic metabolism, renal excretion (65%), $T_{1/2}$ ~3 d
- **AEs: Cerebrovascular and ischemic cardiovascular events,** seizure, fatigue, arthralgia, rash, decreased appetite, fall, weight decreased, hypertension, hot flush, diarrhea, & fracture
- **DDI:** CYP2C8 & 3A4 inhibitors/inducers (↑/↓ conc. of apalutamide), a strong inducer of CYP3A4 & CYP2C19, & a weak inducer of CYP2C9, P-gp, BCRP, & OATP1B1
- **Clinical pearls:** Supplied as 60-mg tablet. Can be taken w/ or w/o food

Goserelin (Zoladex)

- **Dosing: Prostate CA (advanced):** 3.6 mg SC every 28 d OR 10.8 mg every 12 wks; **prostate CA (local w/ antiandrogens + RT):** 3.6 mg SC every 28 d × 4 doses or 3.6 mg once followed by 10.8-mg implant; **breast CA:** 3.6 mg SC every 28 d. No renal or hepatic dose adjustments recommended
- **PK/PD:** Estradiol & testosterone suppression w/in 2–4 wks; rapid absorption; slow release × 8 d, then continuous release × 28 d; renal excretion (90% unchanged), $T_{1/2}$ 4 h (males, ↑ to 12 h in renal impairment), 2 h (females)
- **AEs:** Peripheral edema, HA (up to 75% in females), emotional lability/depression (↑ females), acne/seborrhea, hot flashes, ↓ libido, ↓ **BMD,** tumor flare, **hyperglycemia,** vaginal dryness
- **DDI:** No known significant drug interactions
- **Clinical pearls:** Tumor flare can be alleviated w/ concomitant antiandrogen Rx, consider Ca & vit D supplementation while on goserelin. Potential ↑ in CV dz risk w/ androgen deprivation Rx

Leuprolide (Lupron, Lupron Depot, Eligard)

- **Dosing: Prostate CA:** Lupron (IM), Eligard (SC): 7.5 mg every mo, 22.5 mg every 12 wks, 30 mg every 16 wks, 45 mg every 24 wks; **breast CA:** 3.75 mg every 28 d OR 11.25 mg every 3 mos, continue up to 24 mos. No renal or hepatic dose adjustments recommended
- **PK/PD:** Testosterone suppression w/in 2–4 wks, ~45% protein bound
- **AEs:** Injection-site pain, edema, HA, fatigue, depression, hot flashes, ↓ libido, vaginitis, ↓ BMD, ↑ glc
- **DDI:** Antidiabetic agents (potential ↑ glc & insulin resistance)
- **Clinical pearls:** Tumor flare can be alleviated w/ concomitant antiandrogen Rx, consider Ca & vit D supplementation while on goserelin. Potential ↑ in CV dz risk w/ androgen deprivation Rx

Degarelix (Firmagon)

- **Dosing:** Loading dose: 240 mg (2–120 mg injections) SC × 1; maintenance dose: 80 mg SC every 28 d. Use w/ caution in CrCl <50 mL/min & in sev. hepatic impairment.
- **PK/PD:** Biphasic release, rapid onset of action (w/in 3 d), ~90% protein bound, hepatobiliary metabolism via hydrolysis, mod. renal excretion (~30%), $T_{1/2}$ ~53 d
- **AEs:** Hot flashes, injection-site rxns, ↑ LFTs, Ab formation, wt gain, arthralgia
- **DDI:** QTc-prolonging agents (↑ QTc prolongation)
- **Clinical pearls:** Consider Ca & vit D supplementation while on degarelix

Anastrozole (Arimidex)

- **Dosing:** 1 mg oral daily. No renal dose adjustment recommended. Use caution in sev. hepatic impairment
- **PK/PD:** 40% protein bound; extensive hepatic metabolism (~85%); onset of estradiol reduction 70% after 24 h, 80% after 2 wks; $T_{1/2}$ 50 h
- **AEs:** Vasodilation, HTN, fatigue, HA, hot flashes, mood disturbance, ↓ **BMD,** ↑ **cholesterol (↑ CV risk), arthralgia,** weakness, fatigue, peripheral edema, ↑ LFTs, insomnia
- **DDI:** Estrogen derivatives (↓ anastrozole effect), tamoxifen (↓ efficacy of anastrozole, conc. ↓ by 27%)
- **Clinical pearls:** Can be taken w/ or w/o food, consider Ca & vit D supplementation while on anastrozole

Letrozole (Femara)

- **Dosing:** 2.5 mg oral daily. No renal dose adjustment recommended. Sev. hepatic dysfunction (Child–Pugh class C) & cirrhosis: 2.5 mg oral every other d
- **PK/PD:** Rapid absorption, hepatic metabolism via CYP3A4/2D6, renal excretion (90%), $T_{1/2}$ 2 d
- **AEs:** Edema, HA, ↑ **cholesterol,** hot flashes, weakness, **arthralgia,** ↓ **BMD,** diaphoresis, fatigue, dizziness
- **DDI:** CYP2A6 substrates (↑ conc. of substrate), tamoxifen (↓ conc. of letrozole by 38%)
- **Clinical pearls:** Can be taken w/ or w/o food, consider Ca & vit D supplementation while on letrozole

Exemestane (Aromasin)

- **Dosing:** 25 mg oral daily. Use caution in pts w/ mod.-to-sev. renal or hepatic dysfunction. Concomitant CYP3A4 inducer: 50 mg oral daily
- **PK/PD:** 40% ↑ absorption w/ high-fat meal, 90% protein bound, extensive tissue distribution, hepatic oxidation via CYP3A4, mod. renal excretion (~40%), $T_{1/2}$ 24 h
- **AEs:** HTN, fatigue, insomnia, HA, depression, **hyperhidrosis,** hot flashes, nausea, arthralgia, ↑ alk phos, edema, dizziness, ↓ BMD
- **DDI:** CYP3A4 inducers (↓ conc. of exemestane), no effect of CYP3A4 inhibitors
- **Clinical pearls:** Administer after a meal, consider Ca & vit D supplementation while on exemestane

Fulvestrant (Faslodex)

- **Dosing:** 500 mg IM d 1, 15, 29, then 500 mg IM monthly. No renal dose adjustment recommended. Hepatic: Child–Pugh class B: ↓ initial & maintenance dose to 250 mg; Child–Pugh class C: caution advised
- **PK/PD:** Steady state achieved ~1 mo, 99% protein bound, hepatic metabolism (CYP3A4 involved but contribution unknown), $T_{1/2}$ ~40 d
- **AEs:** Hot flashes, ↑ LFTs, joint disorders, injection-site pain, bone pain, arthralgia, fatigue, HA, nausea, vasodilation, pharyngitis

- **DDI:** No known significant drug interactions
- **Clinical pearls:** IM administration ONLY. Each 500-mg dose requires 2 IM injections

Raloxifene (Evista)

- **Dosing: Breast CA risk reduction:** 60 mg oral daily × 5 y. Use caution w/ mod.-to-sev. renal impairment. Use caution in hepatic impairment (↑ conc. in hepatic impairment).
- **PK/PD:** Rapid absorption, bioavailability ~2%, onset 8 wks, >95% protein bound (albumin & α-glycoprotein), hepatic metabolism, extensive 1st-pass metabolism, $T_{1/2}$ 28–33 h
- **AEs: ↑ VTE risk (BBW), ↑ risk of stroke (BBW),** peripheral edema, hot flashes, arthralgia, leg cramps, flu-like syndrome
- **DDI:** Levothyroxine (↓ effects of levothyroxine), bile acid sequestrants (↓ absorption of raloxifene)
- **Clinical pearls:** Can be taken w/ or w/o food

Tamoxifen (Nolvadex, Soltamox)

- **Dosing:** 20 mg oral daily. No renal or hepatic dose adjustments recommended
- **PK/PD:** Well absorbed, distributes well into uterine, endometrial, & breast tissue, 99% protein bound, hepatic metabolism via CYP2D6 & CYP3A4/5, min. renal excretion (~10%), $T_{1/2}$ (tamoxifen) 5–7 d, (metabolite) ~14 d
- **AEs:** ↑ uterine/endometrial CA (BBW), ↑ **VTE risk (BBW),** flushing, vasodilation, skin changes, hot flashes, fluid retention, amenorrhea, nausea, wt loss, vaginal d/c, weakness, arthralgia
- **DDI:** CYP2D6 inhibitors (↓ conc. of tamoxifen, risk ↑ breast CA recurrence), SSRI (↓ tamoxifen efficacy, esp. fluoxetine, paroxetine, sertraline) (*J Clin Psychiatry* 2009;70:1688), QTc-prolonging agents (↑ QTc prolongation), P-gp substrates (↓ conc. of substrates), CYP3A4 inhibitors/inducers (↑/↓ conc. of tamoxifen), CYP2C9 inhibitors/inducers (↑/↓ conc. of tamoxifen), grapefruit juice (↓ metabolism of tamoxifen)
- **Clinical pearls:** CYP2D6 poor metabolizers (↓ endoxifen conc. & efficacy), can be taken w/ or w/o food

Info based on publicly available drug inserts from Abbott, Astellas, AstraZeneca, Eli Lilly, Janssen, Novartis, Schering, and Sanofi-Aventis.

BONE-MODIFYING AGENTS

Drug Class	Agents	Mechanism
Bisphosphonate	Alendronate Etidronate Ibandronate Risedronate Pamidronate Zoledronate	Inhibit osteoclast-mediated bone resorption & promote bone mineralization
Monoclonal Ab	Denosumab	RANKL inhibitor to receptor activator of RANKL → inhibits osteoclasts to promote bone mineralization

Alendronate (Fosamax)

- **Dosing:** Ppx: 35 mg oral weekly or 5 mg oral daily. Tx: 70 mg oral weekly or 10 mg oral daily. CrCl <35 mL/min: Use not recommended. No hepatic dose adjustments
- **PK/PD:** Poor bioavailability (fasting 0.6%, ↓ up to 60% w/ food), 78% protein bound, fecal & urinary excretion (unabsorbed drug), $T_{1/2}$ 10 y
- **AEs:** ONJ, ↓ Ca, GI irritation & esophageal erosion (pts should remain upright ≥30 min post dose), & muscle pain
- **DDI:** Antacid/PPI/mineral-containing medications (↓ absorption of oral bisphosphonate), NSAIDs & aspirin (↑ GI irritation)
- **Clinical pearls:** Take w/ water in AM, ≥30 min prior to medications or food, & do not lie down ≥30 min post dose. Not indicated for malignant hypercalcemia. Use concurrent Ca & vit D supplements for indications other than hypercalcemia. Ensure good oral health before starting Rx

Etidronate (Didronel)

- **Dosing:** 5–20 mg/kg/d orally. Use w/ caution & consider dose reduction in renal & hepatic impairment
- **PK/PD:** 3% oral absorption, fecal & urinary excretion
- **Adverse effect:** GI upset, ONJ, ↓ Ca, esophageal erosion (pts should remain upright ≥30 min post dose), muscle pain
- **DDI:** Antacid/PPI/mineral-containing medications (↓ absorption of oral bisphosphonate), NSAIDs & aspirin (↑ GI irritation), warfarin (↑ bleeding risk)
- **Clinical pearls:** Take w/ water in AM, ≥30 min prior to medications or food, & do not lie down ≥30 min post dose. Not indicated for malignant hypercalcemia. Use concurrent Ca & vit D supplements for indications other than hypercalcemia. Ensure good oral health prior to Rx

Ibandronate (Boniva)

- **Dosing:** Osteoporosis: 150 mg oral monthly or 3 mg IV every 3 mos. Hypercalcemia (unlabeled use): 2–6 mg IV infused over 1–2 h once or every 3–4 wks for bone met in breast CA. CrCl <30 mL/min: Use is not recommended. No hepatic dose adjustments recommended
- **PK/PD:** Min. absorption (90% ↓ post breakfast), 86–99.5% protein bound, fecal & urinary excretion, $T_{1/2}$ (IV) 5–25 h, (oral) 37–157 h
- **AEs:** GI, back pain (<14%), ONJ, esophageal erosion (pts should remain upright ≥30 min post dose)
- **DDI:** Antacid/PPI/mineral-containing medications (↓ absorption of oral bisphosphonate), NSAIDs, & aspirin (↑ GI irritation)
- **Clinical pearls:** Oral form not indicated for malignant hypercalcemia. IV can be used off label in oncology. Take w/ water in AM, ≥30 min prior to medications or food & do not lie down ≥30 min post dose. Use concurrent Ca & vit D supplements for indications other than hypercalcemia

Risedronate (Actonel)

- **Dosing:** 5 mg oral daily or 35 mg weekly or 150 mg monthly. CrCl <30 mL/min: Use not recommended. No hepatic dose adjustments recommended
- **PK/PD:** Poor bioavailability, 24% protein bound, fecal & urinary excretion, $T_{1/2}$ up to 456 h

- **AEs:** HTN (11%), HA (<18%), rash (<12%), peripheral edema (8%), GI, arthralgia (<33%), UTI (11%), other infxn ≤31%, ONJ, esophageal erosion (pts should remain upright ≥30 min post dose)
- **DDI:** Antacid/PPI/mineral-containing medications (↓ absorption of oral bisphosphonate), NSAIDs, & aspirin (↑ GI irritation)
- **Clinical pearls:** Take w/ water in AM, ≥30 min prior to medications or food, & do not lie down ≥30 min post dose. Not indicated for malignant hypercalcemia. Use concurrent Ca & vit D supplements for indications other than hypercalcemia. Ensure good oral health before starting Rx

Pamidronate (Aredia)

- **Dosing:** Hypercalcemia: 60–90 mg IV once, may repeat every 7 d. Myeloma & breast CA: 90 mg IV over 2 h monthly. CrCl <30 mL/min or SCr >3 mg/dL: Myeloma: infuse over 4–6 h &/or use ↓ dose. Other indications: Not recommended or use w/ extreme caution
- **PK/PD:** Up to 24 h for ↓ in albumin-corrected serum Ca; max effect up to 7 d, urinary excretion w/in 120 h, $T_{1/2}$ 21–35 h
- **AEs: Acute renal** tox (esp. in myeloma pts), electrolyte imbalances (↓ K, phos, Mg, Ca), fevers (<39%), HA, fatigue, ONJ
- **DDI:** Thalidomide (↑ nephrotoxicity), other nephrotoxic agents
- **Clinical pearls:** Check SCr before each dose. Longer infusion (>2 h) may ↓ risk of renal tox. Ensure good oral health prior to Rx

Zoledronate (Zometa, Reclast)

- **Dosing:** Zometa (Oncology): Malignant hypercalcemia 4 mg IV once, may repeat after 7 d. Myeloma: 4 mg IV monthly. Reclast (osteoporosis): 5 mg IV yearly or every 2 y. Nononcology use: CrCl <35 mL/min: Use is not recommended. Myeloma or bone mets: CrCl 50–60 mL/min: 3.5 mg; 40–49 mL/min: 3.3 mg; 30–39 mL/min: 3 mg; <30 mL/min: use not recommended. Malignant hypercalcemia: Sev. renal impairment (SCr >4 mg/dL): Use w/ extreme caution
- **PK/PD:** Low protein binding (28–53%), urinary excretion w/in 24 h, $T_{1/2}$ 146 h
- **AEs:** Acute infusion rxn (flu-like sx) w/in 3 d post infusion (up to 44%), **acute renal** tox (esp. in myeloma pts), alopecia, ONJ, electrolyte disturbances (↓ K, phos, Mg, Ca)
- **DDI:** Thalidomide (↑ nephrotoxicity), other nephrotoxic agents
- **Clinical pearls:** Check SCr before each dose. ↑ infusion time may ↓ renal tox. APAP prior & 72 h post infusion may ↓ incidence of infusion rxn. Ensure good oral health prior to Rx

Denosumab (Xgeva, Prolia)

- **Dosing:** Prevention of **skeletal events** in solid tumors **(Xgeva):** 120 mg SC every 4 wks. Prevention of **bone loss (Prolia):** 60 mg SC every 6 mos. Prolia: No renal dose adjustment. Xgeva: Not studied in renal impaired pts. Hepatic impairment: Not studied
- **PK/PD:** 60% SC bioavailability, $T_{1/2}$ 25–28 d
- **AEs:** ONJ, rash, fatigue, flu-like sx, ↓ calcium, ↓ phos, GI tox, infxn, & peripheral edema
- **DDI:** No formal studies have been conducted
- **Clinical pearls:** Oral exam prior to Rx. Monitor for s/s of infxn. May cause fetal harm

Info based on publicly available drug inserts from: Merck, Procter & Gamble, Genetech, Warner Chilcott, Novartis, & Amgen. Accessed February 17, 2013.

NOVEL ORAL ANTICOAGULANTS (NOAC)

NOAC Targets	
Apixaban (Eliquis)	Factor Xa
Dabigatran (Pradaxa)	Factor IIa
Edoxaban (Savaysa)	Factor Xa
Rivaroxaban (Xarelto)	Factor Xa

Apixaban (Eliquis)

- **Dosing:**
  - VTE tx: 10 mg PO BID d 1–7, then 5 mg PO BID → 2.5 mg PO BID after ≥6 mos
  - Nonvalvular atrial fibrillation: 5 mg PO BID
  - DVT prophylaxis following hip/knee replacement surgery: 2.5 mg PO BID 12–24 h postsurgery
- **Dose adjustments:**
  - *General:* 2.5 mg PO BID for pts w/ ≥**2** of the following: ≥80 yo, ≤60 kg, serum creatinine ≥1.5 mg/dL
  - *Concomitant dual CYP3A4 & P-gp Inhibitors:* 5–10 mg PO BID ↓ dose by 50%; *avoid* use if current dose is 2.5 mg PO BID
- **PK/PD:** Food does not affect bioavailability, extensively metabolized via CYP3A4 & substrate of P-gp. Renal excretion accounts for ~27% of total clearance. $T_{1/2}$ of 12 h
- **DDI:** Inhibitors of CYP3A4 & P-gp (eg, amiodarone, ritonavir) ↑ exposure to apixaban. Inducers of CYP3A4 & P-gp (eg, phenytoin, rifampin) ↓ exposure to apixaban
- **Clinical pearls:** 5-mg & 2.5-mg tablets may be crushed & suspended in apple juice, applesauce, or water (stable for up to 4 h). No commercially available reversal agent. PT, INR, & aPTT will be prolonged but are NOT useful for therapeutic monitoring. Conversion from non-warfarin anticoagulant (parental & oral): Start apixaban at the time of next scheduled dose. Conversion from warfarin: Stop warfarin & start apixaban when INR <2.0

Dabigatran Etexilate (Pradaxa)

- **Dosing:**
  - VTE tx/reduction in risk of recurrence:
    - CrCl >30 mL/min: 150 mg PO BID
    - CrCl ≤30 mL/min or dialysis: No recommendation
    - CrCl <50 mL/min + concomitant P-gp inhibitor: Avoid combination
  - Nonvalvular atrial fibrillation:
    - CrCl >30 mL/min: 150 mg PO BID
    - CrCl 15–30 mL/min: 75 mg PO BID
    - CrCl <15 mL/min or dialysis: No recommendation
    - CrCl 30–50 mL/min + concomitant P-gp inhibitor: 75 mg PO BID
    - CrCl <30 mL/min + concomitant P-gp inhibitor: Avoid combination
  - VTE prophylaxis following hip replacement surgery:
    - CrCl >30 mL/min: 110 mg PO on 1st d, then 220 mg PO once daily
    - CrCl ≤30 mL/min or dialysis: No recommendation
    - CrCl <50 mL/min + concomitant P-gp inhibitor: Avoid combination
- **Dose adjustments:** As above per indication
- **PK/PD:** Prolongs aPTT (provides approximate anticoagulation effect), **1**° renal clearance, $T_{1/2}$ 12–17 h, prodrug converted to dabigatran
- **DDI:** P-gp inducers (rifampin) ↓ exposure to dabigatran; P-gp inhibitors (dronedarone, ketoconazole) ↑ exposure to dabigatran
- **Clinical pearls:** Take w/ or w/o food; specific reversal agent (idarucizumab) available for dabigatran reversal for emergent surgery/urgent procedures or in life-threatening/uncontrolled bleeding; conversion from parenteral anticoagulants → start dabigatran etexilate 0–2 h before next scheduled dose; conversion from warfarin → stop warfarin & start rivaroxaban when INR <2.0

Edoxaban (Savaysa)

- **Dosing:**
  - VTE tx:
    - CrCl >50 mL/min: 60 mg PO daily
    - CrCl 15–50 mL/min or <60 kg or verapamil, quinidine, or dronedarone: 30 mg PO daily

- Nonvalvular atrial fibrillation:
  - CrCl >95 mL/min: AVOID use
  - CrCl >50–≤95 mL/min: 60 mg PO daily
  - CrCl 15–50 mL/min: 30 mg PO daily
- **Dose adjustments:** As above per indication
- **PK/PD:** Metabolism via hydrolysis CYP3A4. Renal & biliary elimination. $T_{1/2}$ 10–14 h
- **DDI:** Rifampin, ketoconazole, digoxin, verapamil, cyclosporine, amiodarone
- **Clinical pearls:** PT, INR, & aPTT will be prolonged but NOT useful for therapeutic monitoring. Conversion from non-warfarin anticoagulant (parental & oral): Start edoxaban at time of next scheduled dose. Conversion from UFH heparin: Start edoxaban 4 h post infusion discontinuation. Conversion from warfarin: Stop warfarin & start edoxaban when INR ≤2.5

Rivaroxaban (Xarelto)

- **Dosing:**
  - VTE tx: 15 mg PO BID × 21 d, followed by 20 mg PO once daily
  - Reduction in risk of VTE recurrence: 20 mg PO once daily
  - Nonvalvular atrial fibrillation:
    - CrCl >50 mL/min: 20 mg PO once daily w/ evening meal
    - CrCl 15–50 mL/min or dialysis: 15 mg PO once daily w/ evening meal
  - VTE prophylaxis following hip/knee replacement surgery:
    - Hip replacement: 10 mg PO once daily × 35 d
    - Knee replacement: 10 mg PO once daily × 12 d
- **Dose adjustments:**
  - General: As above per indication, avoid in CrCl <30 mL/min
  - Concomitant dual CYP3A4 & P-gp inhibitors: Avoid concomitant use w/ ketoconazole, itraconazole, lopinavir/ritonavir, indinavir, conivaptan
  - Concomitant dual CYP3A4 & P-gp inducers: Avoid concomitant use w/ carbamazepine, phenytoin, rifampin, St. John's wort
- **PK/PD:** Dose-dependent prolongation of PT/aPTT; metabolized by CYP3A4/5 & CYP2J2; renal elimination; $T_{1/2}$ 5–9 h
- **DDI:** Dual CYP3A4/P-gp inhibitors & dual CYP3A4/P-gp inducers
- **Clinical pearls:** Take w/ food; 10-mg, 15-mg, or 20-mg tablets may be crushed & mixed w/ applesauce (stable 4 h); 10-mg, 15-mg, or 20-mg tablets may be crushed & suspended in 50-mL water & administered via NG/gastric feeding tube (stable 4 h); conversion from non-warfarin anticoagulants: Start rivaroxaban 0–2 h prior to next scheduled dose; conversion from warfarin: Stop warfarin & start rivaroxaban when INR <3.0

Information based on publicly available drug inserts from Janssen, Bristol-Myers Squibb, & Boehringer Ingelheim, & National Comprehensive Cancer Network (NCCN) Cancer-Associated Venous Thromboembolic Disease guidelines V.2016.

GROWTH FACTOR THERAPY

Proposed clinical utility

- **Preventative:** Shorten duration of expected nadir (myeloid, erythroid, megakaryocytic)
- **Therapeutic:** ↑ values out of range (neutropenia) or ↓ transfusion burden (erythroid & megakaryocytic)

Myeloid Growth Factors	
Granulocyte-colony–stimulating factor (G-CSF—Neupogen) "Biosimilar/alternatives": Filgrastim-sndz (Zarxio), tbo-filgrastim (Granix)	
Adult dosing	**Postchemo:** 5 mg/kg SC qd (often rounded to vial size—300/480 mcg) Duration: Until ANC recovery & past nadir or as directed per chemo regimen. **Post-BMT:** 10 mg/kg SC qd Duration: Per institution guidelines **Mobilization:** 10 mg/kg SC qd Duration: Per institution guidelines **Sev. chronic neutropenia:** 5 mg/kg SC qd Duration: As needed **Role in febrile neutropenia:** See ASCO guidelines for risk factors No renal or hepatic adjustments
Pegylated G-CSF (Pegfilgrastim—Neulasta, Neulasta Onpro)	
Adult dosing	**Postchemo:** 6 mg SC once per cycle; no renal or hepatic adjustments

Erythroid Growth Factors	
Epoetin alfa (Epogen/Procrit)	
Adult dosing (HD/ non-HD pts)	Start 50–100 units/kg SC/IV TIW Duration: Target Hb >10 mg/dL; frequency & duration can vary widely (see prescribing information). Peak Hb effect w/in 2–6 wks WARNING: Has been associated w/ MORTALITY, tumor progression or relapse, & serious CV & thromboembolic events Restricted distribution: www.esa-apprise.com for more info
Darbepoetin (Aranesp)	
Adult dosing	HD pts: Start 0.45 mg/kg SC/IV qwk Non-HD pts: Start 0.45 mg/kg SC/IV q4wk Duration: Target Hb >10 mg/dL; frequency & duration can vary widely WARNING: Has been associated w/ MORTALITY, tumor progression or relapse, & serious CV & thromboembolic events Restricted distribution: www.esa-apprise.com for more info

Megakaryocytic Growth Factors	
Eltrombopag (Promacta)	
Adult dosing	**Chronic ITP:** Start 50 mg PO daily (max: 75 mg); start 25 mg daily in pts of East-Asian ethnicity Duration: Lowest effective dose to keep plt >50 but <400; stop if no improvement in 4 wks WARNING: Has been associated w/ hepatotoxicity. Has *not* been approved for use in chemotherapy-induced thrombocytopenia.
Romiplostim (Nplate)	
Adult dosing	**Chronic ITP:** Start 1 mg/kg SC qwk (Max: 10 mg/kg) Duration: Lowest effective dose to keep plt >50 but <400; stop if no improvement in 4 wks WARNING: Has not been approved for chemotherapy-induced thrombocytopenia.

Info based on publicly available drug inserts from Amgen Inc., Sandoz Inc., Teva Pharmaceuticals, Janssen Products, Novartis Pharmaceuticals.

MISCELLANEOUS AGENTS

Drug Class	Agents	Mechanism
Differentiating agents	ATRA, ATO	Induction of differentiation of APL cells, damages or degrades the fusion protein PML-RARalpha
Enzymes	Erwinia asparaginase, pegaspargase, calaspargase pegol-mknl	Inhibition of protein synthesis by hydrolyzing asparagine to aspartic acid & ammonia (G1 phase specific)
Hematopoietic agents	Luspatercept-aamt	Inhibition of TGF-β superfamily results in increased differentiation and proliferation of erythroid precursors

Devita, Hellman, and Rosenberg's Cancer: Principles and Practice of Oncology. 9th ed. 2011.

All-Trans Retinoic Acid, ATRA, Tretinoin (Vesanoid)

- **Dosing:** 45 mg/m^2/d in 2 divided doses. No renal dose adjustments recommended. Hepatic: AST/ALT 5× ULN: Hold
- **PK/PD:** Good oral absorption (↑ absorption w/ food), does not cross BBB, hepatically metabolized, renal excretion (63%), $T_{1/2}$ 0.5–2 h
- **AEs:** APL differentiation syndrome (**BBW,** 25%, fever, dyspnea, ↑ wt, pulm infiltrates), leukocytosis (**BBW,** 40%), peripheral edema, HA, dry skin, rash, ↑ cholesterol, ↑ LFTs, pseudotumor cerebri
- **DDI:** Oral contraceptives (↓ effect of oral contraceptives)
- **Clinical pearls:** APL differentiation syndrome tx: high-dose steroids, (dexamethasone 10 mg IV every 12 h for 3–5 d), consider holding ATRA temporarily if sev./life-threatening; pseudotumor cerebri tx: acetazolamide; plasma conc. may ↓ w/ continued administration (induces own metabolism)

Arsenic Trioxide, ATO (Trisenox)

- **Dosing:** 0.15 mg/kg/d IV until BM remission (max: 60 doses), Same dose for consolidation but typically administered 5 d/wk. No initial hepatic adjustments, hold for grade 3 hepatotoxicity. CrCl <30 mL/min: Use w/ caution
- **PK/PD:** Widely distributes into body & CNS, hepatically metabolized, renal excretion (15% as unchanged drug), $T_{1/2}$ 10–14 h
- **AEs:** APL differentiation syndrome (**BBW,** fever, dyspnea, wt gain, pulm infiltrates), QT prolongation (**BBW**), ↓ K/Mg, ↑ glc, ↑ WBC, neuropathy, rash, headache, ↑ LFTs, hearing loss, myelosuppression
- **DDI:** QTc-prolonging agents (↑ QTc interval)
- **Clinical pearls:** Baseline then weekly 12-lead ECG (QTcF preferred). Monitor electrolytes & LFTs. APL differentiation syndrome tx: High-dose steroids (dexamethasone 10 mg IV every 12 h for ≥3 d); most pts may continue ATO

Pegaspargase (Oncaspar)

- **Dosing:** 2,500 units/m^2 IM/IV, no more than every 14 d
- **PK/PD:** Slow IM absorption, systemically degraded, $T_{1/2}$ ~5.5–6 d (IM) & 5.3–7 d (IV). $T_{1/2}$ is typically longer in asparaginase-naïve adults
- **AEs:** HSR (no prior asparaginase HSR: 1–10%; prior HSR: 32%), coagulopathy (7%), ↑ glc, edema, pancreatitis, thrombosis, ↑ bilirubin
- **DDI:** May decrease efficacy of UFH & LMWH (↓ antithrombin III)
- **Clinical pearls:** Asparaginase activity level monitoring is recommended to assess for neutralizing antibodies ("silent inactivation"). May cause ATIII depletion (monitoring & repletion are controversial). Monitor amylase/lipase, TGs, fibrinogen, PT/PTT, bilirubin

Erwinia asparaginase (Erwinaze)

- **Dosing:** 25,000 units/m^2 3 times weekly for 6 doses for each planned asparaginase dose
- **PK/PD:** $T_{1/2}$ ~16 h (IM), ~7.5 h (IV)
- **AEs:** HSR (grade 3–4: 5%), coagulopathy, ↑ glc, seizures, pancreatitis, thrombosis, ↑ liver transaminases
- **DDI:** Dexamethasone (↑ serum conc. of dexamethasone)
- **Clinical pearls:** Indicated for pts w/ grade 3–4 HSR &/or demonstrate silent inactivation w/ pegaspargase. Contraindicated for history of pancreatitis w/ prior asparaginase therapy

Calaspargase pegol-mknl (Asparlas)
- **Dosing:** 2,500 units/m^2 IV, no more than every 21 d. No hepatic/renal adjustments
- **PK/PD:** $T_{1/2}$ ~16.1 d
- **AEs:** HSR (grade 3–4: 7–21%), pancreatitis (12-16%), thrombosis (9–12%), hemorrhage, hepatotoxicity
- **DDI:** Oral contraceptives (hepatic metabolism may be decreased)
- **Clinical pearls:** Similar s/e profile & monitoring as pegaspargase. FDA approved for pediatric ALL pts age 1 mo–21 y

Luspatercept-aamt (Reblozyl)
- **Dosing:** Starting dose: 1 mg/kg subQ q3wks (MDS). May increase to 1.33 mg/kg q3wks if no RBC response after 2 doses. Max dose = 1.75 mg/kg subQ q3wks. No hepatic/renal adjustments
- **PK/PD:** $T_{1/2}$ ~13 d
- **AEs:** Myalgia/arthralgias, HTN, diarrhea, cough, ↓ CrCl, ↑ LFTs
- **DDI:** No known clinically significant DDIs
- **Clinical pearls:** FDA indications include pts with MDS/MPN with ring sideroblasts and thrombocytosis or MDS with ring sideroblasts (MDS-RS) who have anemia (needing 2+ units pRBC w/in 8 weeks) with failure of an erythropoiesis stimulating agent

Info based on publicly available drug inserts from Roche, Cephalon, Lundbeck, Jazz Pharmaceuticals, Bristol Meyers Squibb, Shire & Enzon Pharmaceuticals.

Drug Class	Agents	Mechanism
Proteasome inhibitors	Bortezomib, carfilzomib	Reversible (bortezomib) & irreversible (carfilzomib) inhibition of chymotrypsin-like activity at 26S proteasome → apoptosis
mTOR inhibitors	Everolimus, temsirolimus	Inhibition of mammalian target of rapamycin (mTOR) → ↓ protein synthesis & cell proliferation
Antiangiogenic agent inhibitor	Bevacizumab, ziv-aflibercept	Inhibits/traps VEGFR → ↓ activation of receptors → ↓ angiogenesis
Radiopharmaceutical	Radium-223 dichloride	Alpha-emitting isotope w/c targets bone mets; mimics Ca^{2+} to form complexes w/ bone mineral → induces double strand DNA breaks in adjacent cells

Devita (2011). 9th ed. 166, 339.

Bortezomib (Velcade)
- **Dosing:** 1.3 mg/m^2 SC or IV twice weekly (d 1, 4, 8, 11) for 21-d cycle or longer for 42-d cycle. No renal or hepatic dose adjustments recommended
- **PK/PD:** Distributes to peripheral tissues; hepatically metabolized via CYP2C19 & CYP3A4; $T_{1/2}$ single dose 9–15 h, multiple doses 76–108 h
- **AEs:** Myelosuppression (nadir d11), herpes reactivation, peripheral neuropathy, constipation/diarrhea, ↓ BP, HF (<1%)
- **DDI:** CYP3A4/2C19 inhibitors/inducers (↑/↓ conc. of bortezomib), ascorbic acid & green tea (↓ bortezomib effect)
- **Clinical pearls:** ↓ peripheral neuropathy w/ SC route

Carfilzomib (Kyprolis)
- **Dosing:** 20 mg/m^2 IV × 2 consecutive d every wk × 3 wks, then 27 mg/m^2 IV × 2 consecutive d every wk × 3 wks. No renal or hepatic dose adjustments recommended
- **PK/PD:** Extensive metabolism via hydrolysis (little metabolism via CYP450)
- **AEs:** Myelosuppression, HSR (w/in 24 h of infusion), peripheral edema, HTN, peripheral neuropathy, herpes reactivation, N/V (mod. emetogenic potential), ↓ K/Mg, ↑ SCr & AST
- **DDI:** P-gp inhibitors/inducers (↑/↓ conc. of carfilzomib)
- **Clinical pearls:** Less peripheral neuropathy (14%) compared to bortezomib. Hydrate w/ 250–500 mL NS & premedicate w/ dexamethasone in cycle 1

Everolimus (Afinitor, Zortress)
- **Dosing:** 10 mg PO daily. No renal or hepatic dose adjustments recommended.
- **PK/PD:** Fast absorption, extensive hepatic metabolism (CYP3A4), $T_{1/2}$ 30 h
- **AEs:** Myelosuppression, edema, mucositis, HTN, rash, ↑ cholesterol/TG/glc, electrolyte imbalances

- **DDI:** Strong CYP3A4 inducers (avoid use, ↓ conc. of everolimus), strong CYP3A4 & P-gp inhibitors (avoid use, ↑ conc. of everolimus)

Temsirolimus (Torisel)

- **Dosing:** 25 mg IV weekly. No renal dose adjustments recommended. Hepatic: Tbili >1–1.5 × ULN or AST > ULN: 15 mg weekly, Tbili >1.5 × ULN: contraindicated
- **PK/PD:** Hepatically metabolized via CYP3A4 to active metabolite (sirolimus)
- **AEs:** Myelosuppression, HSR, edema, mucositis, HTN, rash, ↑ cholesterol/TG/glc, electrolyte imbalances
- **DDI:** Strong CYP3A4 inducers (avoid use, ↓ conc. of temsirolimus), strong CYP3A4 & P-gp inhibitors (avoid use, ↑ conc. of temsirolimus)
- **Clinical pearls:** Premedicate w/ H1 antagonist 30 min prior to infusion

Ziv-Aflibercept (Zaltrap)

- **Dosing:** 4 mg/kg IV every 2 wks. No renal or hepatic dose adjustments recommended
- **PK/PD:** $T_{1/2}$ ~6 d
- **AEs: GI perforation (BBW), hemorrhage (BBW), impaired wound healing (BBW),** proteinuria, HTN, thromboembolism, ↑ LFTs
- **DDI:** Contraindicated w/ clozapine (↑ risk of agranulocytosis)
- **Clinical pearls:** Monitor CBC, urine protein, BP, & signs of bleeding. Hold Rx at least 4 wks prior & 4 wks after major elective surgery

Radium-223 (Xofigo)

- **Dosing:** 55 kBq/kg q4wks × 6 doses. No renal or hepatic dose adjustments recommended. Doses should be held if hematologic tox occurs
- **PK/PD:** $T_{1/2}$ elimination: 11.4 d; excretion: feces (13%); urine (2%)
- **AEs:** Peripheral edema; nausea (36%); vomiting (19%); diarrhea (25%); thrombocytopenia (31%; grades 3/4: 1–6%), neutropenia (18%; grades 3/4: 1–3%); anemia (93%; grades 3/4: 6%)
- **DDI:** No formal clinical drug interaction studies have been performed
- **Clinical pearls:** Monitor CBC; therapy adjustment may be required for ANC <1,000 & platelets <50K. Resume drug when counts recover. If suppression still occurs at least 6 wks out, tx may be discontinued

Info based on publicly available drug inserts from Millennium Pharmaceuticals, Onyx Pharmaceuticals, Novartis Pharma, BDI Pharma, Bayer HealthCare, Janssen, & Sanofi-Aventis.

TUMOR LYSIS SYNDROME

Definition

TLS is an oncologic emergency caused by electrolyte abnormalities a/w spontaneous &/or tx-induced cell death that can be potentially fatal

4 key electrolyte abnormalities 2° to excessive tumor/cell lysis:

- Hyperkalemia • Hyperphosphatemia • Hypocalcemia • Hyperuricemia (2° to catabolism of nucleic acids)

Presentation

Nausea, vomiting, diarrhea, constipation, oliguria/low UOP, wt gain, AKI, weakness cramps, seizures, tetany, or dysrhythmias

Cairo–Bishop definition with the Howard modification for TLS

TLS may be subclassified as laboratory &/or clinical TLS (*NEJM* 2011;364:1844)

Laboratory TLS defined as ≥2 above abnormalities w/in 3 d before or 7 d after treatment in the setting of hydration & use of a hypouricemic agent OR not directly related to a therapeutic agent

Clinical TLS is defined as laboratory TLS plus end-organ manifestation

- Serum creatinine ≥1.5 ULN • Seizure • Cardiac arrhythmia, sudden cardiac death
- Symptomatic hypocalcemia

Risk factors

↑ TLS risk w/ baseline renal dysfunction, hyperuricemia, hyperkalemia, hyperphosphatemia, volume depletion, & (in some dzs) ↑ LDH (*Haematol* 2008;93:67)

High risk: >5% chance of clinical TLS; Intermediate: 1–5%, Low: <1% (*BJH* 2010;149:578)

- Prevention & management of TLS depends on risk level
- Greatest concern w/ heme malignancies, but highly chemotherapy-sensitive solid tumors (neuroblastoma, germ cell tumor, small-cell lung CA) are considered intermediate risk*

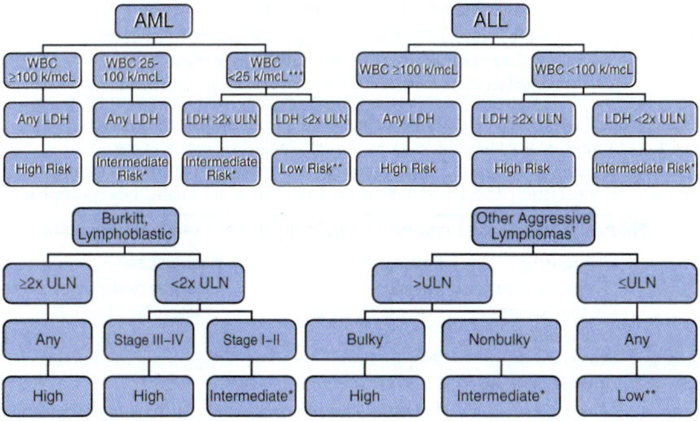

- CLL risk stratification depends on factors incl. lymph node size, tx, baseline renal dysfunction, electrolyte derangements; see NCCN guidelines for CLL/SLL (v1.2022)

†Examples include ATLL, DLBCL, mantle cell lymphoma w/ blastoid or pleomorphic morphology, PTCL, large cell transformation of indolent lymphoma.

*High risk if baseline renal dysfunction, hyperuricemia, hyperkalemia, or hyperphosphatemia present.

**Intermediate risk if baseline renal dysfunction present.

***AML on venetoclax combos may be monitored outpt if WBC <25, nl CrCl, good PS, tx w/ allopurinol (*Blood* 2019;133:7), but CLL/lymphoma are higher risk w/ venetoclax.

Prevention of TLS in patients w/ hematologic malignancies

Monitoring	
Risk Group	**Monitoring**
Low	Electrolytes[a] prior to starting therapy & at least daily after starting therapy initially in those w/ more than minimal risk
Intermediate	Electrolytes[a] prior to starting therapy & every 8–12 h after starting therapy (for 1st 48–72 h)

High	Electrolytes[a] prior to starting therapy, at 4–6 h after starting therapy, & every 6–8 h thereafter initially (for 1st 48–72 h)

[a]Electrolytes: Basic metabolic panel, UA, phosphorus, calcium.
Note: If tx w/ rasburicase, UA must be drawn in prechilled tubes & placed on ice.

Prophylaxis			
Risk Group	**Intravenous Hydration[a]**	**Xanthine Oxidase Inhibitor**	**Prophylactic Rasburicase**
Low	Rec for inpts w/ more than minimal risk	Consider	No
Intermediate	Yes	Yes	No
High	Yes; 2–3 $L/m^2/d$ initially (Urine output 80–100 $mL/m^2/h$)	Yes; delay by 48–72 h if administering rasburicase	Consider

Note: No indication for alkalinization of urine unless concomitant metabolic acidosis.
[a]Isotonic fluids preferred (avoid fluids containing electrolytes associated with TLS). Diuretics may be considered if volume overloaded or to maintain adequate urinary output.

Management of TLS

Electrolyte	Management
Hyperkalemia	EKG, if hyperkalemia assoc changes, calcium gluconate 1–2 g IV × 1 Other acute mgmt: Regular insulin 10 U IVP plus 25–50 g D50, Sodium Bicarb 50–100 mEq IV, albuterol neb 10–20 mg Consider potassium-binding agents. Implement prevention/monitoring
Hyper-phosphatemia	IV fluids +/– diuretics to promote excretion Non–calcium-containing phosphate binders
Hypocalcemia	Use minimum necessary dose of calcium for symptomatic hypocalcemia to alleviate sxs (avoids Ca-Phos crystal formation)
Hyperuricemia	Rasburicase 3 mg IV × 1, 7.5 mg × 1 if ≥12 mg/dL. Repeat dose in 24 h if remains >8 mg/dL (check **G6PD** as below) Hold xanthine oxidase inhibitors for 48–72 h post rasburicase administration

Renal replacement therapy should be considered in the following scenarios:
- Oliguira/anuria • Volume overload • Hyperkalemia • Severe acidemia
- Ca-Phos product >70 mg^2/dL^2 in selected cases • Symptomatic hypocalcemia
- Inability to administer phosphate binders for severe or symptomatic hyperphosphatemia

Medical Therapy for Prevention and Management of Hyperuricemia			
	Allopurinol	**Febuxostat**	**Rasburicase**
MOA	Xanthine oxidase competitive inhibitor	Selective inhibitor of xanthine oxidase	Catalyzes oxidation of UA to allantoin
Benefits	Relatively cheap Readily available	If intolerant to allopurinol	Rapidly reduces UA w/in h
S/e	Allergy/SJS ↑ levels can lead to renal failure d/t xanthine nephrolithiasis	↑ levels can lead to renal failure d/t xanthine nephrolithiasis	Risk of **hemolytic anemia & methemoglobinemia** in **G6PD-deficient pts** Anaphylaxis
Other	Doesn't lower pre-existing UA CrCl dosage Can lead to ↑ UA in short term Take >24 h	Doesn't lower pre-existing UA Favorable UA control in RCT vs. allopurinol (*Ann Oncol* 2015;26:2155)	**Test for G6PD:** If qualitative screen indeterminate, send quantitative UA lab sent in prechilled tube, on ice (post-rasburicase)

METABOLIC EMERGENCIES

Hypercalcemia: Overview

- **Epidemiology:** 10–30% of all pts w/ malignancy
- **Definition:** Normal values: 9–10.5 mg/dL, mild = elevated but <12; mod. = 12–14; sev. >14
  "Corrected" Ca (mmol/L) = Ca measured (mmol/L) + 0.02*(40 – albumin [g/L])
  (note: may be inaccurate in pts w/ renal dysfunction)
- **Pathogenesis:** Tumor secretion of PTHrP (80%); local destruction from bone met paracrine factors (20%), ectopic production of 1,25-vit D, (rarely) PTH or calcitriol (<1%)
  - Humoral mechanisms: ~80% of all hyperCa of malignancy (esp SCC of lung, head/neck, renal, bladder, NHL, leukemias, HL [calcitriol]). PTHrP (shares same amino acid terminus as PTH) & less commonly calcitriol secreted by tumor → ↑ bone turnover & ↑ renal Ca reabsorption
  - Osteolytic bone lesions: ~20% of all hyperCa of malignancy (esp breast, lung, MM, renal, less likely prostate [osteoblastic]). Tumor mets to bone → express PTHrP locally (paracrine) → activate osteoclasts via RANKL–RANK interaction → bone resorption → ↑ Ca
- **Sxs:** Neurologic (lethargy, weakness, hyporeflexia, rarely coma/seizure), cardiac (↓ QTc, widened T waves, heart block), renal (polyuria/polydipsia, hypovolemia, nephrocalcinosis), dermatologic (pruritis)
- **Workup: H&P:** Bone pain, meds/diet (thiazides/Li, vit supplements, volume status, familial hypercalcuric hypercalcemia)
- **Labs:** CMP (Ca, Cr, alb, phos), **iCa, iPTH,** if unclear source → PTHrP & vit D (1,25 & 25-OH), still unclear → SPEP/UPEP/FLC, still unclear → CXR/vit A/endocrine workup

Hypercalcemia: Treatment

- Medication, supplement, & diet review; stop offending agents, if possible
- **Tx underlying malignancy** = the only definitive tx, all others are temporizing
- **IVF** essential to correct hypovolemia & promote calciuresis; >5 L deficit common. If no ESRD/CHF, bolus 1–2 L followed by 200–250 cc/h. If CHF/ESRD, may need HD
- **Osteoclast inhibition:** Modern cornerstone of tx w/ IVFs
  Bisphosphonates: Pamidronate (60–90 mg IV) & zoledronic acid (4 mg IV). ZA may be more effective than pamidronate (*J Clin Oncol* 2001;19:558), but ↑ risk of AKI (contraindicated in CrCl <35). Either acceptable. Both ↑ risk of hypoCa
  RANK-L inhibitor: Denosumab approved for hyperCa of malignancy refractory to bisphosphonates, ↑ risk of hypoCa, esp if recent bisphosphonate or prostate CA w/ blastic lesions
- **Loop diuretics:** No role unless needed for volume overload (*Ann Int Med* 2008;149:259)
- **Calcitonin:** Rapid, temporary ↓ Ca, monitor for hypoCa, HSR, & tachyphylaxis (>48 h)
- **HD:** If all above fail → AKI progresses → sev hypervolemia

Hypercalcemia Treatments

Agent	Rapidity	Duration	Notes
IVF	min–h	h	Goal UOP 100–200 mL/h
Bisphosphonates	D	wk	Adjust for Cr; caution if CrCl <35
RANK-L Inhibitor	D	wk	120 mg SC weekly for 4 doses then monthly
Calcitonin	4–6 h	h	Not intranasal; no effect >48 h
Corticosteroids	**h–d**	**d**	↓ calcitriol; 1,25-vit D production a/w HL, NHL, & granulomatous dz

Hypercalcemia Management

Corrected Ca (mg/dL)	Severity	Usual Tx
10.5–12	Mild	IVFs, consider bisphosphonate
12–14	Mod.	IVFs, bisphosphonate
>14	Sev.	IVFs, calcitonin, bisphosphonate, consider HD

Hyponatremia (serum Na ≤135)

- **Etiology:** Disturbances in TBW, often **multifactorial:** ↓ PO intake, SIADH, renal loss (esp drug-induced), & GI loss. Rarely: ANP secretion, cerebral salt-wasting. R/o pseudohypoNa (↑↑ TGs, ↑↑ protein). R/o hypertonic hypoNa (↑↑ serum glu/mannitol), post–CAR-T cells (see CAR-T cell chapter, a/w ↑ IL-6, *Clin Nephrol* 2020;93:42–46)
- **S/S:** Severity based on degree of hypoNa & rapidity of decline. Anorexia, nausea, weakness, or confusion/AMS from cerebral edema → seizures, coma, death

- **Workup: H&P:** New meds/chemo, changes in fluid intake/output (GI loss, renal loss, ↑ fluids, ↓ PO, tea & toast, etc.), exam to assess fluid status (VS, orthostatics, turgor, edema)
- **Labs:** BMP, serum & urine Osm, urine Na/urea (if on diuretic). Consider TSH, cortisol

Figure 10-1 Focused differential diagnosis of hyponatremia etiology in oncology patients. FE_{Na}, FE_{Urea} = fractional excretion = $(U_x/plasma_x)/(U_{Cr}/plasma_{Cr}) \times 100$.

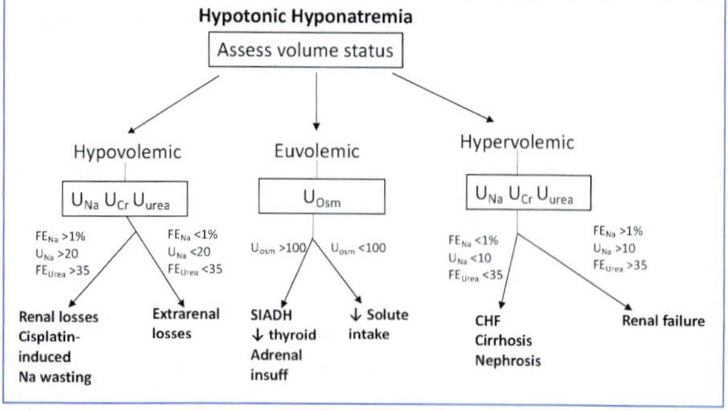

Hyponatremia: Treatment

- Based on underlying etiology (algorithm above) & chronicity
- Regardless of etiology, free water & hypotonic fluid intake must be restricted
  - Hypovolemic: Isotonic fluid resuscitation (↓ stimulus for ADH release)
  - Cerebral salt wasting: Hypertonic saline ± fludrocortisone
  - Hypervolemic: Loop diuretics, dialysis, or both
  - Euvolemic: Free water restriction
  - Pseudohyponatremia: No therapy except confirmation w/ lab
  - Translocational hyponatremia: Glucose control, discontinue mannitol (if possible)
- Chronic hyponatremia → brain cells adapt → **overly rapid correction** → brain cells swell → **osmotic demyelination syndrome** (formerly central pontine myelinolysis)
- If onset of hyponatremia unknown, gradually correct/treat as chronic: 6–8 mEq/24 h
  1. **Calculate Na deficit** = **TBW** (50% of total mass in women & 55% of total mass in men) (**desired Na – actual Na**)
  2. Delivery rate = (Goal mEq rise in 24 h)/([(IVF mEq)/vol. in mL]/24 h) = rate mL/h
- **Severe S/S, AMS, or seizures**—3% hypertonic saline for rapid correction until sx abate **regardless of chronicity**

Syndrome of inappropriate antidiuretic hormone secretion (SIADH)

- **Etiology:** Paraneoplastic or complication of tx/meds
  - Ectopic production by tumor: 15% of all SQCLC, 3% of head/neck, rarer in hematologic malignancies or NSCLC
  - Chemotherapy-induced: Alkylators (cyclophosphamide, ifosfamide); vinca alkaloids; platinum agents; proteasome inhibitors (bortezomib)
  - Drug-induced: TCAs, AEDs (carbamazepine, valproic acid, oxcarbazepine), antipsychotics
  - Other: Infxn, esp PNA; nausea, pain
- **Clinical manifestations:** Hypoosmolar/dilutional hyponatremia w/ excess diuresis. ↓ serum Osm w/ inappropriate ↑ urine Osm, in the setting of normal renal fxn
- **Treatment:**
  1st-line: **Free water restriction, salt tabs w/ or w/o loop diuretics**
  2nd-line: **V2 antagonists:** Tolvaptan or conivaptan—directly inhibit water reabsorption in collecting duct → dilutes urine; demeclocycline causes nephrogenic DI, urea (available through compounding pharmacies).
  AMS, seizure, other severe s/sx: 3% hypertonic saline
  (If no response, send ADH & ANP levels, may be ANP-secreting tumor, different tx)

Lactic acidosis with normal tissue perfusion

- **Etiology:** Often seen w/ liver mets or rapidly progressive heme malignancies
- **Tx:** Directed toward underlying malignancy & aggressive hemodynamic support
- **High mortality** despite aggressive tx

SVC SYNDROME

Definition

- Obstruction of the SVC causing incr. venous pressure resulting classically in edema, plethora, venous distension, & dyspnea (see below)

Epidemiology

- ~15,000 new cases dx'd in the United States annually
- 60–80% a/w malignancy

Differential diagnosis

- Thrombus, infxn, fibrosing mediastinitis, postradiation fibrosis, aortic aneurysm

Malignant Causes of SVC Syndrome		
Tumor Type	**% (Range)**	**Suggestive Clinical Features**
NSCLC	50 (43–59)	H/o smoking; often age >50
SCLC	22 (7–39)	H/o smoking; often age >50
Lymphoma	12 (1–25)	LAN outside the chest; often age <65
Met ca	9 (1–15)	H/o solid tumor; 2/3 breast ca
Germ cell ca, Thymoma, Mesothelioma, Other	7 (0–13)	

Adapted & reproduced with permission from *NEJM* 2007;356:1862.

Clinical Manifestations of SVC Syndrome	
Sx	**% Affected**
Facial edema	82
Pleural effusion	66
Distended neck veins	63
Dyspnea	54
Cough	54
Distended chest veins	53
Arm edema	46
Facial plethora	20
Hoarseness	17
Syncope	10
Stridor	4

Adapted and reproduced with permission from *NEJM* 2007;356:1862.

Diagnosis

- Clinical dx, confirmed w/ imaging
- If severe, life-threating sxs → **Venography**
- If mild/moderate sxs → **CT + contrast or MRI** if cannot give contrast; **Duplex US** may be helpful though generally cannot visualize SVC itself directly
- Tissue bx may be **needed to confirm malignancy**

Severity

Proposed Grading System			
Grade	**Category**	**~Incidence (%)**	**Definition**
0	Asx	10	Radiographic SVC obstruction; no sxs
1	Mild	25	Edema in head/neck, cyanosis, plethora
2	Moderate	50	Edema in head/neck + functional impairment (dysphagia, cough, visual disturbance, movement of head/jaw/eyelid impairment
3	Severe	10	Mild/moderate cerebral edema (HA, dizziness) or mild/moderate laryngeal edema or diminished cardiac reserve (syncope after bending)
4	Life-threatening	5	Significant cerebral edema (confusion, obtundation) or significant laryngeal edema (stridor) or significant hemodynamic compromise (hypotension, syncope, renal injury)
5	Fatal	<1	Death

Adapted and reproduced from *JTO* 2008;3(8):811–814.

Management

- Determined by: Severity, rapidity of onset, & underlying cause
- In general, obtain bx before RT or chemotherapy (*J Clin Oncol* 1997;9:83)
- **Emergent tx:** Endovascular recanalization + stent (+/– fibrinolytic & AC if thrombus), for pts w/ central airway obstruction, severe laryngeal edema or coma from cerebral edema
- **Nonemergent tx options:**
  - Supportive: Elevate head of bed ± loop diuretics ± steroids (lymphoma & some thymomas steroid-sensitive; steroids prior to tissue bx for lymphoma may affect yield)
  - Chemo: Especially if tumor likely rapidly responsive (see below)
  - RT for radiosensitive tumors, not responsive to chemo
  - Intravascular stent: Pts requiring tissue dx (*Vascular* 2007;15:314) or pts w/ malignancy thought unlikely to respond quickly to RT or chemo (see above) or in case of thrombosis
  - Surgical bypass graft infrequently used, can be part of attempted curative multimodality tx if caused by thymoma/thymic carcinoma
- **If thrombus:** Fibrinolytic + AC, consider removing any assoc indwelling catheter
- SVC syndrome does not change the likelihood of cure of an underlying malignancy & **should not compromise the choice of curative tx**

Variable Responsiveness of Malignancies to Chemotherapy
Usually highly responsive (in order of responsiveness)
Lymphoma
SCLC
Germ cell tumors
NSCLC (relief of sx of obstruction of SVC usually results from tx of the CA w/ chemo [stage IV] or chemo + RT [stage III] but degree & rapidity of response is less so than above) (*JAMA* 1983;250:71)
Usually resistant to chemo or RT (ie, unlikely to rapidly decrease in size)
Mesothelioma
Malignant thymoma
Thymic carcinoma

SPINAL CORD COMPRESSION

Definition/risk factors

- **Neuro-oncologic emergency**
- Vertebral metastases invade the epidural space → thecal sac compression → ESCC → spinal cord infarction & irreversible neurologic damage
- Graded w/ ESCC score of 0–3 (see Fig. 10-2 [*J Neurosurg Spine* 2010;3:324])
- **Conus medullaris syndrome (UMN & LMN involvement):** Symmetric saddle anesthesia, bladder & bowel dysfunction, absent bulbocavernosus & anal reflexes
- **Cauda equina syndrome (LMN only):** Severe back & radicular pain, leg weakness, sensory loss ± decr lower extremity reflexes; can spare bowel & bladder fxn
- Metastatic tumor from any 1° site can cause ESCC; most common histologies include lung, breast, prostate, RCC, NHL, MM

Figure 10-2 Epidural spinal cord compression (ESCC) grading scale. Grade 0: Bone only. Grade 1 **A:** Epidural extension without abutting dura. Grade 1 **B:** Dural sac deformation without cord abutment. Grade 1 **C:** Deformation of sac with cord abutment but no cord compression. Grade 2: Cord compression with visible CSF surrounding cord. Grade 3: Cord compression with obliteration of CSF space.

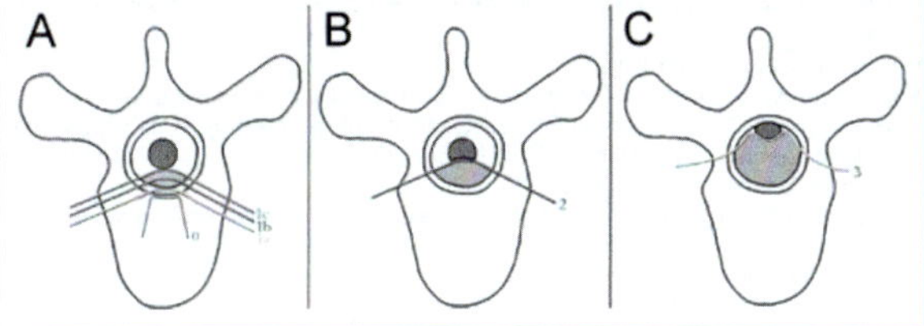

Anatomy

- Tip of the spinal cord lies at ~L1 vertebral level
- Below L1, the lumbosacral nerves form the cauda equina
- Conus medullaris: Terminal end of the spinal cord at L1/L2
- Sites of ESCC involvement: **Thoracic (70%),** lumbar (20%), cervical (10%)

Clinical manifestations

- S/S depend on location & degree of thecal sac compression
- **Back pain (80–95%) is an early sx & can precede dx by 4–7 wks; typically worse at night or in the early morning** (*Eur J Cancer* 1994;30A(3):396)
- Lower extremity weakness (or upper extremity weakness w/ cervical cord compression) → gait instability→ paralysis
- Anterior column compression is more common & a/w compression of spinothalamic tracts leading to numbness
- Posterior column (30%) compression leads to loss of proprioception & ataxia
- + Babinski responses (upgoing toes)
- Sensory loss is an early sx, ascending numbness/paresthesia (legs/perineum)
- Autonomic dysfunction (urinary retention/incontinence, decr anal sphincter tone → bowel incontinence) is typically a late finding
- Note: Pain w/ movement suggests spinal instability & abrupt worsening of pain may indicate a pathologic compression fracture

Diagnostic evaluation

- **Do not wait for neurologic signs to develop**
- Most important prognostic factor for regaining neurologic fxn is pretreatment neurologic status (*Spine* 2016;15:41)
- Obtain a **STAT whole spine MRI w/ & w/o gadolinium** as multiple noncontiguous spinal levels may be involved (*AJR* 1987;149:1241); if MRI contraindicated, obtain a CT myelogram
- Other diagnostic radiographic modalities: CT whole spine, plain spine films, bone scans
- If sxs of headache or meningismus, obtain CSF for evaluation; however, spinal cord compression evaluation takes precedence over investigation of leptomeningeal involvement

- Consult radiation oncology & neurosurgical services (see Fig. 10-3)

Figure 10-3 Workflow for suspected cord compression.

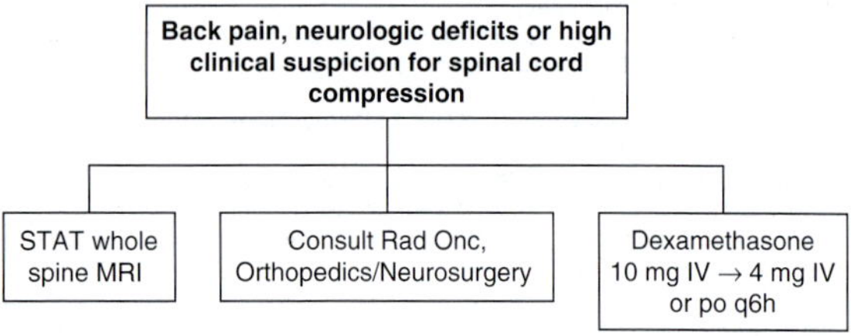

Treatment

- **Initiate tx immediately** while awaiting imaging if back pain & neurologic deficits
- **Dexamethasone 10 mg IV followed by 4 mg IV or PO q6h** (*Clin Spine Surg* 2017;30:156)
- Reserve dexamethasone doses of 100 mg for pts w/ severe neurologic dysfunction followed by rapid taper, as there is unclear benefit & may be a/w incr. toxicity (*J Neurooncol* 1992;12:141)
- Pain control w/ opioid analgesics
- Emergent RT or surgical decompression → postop radiation (Consensus Guidelines – *J Neurosurg Spine* 2017;26:3) depending on neurologic, oncologic, mechanical stability, & systemic factors (see Fig. 10-4 for NOMS framework—*Oncologist* 2013;6:744) if confirmed compression/neurologic deficits
- Radiation oncology service should be consulted for pts w/ radiosensitive tumors, ESCC Grade 1–2, & poor surgical candidates (Fig. 10-4)
  - Hypofractionated SBRT of 1–5 fractions provides durable local tumor control of 80–90% at 1 y (*JAMA Oncol* 2020;6:567)
- Neurosurgery + postop RT (vs. RT alone) results in improved neurofunction (incl. ability to walk, continence, muscle strength) for solid tumors (*Lancet* 2005;366:643)

Figure 10-4 Reproduced from *Oncologist* 2013;6:744. NOMS decision-making framework for the management of malignant cord compression. **Patients with mechanically stable disease should follow remaining workflow as above.*

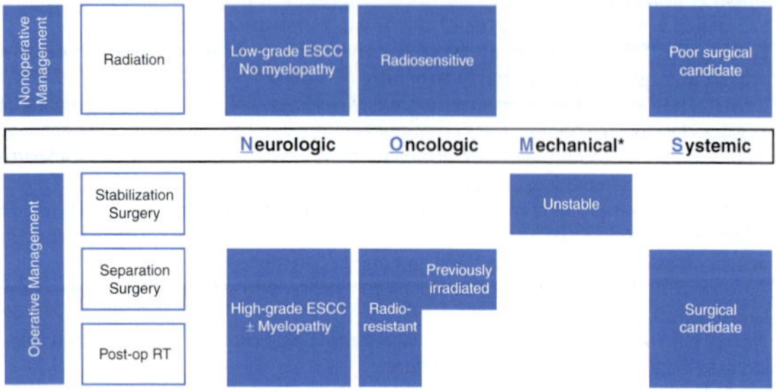

TIPS FOR ON-CALL FELLOWS

Symptoms

- **Fever:** If the pt received chemotherapy in the last 28 d (+3–28), obtain a CBC to assess for neutropenia. See **infectious disease section.** Notable drugs a/w noninfec fever: gemcitabine (w/in 72 h), dabrafenib, mAbs (w/in h). Some targeted tx a/w neutropenia: PARPi, CDK4/6i
  - High-risk pts: BMT, germ cell tumors, DLBCL
- **Nausea: (Refer to nonpain symptom management section),** confirm QTc in chart. 1st line: ondansetron. 2nd line: prochlorperazine, metoclopramide, olanzapine, dronabinol, lorazepam, dexamethasone. Consider leveraging s/e profile. If constipated, consider metoclopramide. If difficulty sleeping, consider olanzapine. If anxiety, consider lorazepam. If edema/pain & not on IO, consider dexamethasone. Discuss adjusting prechemo antiemetic ppx w/ 1° oncologist
- **Vomiting:** If bloody-> ER. Treat nausea. Check if pt is adequately hydrating (if no, send to ER). Consider bowel obstruction if pt at risk (abd malignancy, prev sx) **(refer to malignant bowel obstruction chapter)**. Pts on VEGF inhibitor are at risk for bowel perf. Consider CNS causes of vomiting (↑ ICP d/t tumor or leptomeningeal dz)
- **Mucositis:** Supportive mgmt includes NaCl/$NaHCO_3$ rinses, dexamethasone rinse (may need compounding pharmacy), lidocaine swish & spit, good dental hygiene. Consider thrush on ddx
- **Constipation: (Refer to constipation in Nonpain Symptom Management chapter)** common, r/o obstruction. Do not use supp/enema in pt at risk for neutropenia. Vincristine may cause fecal impaction, intestinal necrosis. Numerous supportive meds
- **Dyspnea: (Refer to dyspnea in Nonpain Symptom Management & Toxicities of Immune Checkpoint Inhibitors chapters)** if uncertain etiology, likely requires eval. Possible causes include anemia, mass, pneumonitis, effusion, infxn, PE. If on immunotherapy, consider pneumonitis, req CT to eval
- **Pain: (Refer to Pain Medications chapter)** consider emergencies which include spinal cord compression, pain crisis, end of life. Consider renal & hepatic function in opioid choice. If new pain of unexplained etiology, ER eval
- **Edema:** Consider DVT, chemo tx–related etiologies, new unilateral LE edema requires immediate eval
- **Headache:** Sudden severe HA req immediate eval. Consider elevated ICP (tumor, bleeding). If on immunotherapy, consider hypophysitis (check cortisol). Consider leptomeningeal dz, venous sinus thrombosis
- **Diarrhea:** R/o infxn causes; consider AE of tx (can be an irAE as well)

Special cases by drug family

- **Refer to pharmacology section for expected adverse effects & clinical pearls**
- **TKIs/VEGF inhibitor:** HTN (discontinue for uncontrolled HTN), increased risk of thrombosis, CVA, MI. Can be a/w skin tox, manage supportively (moisturize)
- **Immunotherapy (refer to Toxicities of Immunotherapies chapters):** Important to be aware that irAEs are broad & communicate concerns to nonspecialist providers
- **Venetoclax:** Pts w/ recent start can be high risk for TLS **(refer to TLS chapter)**
- **Pegaspargase:** Affects hepatic synthetic fxn w/ risk of **bleeding** (↓ clotting factors & fibrinogen, ↑ PT/aPTT) or **thrombosis** (incl. in CNS), ↑ triglycerides, pancreatitis
- **Clinical trial pts:** Involve attending provider early

Special cases by laboratory values

- **Electrolyte derangements: Refer to TLS/metabolic emergencies chapters**
- **Positive blood culture:** Generally, refer to ER for treatment
- **New coagulopathy:** Consider DIC, if new leukemia, consider APL & treat urgently **(refer to AML chapter)**
- **LFT derangements:** Review medication AE, acetaminophen use, supplement use. Significant derangements, consider ER referral & imaging

Special cases by patient population

- **BMT pts (refer to stem cell transplantation & infectious disease sections):** Pts at risk for infxn & GvH dz. Low threshold to involve attending & refer to ER for evaluation. Attempt eval at transplant center
- **CAR T-cell recipients (refer to CAR-T Cell Therapy chapter):** Involve attending early, potential for CRS, neurologic tox & sz. Low threshold to refer to ER for eval at CAR T-cell center

PRINCIPLES OF PALLIATIVE CARE

What is palliative care?

"Pt & family-centered care that **optimizes QoL** by anticipating, preventing, & treating suffering. Palliative care **throughout the continuum of illness** involves addressing physical, intellectual, emotional, social, & spiritual needs **to facilitate pt autonomy, access to information, & choice"** (Center for Medicare and Medicaid Services, Code of Federal Registrar 79 FR 50509, 2014; qtd in: National Consensus Project for Quality Palliative Care Guideline (nationalcoalitionhpc.org). See also: National Palliative Care Research Center (npcrc.org) & Center to Advance Palliative Care (capc.org)

Integration of palliative care into standard oncology care

- Several **RCTs have supported the integration of palliative care w/ oncologic care,** but specific interventions & models of care have varied
- **NCCN guideline** (Palliative Care Version 2.2021): Initiated by oncologist, who arranges collaboration w/ palliative care & interprofessional specialists. Continued serial screening for palliative care needs begins at initial visit
- **ASCO guideline:** "Inpts & outpts w/ advanced CA should receive dedicated palliative care services, early in the dz course (w/in 8 wks of dx), concurrent w/ active tx. Referral of pts to interdisciplinary palliative care teams is optimal, & services may complement existing programs" (*J Oncol Practice* 2017;13:119–121; ASCO.org)

Essential components of palliative care (ASCO, *J Oncol Practice* 2017;13:119–121)

- Rapport & relationship building w/ pts & family caregivers
- Symptom, distress, & functional status mgmt (eg, pain, dyspnea, fatigue, sleep disturbance, mood, nausea, or constipation)
- Exploration of understanding & education about illness & prognosis
- Clarification of tx goals
- Assessment & support of coping needs (eg, provision of dignity therapy)
- Assistance w/ medical decision making
- Coordination w/ other care providers & provision of referrals as indicated

Criteria for consultation with a palliative care specialist (NCCN V2.2021)

- Pt characteristics: Limited anti-CA tx options, high sx burden, uncontrolled pain, frequent ER visits or readmissions, complex ICU care, communication barriers, assistance w/ advanced care planning, poor performance status, request for hastened death
- Social circumstances: Inadequate caregiver/social support, limited access to care, family discord, concerns about care of dependents, spiritual/existential crisis
- Staff issues: Complex care coordination, compassion fatigue, moral distress, burnout

Useful communication tips

- Use open-ended questions to elicit pt concerns. Clarify how much pt would like to know
- Use an **Ask-Tell-Ask** approach when delivering information
  - Ask: "What do you understand about your illness?"
  - Tell: "That is correct, the CA has spread to…."
  - Ask: "What questions does this information raise for you?"
- Be clear when the medical situation has changed by saying **"we're in a different place"**
- Focus on **what can be done** (not just what can't be done)
- Use the phrase **"allow natural death"** when discussing resuscitation preference
- Remove the phrase "do everything" from your medical vocabulary
- Align w/ pt goals by using **"I wish"** statements
- Redefine hope by supporting realistic & achievable goals
- Recognize emotional cues & use the **NURSE** mnemonic to **make empathy explicit**
- www.VitalTalk.org has resources/app for practicing key communication skills

NURSE	Example Statement
Name the emotion	"You seem worried"
Understand the emotion	"I can see why you are concerned about this"
Respect the emotion	"You have shown a lot of strength"
Support the pt	"I want you to know that I will still be your doctor whether you have chemotherapy or not"
Explore the emotion	"Tell me more about what is worrying you"

Cancer 2008;113(7 Suppl):1897; *J Palliat Med* 2014;17:1019. See: Vitaltalk.org (accessed 10/2021).

Care for caregivers

- Nurses, social workers, or other members of the interdisciplinary care team should initiate caregiver-tailored palliative care support
- Caregiver support includes coaching, education, referrals, & face-to-face meetings. For family caregivers who may live in rural areas &/or are unable to travel to clinic, telephone or televisit services should be offered
- Common stressors of caregivers include practical assistance (transportation, meal preparation, home care), physical care (bathing, toileting, transferring), medical care, social care, advocacy, & financial distress (costs of care, lost work, insurance, &/or opportunity costs)
- RFs for caregiver burden include female sex, low educational attainment, residing w/ the care recipient, hx of depression, social isolation, financial distress, higher number of hours spent caregiving, & lack of choice in being a caregiver (*J Palliat Med* 2021;24(8):1246–1247)
- Beyond just attending to the needs of the seriously ill pt, clinicians should explore the caregiver's sense of well-being, their confidence in providing care, & their need for additional support, esp. during care transitions

Care at the end of life (EOL)

- Recognize the dying process; respect pt/family values & preferences
- Continue only those medications & interventions directly contributing to pt comfort
- Review nutrition & hydration. Overhydration may contribute to fluid overload, causing incr. respiratory distress & anasarca
- Understand nonverbal signs of pain & distress incl. body language, respiratory status, & position. Tools such as the Checklist of Nonverbal Pain Indicators are available (*Pain Manag Nurs* 2000;(1):13)
- Alleviate pain & other physical sxs (nausea, constipation, anorexia, dyspnea, fatigue, & delirium) as discussed in the following sections of this chapter
- Manage agitation by reorientation, addressing any comfort needs such as urinary retention, constipation, & uncomfortable positions
- Provide pt & family w/ respectful space & uninterrupted time together
- Ask about nonphysical forms of distress, such as spiritual or existential conflicts
- Offer anticipatory bereavement support; consider social work & chaplaincy consults
- Most common complaints about EOL care by bereaved caregivers are about the quality & quantity of communication
- Bereavement care also protects physicians who grieve, & reduces their sense of guilt

Medicare hospice benefit

- Eligibility: Pt must be entitled to Medicare Part A, certified by 2 physicians to have a life expectancy <6 mos, & sign a statement choosing to forego dz directed Rx
- Levels of care: Routine home care, continuous home care (crisis mgmt in home), general inpt care (short-term to control acute sxs), respite care
- Services provided: Doctors' services, nursing care, medical equipment & supplies, prescription drugs, counselors, social work, PT & OT, speech language pathologists, dietary counseling, hospice aides, homemakers/HHA & volunteers, grief & loss counseling
- Not covered: Continuous nursing assistance; nursing home room & board charges

Disparities in EOL care

- Gender, race, age, & ethnic disparities are notable in EOL care (*JAMA* 2021;325:423–424) Not all pts prefer to die at home, & caregiver ability is important to assess
- Barriers to quality EOL care include provider comfort, socioeconomic status, pt living arrangements, insurance status, & access to local resources

PAIN MEDICATIONS

Types of pain

1. **Nociceptive pain**
   a. Somatic pain: Cutaneous or musculoskeletal tissue (ie, bone, soft tissue metastases). Usually well localized, incr. w/ use/movement
   b. Visceral pain: Compression, obstruction, infiltration, ischemia, stretching, or inflammation of solid & hollow viscera. Diffuse, nonfocal
2. **Neuropathic pain:** Direct injury/dysfunction of peripheral or CNS tissues. Typically burning, radiating, may increase at rest or w/ nerve stretching

Pain emergencies

- DDx: Spinal cord compression, fracture, bowel obstruction, severe mucositis, acute severe s/e of opioids (addiction crisis, delirium, respiratory depression), severe pain in imminently dying pt
- Pain crisis: Pt reports severe, uncontrolled pain causing distress for pt &/or family members; requires aggressive assessment & intervention
- Pain mgmt at the EOL is a moral obligation to alleviate pain & unnecessary suffering & is not euthanasia (Vacco v. Quill, U.S. Supreme Court, 1997).
- Guidelines: NCCN Adult Cancer Pain V2.2021

Pain assessment scales

- Pt report is the gold standard
- Measures include numeric scales, verbal ratings, visual analog scales (eg, Baker–Wong), important to include functional outcomes/pain interference (eg, Brief Pain Inventory)

The World Health Organization (WHO) analgesia ladder, depending on pain

- Step 1 (mild): Nonopioid therapy: acetaminophen, NSAIDs, adjuvant analgesics
- Step 2 (mod.): Add lower-potency/dose opioid
- Step 3 (mod.–sev.): Use high-potency opioids (morphine, hydromorphone, etc.)

Opioid treatment guidelines

1. For mod.–sev. CA pain (w/ close supervision), add PRN opioid:
   - **Route:** PO opioids q2–4h depending on tx/pt, IV opioid q15–30min (if in crisis)
   - In **opioid naïve,** hydromorphone 0.2–0.4 mg IV, 2–4 mg PO; morphine 2.5–5 mg IV, 7–15 mg PO; or oxycodone 5–10 mg PO. Dose reduce by 50% for elderly pts/severe renal/liver/lung dz & titrate up as needed & as tolerated
   - In **opioid-tolerant,** add 10–20% of the total 24 h every 15–30 min IV or every 1–3 h PO
2. After determining new effective & tolerated 24-h dose, change this dose to extended-release (ER) formulation & give 10–20% total daily dose q2–3h PRN as immediate-release (IR) formulation
3. Dose reduce by 50% for elderly pts/severe renal/liver/lung dz & titrate up as needed & as tolerated
4. Pt education: Importance of using, storing, & disposing opioids safely
5. Consider pain/palliative consult when starting or titrating methadone
6. Avoid codeine & meperidine unless familiar w/ their metabolism

Opioid adverse side effects

- Constipation (no tolerance, treat when initiating opioids), N/V (tolerance develops in 3–7 d), hypogonadism, urinary retention, sedation, respiratory depression/arrest (only after the onset of sedation), myoclonus, delirium, seizures, addiction, diversion

Opioid withdrawal syndrome

- Flu-like sx incl. sweating, anxiety, N/V, diarrhea, chills, pupillary dilation, piloerection, yawning, lacrimation.
- Usually self-limited & not life-threatening

Opioid overdose

- Manifestations: Sedation w/ respirations <6–8/min, constricted pupils, skeletal muscle flaccidity, cold or clammy skin
- Tx:
  1. Naloxone—0.4 mg diluted in 10 mL NS, give 1 mL q30s to reverse respiratory depression/severe sedation; may need an infusion to counteract the effect of extended release opioids incl. methadone & fentanyl patch
  2. Stay w/ the pt until stable
  3. Stop/decrease opioids & then titrate up as needed for pain & to prevent withdrawal
- Acetaminophen: Opioid sparing; s/e: Hepatotoxicity in high doses
- NSAIDs: For bone pain or as opioid-sparing agent; s/e: GI & renal tox

- Antidepressants (TCA, SSRI, etc.): For visceral & neuropathic pain, time to effect 3–7 d after reaching therapeutic dose (eg, amitriptyline 75–125 mg/d)
- Anticonvulsants (gabapentin, pregabalin): For neuropathic pain, long titration, time to analgesia 3–7 d after reaching therapeutic dose (eg, gabapentin 2,700–3,600 mg/d)
- Steroids: For pain from ICP, liver capsule, or bone pain; s/e: GI tox, osteoporosis, insomnia, wt gain, infxn
- Ketamine: Used in selected cases at subanesthetic doses
- Nonpharmacologic tx: Nerve blocks, PT, psychological interventions (eg, CBT)

	Chronic Opioid Administration Equianalgesic Single Dose*		
Medication	**IM/IV onset 15–30 min**	**PO onset 30–60 min**	**PAIN**
Morphine	10 mg	30 mg	MODERATE TO SEVERE
Oxycodone	NA	20 mg	
Hydromorphone	1.5 mg	7.5 mg	
Fentanyl	250 mcg	NA	
Hydrocodone	NA	30 mg	MILD TO MODERATE

*Adapted from *Drug Facts and Comparisons* 2008, 62nd ed., by Facts and Comparisons, 2007, Philadelphia, PA: Lippincott Williams and Wilkins; *Principles of Analgesic Use in the Treatment of Acute Pain and Cancer Pain,* 6th ed., by the American Pain Society, 2009, Glenview, IL: American Pain Society.

Methadone

- Long-acting opioid (see following table)
- For pain, can be prescribed by any opioid prescriber
- For medication-assisted tx (MAT) of addiction, must be prescribed by certified addiction psychiatrist

Oral Morphine Equivalent Per Day	Morphine (PO): Methadone (PO)	Unique Characteristics
<60 mg or opioid naïve	≤7.5 mg daily	Long & unpredictable half life
60–199 mg & pt <65 y	10:1	May prolong QTc
≥200 mg & pt >65 y	20:1	May cause hypoglycemia

Adapted from *J Pain Symptom Manage* 2019;57(3):635–645.

Buprenorphine

- Only partial opioid agonist used in clinical practice
- Reported to have less severe s/e profile (incl. nausea, emesis, constipation, respiratory depression) compared to full opioid agonists
- If opioid-tolerant pt is rotated to buprenorphine, opioid withdrawal syndrome likely

Cancer pain management in opioid and substance use disorder (SUD)

- Use appropriate terminology: "Persons w/ SUDs," "use/misuse" rather than "abuse"
- Consider risk of relapse & prepare for it, use multidisciplinary team approach & consultation w/ an SUD specialist
- Methadone & buprenorphine for MAT should be continued during hospitalizations/transitions of care, contact the program to coordinate care; anticipate these pts will need higher doses of rescue

Nausea and vomiting

Pathways of Nausea and Vomiting		
Pathway Affected	**Triggers**	**Therapeutic Agents**
Cerebral cortex	↑ ICP, meningeal irritation, anxiety, memory (eg, smell)	H1 antagonist 5HT2 antagonist Steroids AchM antagonist
Vestibular apparatus	Motion sickness, vestibular dz; opioids	H1 antagonist AchM antagonist
Chemoreceptor trigger zone	Drugs (incl. CINV, opioids), uremia, hypercalcemia	D2 antagonist 5HT3 antagonist NK1 antagonist
Peripheral pathway: Chemo/ mechanoreceptors in GI tract	Gastric irritation (incl. radiation induced), intestinal distension, opioids	5HT3 antagonist D2 antagonist (peripheral)

- **Antiemetic Rx:** Select agent based on trigger & receptor as above. Start dosing as PRN & ↑ to standing if needed; if inadequate, add agent from another class

Antiemetics		
Category	**Medication Name**	**Dosing and Frequency (all PRNs)**
H1 antagonist	Promethazine	12.5–25 mg PO q4–6h or 25 mg suppository PR q6h
D2 antagonist	Metoclopramide (peripheral)	10–20 mg PO/IV q4–6h
	Prochlorperazine (central)	10 mg PO/IV q6h or 25 mg suppository PR q12h
	Haloperidol (central)	0.5–2 mg PO/IV q4–6h
AchM antagonist (anti-acetylcholine)	Scopolamine	1.5 mg transdermal q72h
5HT2 antagonist	Olanzapine	5–10 mg PO q24h
Cannabinoids	Dronabinol	5–10 mg PO or 2.1–4.2 mg/m² oral solution q6–8h
	Nabilone	1–2 mg PO BID
Benzodiazepines	Lorazepam	0.5–2 mg PO/SL/IV q6h

- **Chemo-induced N/V**—3 distinct types:
  - Acute; begins 1–2 h after chemo & peaks at 4–6 h
  - Delayed; begins at 24 h & peaks at 48–72 h
  - Anticipatory; conditioned response to nausea a/w previous cycles of chemo
- **Classifying risk of CINV—**based on %frequency of associated nausea/emesis, chemotherapeutic agents are classified into risk classes:
  - High risk: >90%; common agents: Cisplatin, high-dose cyclophosphamide, anthracycline/ cyclophosphamide (AC) regimens
  - Mod. risk: <90% & >30%; eg, doxorubicin, low-dose cyclophosphamide
  - Low risk: <30% & >10%; eg, docetaxel, trastuzumab, gemcitabine
  - Minimal risk: <10%; eg, vincristine, rituximab

CINV Prophylaxis and Tx			
Tx for IV chemo w/ Mod. and High Emetogenic Risk			
Category	**Medication Name**	**D 1 (start before chemo)**	**D 2, 3, & 4**
5HT2 antagonist	Olanzapine	5–10 mg PO	5–10 mg PO daily
5HT3 antagonist	Dolasetron	100 mg PO	100 mg PO daily
	Granisetron	2 mg PO or 0.01 mg/kg (max 1 mg) IV or 3.1 mg/ 24-h transdermal patch applied 24–48 h prior	1–2 mg PO or 1 mg PO BID or 0.01 mg/kg IV daily
	Ondansetron	16–24 mg PO or 8–16 mg IV (max 32 mg daily)	8 mg PO BID or 16 mg PO daily or 8 mg (max 32 mg daily) IV
	Palonosetron	0.25 mg IV (d 1 only)	
Corticosteroids	Dexamethasone	12 mg PO or IV	8–12 mg PO or IV daily
Neurokinin 1 antagonists	Aprepitant	125 mg PO	80 mg PO daily (d 2,3) ± dexamethasone 8 mg
	Fosaprepitant	150 mg IV (d 1 only)	
Neurokinin 1/ 5HT3 antagonist	Netupitant/ Palonosetron	300 mg/0.5 mg PO (d 1 only)	
	Fosnetupitant/ Palonosetron	235 mg/0.25 mg IV (d 1 only)	

5HT3 antagonists, NK1 antagonists, & corticosteroids doses generally lower outside of CINV or in less emetogenic regimens. Adjunctive medications include—Lorazepam 0.5–2 mg PO or IV or sublingual q6h, H2 blockers &/or PPI.

Constipation

- **Frequency—**affects 60–90% of advanced CA pts on opioid tx (*Curr Treat Options Oncol* 2019;20(12):91); other contributors: Malignant obstruction, ↓ PO/fluid intake, inactivity, anticholinergics, electrolyte imbalance
- **Goal—**easily passed bowel movement (BM) q1–2d; initiate PPx when opioids are started
- **Evaluation**—R/o obstruction & fecal impaction; if impacted, administer glycerol suppositories ± mineral oil enema. Consider disimpaction if no contraindications; consider premedication w/ analgesic ± anxiolytic prior to procedure. Avoid PR meds w/ neutropenia
- **Nonpharm Tx,** if able: ↑ fluid intake, ↑ activity/exercise, ↑ dietary fiber or supplementation
- **Prophylactic Tx:** Stimulant laxative ± osmotic laxative; eg, senna 8.6 mg tab, 2 tabs (17 mg) qhs ± polyethylene glycol 17 g/d; if not on opioids, may start polyethylene glycol as initial agent if can tolerate volume
- **Step up Rx**—add to initial w/ bisacodyl, titrate to 10–15 mg PO daily-TID. If persistent, consider bisacodyl suppository, 1 suppository PR daily-BID (avoid in neutropenia); titrate polyethylene glycol, 1 capful/ 8 oz water PO BID (max 34 g/d); lactulose 30 mL PO BID-QID or 60 mL daily; sorbitol, 30 mL PO q2h ×3, then PRN; magnesium hydroxide, 30–60 mL PO daily-BID; or magnesium citrate, 8 oz PO/PR daily
- If opioid-induced constipation is refractory to standard Rx, consider peripherally acting μ-opioid receptor antagonist (PAMORA) methylnaltrexone, 8 or 12 mg/dose SC no more than once daily or naloxegol, 12.5–25 mg/d PO; **must r/o obstruction before initiating methylnaltrexone**

Anorexia/cachexia syndrome

- Definitions: **Anorexia**—loss of appetite & ↓ caloric intake
  - **Starvation**—loss of wt w/ relative preservation of muscle mass until end stages
- **Cancer cachexia syndrome—**multifactorial syndrome defined by loss of skeletal muscle mass not fully reversed by nutritional support → progressive functional impairment (*Lancet Oncol* 2011;12(5):489)
- **Pathophysiology—**chronic inflammation w/ ↑ cytokine activity (TNFα, IL-1β, IL-6) → dysregulated metabolism w/ ↑ proteolysis & ↓ appetite
- **Diagnosis—**≥5% involuntary wt loss over 6 mos (in absence of simple starvation) or ≥2% wt loss in pt w/ initial BMI <20 or sarcopenia & any degree of wt loss ≥2%

- **Evaluation—**screen for reversible potential contributors (eg, dysgeusia, mucositis, pain, N/V, dyspnea, constipation/bowel obstruction, mucositis, xerostomia, oral candidiasis, depression, anxiety, delirium, fatigue)
- **Interventions—**pt/caregiver education, dietary/modular nutritional supplementation or support, exercise program, nutritional counseling or registered dietician consult, consider swallow evaluation
- **Pharmacology**—appetite stimulants:
  - **Corticosteroids:** Dexamethasone 4–8 mg/d or prednisone 20–40 mg/d. Use & benefit limited by s/e w/ long-term use, indicated primarily for short courses (<6 wks) in advanced dz
  - **Progesterone analogs:** Megestrol acetate 400–800 mg/d if life expectancy at least mos to wks (more efficacious at higher doses)—appetite ↑ in ~1 wk, wt gain takes several wks; fewer s/e than steroids w/ similar efficacy, & include ↑ risk of VTE, suppression of hypothalamic–pituitary axis; consider olanzapine 5 mg PO as alternative
  - **Cannabinoids:** Dronabinol may ↑ appetite, less wt gain, s/e include sedation & confusion. Evidence for efficacy limited in advanced CA pts
  - If concurrent depression/anorexia, consider mirtazapine 7.5–30 mg PO qhs
  - If concurrent gastroparesis (early satiety), consider metoclopramide 5–10 mg PO QID 30 min before meals & at bedtime
  - No evidence for prophylactic use of any pharmacologic agents

Dyspnea

- **Etiology**—multifactorial, various causes: Space-occupying masses or pleural effusions; anemia; comorbid COPD or CHF, PE, PNA, hypoxia or hypercarbia; thick secretions; & respiratory muscle weakness
- **Tx**—target specific etiologies & direct Rx to these (eg, thoracentesis for pleural effusion, bronchodilators for bronchospasm, CA-directed tx for underlying dz)
- **Supplemental O_2**—clear utility in hypoxia; in nonhypoxemic pts may have some benefit but no more efficacious than room air by nasal cannula
- **Nonpharmacologic approaches**—airflow or fan, supplemental O_2 if hypoxemic, self-mgmt strategies, breathing postures & techniques, physical therapy, acupressure or reflexology, pt/caregiver education & support (*J Clin Oncol* 2021; 39:12)
- **Pharmacologic approach**—for 1° tx of dyspnea in advanced dz:
  - Opioids—1st-line Rx for dyspnea
    - Initial doses: Opioid naïve pt—PO morphine sulfate 2.5–10 mg q2h PRN or 1–3 mg IV q2h PRN
    - If opioid tolerant, increase dose by 25% or use efficacious dose of currently used opioid
    - If dyspnea intermittent, use PRN; if constant, consider regularly scheduled dosing or starting a long-acting medication
    - More aggressive titration warranted w/ acute, progressive dyspnea or for opioid tolerant pts
  - Benzodiazepines—2nd-line Rx, 1° efficacy is in combination w/ opioids. For intermittent mgmt, use short-acting benzo (eg, lorazepam 0.25–1 mg PO q4h PRN if benzo naive); for persistent, consider long-acting benzo (eg, clonazepam 0.25 mg q12h)

Fatigue

- **Prevalence/screening**—occurs in up to 75% of all solid tumor pts & up to 99% of CA pts receiving multimodal tx. Providers should screen for fatigue at initial visit, at dx of advanced dz & w/ each chemo visit; should assess for depression & insomnia w/ new dx of fatigue
- Tx contributing factors—pain, depression, anxiety, sleep disturbance, nutritional deficits, decreased functional status
- **Tx**—cognitive–behavioral Rx incl. teaching & counseling, education, exercise (unless contraindicated), energy conservation strategies, referral to appropriate specialist or supportive care provider
  - Pharm—stimulants: Limit to pts w/ mod.-to-sev. fatigue when nonpharm methods unsuccessful; optimal dosing not yet established
  - Methylphenidate—initial dose 5–10 mg PO in AM ± 5 mg at noon
  - Modafinil—200 mg in AM ± 100 mg at noon (max 400 mg/d)
  - Corticosteroids—use in setting of concurrent sx, incl. anorexia or nausea
- Common 2° causes to eval & target include anemia (most common), thyroid or adrenal insufficiency, hypogonadism

Definition

- Any process, mechanical or functional, preventing the forward propulsion of bowel contents
- **Can be partial or complete, single or multifocal** & **is a medical emergency**

RFs & prevalence

- Common complication in pts w/ **abd or pelvic CAs**
- Ovarian > colorectal > gastric
- Frequency as high as 42% of advanced ovarian cas
- Small bowel (extraluminal peritoneal mets) > large bowel involvement (intraluminal colorectal)

Clinical manifestations

- **Nausea (most common), vomiting, abd pain, absence of stool/flatus,** ± **abd distention**
- Absent bowel sounds, hypoactive or high-pitched → impending obstruction
- Vomiting occurs early in proximal obstructions, late in distal
- Abdominal pain may be continuous (90%), colicky (80%)

Diagnosis

- **Hx** → **prior abd surgery or malignancy must be sought**
- PE → fever, tachycardia, abd distention, paucity of bowel sounds, surgical abd scars. Rectal exam may reveal empty vault, mass, or blood PR.
- Imaging → **AXR** demonstrating dilated proximal colon, no distal air, presence of air–fluid levels; **CT** demonstrating transition point
- Pneumoperitoneum → surgical emergency

Management

Interventional Management		
Intervention	**Indication**	**Notes**
NGT + IVF	Initial resuscitative measures, short-term GI compression (<8 d)	Uncomfortable & a/w nasal cartilage erosion, sinusitis, aspiration PNA, & bleeding (*Curr Oncol Rep* 2009;12:520) Only 20% effective (*Oxford Handbook of Pall Care*. 2nd ed. 2009)
Surgery	Localized dz, good PS, >2 mos estimated survival	High postop morbidity & mortality w/ short survival (*JAMA Surg* 2014;149:383)
Stent	High-risk surgical pt, single obstruction in proximal & colorectal obstruction	Well tolerated, improves sxs in >75% (*Ann of Med and Surg* 2015;4:264; *Cancer Manag Res* 2012;4:159)
PEG	Intractable N/V, long-term bowel decompression	May allow intermittent PO intake (*Palliat Med* 2002;16:520)

Medical Management	
Category	**Medication**
Analgesics	**Opioids**—follow institutional opioid guidelines & titrate to effect. Parenteral route preferred
Steroids	**Dexamethasone**—consider in inoperable cases w/ intractable sxs, 6–18 mg IV daily, may resolve obstruction, no significant difference in mortality (*Cochrane Database Sys Rev* 2000(2):CD001219)
Antiemetics	**Olanzapine**—2.5–10 mg PO/IM once daily (*J Pain Symptom Manage*. 2012;44(4):604) **Haloperidol**—1–2 mg IV/SC q6–8h (*Anesthesiology* 2004;101:1454) **Metoclopramide**—for functional obstruction; 10–20 mg IV/SC q6h or 2–4 mg/h IV (*Support Care Cancer* 2004;12:432)
Antisecretory	**Octreotide (preferred)**—0.25–0.5 mg/d IV/SC titrate daily to 0.75 mg/d (*J Pain Symptom Manage* 2010;40:1) **Scopolamine**—0.1 mg/h IV/SC or 0.1–0.2 mg/h TD patch (*J Pain Symptom Manage* 2000;19:23) **Glycopyrrolate**—0.2–0.4 mg IV/SC or 0.02 mg/h IV/SC (*J Pain Symptom Manage* 1999;18:153)

Hydration

- Most pts w/ bowel obstruction are dehydrated → ↑ secretion of water into bowel ↓ PO of fluids
- **No correlation between intensity of thirst, dry mouth, & quantity of hydration administered** (*J Pain Symptom Manage* 1995;10:192)
- Sx of dry mouth can be addressed w/ **sips of water, ice chips, & meticulous oral care** (*J Pain Symptom Manage* 2000;19:23)
- Indications for hydration in terminally ill CA pts:
  Prevent dehydration-induced agitation/confusion
  Prevent prerenal failure w/ resulting delirium, myoclonus, & seizures
- **Limit PO to volume of UOP/24 h + 500 mL for insensible losses**

Total parental nutrition

- Avoid routine use of TPN—controversial use in advanced incurable CA pts (*Nutrition* 1996;12:163; *Eur J of Cancer* 2008;44:1105)
- **Selection of appropriate pts the most critical decision**
- Consider social, cultural, emotional, existential, spiritual, & ethnic background & needs
- **Will not correct CA-induced cachexia**
- <50% of terminally ill CA pts experience sensation of hunger or thirst. **Select pts at EOL—sips of water, soup, or ice chips may be offered for pleasure if tolerated**
- Nutritional benefits limited if delivered only for very short time
- Requires full discussion w/ pt & family regarding risks, benefits, & triggers for discontinuation of TPN
- Concurrent chemo + TPN: Low efficacy, high morbidity & mortality (*Nutr Clin Prac* 1994;9:91)

Total Parenteral Nutrition	
Indication	Maintain or restore nutritional status & prevent malnutrition-related sx
Selection	KPS >50 (*Nutrition* 2006;22:355) Predicted survival >3 mos (*J Parenter Enter Nutr* 1997;21:339)
Benefits	Prevent further nutritional deterioration Correct some manifestations of malnutrition QoL benefit in selected pts (*Cancer Med* 2017:1799:1806)
Risks	Central line–associated pneumothorax, thrombosis, & sepsis (*J Pain Symptom Manage* 1997;13:104) TPN-associated electrolyte abnormalities, liver failure, & hyperglycemia ↑ fluid intake → ↑ GI & pulmonary secretions, peripheral edema
Considerations	Permanent invasive central venous access required—cannot use a peripheral IV Requires training to maintain TPN at home—sometimes wk (*Support Care Cancer* 2001;9:223) Frequent electrolyte & hydration assessment needed **May prolong survival at cost of prolonged suffering**—relevant in pts w/ no further chemo tx options

What is adolescent and young adult (AYA) oncology?

- **Pts 15–39 yo** have unique needs & inferior outcomes, potentially d/t biology, later dx, lower clinical trial accrual, inferior adherence, unclear standards of care & inconsistent use of supportive services
- Unique biopsychosocial needs/developmental stages & maturity make tailoring of CA care important, ideally in a center w/ AYA-specific expertise/resources. Guidelines: *NCCN Clinical Practice Guidelines (Adolescent and Young Adult Oncology (V2.2018))*
- **Common AYA CA:** Leukemias, lymphomas, sarcomas, testicular, germ cell, thyroid, melanoma, CNS. Other CAs have also been occurring earlier (early-onset) (eg, breast, cervical, CRC)

Fertility

- Discuss contraception, risks of **infertility,** & options for fertility preservation (male: Sperm banking +/– testicular sperm extraction/electroejaculation; female: Embryo/oocyte or ovarian tissue cryopreservation) as soon as possible, preferably prior to therapy initiation. Care incl. mental health & social services support **(see also Cancer Survivorship chapter on fertility)**
- Consider menstrual suppression for expected cytopenias or oophoropexy for planned RT

Genetics

- Consider referral to genetic counselor, as nearly **10% of AYAs will have a germline mutation in a CA-predisposing gene** (*NEJM* 2015;373:2336)
- Consider germline &/or somatic genomic analysis for all pts

Psycho-oncology and supportive care

- Evaluate individual's support system & preferred extent of involvement of support system, incl. role of parents & significant other
- Provide resources for ongoing educational & vocational support
- Assess gender expression & identity, sexual identity, & chosen name/pronouns
- Prepare for changes in body image, identity, goals & perceptions of future
- Understand role of spirituality & religion in individual's life
- Connect w/ peer support groups, both virtual & in person, where safe & available
- Obtain detailed social hx, incl. substance use/abuse, sexual health, physical activity & diet, & sleep patterns
- Explore role of complementary/alternative medicine & integrative therapies

Clinical trials and treatment

- Given inferior outcomes for AYAs w/CA, offer clinical trials in specific dzs if eligible & appropriate
- Consider the use of pediatric-adapted protocols for AYAs when available
- Discuss late-term & long-term tx effects & toxicities as aggressive txs can compromise long-term fxn & QoL; monitor cumulative doses
- Screen for cardiotoxicity, nephrotoxicity, ototoxicity, neurotoxicity, & endocrinopathies

Vulnerable subpopulations

- **LGBTQ+:** Significant comorbid psychosocial stressors that can affect adherence
- Socioeconomically disadvantaged: May lack access to AYA programs & centers

Survivorship

- Develop a **CA tx summary & survivorship care plan** **(see also survivorship section)**

Miscellaneous

- Discuss advanced directives, medical power of attorney & living will early during tx
- Consider caregiver & **parent/spouse burden & needs of children**
- Recognize role of culture & heritage in decision making & EOL care
- Acknowledge **financial burden & toxicity** & discuss insurance
- **Provide resources** for transportation, food scarcity, & accommodations when possible

OLDER ADULT ONCOLOGY

Definition of older adult

- Based on **functional status & age** (generally >65 yo); significant % of pts w/ CA (*J Clin Oncol* 2009;27(17):2758–2765)

Why approach older adults differently?

- Biologic characteristics of certain CAs & how they respond to tx may be different
- Physiologic changes w/ aging may affect ability to tolerate chemo &/or other CA txs
- Older adults are underrepresented in clinical trials → data lacking
- Consider life expectancy & risks of testing, over-dx & over-tx before recommending CA screening, incl. for breast, colorectal, & prostate CA (see American Board of Internal Medicine [ABIM]/American Geriatrics Society [AGS] 2021 guidance on ChoosingWisely.org)

When to consult geriatrics?

- If + on formal screening tools (eg, G8, TRST, VES-13)—assesses need w/ Comprehensive Geriatric Assessment (see *J Clin Oncol* 2014;32(24):2595–2603; *J Natl Compr Canc Netw* 2021;19(9): 1006–1019)
- In the presence of:
  - Cognitive impairment
  - Functional or physical impairment
  - Multiple comorbidities (incl. vision & hearing)
  - Polypharmacy
  - High-risk procedure/txs (eg, HSCT)
  - Presence of geriatric syndromes such as frailty, osteoporosis, pressure ulcers, incontinence, neglect, or abuse
  - Wt loss/compromised nutritional status
  - Socioeconomic stressors
  - Psychosocial distress (eg, depression)

Approach to cancer treatment decision making

- Assess **decisional capacity**
  - If capacity: Assess if pt goals/values in line w/ anti-CA tx
  - If no capacity: Proxy/advanced directive/family meeting/sw & other support
- **Surgery:** For older adults undergoing surgery, refer to AGS/American College of Surgery (ACS) guidelines
  - Incr. functional requirements preop —> incr. postop complications, hospital stay & mortality
  - Prehabilitation &/or collaboration w/ geriatricians may improve outcomes of frail pt
- **Systemic therapy:** Tools to assess risks of chemo toxicity in older population:
  - Cancer & Aging Research Group (CARG)—Demographics, CA type, chemo risk, laboratory values, functional status, hearing
  - Chemotherapy Risk Assessment Scale for High-Age Patients (CRASH)—Risk according to regimen, hematologic RFs, nonhematologic RFs
  - Approach steroids w/ caution d/t incr. risk of cognitive s/e

Special considerations for older adults

- **Hearing loss:** Monitor & avoid neurotoxic agents
  - Amplifying devices include hearing aids, pocket-talker
- **Falls:** Periodic fall assessments throughout tx
- **Insomnia:** Avoid benzos & sedative hypnotics as 1st-line tx, trial nonpharm mgmt
- **Optimizing communication:** Avoid medical terminology, rephrase rather than repeat, use teach back for major concepts
- **Improving adherence:** Synchronize med refills w/ pharmacy, prepare pt for anticipated s/e, provide written instructions, engage family/care providers

PSYCHO-ONCOLOGY

Interdisciplinary field; addresses biopsychosocial, behavioral, & physical aspects of CA during all phases of dz for pts & caregivers. CA occurs in pts w/ mental illness & mental illness occurs in pts w/ CA.

Screening tools

- May identify pts who benefit from further evaluation for psycho-oncologic illness, but tx should not be initiated solely based on screening instrument
- **Psychological distress:** Rescreening at regular intervals & "at pivotal medical visits"
- **Distress thermometer (DT):** 10-point self-reported scale for clinically significant distress
- **Delirium:** Multiple screening tools, eg, Delirium Rating Scale (DRS) (*Psychiatry Res* 1988;23:89–97); Confusion Assessment Method (CAM) (*Ann Intern Med* 1990;113:941–948)

Delirium

- Common & underdiagnosed neuropsychiatric complication, esp. in elderly pts. Can lead to incr. length of hospitalization & higher mortality & morbidity
- Delirium subtypes include **hyperactive, hypoactive, & mixed delirium**
- RFs: **Advanced age,** severity of illness, cognitive impairment, immobility, sensory impairment, pain, poor nutritional status
- Identify & treat underlying causes (eg, infection, intoxication, withdrawal, pulmonary embolism, acute neurologic event, etc.)

Medications Used for Delirium in Cancer Patients

Class	Name	Dose and Route	Side Effects
Antipsychotics "typical"	Haloperidol—1st-line agent	Mild to moderate: 0.5–2 mg every 8–12 h; PO/IV/IM/SC Severe: 0.5–2 mg IV q1–4h PRN	Sedation QT prolongation Need EKG at baseline & w/ dosing changes Greater risk w/ typical agents & parenteral admin Extrapyramidal sx (typical > atypical) Wt gain, metabolic syndrome (atypical > typical)
	Chlorpromazine	Severe: 25–100 mg PO/PR/IV q4h PRN for bedbound pts	
Antipsychotics "atypical"	Olanzapine	Mild to moderate: 5–20 mg every 24 h; PO Severe: 2.5–7.5 mg PO/SL q2–4h PRN (max dose: 30 mg/d)	
	Risperidone	0.5–2 mg every 12 h; PO, oral disintegrating	
	Quetiapine	25–200 mg every 12–24 h; PO/SL	

Depression

- Common in CA pts & confounded d/t sxs of CA &/or CA tx
- High prevalence of depressive disorders in pancreas, head & neck, breast, lung CA
- Recognition/tx mitigates sxs, improves QoL. SSRIs & psychosocial interventions are considered 1st-line tx as listed in the following table
- Choice of antidepressant—largely based on s/e profile & drug–drug interaction. Usually start at low doses & gradually titrate up to effective dose
- Psychostimulants: Sometimes used for fatigue/psychomotor retardation at EOL d/t quick onset, but currently no strong evidence supports this. Activating antidepressants (eg, bupropion, duloxetine, etc.) may increase anxiety/exacerbate sleep disturbance

Anxiety

- Common/expected reaction to CA, esp. at initial dx, relapse, high sx burden, EOL, etc.
- Maladaptive & debilitating anxiety should be addressed & treated

- Psychotherapeutic & behavioral interventions can also be very helpful
- Pts may not be able to accurately describe anxiety. Pain refractory to escalating opioids may represent anxiety & may benefit from a benzodiazepine (benzo)
- Benzos, esp. in combination w/ opioids, may result in severe suppression of the respiratory drive. Use w/ caution & consider naloxone prescription for opioid overuse if this is compatible w/ goals of care
- Benzos may be insufficient for anxiety of sev. respiratory distress. Opioids should be used

Medications Used for Depression in Cancer Patients			
Class	**Name and Benefit**	**Dose and Route**	**Side Effects**
SSRI (most commonly used are Sertraline, Escitalopram, Citalopram)	**Sertraline** Least CYP450 drug interaction	25–150 mg/day PO—Available in liquid form	GI s/e, bleeding risks, hyponatremia, sexual dysfunction Citalopram & Escitalopram can prolong QTc esp. when combined w/ other QTc prolonging agents
	Citalopram Preferred in hepatic dz	10–20 mg/day PO—Available in liquid form	
	Escitalopram Least CYP450 drug interaction	5–10 mg/day PO—Available in liquid form	
SNRI	**Venlafaxine** Least interaction w/ Tamoxifen	37.5–225 mg/day PO, XR once a day formulation available	Dose-dependent increase in diastolic BP, withdrawal sxs, urinary retention
	Duloxetine Useful for pts w/ neuropathic pain	20–60 mg/day PO	Urinary retention, dry mouth, nausea
Other agents	**Mirtazapine** Helps w/ insomnia, antiemetic, & appetite	7.5–45 mg/day PO, SolTab available	Sedation, wt gain, constipation, vivid dreams
Medications Used for Anxiety in Cancer Patients			
Class	**Name and Benefit**	**Dose and Route**	**Side Effects**
Benzodiazepine	**Alprazolam** Acute onset of action	0.25–1 mg PO q4–24h	Respiratory depression, paradoxical effect in the elderly causing agitation & delirium. Potential cause of abuse
	Clonazepam	0.25–1 mg PO q12–24h	
	Diazepam	2–10 mg PO/IV q6–q24h	
	Lorazepam	0.25–2 mg PO/IM/IV q2–q24h	

Suicide

- Incidence of suicide ↑ in pts w/ CA compared to the general population; up to 17% of pts w/ CA have suicidal thoughts at some point (*J Psychosoc Oncol* 2008;26:49–62)
- Higher rates in some CAs (lung, GI, head & neck)
- RFs include male sex, white race, unmarried status, hx of suicide attempt or self-injurious behavior, psychiatric dx, high sx burden, & undertreated pain (*J Clin Oncol* 2008;26:4731–4738)
- Thoughts of or wish to talk about death are not unusual w/ advanced illness & may not represent mental illness or suicidality. Pts may have difficulty raising the topic or meet resistance from supports who are uncomfortable w/ EOL issues. Thoughtful/compassionate exploration can avoid psychiatric referral in some

Supportive psychotherapy

- Providers of all specialties can deliver interventions such as reassurance, education, encouragement, & facilitating emotional expression
- Education regarding tx options at EOL can help relieve distress

CANCER SURVIVORSHIP

Overview

- W/ improvement in dx & tx of CA, there are millions of CA survivors & this # is ↑
- Pts experience nl issues of aging, compounded by long-term effects of CA & CA tx
- CA survivors are at ↑ risk of developing morbidity at younger age than general population d/t their CA tx

Key components of survivorship care (ASCO.org)

- Ensure screening for CA (incl. genetic testing referrals as necessary) & assessing for recurrent dz
- Implement prevention programs (incl. education regarding healthy lifestyle)
- Monitor side effects & psychosocial effects, & ensure access to services (eg, fertility counseling, financial services)
- Encourage advocacy & education

Survivorship care plan

- **Comprehensive care summary & clear follow-up plan should be completed after 1° tx for all pts**
- **Tx summary should include the following:**
  CA type
  Tumor characteristics (site, pathology, stage, grade)
  Tx received: Surgery, chemo, biologic, hormonal rx, transplant, radiation (include agents, dose, sites, dates)
  Care provider & institution contact info
- **Survivorship care plan should include the following:**
  Timing & type of surveillance rec; recommendations for preventive practices & monitoring of potential consequences of tx; address potential psychosocial concerns

Secondary cancer risks of treatment

Secondary Primary CA	RFs
Hematologic (MDS, leukemia, lymphoma)	Alkylating chemo RT exposure
Solid tumors	RT to specific tissue *(NEJM 2003;349:640)* 1. Breast CA w/ RT, ↑ risk in women exposed to RT <30 y 2. Lung CA w/ RT, alkylating chemo, ↑↑ risk w/ tobacco 3. Bone & soft tissue sarcoma w/ RT 4. Colon CA & esophageal CA w/ RT to those fields 5. Thyroid CA w/ RT

Cancer screening recommendations as per ACS guidelines:
(https://www.cancer.org/healthy/find-cancer-early/american-cancer-society-guidelines-for-the-early-detection-of-cancer.html)

Colorectal: Colonoscopy starting at age 45 for those considered at standard risk, repeat every 5–10 y/based on findings & gastroenterologist recommendations

Cervical cancer: Starting age 25 PAP Smear, +HPV screening per GYN/ACS guidelines

Breast: Annual MMG. Add'l screening rec for high-risk individuals per ACS-family hx, genetic predisposition

*Women exposed to chest RT< age 30 should have MMG & breast MRI 8 y after RT or at age 35, whichever comes 1st

Prostate: PSA monitoring w/ PCP or urologist as per ACS guidelines

Lung: Pts aged 55–80 who have been CA free for 5 y & have a h/o smoking at least 1 ppd × 30 y who currently smoke or quit w/in past 15 y should have screening low-dose CT chest annually × 3 y.

Long-term complications of cancer treatment

Complications by System	Risk Factors/Recommendations
CV dz CHF	**Anthracyclines** (cumulative dose-dependent >300 mg/m^2, ↑ risk w/ concurrent RT, younger age at tx) (*NEJM* 1998;339:900) & for pts w/ other RFs for cardiac dx (eg, smoking, obesity, HTN, HLD, T2DM, strong family hx) (*JCO* 2017;35:893–911) For high-risk survivors, recommend screening for HF (echo w/ strain rate) consider referral to cardiology (*BMC Cancer* 2015;15:366) HER2-targeted therapies (eg, trastuzumab)
Vasospasm	Fluoropyrimidines (eg, fluorouracil, capecitabine)
CAD	RT-related CAD (*Blood* 2007;109:1878)
GI Dysmotility, malabsorption, bowel dysfunction	RT, surgery (eg, gastrectomy), vinca, antitubule drugs
Hepatic dysfunction	MTX, carmustine (*NEJM* 2018; 379:2438–2450)
Impaired immune fxn	Steroids, rituximab, alemtuzumab, SCT, splenectomy, CAR-T Monitor for chronic sinopulmonary infxns, monitor IgG levels prn. Consider IVIG/referral to immunologist, implications for vaccine effectiveness post tx
Lymphatic	RT, LN dissection
Lymphedema	Referral for compression sleeve/lymphedema therapy
Musculoskeletal Bone & soft tissue damage Osteoporosis Osteonecrosis	Low BMI, personal or parental h/o nontraumatic fx, current smoking, >3 alcoholic drinks/day. Menopause Antiandrogens (prostate CA) Aromatase inhibitors (breast CA) Prolonged steroid use (leading to avascular necrosis) Radiation fibrosis (2/2 RT) DEXA screening, adequate dietary vitamin D3 & calcium. Monitor vitamin D level, rec wt-bearing exercises. Bisphosphonates, RANKL-inhib considered w/ high-risk pts (*JCO* 2012;30:3665–3674)
Neurologic Cognitive changes, fatigue	WBRT; chemo, hormonal agents Older age, prolonged intensive chemo, anxiety, depression, fatigue, intrathecal chemo (*Neurosci Biobehav Rev* 2017;83:417–428) Neurocognitive assessment. R/o other reversible causes (eg, depression) Tx: CBT, compensatory strategies for executive fct deficits, physical activity
Pulmonary complications: Pneumonitis, COP Chemo lung tox Long-term respiratory sxs	Radiation-induced changes Bleomycin, taxanes, gemcitabine, TKIs, trastuzumab, CPIs Surgical resection Consider obtaining PFTs post tx
Renal Impaired kidney fxn	Cisplatin, MTX, nitrosoureas, RT Monitor at-risk pts w/ BUN/Creatinine/GFR & UA annually
Reproductive Ovarian failure, premature menopause, or azoospermia 2° chemo	SERMs, aromatase inhibitors; GnRH agonists, ADT Chemo, pelvic radiation, surgery (ooph/hyst/orchiectomy) Referral for further eval w/ reproductive endocrinologist
Psychiatric	H/o mental illness, sedentary lifestyle, lack of social support, financial concerns, prior trauma, chronic pain, CA tx that causes physical limitations (*J Natl Compr Canc Netw* 2007;5:3–7)
Anxiety/depression PTSD Fear of recurrence	All survivors should be screened at all visits for anxiety, depression, distress (*JCO* 2014; 32:1605) Pharmacologic interventions: Antidepressants/anxiolytics, etc. (*Med Clin North Am* 2017;101:1099–1113)
Return to work/ financial issues	Nonpharm interventions: CBT, mindfulness, physical activity, psychotherapy
Thyroid Hypothyroidism Thyroid nodules	Neck radiation (dose-dependent) Annual thyroid exam, TSH, free T4 for pts w/ h/o neck RT

Sexual dysfunction	Chemo, tamoxifen, aromatase inhibitors, antiandrogens, prostatectomy/RT for prostate CA, pelvic surgery & RT Women: Vaginal moisturizers, intravaginal estrogens, tx of vasomotor sxs, vaginal dilators, antidepressants Men: 5-phosphodiesterase inhibitors, alprostadil inj or suppository, tx of vasomotor sx, penile implants Couples counseling, physical activity, pelvic floor physical therapy (*JCO* 2018;36:492–511)
Peripheral neuropathy	Taxanes, platins, vinca alkaloids, proteasome inhibitors, antitubule ADCs (eg, brentuximab, polatuzumab) Dose dependent, duloxetine, gabapentin, topical agents. Nondrug interventions: Frozen gloves, socks, supportive shoes (*JCO* 2014;32:1941)
Chronic pain	CA-related & tx-related causes Pharmacologic & nonpharmacologic interventions available
Fatigue	Chemo/RT/IO & BMT Pharmacologic interventions/CBT, exercise, psychotherapy (*JCO* 2014;32:1840–1850)
Insomnia	Chemo, vasomotor sxs, RT, HDC, BMT Sedatives, hypnotics, melatonin, tx of vasomotor sxs, sleep hygiene, physical activity, CBT
Metabolic syn	Cranial irradiation, advanced prostate CA, prostate CA w/ higher Gleason scores Inflammation, obesity, insulin resistance Tx of DM, HTN, & HLD. Healthy diet & exercise (*Cancer* 2016;7:289–295)

Health promotion (NCCN guidelines, Survivorship 3.2021)

- Diet: Plant-based, limit refined sugars & red meat, ≤3 servings of soy foods. ↑ omega 3's (protective measures against 2nd malignancies) (*Nutr Rev* 2016;74(12):737–748)
- Exercise 150 min/wk (Studies in colon/breast CA found reduced risk of recurrence). Linked w/higher QoL for CA survivors (*Cancers* 2017;9(5):E53)
- Wt mgmt: Obesity linked to CA risk & outcomes (*JCO* 2014;32:3568–3574)
- Smoking cessation: Referral to smoking cessation program
- Reduce alcohol consumption: Limit: 2 drinks/d for men, 1 drink/d for women (*JCO* 2018:36: 83–93)

Older survivors

- % of CA survivors over 65 y is ↑ ing. Older CA survivors may not have the same goals as younger adult survivors. Rec no longer screening pts for 2nd CA once life expectancy is <10 y (*Am Fam Physician* 2016;93(8):659–667)

Vaccines

- Annual flu
- PNA: All pts >65 yo. Pts aged 19–64 y w/ immunocompromising conditions, ie, generalized malignancy (CDC). 1 dose PCV13, 1 dose PPSV23 at least 8 wks later, then PPSV23 5 y later & at age 65 y
- Shingrix age >50 y. 2 doses given 2–6 mos apart
- SARS-CoV-2 vaccination for all survivors regardless of immunocompetency

Resources for providers and patients

National Coalition of Cancer Survivorship (www.canceradvocacy.org); LIVESTRONG (www.livestrong.org); ACS Survivorship Resource Center (www.cancer.org/survivorshipcenter); CDC guidelines—Recommended Vaccines for adults (https://www.cdc.gov/vaccines/adults/rec-vac/index.html); NCI—Office of Cancer Survivorship (http://cancercontrol.cancer.gov/ocs/)

FERTILITY PRESERVATION

Adult cancer patient population

- ~327,430 male & ~416,840 female CA survivors <40 yo (*Cancer Treatment and Survivorship Facts and Figures 2019–2021*, ACS)
- Fertility is important to survivors & many CA therapies pose a risk to future fertility. Providers caring for pts (adult & pediatric) dx'd w/ CA should address the possibility of infertility *before* tx begins

Risk factors for impaired fertility

Treatment (*JCO* 2018;36:1994; *Fertil Steril* 2019;112:1022)

- Surgery resulting in resection of or damage to reproductive structures
- Chemo destroying spermatogonia or oocytes (alkylating chemo highest risk; platinum & anthracyclines intermediate risk; risk varies based on agents & cumulative dose)
- RT w/ reproductive structures in tx field (risk based on volume of organ exposed & dose)
- Damage to hypothalamic–pituitary–gonadal axis from cranial surgery or radiation
- Effects of targeted & immunologic agents are largely unknown; however, limited evidence indicating bevacizumab may cause ovarian failure

Pt characteristics

- Age (risk increases w/ age d/t decr ovarian reserve)
- Dx (men w/ testicular CA, lymphoma, & leukemia may have impaired sperm production pretx) (*J Natl Cancer Inst Monogr* 2005:9)
- Obesity, tobacco smoking, excess alcohol intake, & use of recreational drugs are a/w impaired fertility
- H/o unrelated fertility problems (eg, PCOS)

Potential effects of cancer treatment on fertility (*JCO* 2018;36:1994; *Fertil Steril*, 2019; 112:1022)

Females

- Premature ovarian failure (infertility & early-onset menopause)
- Inability to carry a pregnancy
- Disruption of hypothalamic–pituitary–ovarian axis

Males

- Impaired spermatogenesis (low sperm count, azoospermia)
- Impaired transport of sperm (eg, erectile dysfunction, ejaculatory dysfunction)
- Disruption of hypothalamic–pituitary–testicular axis

Fertility preservation options for males (*JCO* 2018;36:1994; *Fertil Steril* 2019;112:1022)

Semen cryopreservation

- *Definition:* Freezing of semen obtained through masturbation, electroejaculation (if unable to ejaculate through masturbation), testicular sperm extraction (if no sperm found in semen); technique for future use depends on sperm concentration & motility but most commonly requires in vitro fertilization
- *Comment:* Recommend 3 collections w/ 2–5 d of abstinence b/w collections; can collect on consecutive days if tx is urgent

Fertility preservation options for females (*JCO* 2018;36:1994; *Fertil Steril* 2019;112:1022)

Embryo cryopreservation

- *Definition:* Freezing of embryos obtained following ~10 d of ovarian stimulation, transvaginal retrieval of mature eggs, & in vitro fertilization; embryos are subsequently thawed & transferred to the uterus when ready to attempt pregnancy
- *Comment:* Most established technique. Requires a male partner or donor sperm

Oocyte cryopreservation

- *Definition:* Freezing of unfertilized eggs obtained following ~10 d of ovarian stimulation & transvaginal retrieval of mature eggs; eggs are thawed & fertilized w/ sperm to create embryos to be transferred to the uterus when ready to attempt pregnancy
- *Comment:* Does not require a male partner or sperm donor at the time of freezing. Success decreases w/ incr. age; most successful in women <35 yo

Ovarian transposition

- *Definition:* Surgical repositioning of the ovaries outside of a RT field
- *Comment:* Embryo or egg freezing should be offered 1st if female wants to have a biologic child in the future; if fallopian tubes are dissected, pt cannot conceive naturally

Ovarian tissue cryopreservation

- *Definition:* Freezing of ovarian tissue obtained by unilateral or partial oophorectomy; tissue may be thawed & reimplanted when ready to attempt pregnancy
- *Comment:* There is a potential for reseeding of CA cells in certain tumor types (eg, leukemia) w/ reimplantation

Ovarian suppression

- *Definition:* The use of GnRH analogs (eg, leuprolide) during chemo to suppress recruitment of follicles & egg maturation
- *Comment:* Controversial regarding efficacy, considered experimental. Should not replace more established fertility preservation methods

Alternative tx for early-stage gynecologic CAs

- Cervical CA: Radical trachelectomy
- Ovarian CA: Unilateral oophorectomy
- Endometrial CA: Progestin therapy
- Comment: Only appropriate for select pts w/ early-stage dz

Post-treatment considerations

- Advise pts to wait at least 1 y post tx before attempting pregnancy, for clearance of gametes exposed to chemo or radiation during maturation
- Pts may be advised to wait a full 2–3 y post tx before attempting pregnancy depending on individual risk of recurrence
- Alternative options for family building include use of donor sperm, donor eggs, & donor embryos. Woman unable to carry a pregnancy can consider surrogacy w/ a gestational carrier (or adoption)

Resources for patient education

American Cancer Society (ACS)

Fertility and Men with Cancer (www.cancer.org/treatment/treatmentsandsideeffects/physicalsideeffects/sexualsideeffectsinmen/fertilityandmenwithcancer/index)

Fertility and Women with Cancer (http://www.cancer.org/treatment/treatmentsandsideeffects/physicalsideeffects/sexualsideeffectsinwomen/fertilityandwomenwithcancer/index)

CancerNet (ASCO)

Fertility Preservation (www.cancer.net/publications-and-resources/what-know-ascos-guidelines/what-know-ascos-guideline-fertility-preservation)

Livestrong/Fertility

Brochures available for free in English & Spanish (http://assets.livestrong.org/we-can-help/LIVESTRONG-Fertility-Brochure.pdf?_ga =1.205086739.226511752.1413988424)

Oncofertility Consortium of Michigan State University

https://oncofertility.msu.edu/for-patients SaveMyFertility (www.savemyfertility.org)

THE HIGH-RISK ONCOLOGY PATIENT

Background: Risk assessment and categories

Infxn risk depends on pt characteristics, underlying malignancy & CA tx. NCCN categories of risk help guide antimicrobial ppx (see following tables). *(NCCN 2.2020. Prevention and Treatment of Cancer-Related Infections)*

Infection Risk Categories (NCCN 2.2020).

Infection Risk	Examples
Low	Most solid tumors on standard chemo Expected neutropenia duration <7 d
Intermediate	Lymphoma, MM, CLL Purine analogs (eg, fludarabine, clofarabine) auto-HCT Expected neutropenia duration 7–10 d
High	AML or ALL induction, consolidation, maintenance allo-HCT GVHD on high-dose steroids Alemtuzumab Expected neutropenia duration >10 d

Predisposing diseases and therapies

Diseases

- *AML, ALL, MDS, lymphoma:* Leukopenia from marrow dysfunction or leukemic infiltration
- *CLL, MM:* Hypogammaglobulinemia predisposes to infxn w/ encapsulated organisms
- *Refractory CA:* Marrow infiltration or poor marrow fxn d/t prior therapies
- *Bulky tumor:* Anatomy disruption may cause stasis &/or fistulas. Assoc necrosis may serve as infectious nidus

Therapies

- *Chemo:* Neutropenia + disruption of mucosal barrier predisposes to bacteremia
- *Other immunosuppressants:*
  - Purine analogs (eg, fludarabine, pentostatin): Listeria, PJP, mycobacteria, opportunistic viral & fungal pathogens
  - Temozolomide (when combined w/ RT): PJP (ppx indicated)
  - High-dose corticosteroids: PJP, nocardiosis
  - Immune-targeted agents: Certain agents increase risk of infxn. Screening, monitoring, & prophylactic strategies may be indicated (see following table)
- RT: Disruption of mucosal barrier, delayed BM recovery (RT to pelvis, spine, long bones), functional asplenia (RT to spleen)
- *Transplantation:* Higher risk w/ allo-HCT vs. auto-HCT & w/ T-cell depleted, cord or haploidentical transplants, myeloablative regimens, GVHD. Functional asplenia in allo-HCT

Screening

- *HIV, HBV, HCV:* Pts who will receive chemo, immunosuppressive therapy, certain immune-target agents (see following table)
- *LTBI:* CD52, mTOR, JAK inhibitors, high-dose steroids
- For screening prior to HCT, see "Infections in the Transplant Host" chapter

Strategies for antimicrobial use

- **Prophylactic:** ABX to prevent infxns in intermediate or high-risk pt
- **Preemptive:** ABX for asx pt w/ laboratory markers of viremia
- **Therapeutic:** ABX to treat established infxn

Fever and neutropenia

Definitions: *Fever:* Single oral temperature ≥38.3°C or ≥38.0°C over 1 h; *Neutropenia:* ANC ≤500 or ANC ≤1,000 + expected to ↓ to ≤500 during next 48 h; *Profound neutropenia:* ANC ≤100; *Prolonged neutropenia:* Neutropenia >7 d

Antimicrobial Prophylaxis Considerations According to Risk Categories			
Host Risk	**Bacterial ppx**	**Fungal ppx**	**Viral ppx**
Low	None	None	If prior episode of HSV
Intermediate	During neutropenia: 1st line: FQ. If allergic or intolerant: Oral 3rd-generation cephalosporin or TMP-SMX	Fluconazole or micafungin during neutropenia or if mucositis anticipated *PJP*: 1st line: Bactrim. Alternatives: Atovaquone, pentamidine IV or aerosolized – Until CD4 >200 or 3–6 mos post auto-HCT	*HSV*: During active chemo, possibly longer *VZV*: 6–12 mos post auto-HCT
High	During neutropenia: 1st line: FQ If allergic or intolerant: Oral 3rd generation ceph-alosporine, TMP-SMX Allo-HCT w/ GVHD: Penicillin or Bactrim	Fluconazole or micafungin: ALL during neutropenia, Allo-HCT for at least 75 d posttransplant Posaconazole: MDS/AML during neutropenia HCT w/ GVHD on immunosuppressant until resolution *PJP*: 1st line: Bactrim. Alternatives: Atovaquone, pentamidine IV or aerosolized – Allo-HCT- until 6 mos post HCT + while on immuno-suppressant – Alemtuzumab-min 2 mos after stopping or until CD4 ≥200	*HSV*: AML/ALL during chemo Alemtuzumab (minimum 2 mos after stopping or until CD4 ≥200) Allo-HCT GVHD on steroids *VZV*: Alemtuzumab Allo-HCT for at least 1 y post HCT GVHD on steroids Proteasome inhibitors *CMV*: Routine surveillance PCR if on alemtuzumab or allo-HCT. If positive, preemptive tx w/ valganciclovir or ganciclovir Consider letermovir for allo-HCT CMV+ recipient

Prophylactic and Screening Considerations for immune/targeted Agents						
Target	**Bacterial ppx**	**Azole ppx**	**PJP ppx**	**Acyclovir ppx**	**CMV Monitoring**	**HBV Screen/ Treat**
BTK			✓	✓		
PI3K			✓		✓	
BCR-ABL						✓
mTOR			✓			✓
JAK			If add'l risk	✓		✓
CD19			✓	✓		✓
CD20			If add'l risk	✓		✓
CD30			✓	✓	✓	If combined regimen
CD38			✓	✓		
CD52			If CD4 <200	✓	✓	
CD19 CAR-T	✓	✓	B-ALL or if add'l risk	✓		✓

Fever & neutropenia (F&N) syndromes
- *Unexplained:* F&N w/o clinical focus or isolated pathogen
- *Clinically documented infxn:* F&N + clinical focus of infxn
- *Microbiologically documented infxn:* F&N + clinical focus of infxn + isolation of pathogen

Epidemiology (*Clin Infect Dis* 2011;52:e56)
- 10–50% of pts w/ solid tumors & >80% of pts w/ hematologic tumors
- Clinically documented infxn in only 20–30%
- Common sites of infxn: Blood, lungs, skin, & GI tract
- Tx should be started w/in 2 h of fever onset which improves outcomes

Risk stratification: Validated scores help identify low-risk & high-risk pts. The latter benefit from hospitalization. These include:
- Multinational Association for Supportive Care in Cancer (MASCC)
- Clinical Index of Stable Febrile Neutropenia (CISNE) (*JCO* 2000;18:3038; *JCO* 2015;33:465; NCCN 2.2020)

Neutropenic Host at High Risk for Complications
Adv age & poor performance status
Severe prolonged neutropenia
Hemodynamic instability or significant comorbidities
Severe oral &/or GI mucositis
Inpt status or hemodynamic instability
Allo-HCT or alemtuzumab
Refractory/progressive CA
Pneumonia or complex infxns
Hepatic (AST/ALT ↑ >5 ULN) or renal (CrCl of <30 mL/min) insufficiency
MASCC ≥21 or CISNE <3

Antibiotic therapy of fever and neutropenia

Initial therapy
- Low-risk (no high RFs, MASCC ≥21): PO ABX (eg, ciprofloxacin + amoxicillin-clavulanate) OR IV ABX at home OR daily long-acting IV +/- PO ABX
- High-risk: Monotherapy w/ antipseudomonal β-lactam ABX (eg, ceftazidime, cefepime, piperacillin–tazobactam, carbapenem)
- Penicillin allergy: ID consultation, consider vancomycin + aztreonam if severe allergy
- Consider modifications to ABX if hemodynamic instability, h/o MDRO, focus of infxn

Add'l antibiotic coverage
- Vancomycin or other gram-positive coverage: Suspected SSTI, MRSA pneumonia, catheter-assoc infxn, hemodynamic instability
- Anaerobic coverage (if not already receiving): Intra-abdominal/perirectal process, hemodynamic instability
- Atypical coverage (azithromycin, doxycycline, fluoroquinolone): Lung infiltrates

Figure 13-1 Empiric Antimicrobial Therapy of Fever and Neutropenia in High-Risk Patients

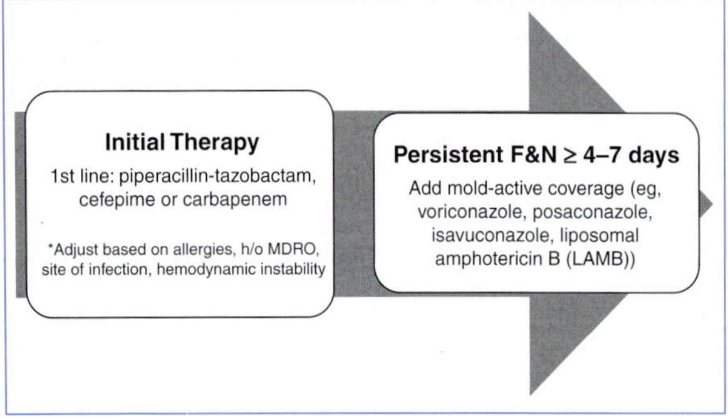

- **Empiric fungal coverage**
  - -Pts w/ thrush or esophagitis (azole or echinocandin), sinus/nasal infxn in high-risk pts (LAMB), lung infiltrates in high-risk pts (mold-active) OR
  - -Not clinically responding after 4–7 d after broad-spectrum antibiotics (see Figure 13-1)

Background

Cause of death in 8% of auto-HCT & up to 21% of allo-HCT recipients (*Biol Blood Marrow Transplant* 2009;15:1143; *OFID* 2017;4:2)

Higher-risk characteristics (*N Engl J Med* 2006;354(17):1813; *Infect Dis Clin N Am* 2010;24:257–272)

- Transplant type: Allo-HCT (slow immune reconstitution)
- Donor type: Unrelated, mismatched, haploidentical (slow immune reconstitution, GVHD risk)
- Graft: Cord blood transplant (slow engraftment)
- Manipulation: T-cell depletion (slow immune reconstitution)
- Conditioning: Myeloablative regimens (mucosal injury, long duration of neutropenia)
- Immunosuppressive regimen: ATG (T-cell deficiency), methotrexate (mucosal injury)
- Other: CVCs (skin breakdown), GVHD, adv dz prior to transplant

Transplant phases and related infections

Based on myeloablative conditioning. Degree of immunosuppression may vary & is based on several factors as mentioned above (*Biol Blood Marrow Transplant* 2009;15:1143; *Infect Dis Clin N Am* 2010;24:257–272)

Transplant Phase	Predisposing Factors	Common Infections
Phase I: Pre-engraftment (<15–45 d)	**Neutropenia** Expected duration: -Auto-HCT: 10–14 d -Allo-HCT (myeloablative): 15–30 d -Allo-HCT (nonmyeloablative): 5–7 d **Barrier breakdown** Mucosal injury from conditioning CVCs	**Bacterial: (GI, Skin flora)** • Gram-neg rods (inclu. *Pseudomonas*) • Gram-positives (CoNS, *Enterococci, Streptococci*) • *C. difficile* **Fungal:** • Mainly Candida spp • Aspergillus spp. if neutropenia is prolonged **Viral:** • Mainly HSV • Seasonal respiratory & enteric viruses
Phase II: Early Post-engraftment (Day 15–45 to Day 100)	**Impaired cellular immunity** • Acute GVHD & immunosuppressants **Impaired humoral immunity** **Barrier breakdown** Mucosal injury (GI GVHD) CVCs	**Bacterial:** Same as above but less frequent **Viral:** • CMV • HSV • EBV (PTLD) • Seasonal respiratory & enteric viruses • HHV 6 **Fungal:** • *Pneumocystis jiroveci* • *Aspergillus spp* • *Mucorales* **Parasites:** • *Toxoplasma* • *Strongyloides*
Phase III: Late Post-engraftment (>100 d)	**Impaired cellular immunity** • Chronic GVHD & immunosuppressants **Impaired humoral immunity**	**Bacterial:** Encapsulated bacteria, Nocardia, Mycobacteria **Viral:** • VZV • CMV, HSV • HHV 6 • EBV-related (PTLD) • Seasonal respiratory & enteric viruses **Fungal:** • *Pneumocystis jiroveci* • *Aspergillus spp* • *Mucorales*

Bacterial infections

- Bacteremia: Common during conditioning & preengraftment phase
  - RFs: Intestinal domination by single bacteria (eg, VRE, GNR) (*Clin Infect Dis* 2012;55:905)
  - Consider antibacterial ppx (see "The High-Risk Oncology Patient" chapter)
- *C. difficile* colitis: Dx: Unexplained new-onset diarrhea (≥3 episodes/24 h) AND + stool test. Tx of initial nonsevere infxn: PO vancomycin or fidaxomicin (*Clin Infect Dis* 2018;66:987)
- Encapsulated organisms (*S. pneumoniae*, *H. influenzae*): Mainly in late postengraftment
  -Ppx: Antibacterial ppx for chronic GVHD or low IgG. IVIG for severe hypogammaglobulinemia if no contraindications Immunizations as indicated (*Biol Blood Marrow Transplant* 2009;15:1143–1238)
- Intracellular organisms:
  -Nocardia (if on immunosuppressants)—can cause nodular lesions in lungs, skin, & CNS
  -Legionella (if not on levofloxacin ppx)—lung is affected in the majority of cases (sometimes causes nodular infiltrate); extrapulmonary manifestations possible
  -Listeria (steroids increase risk)—can cause diarrhea, sepsis, or meningoencephalitis

Viral infections

- **CMV**:
  -Viremia: Recovery of CMV DNA from blood
  -Dz: End-organ damage (eg, pneumonitis, hepatitis, colitis, chorioretinitis, encephalitis)
  -RFs: High-dose steroids, MMF, anti–T-cell therapies (eg, fludarabine, alemtuzumab, T-cell depleted graft, seropositive recipient or donor; chronic GVHD)
  -Ppx: **See high-risk oncology patient chapter**
  -Surveillance: Weekly PCR from time of engraftment until day +100 or longer
  -Preemptive therapy: 1st line: Ganciclovir or valganciclovir, 2nd line: Foscarnet, cidofovir Duration: At least 2 wks. If PCR still positive, continue maintenance therapy until neg
- **HSV/VZV** reactivation can occur at any stage of HCT
  -Ppx: Acyclovir for all HCT pts during conditioning & until engraftment or resolution of mucositis, whichever is longer
- **EBV** reactivation correlates w/ PTLD
- **HHV-6** reactivation occurs early in about half of allo-HCT recipients & may be a/w acute GVHD (*Transpl Infect Dis* 2014;16:440–449)
  -Manifestations: Encephalitis, engraftment delay, cutaneous
- **Adenovirus** reactivation can be fatal. 1° infxn is common in children (*Curr Opin Infect Dis* 2019;32:591–600)
  -RFs: GVHD, T-cell depletion, haploidentical grafts
  -Manifestations: Gastroenterocolitis, pneumonitis, cystitis, nephritis, hepatitis, encephalitis, dermatitis, disseminated dz
  -Tx: Reduce immunosuppression if possible. Cidofovir is commonly used but limited by nephrotoxicity. Adenovirus-specific CTLs are under study

Fungal infections

- **Invasive aspergillosis:** 1st line tx: Voriconazole. Alternatives: Isavuconazole & posaconazole (*CID* 2016;63(4):e1–e60; *Lancet* 2016;387:760; *Lancet* 2021;397(10273):499)
- **Other fungi:** *Candida spp*, non-*Candida* yeasts, & non-*Aspergillus* molds
- **PJP:** Presentation often acute & severe. 1st line tx: TMP/SMX preferred; alternative agents depend on dz severity
- Antifungal ppx: **See high-risk oncology patient chapter**. Some centers consider mold-active ppx for higher risk allo-HCT pts

Parasitic infections

- ***Toxoplasma gondii:***
  Manifestations: Can cause encephalitis, pneumonitis, chorioretinitis, disseminated dz. Early onset (<d 60) dz has worse prognosis (*Clin Infect Dis* 2000;31:1188); Dx may be difficult & requires a ↑ degree of suspicion
  Ppx: Consider prophylactic drug or PCR surveillance if IgG positive

Strongyloides stercolaris: Hyperinfxn syn carries high mortality; screen pts w/ eosinophilia or from endemic areas. Pts w/ positive screen or pts w/ unexplained eosinophilia & travel to endemic area should be treated. 1st line: Ivermectin (if no concern for loiasis)

Screening prior to HCT

HIV Ag/Ab, HBV surface Ag/Ab & core Ab +/- PCR, HCV Ab +/- PCR, CMV IgG, Toxoplasma IgG, LTBI screen (allo-HCT), *Strongyloides* Ab (unexplained eosinophilia or endemic area), *T. cruzi* Ab (h/o blood transfusion or living in endemic areas), Malaria (if from endemic area)

Background

No data to suggest incidence of COVID-19 differs b/w CA vs. non-CA pts

In pts hospitalized d/t COVID-19, all-cause mortality rate is approximately 25% in CA pts (*Lancet Oncol* 2020;21(10):1309–1316; *Eur J Cancer* 2020;139:43–50) compared to 17.1% in the general population (*Ann Epidemiol* 2021;57:14–21)

Risk Factors for Mortality in Cancer Patients with COVID-19
Advancing age
Male sex
Hematologic malignancy (↑ leukemia, lymphoma, multiple myeloma)
Presence of cardiovascular comorbidities (HTN, previous CHF)

Who to test (varies by institution)

- Any symptomatic pt
- Asx immunocompromised pts at time of hospital admission
- Asx pts before initiation of immunosuppressive therapy or transplantation

Transmission

Median incubation time is 4–5 d after exposure & 97.5% of people develop sxs w/in 11.5 d (*Lancet* 2020;395:507–513)

Transmission from asx & presymptomatic pts is a major hallmark of this pandemic

In the general population w/ mild–mod. infxn, replication-competent virus has generally not been recovered beyond 10 d from sx onset despite any lingering PCR positivity (*Nat Commun* 2021;12:267)

In pts w/ severe infxn & severe immunocompromise (see below), shedding of replication-competent virus has been observed for >2 mos (*NEJM* 2020; 383:2586–2588), which has infxn control implications

PCR positivity may persist for up to 12 wks even in nonimmunocompromised pts, but this does not necessarily imply contagiousness

Severely Immunocompromising Conditions Predisposing to Prolonged Infectivity
HSCT
Lymphoma & CLL
Acquired hypogammaglobulinemia
CAR-T therapy
Untreated HIV w/ CD4 <200
Prednisone ≥20 mg/d for ≥14 d (or equivalent)

Cancer treatment considerations

Data on course of COVID-19 after recent chemo or immunotherapy are mixed. The American Society of Clinical Oncology recommends (*ASCO, July 29 2021*):

- Chemo: Balance risk of interrupting chemo w/ the "poorly defined risk of adverse COVID-19 outcomes in pts receiving active CA tx"
- Immune checkpoint inhibitors: If reasonable, dose less frequently in pts w/ active COVID-19
- BMT/SCT: If infected prior to transplant + pt is able to be managed conventionally, can delay transplant up to 3 wks & until sxs resolve
- Radiation: Per American Society for Therapeutic Radiology and Oncology, hypofractionated radiation schedules can be considered if CA is not rapidly progressing & is potentially curable (*ASTRO, 2021*)
- COVID-19 vaccination is widely available & rec to all people 12 y & older, given their high effectiveness in decreasing risk of hospitalization & death (*CDC.gov, 2021*)
- Studies have shown lower vaccine effectiveness in immunosuppressed pts (*medRxiv 2021 Jul 8;2021.07.08.21259776*). Based on this evidence, CDC recommends an add'l mRNA vaccine dose following a 2-dose 1° series (*CDC.gov, 2021*). Guidelines are evolving quickly

LOCALIZED PROSTATE CANCER

Epidemiology

- Incidence: ~248,500, leading cause of CA in men (*CA Cancer J Clin* 2021;71(3):209). Annual Mortality: ~34,000, 2nd highest cause of CA death in men in the U.S. (*CA Cancer J Clin* 2021;71(1):7). Declining mortality: 1992 was 39 & 2017 was 19/100,000
- RFs: Age (rare before 40 y), Black race, 1st-degree relative <65 y w/ prostate CA, *BRCA2, ATM*, Lynch syn

PSA screening

- Aim is to reduce dz-specific morbidity &/or mortality. 3 RCTs: PLCO, ERSPC, CAP. In men 55–69 y may prevent ~1.3 dz-specific deaths over ~13 y & 3 cases of metastatic prostate CA per 1,000 men screened (*JAMA* 2018;319:1901). Note methodologic flaws in screening trials. PSA screening increases detection, small benefit in reducing prostate CA mortality, no benefit in reducing overall mortality. Encourage shared decision making—potential benefits & harms (false positive, overdx, bx, anxiety)
- Digital Rectal Exam (DRE) generally not used as a screening test—warranted if sxs or abnormality

Society/task force recommendations

- ACS: Discussion of PSA screening, if life expectancy >10 y, starting at 50 y for avg risk, at 45 y if Black or 1st-degree relative w/ prostate CA <65 y, or at 40 y w/ multiple 1st-degree relatives w/ prostate CA <65 y (yearly if PSA ≥2.5 ng/mL, otherwise every 2 y). Informed decision making (*CA Cancer J Clin* 2010;60:70)
- AUA: Shared decision making for men 55–69 y, w/ option for 2+ y interval for men who decide on PSA screening. Recommends against PSA screening in: Men <40 y, avg risk men 40–54 y, >70 y, or w/ <10–15 y life expectancy (*J Urol* 2013:190:419, confirmed 2018)
- USPSTF: Shared decision making for men aged 55–69 y (*JAMA* 2018;319:1901)

Initial workup

- Interpret abnl PSA (≥4 ng/mL) in context (incl.: Age, benign prostatic hypertrophy (BPH), recent prostatitis, urinary retention, urethral instrumentation, transurethral resection of prostate (TURP), bx hx, use of 5α reductase inhibition). Consider verification w/ repeat draw, risk calculators pre-bx
- DRE—may detect nodules, induration, asymmetry of posterior or lateral prostate
- Novel serum (eg, 4K, Prostate Health Index (PHI)) & urine biomarkers (eg, PCA3) may inform bx decision
- Optimal diagnostic prostate bx should systematically sample ≥12 cores incl. apical & far-lateral cores under U/S guidance (*J Urol* 2013:189:2039)
- Decision to bx (transrectal, sometimes transperineal) based on clinical suspicion of detecting significant dz (Gleason grade ≥7)
- If available, consider prostate multiparametric MRI (mpMRI) esp in the setting of prior neg bx & persistent clinical suspicion for prostate CA (anterior &/or aggressive CA). PI-RADS version 2 category 3–5 should prompt image-guided bx (TRUS-MRI fusion, in-bore MRI-targeting) w/ at least 2 cores from each MRI target w/ or w/o concurrent systematic sampling (*J Urol* 2016:196:1613). MRI-targeted bx is noninferior to standard bx (*NEJM* 2021;385:908)
- Gleason grade reflects growth/differentiation pattern & ranges from 1 to 5, from most differentiated to least differentiated. Gleason score is the sum of 1° & 2° grades, w/ predominant pattern listed 1st (eg, grade 4 is 1° in 4 + 3 = 7 dz & 2° in 3 + 4 = 7)

TNM Staging (AJCC 8th Edition, 2017)	Simplified AJCC Prognostic Groups					
T1: Clinically inapparent T2: Palpable, prostate contained	I:	T1–2	N0	M0	PSA <10	Gleason ≤6
T3: Extends through prostatic capsule T4: Fixed, or invades locally beyond seminal vesicle: bladder, levators, pelvic wall	IIA: IIB: IIC:	T1–2c T1–2 T1–2	N0 N0 N0	M0 M0 M0	PSA ≥10<20 PSA <20 PSA <20	Gleason ≤6 Gleason 3+4 Gleason 4+3
N1: Regional LN (s) M1a: Nonregional LN(s) M1b: Bone(s)	IIIA: IIIB:	T1–2 T3–4	N0 N0	M0 M0	PSA ≥20 Any PSA	Gleason 6–8 Gleason 6–8
M1c: Other sites, w/ or w/o bone	IVA: IVB:	Any T Any T	N1 or N	M0 M1	Any PSA Any PSA	Any Gleason Any Gleason

Staging workup: Imaging

- mpMRI: Consider if low risk → establish not missing higher-risk dz & candidacy for surveillance. mpMRI to evaluate extracapsular extension (ECE) can inform decision making for nerve-sparing RP (*J Urol* 2014:192:82)
- Bone scan: T2 + PSA >10; high risk; very high risk
- Pelvic CT: Intermediate risk + predicted LN involvement >10%; high risk; very high risk
- If above are equivocal, consider C-11 choline PET, or PSMA-PET, if available

Prognosis

- Validated nomograms & prediction tools should be employed to estimate individualized prognosis & likelihood of LN involvement, ECE, seminal vesicle invasion, etc.
- Germline genetic testing rec for prostate CA with any of: (i) high risk, very high risk, regional, or metastatic; (ii) Ashkenazi Jewish ancestry; (iii) Positive FHx (*Can J Urol* 2019; 26(5 Suppl 2):34)
- Risk assessment may be supplemented by tumor molecular characteristics (eg, testing with Oncotype DX, Prolaris, ConfirmMDx, Decipher)

Initial treatment (by risk group) of localized disease (NCCN risk groups: v1.2022)

Very Low (All of the following) • T1c • Gleason ≤6 • PSA <10 • <3 bx cores w/ ≤50% CA/core • PSA density <0.15		Life expectancy <10 y: Observation Life expectancy 10–20 y: Active surveillance (w/ PSA ≥q6mo, DRE ≥q12mo, bx ≥q12mo, mpMRI ≥q12mo unless clinically indicated Life expectancy ≥20 y: Active surveillance (preferred) or RT or radical prostatectomy (RP)
Low (All of the following) • T1–2a • Gleason ≤6 • PSA <10		Life expectancy <10 y: Observation Life expectancy ≥10 y: Active surveillance, or RT (EBRT or brachytherapy), or RP
Intermediate • T2b–c • Gleason 7 • PSA 10–20	Favorable Intermediate (FI) Unfavorable Intermediate (UI)	Life expectancy <10 y: Observation (preferred) or EBRT ± (if UI) brachytherapy± ADT (4–6 mos) Life expectancy ≥10 y: RP ± PLND if probability of LN met ≥2% ± Adjuvant therapy or EBRT± brachytherapy ± ADT (4–6 mos) or active surveillance (only if FI)
High (1 of the following) • T3a or • Gleason 8–10 • PSA >20		EBRT + ADT (1.5–3 y) or EBRT + brachytherapy + ADT (1–3 y) or RP + PLND ± Adjuvant therapy or If life expectancy <5 y: Observation or ADT or EBRT
Very high (1 of the following) • T3b–T4 • 1° Gleason 5 • 2 or 3 high-risk features • >4 cores Gleason 8–10		EBRT + ADT (1.5–3 y) ± docetaxel or EBRT + brachytherapy + ADT (1–3 y) or RP + PLND ± Adjuvant therapy or If life expectancy <5 y: Observation or ADT or EBRT

- When randomized to RP, RT + ADT (3–6 mos), or active monitoring among localized prostate CA, 10 y overall & prostate CA-specific mortality equivalent. Incidence of metastases is significantly greater w/ active monitoring, longer-term survival data needed (*NEJM* 2016;375:1415). Sexual fxn & urinary continence worse w/ RP. Bowel fxn, urinary voiding, & nocturia worse w/ RT + ADT, but considerable recovery (other than increasing frequency of bloody stools) (*NEJM* 2016;375:1425)
- Pelvic LN dissection using extended technique if ≥2% probability of nodal metastases based on MSKCC nomogram (NCCN recommendation) (*J Urol* 2003:170:1798)
- Focal therapies (eg, HIFU, cryoablation) for small, localized tumors are under investigation. Inadequate long-term data to consider these to be standard approaches
- Next-generation androgen-directed drugs (eg, abiraterone, enzalutamide) as a component of tx for localized dz are under investigation & may be a clinical trial option

Management of adverse findings following surgery

• **Positive margins, seminal vesicle Invasion, ECE**	EBRT, or Observation
• **LN metastasis**	ADT ± EBRT, or Observation

Monitoring

- **After definitive Rx:** PSA q6–12mo × 5 y then q12mo; DRE q12mo, may be omitted if PSA undetectable (rare instances of local recurrence may occur w/o PSA)

Biochemical recurrence (BCR)

Definition

- **Rising PSA after definitive RP:** Undetectable PSA after RP w/ subsequent detectable PSA (≥0.2 ng/mL) that is confirmed on at least 2 subsequent determinations (*J Urol* 2007;177(2):540)
- **Rising PSA after definitive RT:** Rise of PSA by 2 ng/mL or more above the nadir PSA (*Int J Radiat Oncol Biol Phys* 2006;65(4):965). Usually confirmed to r/o "PSA Bounce." Nadir may take up to 18 mos post RT to achieve

Workup

- Evaluate risk of metastases or death: Higher risk for PSA doubling time (≤12 mos), Gleason score (≥8), time to biochemical failure ≤18 mos post RT (*Eur Urol* 2019;75(6):896). Consider age, life expectancy, comorbidities
- R/o local recurrence, regional (pelvic LNs most common) or distant metastases (bone most common). Bone scan, CT/MRI/TRUS, C11-Choline PET, prostate bx
- Local recurrence may be detected by MRI: Post RT—aim to bx, if possible. Post RP—role of bx controversial
- Difficult to detect distant dz w/ CT/Bone Scan at PSA <10 ng/mL. If high suspicion & pt a candidate for salvage therapy, consider ^{68}Ga/^{18}F-PSMA PET/CT or ^{18}F-Fluciclovine from PSA ≥0.5 ng/mL, if available

Management

- BCR post RP
  - If no distant mets: Consider salvage RT to prostate bed ± pelvic LN radiation ± ADT
  - If not fit for salvage RT: ADT or observation, consider intermittent ADT
- BCR post RT
  - Local tx options: RP, cryosurgery, high-intensity focused U/S, brachytherapy ± ADT
  - Candidate for salvage surgery if original T1–T2, NX or N0, life expectancy >10 y, current PSA <10 ng/mL
  - If no distant mets identified, prostate bx neg, or not candidate for salvage: Observation vs. ADT, consider intermittent ADT

Metastatic castration sensitive prostate cancer (mCSPC)

Prostate CA that responds to lowering testosterone to castrate levels (<50 ng/dL)

- **N1M0:** RT + long-term neoadjuvant/concurrent/adjuvant ADT (2–3 y) or ADT alone
- **M1:** Evaluate if low volume or high volume

Androgen deprivation therapy (ADT)

- Initial systemic therapy for men w/ advanced prostate CA to suppress testosterone:
  - **GnRH agonists:** Eg, leuprolide. Binds to GnRH receptor in pituitary to cause initial LH & FSH release then fall w/in 3–4 wks. Given w/ antiandrogen, eg, bicalutamide, for at least 7 d to prevent flare related to initial testosterone surge (Figure 14-1)
  - **GnRH antagonist:** Eg, degarelix. Pure GnRH antagonist—does not cause LH/FSH release. Testosterone suppressed w/in 3 d
  - **Bilateral orchiectomy:** Uncommon in the United States
- Can normalize PSA in >90% & cause tumor response in >80%, palliate bone pain & reduce complications 2° to prostate CA. Duration of response is variable
- S/E: Hot flashes, osteoporosis, fracture, obesity, diabetes, hyperlipidemia, coronary artery dz, decr libido, mood lability, possible cognitive impairment. Increase w/ duration of tx

Consider dz risk & volume for combination of ADT w/ 1 of:

- Abiraterone: Given w/ steroid. Consider in high-risk dz (2 of: i. Gleason score ≥8, ii. at least 3 bone lesions, iii. measurable visceral dz). Prolongs OS vs. ADT alone in Phase III RCT (*NEJM* 2017;377(4):338; *NEJM* 2017;377(4):352)
- Docetaxel: Consider in high-volume metastatic dz (visceral mets or ≥4 bone mets w/ ≥1 outside vertebrae & pelvis). ADT+docetaxel 75 mg/m^2 × 6 cycles. Prolongs OS vs. ADT alone. (*NEJM* 2015;373;737; *JCO* 2018;36:1080; *Lancet* 2016;387(10024):1163)
- Apalutamide: Fewer CNS S/E than enzalutamide. OS benefit vs. ADT alone in high volume (visceral mets & 1+ bone lesion, or 4+ bone lesions, at least 1 outside axial skeleton) & low-volume metastatic dz (*NEJM* 2019;381:13; *Lancet Oncol* 2019;20(11):1518)
- Enzalutamide: Delays time to radiographic progression vs. ADT alone in high- & low-volume dz, regardless of prior docetaxel exposure (*JCO* 2019;37(32):2974). OS data not yet mature

Emerging evidence for both metastases directed therapy & prostate directed therapy in this dz state

Castration-resistant prostate cancer (CRPC)

Progressive dz clinically, biochemically, or radiographically despite castrate levels of testosterone (<50 ng/dL). Does not mean independent of androgens; therapy should continue to maintain castrate levels of testosterone

- Germline genetic testing & tumor tissue genetic sequencing for all men w/ metastatic prostate CA who have not already had it
- Neuroendocrine differentiation may emerge after ADT. Rare at initial dx
- Poorer performance status, the presence of visceral mets, use of opioids for pain relief, an ↑ LDH, an ↑ PSA, an ↑ alkaline phosphatase, a ↓ albumin, & a ↓ hemoglobin are a/w shorter OS in men w/ CRPC treated w/ chemo (*J Clin Oncol* 2014;32(7):671)

Agents shown to improve OS in phase III trials CRPC in combination w/ ADT

Choice of therapy depends on prior systemic tx, extent of dz, & presence of sxs. S/e profiles influence choice. Consider clinical trials

- **Cabazitaxel:** Only used post docetaxel—consider in symptomatic or rapidly progressive dz (*Lancet* 2010;376:1147). Less neuropathy than docetaxel
- **Docetaxel:** Consider if symptomatic or rapidly progressive dz (*NEJM* 2004;351:1502; *JCO* 2008;26:242)
- **Olaparib:** PARP inhibition for men w/ germline or somatic DNA mismatch repair mt (*NEJM* 2020;383(24):2345). Those w/ *BRCA2* may benefit most (*Eur Urol* 2019;76(4):452)
- **77-Lu-PSMA-617:** Small molecule delivers β-particle radiation selectively to PSMA positive cells & surrounding microenvironment. Trial required PSMA-positive on PET/CT w/ ^{68}Ga-PSMA-11 (*NEJM* 2021;385:1091)
- **Abiraterone acetate:** W/ steroid. Approved for pre- & postdocetaxel (*NEJM* 2010;364:1995; *NEJM* 2013;368:138). S/e can include hypertension, hypokalemia, fluid retention
- **Enzalutamide:** Approved for metastatic & nonmetastatic CRPC, pre- & postdocetaxel (*NEJM* 2012;367:1187; *NEJM* 2014;371:424)
- **Apalutamide & darolutamide:** Both approved for nonmetastatic CRPC (*Ann Oncol* 2019;30:1813; *J Clin Oncol* 2020;38(suppl):abstr 5514)
- **Radium-223:** α-particle–emitting radiopharmaceutical—bone seeking. OS benefit, for symptomatic bone-only dz (*NEJM* 2013;369:213)
- **Sipuleucel-T:** OS benefit but no change in PSA or tumor burden, appropriate only if asx, ECOG 0–1, no visceral mets, not on: Steroids, RT, chemo, or immunotherapy, & life expectancy >6 mos (*NEJM* 2010;363:411)

Special consideration for bone mets

Denosumab or Zoledronic acid to lower risk of skeletal-related events in castration-resistant dz. If symptomatic: Palliative RT

Figure 14-1 Mechanism of action of antiandrogen therapies.

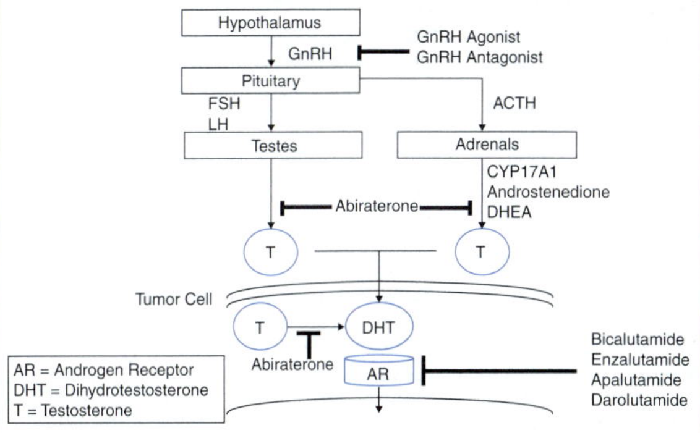

Monitoring

After N1 or M1: Physical exam & PSA every 3 mos. Imaging as clinically indicated

BLADDER CANCER

Epidemiology
- Most common malignancy of the urinary system, ~87,000 pts will be dx'd in the United States in 2021, ~17,000 will die of their dz (*CA Cancer J Clin* 2021;71(1):7)

Etiology and clinical manifestations
- RFs: **Smoking**, aromatic amines, occupational exposures (metal, paint, rubber, leather, textile), chronic infxns, cyclophosphamide, RT; **Hereditary:** Lynch syn
- Presenting sxs: **Painless hematuria** (typically intermittent & gross), irritative voiding sx (frequency, urgency, dysuria), flank or suprapubic pain (symptomatic of locally advanced dz), constitutional sx (fatigue, wt loss, failure to thrive) usually symptomatic of met dz

Pathologic Subtypes	
Urothelial (Transitional Cell) Carcinoma	Most common subtype in the US, Western Europe (90%), men > women, median age at dx 73
SCC	Schistosomal: Most common subtype where infxn w/ **Schistosoma haematobium** are prevalent (up to 75%), men >> women, median age at dx ~40 y
	Nonschistosomal: RFs include **chronic UTIs,** bladder stones, pelvic RT, **chronic indwelling Foley,** men = women, median age at dx ~60 y
AdenoCA	Urachal: Arises from **urachal remnant** at the bladder dome (presents earlier, better outcomes, 59% men).
	Nonurachal: Typically advanced at dx, poor outcome
Other	Sarcomatoid, paraganglioma, melanoma, neuroendocrine, lymphoma,

Workup
- **Evaluation of entire urinary tract:** Cystourethroscopy, consider urine cytology (low sensitivity ~34%, high specificity ~98%) (*Urology* 2003;61:109), abd & upper tract imaging
- Initial cystoscopy includes bimanual exam under anesthesia to assess for locally advanced dz, bladder wash for cytology, visual inspection & tumors biopsied or trans-urethral resection, random bxs if positive urine cytology w/ no visible tumors
- If no muscle in specimen, strongly consider repeat TURBT—aim to correctly identify stage & grade while completely resecting all visible tumors
- UC are either low-grade or high-grade, w/ muscle-invasive dz almost always high-grade

Staging and prognosis

Depth of Invasion	Stage	T, N, M Stage	OS at 5 y
Nonmuscle invasive	**Stage 0**	Ta (noninvasive papillary carcinoma) Tis (carcinoma in situ)	98%
	Stage I	T1 (subepithelial invasion)	88%
Muscle invasive	**Stage II**	T2 (muscularis propria invasion)	63%
Muscle invasive/ locoregionally advanced	**Stage III**	T3 (perivesical fat) or T4a (local structures, prostate, uterus, or vagina) or any N	37%
Advanced	**Stage IV**	T4b (pelvic or abd wall) or any M	15%

- Early-stage prognostic factors: **Stage, histologic grade,** presence of multicentric dz, time to recurrence, tumor size, presence of carcinoma in situ (CIS)
- Met prognostic factors: Poor performance status, visceral mets

Management: Nonmuscle invasive disease
- Depends on T stage & grade: TURBT, followed by either observation for low risk, or intravesical therapy w/ BCG or chemo (mitomycin or gemcitabine) (*Eur Urol* 2021;79(4):480; *J Urol* 2005;174(1):86; *JNCI* 2001;93(8):597)
- Strongly consider reresection if no muscle in TURBT specimen for accurate staging
- The majority (50–80%) of nonmuscle invasive dz will recur if treated by TURBT alone, w/ a proportion (20–25%) progressing to more invasive dz
- Cystectomy considered for residual T1, high-grade or muscle-invasion at reresection

- **BCG:** Unknown exact MOA, but triggers local immune response, given weekly × 6 wks followed by maintenance for 1–3 y based on risk status for relapse.
- Pembrolizumab: Given IV for pts with BCG-unresponsive CIS ± papillary dz who were ineligible for or declined radical cystectomy (*Lancet Onc* 2021;22:919–930)
- Surveillance: Cystoscopy & urine cytology ~3 mos, can be spaced if no recurrent dz

Management: Muscle invasive disease

- **Radical cystectomy** is tx of choice for muscle invasive dz w/ urinary diversion
- **Neoadjuvant cisplatin-based chemo** prior to cystectomy improves OS (*NEJM* 2003;349:859; *Lancet* 2003;361:1927). **Regimens include dose-dense (dd)MVAC** methotrexate, vinblastine, doxorubicin, cisplatin (*JCO* 2014;32:1895; *JCO* 2014;32:1889) or **GC—**gemcitabine, cisplatin (*Clin Genitourin Cancer* 2020;18:387)
- Bladder preservation options include **trimodality tx:** TURBT, followed by concurrent chemoradiation (*NEJM* 2012;366:1477). Pt selection key, w/ up to 40% requiring cystectomy for tx failure or dz recurrence. Criteria: Eligibility for complete TURBT, adequate bladder fxn, UC histology, early stage (T2), no multifocal dz & no hydronephrosis
- No completed prospective RCT establishes adjuvant chemo after radical cystectomy, though meta-analyses show survival benefit (*Eur Urol* 2014;66:42)
- Emerging data in high-risk pts shows ↑ disease free survival (DFS) w/ adjuvant nivolumab (*N Engl J Med* 2021;384:2102)

Management: Metastatic disease

- **Cisplatin-based chemo** is the preferred initial tx **(ddMVAC, GC)**, if eligible 1st line: **GC** preferred over **MVAC** d/t equal efficacy w/ less toxicity (less neutropenia, neutropenic sepsis, mucositis) (*JCO* 2000:18:3068). ddMVAC (q2wk w/ GCSF support) has ↑ RR, ↓ toxicity compared to MVAC (*JCO* 2001;19:2638)
- If **cisplatin ineligible** (CrCl ≤60 mL/min; ECOG PS ≥2; Grade 2 hearing loss/neuropathy; NYHA HF class ≥3) but **platinum eligible**: Use **gemcitabine** + **carboplatin** (*JCO* 2012;30:191) OR if PD-L1 positive: **Pembrolizumab** (*Lancet Onc* 2017;18:1483) or **atezolizumab** (*Lancet* 2017;389:67)
- If **platinum ineligible** (CrCl <30 mL/min; ECOG PS >3; neuropathy grade >3; NYHA HF Class >3; ECOG PS 2 & CrCl <30 mL/min): **Pembrolizumab** or **atezolizumab**
- Maintenance **avelumab** ↑ OS after partial response or stable dz to platinum (*NEJM* 2020;383:1218)
- 2nd line: FDA-approved agents include **pembrolizumab** a/w ↑ OS vs. chemo (*NEJM* 2017;376:1015), **nivolumab** a/w 24% RR (*Lancet Onc* 2016;17:1590), **avelumab** a/w 17% RR (*Lancet Onc* 2018;19:51). If FGFR2/3 genetic alterations, **erdafitinib** can be used post platinum, a/w 40% RR (*NEJM* 2019;381:338), but usually deferred until 3rd or 4th line
- 3rd line: **Enfortumab vedotin** a/w ↑ OS vs. chemo post platinum & PD-1/L1 inhibitor (*NEJM* 2021;384:1125); **Sacituzumab govitecan** a/w RR 27% (*JCO* 2021;39(22):2474)
- Can consider gemcitabine, docetaxel, paclitaxel monotherapy in later tx lines

Cancers of the renal pelvis and ureter

- Upper tract dz can also be multifocal (drop met), Histology: Urothelial CA (>90%) > SCC > adenoCA. Smoking & occupational exposure risks. Can be seen in **Lynch syn**
- Dx w/ direct ureteroscopy & bx (brushings + urine cytology if no obvious 1°)
- Tx of localized dz is **nephroureterectomy** w/ **bladder cuff excision** ± regional LND ± systemic chemo for high-grade/higher T stage
- Neoadjuvant gemcitabine + cisplatin achieved 2-y OS 89% in phase II trial (*J Urol* 2019; 201(Suppl 4):e999)
- Adjuvant **gemcitabine** + **platinum** ↑ DFS in locally advanced dz (*Lancet* 2020;395:1268).
- Any nodal involvement or distant metastasis –> stage IV dz. Tx of metastatic dz is same as metastatic bladder

Molecular biology and targeted therapy

- *FGFR2/3* alterations are only genomic markers currently targeted in clinical practice (*NEJM* 2019;381:338)
- TCGA found frequent mut in potential therapeutic targets: 42% in PI3K/AKT/mTOR, 45% in RTK/MAPK pathway, incl. *FGFR3* & *ERBB2* (*Nature* 2014;507:315). RNA-seq can divide tumors into different subtypes based on expression: Luminal, luminal-papillary, luminal-infiltrated, basal-squamous, & neuronal (*Cell* 2017;171(3):540)
- Potential predictive biomarkers: DNA-damage repair mts (eg, *ERCC2*) predict response to platinum (*Cancer Discov* 2014;4:1140; *Eur Urol* 2015;68:959; *JCO* 2018;36:1949) & to anti–PD-1/L1 (*JCO* 2018;36:1685). Luminal-infiltrated subtype appears more chemoresistant (*Cancer Cell* 2014;25:152) but sensitive to anti–PD-(L)1 (*Lancet* 2016;387:1909). *TGFβ* may mediate resistance to anti–PD-(L)1 (*Nature* 2018;554:544). Data on predictive value of PD-L1 expression are mixed

RENAL CELL CARCINOMA (RCC)

Epidemiology

- ~76,000 new cases & ~13,800 deaths in the United States estimated in 2021 (*SEER. cancer.gov, 2021*)
- Median age at dx 64 y. More prevalent in men
- **RFs:** Tobacco, obesity, hypertension. Familial forms account for ~5% of cases (see below)

Histology and molecular biology

- Clear cell (ccRCC; 80–90% of all RCC). Remainder non–clear cell include papillary, FH-deficient, chromophobe, collecting duct, medullary, TFE3 translocation, & unclassified
- Sarcomatoid is a variant seen w/ any cell type reflecting a phenotype that is more aggressive but possibly more responsive to immunotherapy

Hereditary RCC and germline testing

- There are several RCC-assoc genetic CA syn incl. VHL, HLRCC (FH gene), BAP1 tumor predisposition syn, Birt–Hogg–Dubé (FLCN gene), among others

Consider any of the following for Hereditary RCC gene panel testing & CA Genetics referral:

FHx	Clinical Characteristics	Histopathologic Characteristics
Close relative w/ known pathogenic variant	Dx'd at age ≤46 y	Multifocal papillary histology
≥1 1st- or 2nd-degree relative w/ RCC	Bilateral or multifocal tumors	Histologic features a/w HLRCC or FH deficiency found
	Angiomyolipomas of kidney + 1 other TSC-assoc criterion	BHD syn-related histology (multiple chromophobe, oncocytoma, oncocytic hybrid)
		Succinate dehydrogenase (SDH) deficient histology

Clinical presentation

- Mostly asx & incidental on imaging (minority will present w/ flank pain, hematuria, pyrexia, cachexia, fatigue)
- At presentation: 65% localized dz, 16% locally advanced, 16% met

Staging (TNM classification) and prognosis

- Tumor: **T1:** Tumor <7 cm, **T2:** Tumor >7 cm (both T1 & T2 are confined to the kidney parenchyma), **T3:** Tumor extends into the renal vein or perinephric tissues, **T4:** Tumor extends beyond Gerota fascia to adjacent organs
- Node: (N0 vs. N1) Presence or absence of regional LN involvement
- Met: (M0 vs. M1) Presence or absence of distant met
- OS excellent in early-stage; Median OS for met dz in targeted therapy era ~28 mos

Treatment principles

- **Localized or locally advanced:** Surgery alone (partial or radical nephrectomy) vs. active surveillance/ablative techniques in selected pts. Partial nephrectomy preferred for masses <4 cm
- **Adjuvant therapy:** Few data support adjuvant therapy. Although S-TRAC trial suggested ↑ 1.2 y in DFS w/ sunitinib, ASSURE & PROTECT trials w/ no benefit in DFS for sunitinib, sorafenib, or pazopanib, & ATLAS trial w/ no benefit in DFS for axitinib (*NEJM* 2016;375:2246; *Lancet* 2016;387:2008; *JCO* 2017;35:3916; *Ann Oncol* 2018;29(12):2371). Early data w/ adjuvant immunotherapy. Adjuvant pembrolizumab improves DFS (*NEJM* 2021;385:683)
- **Cytoreductive nephrectomy** in metastatic dz: Benefit depends on pt selection. 2 phase III trials reported in 2001 showed ↑ OS w/ nephrectomy + IFNα vs. IFNα alone (*NEJM* 2001;345:1655; *Lancet* 2001;358:9286). However, the CARMENA trial showed ↑ OS w/ sunitinib alone vs. nephrectomy + sunitinib (*NEJM* 2018;379:417). Best candidates for nephrectomy are intermediate-risk pts w/ limited metastatic burden & low perioperative risk; avoid up-front surgery in pts w/ urgent need for systemic dz shrinkage or where operative complications could delay systemic therapy

Systemic therapy for metastatic clear cell RCC

Algorithm based on risk category for clear cell RCC (*JCO* 1999;17:2530)

- **MSKCC RFs** (Good: 0 RF; Intermediate: 1–2 RF; Poor: ≥3 RF)
  1. LDH level >1.5 × ULN; **2.** Hb < lower limit of nl; **3.** Corrected serum calcium level > ULN; **4.** Interval of less than a year from original dx to the start of tx; **5.** KPS ≤70%

Line of Tx	MSKCC Risk Category	Category 1 or Preferred	Other Options
1st line	Favorable	Cabozantinib+nivolumab Lenvatinib+pembrolizumab Axitinib+pembrolizumab	Sunitinib Pazopanib Ipilimumab+nivolumab Axitinib+avelumab Cabozantinib High-dose IL-2[a] Axitinib[a] Surveillance[a]
	Intermediate/Poor	Cabozantinib+nivolumab Lenvatinib+pembrolizumab Axitinib+pembrolizumab Ipilimumab+nivolumab Cabozantinib	Axitinib+avelumab Sunitinib Pazopanib Axitinib[a] High-dose IL-2[a] Temsirolimus[a]

Preferred systemic therapy regimens in metastatic clear cell RCC.
[a]Useful only in certain circumstances.

Second-line therapies

- **Preferred:** Cabozantinib, nivolumab, or lenvatinib+everolimus
- **Other options:** Any listed in 1st line, everolimus, tivozanib, axitinib+avelumab, sorafenib, or bevacizumab

Combined-modality therapies

**1° endpoint(s) listed below include PFS &/or median OS

- **Axitinib+avelumab** (*NEJM* 2019; 380:1103) vs. sunitinib: PFS: 13.8 mos vs. 8.4 mos (HR: 0.69, *P* <0.001); OS for PD-L1-high 86.3% vs. 84.8% (HR for death: 0.82, *P* = 0.38)
- **Axitinib+pembrolizumab** (*NEJM* 2019;380:1116) vs. sunitinib: PFS: 15.1 mos vs. 11.1 mos (HR: 0.69, *P* <0.001); OS 89.9% vs. 78.3% (HR for death 0.53, *P* <0.0001)
- **Cabozantinib+nivolumab** (*NEJM* 2021;384:829) vs. sunitinib: PFS 16.6 mos vs. 8.3 mos (HR: 0.51, *P* <0.001)
- **Lenvatinib+everolimus** (*NEJM* 2021;384:1289) vs. sunitinib: PFS: 14.7 mos vs. 9.2 mos (HR: 0.65, *P* <0.001)
- **Lenvatinib+pembrolizumab** (*NEJM* 2021;384:1289) vs. sunitinib: PFS 23.9 mos vs. 9.2 mos (HR: 0.39, *P* <0.001)

Tyrosine kinase inhibitors

**1° endpoint(s) listed below include PFS &/or OS at interim analysis

Class S/E: HTN, fatigue, diarrhea, stomatitis, nausea, hand–foot syn, skin/hair color changes ↓ LVEF, ↓ WBC, ↓ PLT, AST/ALT abnormalities, TFT abnormalities

- **Axitinib** (*Lancet* 2011;378:1931) vs. sorafenib: PFS: 6.7 mos vs. 4.7 mos (HR: 0.665, *P* <0.0001)
- **Cabozantinib** (*NEJM* 2015;373:1814) vs. everolimus: PFS 7.4 mos vs. 3.8 mos (HR: 0.58, *P* <0.001)
- **Pazopanib** (*JCO* 2010;28:1061) vs. placebo: PFS: 9.2 mos vs. 4.2 mos (HR: 0.46, *P* <0.0001)
- **Sorafenib** (*NEJM* 2007; 357:203) vs. placebo: OS: 78% vs. 73% (HR for death: 0.72, *P* = 0.02)
- **Sunitinib** (*NEJM* 2007;356:115) vs. IFNα: PFS 11 mos vs. 5 mos (HR: 0.42, *P* <0.001)

Immunotherapies

**1° endpoint(s) listed below include PFS, ORR, OS from time of randomization to death

Class s/e: (see section Toxicities of Immunotherapies)

- **Ipilimumab+Nivolumab** (*NEJM* 2018;378:1277) vs. sunitinib: PFS 11.6 mos vs. 8.4 mos (HR 0.82, *P* = 0.03), OS (int-poor risk) NR vs. 26 mos (HR: 0.63, *P* <0.001), ORR 42% vs. 27% (*P* <0.001)
- **Nivolumab** (*NEJM* 2015;373:1803) vs. everolimus: OS: 25 mos vs. 19.6 mos (HR: 0.70, *P* = 0.002)
- **High dose IL-2:** Yields durable response rarely, but a/w tox, requires specialty center

mTOR inhibitors

**1° endpoint(s) listed below include PFS, OS at interim analysis

Class S/E: Stomatitis, fatigue, rash, edema, pneumonitis, hyperglycemia, hyperlipidemia, ↓WBC, ↓PLT

- **Everolimus** (*Lancet* 2008;372:449) vs. placebo: PFS: 4 mos vs. 1.9 mos (HR: 0.30, *P* <0.0001)
- **Temsirolimus** (*NEJM* 2007;356:2271) vs. IFNα: OS: 10.9 mos vs. 7.3 mos (HR: 0.73, *P* = 0.008)

Non–clear cell histology

- Clinical trial preferred
- Therapy extrapolated from clear cell; anti-VEGF agents w/ ↑RR vs. mTOR inhibitors. Some response to chemo in selected cases

Epidemiology
- ~9,470 new cases of testicular CA in the United States in 2021 (*CA Cancer J Clin* 2021;71(1):7). Most common CA in men 15–40 yo & incidence is rising (*World J Urol* 2015;33:623). More common in young White/Hispanic vs. African American & Asian men
- RFs include cryptorchidism (orchiopexy should be performed prior to puberty), FHx, Klinefelter syn (47XXY), testicular dysgenesis syn

Biology
- 90% of GCTs originate in the testis & 10% are extragonadal (mostly mediastinal & retroperitoneal; retroperitoneal GCTs likely arise from occult testicular GCT & should be managed as if of testicular origin. Pineal/suprasellar site is very rare, but most tumors at this site are GCT)

	Seminoma	Nonseminoma
Median Age	4th Decade	3rd Decade
Common Histologic Types	Pure Seminoma	NSGCT (Embryonal Carcinoma, Yolk Sac, Choriocarcinoma, Teratoma)
Stage Distribution	Stage I: ~80%	Stage I: ~60%
Radiation-Sensitivity	High	Low
Marker Production	hCG, LDH	AFP, hCG, LDH
Estimated 10-y Survival	>95%	>90%

Staging
- Testicular U/S, radical inguinal orchiectomy is the gold standard for dx & initial mgmt of a suspected testicular CA (trans-scrotal orchiectomy is contraindicated), serum tumor markers, CT chest, abdomen & pelvis, discuss sperm banking, brain MRI if sxs or if intermediate/poor risk, hCG levels very high. Brain mets can be asx & usually a/w nonseminoma histology, pulmonary, liver, or bone mets (*JCO* 2015;34:345)
- TNMS Staging System for Testis CA (T = tumor, N = node, M = met, S = postorchiectomy nadir serum tumor marker) (*AJCC Cancer Staging Manual*, vol. 7. Springer New York, 2010)
- 1° Tumor (T): **Tis:** Germ cell neoplasia *in situ*, **T1:** Tumor limited to testis & epididymis, no lymphovascular invasion; **T2:** Lymphovascular invasion present, or invasion through the tunica albuginea into the tunica vaginalis, **T3:** Spermatic cord invasion, **T4:** Scrotal invasion.
- Regional LN(N): Right testis 1° landing zone is the interaortocaval LN. Left testis 1° landing zone is the para-aortic LN
- Serum Tumor Markers (S): Postorchiectomy nadir (LDH, hCG (mIU/mL), AFP (ng/mL)
- AFP: Nonseminomatous germ cell tumor (NSGCT) only (serum half-life: 5–7 d)
- hCG: Both NSGCT & pure seminoma GCTs (serum half-life: 18–36 h)
- LDH: Both NSGCT & pure seminoma GCTs (reflects growth rate & tumor burden)
  S0: Markers w/in nl limits: (LDH ULN: ~250 (lab-dependent)
  S1: AFP <1,000 ng/mL, hCG <5,000 mIU/mL, LDH <1.5 × ULN
  S2: AFP 1,000–10,000 ng/mL, hCG 5,000–50,000 mIU/mL, LDH 1.5–10 × ULN
  S3: AFP >10,000 ng/mL, hCG >50,000 mIU/mL, LDH >10 × ULN

Risk classification
The International Germ Cell Cancer Collaborative Group (IGCCCG) created a risk classification for both seminoma & NSGCTs (*JCO* 1997;15:594)[a]

Risk Category	Seminoma	Nonseminoma
Good risk	Any 1° site & Any markers[b] & No nonpulmonary mets	Testicular or retroperitoneal 1° site & no nonpulmonary mets & ≤S1 markers[c]
Intermediate risk	Any 1° site & Any makers & Nonpulmonary visceral mets	Testicular or retroperitoneal 1° site & no nonpulmonary mets & S2 markers[c]
Poor risk	Does not exist	Testicular or retroperitoneal 1° site & nonpulmonary visceral mets &/or S3 markers. Any mediastinal NSGCT 1° site[c]

[a]*The original risk categorization (1997) remains the standard for treatment decisions in daily practice but there is an updated IGCCCG risk classification nomogram (2021).*
[b]*The IGCCCG 2021 update identified LDH >2.5 times ULN as an adverse prognostic factor within good risk seminoma.*
[c]*IGCCCG 2021 update identified LDH >2.5 times ULN, increasing age, and presence of lung metastases as additional adverse prognostic factors (JCO 2021;39:1553).*

Pathology

About 50% each seminoma & NSGCT; histologic dx is critical to appropriate mgmt

80% of all histologic subtypes have an isochromosome of the short arm of chromosome 12, i(12p), which can be used as a specific genetic marker of GCT (*Cancer Res* 1992;52:2285–2291), & the remaining 20% have excess 12p genetic material

Treatment* (NCCN, Version 2.2021)

Key concepts: See staging for the: role of surgery. No chemo dose reduction or delays >1 wk in GCT; it results in decr CR rate; Carboplatin inferior to cisplatin in treating pts w/ GCT (*JCO* 1993;11:598); Consider prophylactic GF support in pts ≥50 y (*Cancer* 2013;119(14):2574)

Seminoma treatment recommendations

- Stage I: Surveillance (preferred) vs. RT (20 Gy para-aortic field) vs. carboplatin
- Stage IIA/B <3: Chemo [etoposide + cisplatin (EP) × 4 cycles or bleomycin + EP (BEP) × 3 cycles] or RT (30 to 36 Gy para-aortic & ipsilateral iliac LNs). 1° nerve-sparing retroperitoneal lymph node dissection (RPLND) an emerging option which may minimize exposure to chemo & RT (NCT02537548). Good data exists to support chemo for all *proven* IIA (by bx or progression on surveillance) & all IIB seminoma (*JCO* 2011;29:719; *JCO* 2008;26:5416)
- Stage IIB/C or III (good risk): Chemo (EP × 4 cycles or BEP × 3 cycles)
- Stage IIIC (intermediate risk): Chemo (BEP × 4 cycles or VIP × 4 cycles in selected pts)

NSGCT treatment recommendations

- Stage IA: Surveillance (preferred) or nerve-sparing RPLND
- Stage IB: Nerve-sparing RPLND or chemo or surveillance
  After RPLND: ≤2 cm & ≤5 positive LN & no EN invasion: Observation
  >2 cm or ≥6 positive LN or any EN invasion: Chemo (B)EP×2
- Stage IIA-S0: RPLND (preferred) or chemo (rarely)
  After RPLND: ≤2 cm & ≤5 positive LN & no EN invasion: Observation
  >2 cm or ≥6 positive LN or any EN invasion: Adjuvant Chemo (B)EP×2
- Stage IIB-S0: Chemo (EP × 4 cycles or BEP × 3 cycles) or RPLND (in special situations)
- Stage IS, IIA-S1, IIB-S1, IIC, IIIA (good-risk): Chemo (EP × 4 cycles or BEP × 3 cycles) commonly followed by surgery (RPLND & residual dz at other sites, if applicable)
- Stage IIIB (intermediate risk): Chemo (BEP × 4 cycles or VIP × 4 cycles in selected pts) or clinical trial, if available, commonly followed by surgery (RPLND & residual dz at other sites, if applicable)
- Stage IIIC (poor-risk): Chemo (BEP × 4 cycles or VIP × 4 cycles in selected pts)

Salvage therapeutic options

- Up to 30% of pts w/ advanced GCT will either relapse or fail to achieve a CR
- Next-generation sequencing identified an association b/w cisplatin resistance & mutually exclusive alterations in *TP53* & *MDM2* (*JCO* 2016;34:4000)
- 2 major salvage approaches are conventional-dose chemo (CDCT) w/ TIP (*JCO* 2005;23:6549) & high-dose chemo w/ autologous stem cell transplant (HDCT) (*NEJM* 2007;26:340; *JCO* 2010;28:1706)
- The introduction of paclitaxel & varying HDCT regimens have raised the issue of pt selection for CDCT vs. HDCT. The TIGER trial, in which pts stratified by risk criteria are randomized to TIP or HDCT, is testing whether CDCT or HDCT is superior as 1st salvage therapy, & which subgroup(s) require HDCT as 1st therapy.

Toxicity

- Acute: Platinum related: Nephrotoxicity, ototoxicity, peripheral neuropathy, anemia, & arterial & venous thromboembolic events. Bleomycin specific: Pulmonary toxicity & Raynaud phenomenon. Febrile neutropenia related to EP & BEP (*Oncology* 2016;30(7):653)
- Chronic: 20% pts fail to regain nl spermatogenesis (*JNCCN* 2012;10:558); incr. incidence of CV dz (*JNCCN* 2012;10:537); incr. incidence of 2° non-GCT malignancy; incr. risk of CV dz following platinum based chemo & 2° malignancy when both RT & chemo have been given compared to either modality used alone (*JCO* 2007;25:4370)

PENILE CANCER

Epidemiology and risk factors

- Rare (estimated 26,000 cases globally/y), orphan dz designation. More common in less developed nations (*Cancer Incidence in Five Continents* Vol. XI: https://ci5.iarc.fr). Mean age 60 y but trend of earlier onset may be related to HPV prevalence (*Int J Cancer* 2018;142:1586)
- RFs: HPV (30–50% of invasive PSCCs), namely HPV 16,6,18; no circumcision or performed at an older age, phimosis, chronic inflammation, HIV, h/o genital warts, known urethral stricture, penile injury, single, never married, poor penile hygiene, smoking. Mutant **p16** & **p53** a/w development of penile CA. Incr. expression of protein $p16^{INK4a}$, a/w HPV
- Typically presents as a painless lump or ulcer on the penis, majority 1° epithelial SCC. Most occur on mucosal surface glans/prepuce. Precursor lesions: Lichen sclerosis & penile intraepithelial neoplasia (erythroplasia of Queyrat) differentiated & undifferentiated (HPV assoc). Large lesions may obstruct urethral meatus
- Examination of penis for lesion size, location, morphology (papillary, nodular, ulcerating, fungating or flat) & to help determine extent of invasion into the corpus spongiosum or corpus cavernosum, skip lesions & palpation of inguinal LN

Prognostic factors/risk assessment

- Poor differentiation grade, stage, presence of LVI or perineural invasion, palpable LN, LN extracapsular extension (*Urology* 2010;76:S15–S23)

Diagnosis and workup

- Penile bx to include corpus spongiosum for accurate local staging. MRI w/ pharmacologically induced erection to assess extent of 1° lesion. Assess HPV status
- LN assessment based on palpable LAD or high-risk T stage. Staging of inguinal nodes is performed by FNA, SLNB, or superficial inguinal node dissection. If malignant (~50%), warrants consideration of definitive surgical intervention
- Cross-sectional imaging of chest/abdomen/pelvis if inguinal metastases detected to assess for pelvic LNs & distant metastases. Consider 18F-FDG PET/CT

Pathology

Non–HPV-Related Squamous Cell Carcinoma
Usual type (45–75%), papillary carcinoma (2–15%), verrucous carcinoma (3–8%), sarcomatoid carcinoma (1–7%), adenosquamous carcinoma (1–2%), pseudohyperplastic (<1%) pseudoglandular (<1%), cuniculatum (<1%)
HPV-Related Squamous Cell Carcinoma
Warty carcinoma (5–10%), basaloid carcinoma (4–10%), Warty-basaloid carcinoma (4%), clear cell carcinoma (<1%), lymphoepithelioma-like (<1%), papillary-basaloid (<1%) (*Nat Rev Dis Primers* 2021;7:11)

Staging

- **Stage I (T1aN0M0):** Invades stroma, low risk for mets **Stage II (T1b-T3N0M0):** Invade stroma + high risk or involve corporeal tissue or the urethra. **Stage III:** Any positive LN. **Stage IV (T4 or N3 or M1):** Locally invasive 1°, pelvic LNs, or distant spread

Management

Aim to eliminate malignancy while preserving cosmetically acceptable & functional penis. Consider clinical trials

- Organ sparing strategies can be considered, optimally for tumors that are Tis, Ta, or T1 grade 1–2 (topical therapy, laser therapy, WLE, glansectomy, Mohs surgery)
- T1 Grade 3–4: 1 of wide local excision/partial or total penectomy/radiotherapy/chemoradiotherapy
- T2 or greater: Partial or total penectomy/radiotherapy/chemoradiotherapy.
- Positive LN: Cisplatin based neoadjuvant chemo -> inguinal LND (high risk of lymphedema). Consider pelvic LND if detected & response to chemo
- Metastatic: 1–10% of cases de novo. Lack of RCT evidence. Consider clinical trial. TIP = paclitaxel + ifosfamide + cisplatin (*JCO* 2010; 24:3851) or 5-FU+cisplatin (*J Urol* 1999;161:1823). If response, consider consolidation surgery

NON-SMALL CELL LUNG CANCERS

Epidemiology and risk factors

- 200K annual U.S. cases w/ 100K deaths, Lung CA #1 cause of CA mortality, 65% stage III/IV, 25% stage III (*JTO* 2017;12:1109), incidence-based mortality decreasing due to new therapies (*NEJM* 2020;383:940)
- **Cigarette smoking:** 85% of all cases (20× relative risk over nonsmokers), ↑ w/ intensity & dur of smoking, ↓ w/ time since quitting; other risks: Second-hand smoking, previous RT, air pollution, radon, metals, asbestos, synergy w/ smoking + asbestos, germline *TP53* & *EGFR* T790M comprise a small fraction (*Mayo Clin Proc* 2008;83:584)

Pathology

- **AdenoCA (ADCL):** 45% of all NSCLC, most common subtype, ↑ incidence, a/w hypertrophic osteoarthropathy, IHC: +TTF-1 & +Napsin A, –p40
- **Squamous (SQCLC):** 30% of NSCLC, strongly a/w smoking, a/w hyperCa 2° to PTHrP release, IHC: –TTF1, +p40, +p63
- **Others: Adenosquamous (<4%), sarcomatoid (<1%), large cell carcinoma (9%), large cell NEC (<5%), carcinoids (<5%)**

Molecular biology

- ***KRAS* Mt:** 25% of ADCL (*Cancer Discov* 2017;7:596; *CCR* 2018;24:1038), a/w smoking (transversions: G12C 40% of *KRAS* Mt, G12V) but present in 4% of never-smokers (transitions: G12D). Confers worse prog. *KRAS* G12C specific inhibitor available. *Targetable driver oncogenes are generally mutually exclusive in tx-naïve tumors*
- ***EGFR* Mt:** 15% of ADCL, **exon 19 deletions** (LREA) (45%), exon 21 **L858R** (40%), exon 18 (G719X), exon 20 (S768I), exon 21 (L861Q), confer EGFR TKI Sn, initially described in never-smokers, but also present in pts w/ smoking histories (*JCO* 2011;29:2066). **Exon 20 insertions** now targetable driver. Acquired **T790M** Mt confers resistance to earlier generation EGFR TKIs (*NEJM* 2005;352:786)
- ***ALK* fusion:** 4% of ADCL, a/w younger males, never-smoking hx, various *ALK* fusion partners (*EML4-ALK* most common), Sn to ALK kinase inhibitors (*NEJM* 2010;363:1693)
- ***ROS1* fusion:** 1–2% of ADCL, a/w younger, never-smokers, multiple fusion partners (*CD74-ROS1* most common) (*JCO* 2012;30:863; *Nat Rev Clin Oncol* 2020;18:1)
- ***METex14* Mt:** 3–4% of ADCL, Mts lead to exon 14 skipping (ubiquitin-binding site) & persistent activation; a/w sarcomatoid carcinoma. Can be 2° to *EGFR* Mt. Sn to MET inhibitors (*Nat Rev Clin Oncol* 2020;17:569)
- Other actionable alterations: ***BRAF* V600E** 4%, ***RET* Fusion** 1%, ***NTRK1/2/3* Fusion** <1%, ***HER2* Amp/Mt** 3%, High-level ***MET* Amp** <1% (*JAMA* 2014;311:1998)
- Other genomic features: Genome doubling, tobacco-induced mutagenesis (C>A, G>T transversions), tumor suppressor loss-of-function Mt (*TP53, STK11, KEAP1, CDKN2A, NF1*), APOBEC-related subclonal Mt (*Nat Gen* 2018;50:1189; *NEJM* 2016;374:1864)

SQCLCs: Few RTK gene mutations; chr 3q Amp; common: *TP53* (81%), *CDKN2A* loss (72%), *RB1, PIK3CA, PTEN, NFE2L2, KEAP1, NOTCH1, SOX2* Amp, *FGFR1* Amp, *HLA-A* loss (*Nature* 2012;489:519; *J Clin Oncol* 2012;30:abstr 7505)

PD-L1 expression: Scored by % membranous staining of viable tumor cells (TPS), immune cells (IC), reflection of tumor inflammation ↑ a/w ↑ ICI response

Tumor mutation burden (TMB): Nonsynonymous (coding) mutations measured as mutations/megabase (mt/mb) ↑ TMB a/w ↑ ICI response (*Science* 2015;348:124; *Cancer Cell* 2018;33:843) and a/w tobacco-induced mutagenesis

Screening and prevention

- **Annual LDCT:** Recommended for: Age 50–80, 20 pack-y, quit <15 y ago w/ annual LDCT (USPSTF 2021). 20% mortality benefit in National Lung Screening Trial, NNT = 320, high FP rate (*NEJM* 2011;365;395) ↑ screening discussions & wide adoption needed (14% eligible are screened)
- **Smoking cessation:** Most effective method of prevention (incl. 2nd lung 1°). Behavioral support & medical tx rec. Txs include: Nicotine replacement (combining long & short acting more effective), varenicline, & bupropion

Clinical manifestations

- 10% are asx at presentation & detected incidentally by imaging
  - Cough, hemoptysis, dyspnea, postobstructive PNA
  - Regional spread: Pleural effusion, Pancoast syn (apical tumors), SVC syn
  - Extrathoracic mets: LN, brain, bone, liver, & adrenal
  - Paraneoplastic syn: SIADH, hyperCa, hypertrophic pulm osteoarthropathy

Diagnostic and staging evaluation

- **Imaging: CT chest** captures adrenals, **PET scan** to evaluate for distant dz, **MR brain** for pts treated w/ curative intent or sx, preoperative PFTs
- **Tissue:** Depending on site: EBUS-guided bronchoscopic or image-guided bx, thoracentesis (effusion), or video-assisted thoracoscopic surgery (VATS). **Need sufficient tissue in all suspected lung CAs for dx:** Histologic typing, IHC (incl. **PD-L1** expression), & comprehensive **molecular testing** (esp stage IV), tissue-based NGS panel preferred. **ctDNA** ↑ Sn by stage, can be FN, FP clonal hematopoiesis of indeterminate potential (CHIP). Proceeding to surgery w/o bx ok for stage I
  - **Mediastinal evaluation:** Considered for nodes >1 cm on CT or PET+ via EBUS-guided bronchoscopy or mediastinoscopy
  - **Molecular testing:** Actionable alterations in *EGFR, ALK, ROS1, MET, RET, BRAF, HER2, NTRK1/2/3*
- **Stage I:** T1-2N0, **stage IIA:** T2N0, **stage IIB:** T1-2N1, T3N0, **stage IIIA:** T1-2N2 (N2 node, single digit station), T3N1, T4N0-1, **stage IIIB:** T1-2N3, T3-4N2, **stage IIIC:** T3-4N3, **stage IV:** Contralateral lung nodule (M1a), pleural or pericardial met/effusion (M1a), single extrathoracic met (M1b), multiple extrathoracic mets (M1c) (*J Thorac Oncol* 2016;11:39–51)

Prognosis: Overall Survival at 5 y (%), TNM 8th Ed.						
Stage	IA	IB	IIA	IIB	IIIA	IIIB
Clinical	76–92	67	60	33–50	17–34	9–22
Pathologic	81–92	74	65	51–61	34–50	24–40

Management: Pathologic stage I to IIIA (N1)

- **Surgery:** VATS/ robotic-assisted surgery standard where possible, lobectomy w/ mediastinal node dissection preferred. If +margins, reresection preferred over RT
- **RT:** If medically inoperable: SBRT, standard RT (60 Gy), radiofrequency or cryoablation. Multidisciplinary discussion mandatory
- **Adj. Chemo:** Not recommended for stage IA, consider for stage IB (med onc consult mandatory). ↑ OS for stage II–IIIA, CIS doublet for 4 cycles (LACE, *JCO* 2008;26:3552), most studies used CIS/vinorelbine (*NEJM* 2005;352:2589), CIS/peme, & CIS/docetaxel w/ similar efficacy & ↑ tolerability
- **Adj. Targeted Rx:** EGFR TKIs have DFS benefit, OS benefit inconclusive; osimertinib x3y for *EGFR* Mt stage II–IIIA DFS benefit
- **PORT:** Potential benefit if N2 nodes, +margins. Rad onc consultation recommended for N2
- **Multiple 1° Lung CAs:** Different histologies or same histology w/o mediastinal LN involvement or extrathoracic mets—treat by stage as separate primaries (*J Thorac Cardiovasc Surg* 1975;70:606)

Management: Pathologic stage IIIA (N2) to IIIB disease

- Surgery, rad onc, & med onc consults mandatory for **multimodality tx.** Sequence of surgery, RT, & chemo varies
- **Induction:** If resectable, neoadj chemo is best response followed by resection + PORT. Neoadj chemoRT does not improve OS
- Concurrent **ChemoRT:** If unresectable (multiple +N2 LN >3 cm), definitive concurrent chemoRT (*JCO* 1999;17:2692), regimens: CIS/peme, CIS/vinblastine, CIS/etoposide, carbo/paclitaxel
- **Pancoast tumor:** ChemoRT (CIS/etoposide + 45 Gy) followed by surgery (T3N0-1) improves resectability (SWOG 9416, *JCO* 2007;25:313). If unresectable (T4N0-1), chemoRT
- **Adj. checkpoint inhibitor** in IIIB unresectable: ↑ OS w/ durvalumab for 1 y after response to plat doublet w/ definitive RT (*NEJM* 2018;379:2342)

Management: Stage IV metastatic disease

- **Median OS: 6-mo** BSC, **10-mo** plat doublet, **12-mo** plat doublet + Bev (*NEJM* 2006;355:2542), **3-y** *EGFR* Mt EGFR TKI, **5-y+** *ALK* Mt ALK TKI **5y OS: 20%** if PD-L1+, **30%** if PD-L1 ≥50% to checkpoint inhibitor (*JCO* 2019;37:2518), ↑ OS w/ **early palliative care** (*NEJM* 2010;363:733)
- **Initial tx: If sensitizing *EGFR/ALK*,** see Targeted therapy; **If driver neg,** pembrolizumab, atezolizumab, cemiplimab if PD-L1≥50% (RR ~45%) (*NEJM* 2016;375:1823). If PD-L1 <50%, 4–6 cycles of plat doublet+checkpoint inhibitor (RR ~50%) (*NEJM* 2018;378:2078; *NEJM* 2018;379:2040). AdenoCAs: CIS or carbo/peme ± Bev (if eligible: No-SQCLC, no hemoptysis) vs. SQCLC: Carbo/paclitaxel, nab-paclitaxel

- Other initial: Ipi/nivo in TMB ≥10 mt/mb (*NEJM* 2018;378:2093), atezo+carbo/taxol+ Bev in non-SQCLC, *EGFR/ALK* post TKI (*NEJM* 2018;378:2288), ipi/Nivo w/ plat doublet x2cy (*Lancet Onc* 2021;22:198)
- **Maintenance tx:** For CR/PR/SD after 4–6 cycles of plat doublet. D/c plat. Continue peme ↑ OS (PARAMOUNT, *JCO* 2013;31:2895), peme + Bev ↑ PFS (AVAPERL, *JCO* 2013;31:3004), GEM ↑ PFS (*JCO* 2012;30:3516)
- **Subsequent therapies:** Nab-paclitaxel, docetaxel, peme, GEM, vinorelbine, checkpoint inhibitors if not prior: Nivo, pembrolizumab, atezolizumab, ramucirumab + docetaxel (*Lancet* 2014;384:665)
  - **Limited met sites:** (Oligomets): Consider surgery, RT, ablation
  - **RT to symptomatic sites:** Lung, brain (SRS preferred over WBRT), bone lesions, SVC syn
- **Bone Mets:** Denosumab or ZA reduces SRE; symptomatic: Palliative RT
- **Brain Mets:** Multidisciplinary involvement of neuro-oncology/neurology, rad onc/ neurosurgery; symptomatic: Start dexamethasone
- **Leptomeningeal dz:** Consider VP shunt if symptomatic w/ ataxia, encephalopathy, urinary incontinence; WBRT role limited (*JTO* 2012;7:382). If *EGFR* Mt (double dose) osimertinib 180 mg (*JCO* 2020;38:538).
- **Symptomatic pleural effusion:** PleurX w/ talc pleurodesis (*NEJM* 2018;378:1313), thoracic surgery referral for VATS pleurodesis

Targeted therapy

- For this section, approved tx are in bold. Other agents w/ activity listed. All tx apply to stage IV CAs except adj. Osimertinib
- ***EGFR* classical sensitizing mt** (exon 19 deletion or L858R):
  - Initial tx: **Osimertinib** (ORR 80%, PFS 18.9 mos) (*NEJM* 2018;378:113) or **erlotinib & Bev** (ORR 59%, PFS 10.1 mos). Prior care standards: Erlotinib, gefitinib, afatinib, dacomitinib ↑ PFS, improved RR/PFS compared to plat doublet in 1st line (IPASS, *NEJM* 2010;362:2380). S/e: Rash (30–50% pts, Tx: Moisturizers, abx, topical steroids), diarrhea
  - Subsequent tx for ***EGFR* T790M+** (50% resistance cases): **Osimertinib** (if treated w/ erlotinib, gefitinib, afatinib, or dacomitinib) (*NEJM* 2015;372:1689) or progressive CNS dz, chemo if T790M- or continuation of TKI ± local Rx for progression (*JCO* 2013;31:3335)
  - Adj. tx after tumor resection: **Osimertinib**
- ***EGFR* uncommon/atypical mt** (S768O, L861Q, G719X): **Afatinib,** osimertinib
- ***EGFR* exon 20 insertion mt:** 2L+ **amivantamab,** EGFR-MET bispecific (ORR 40%, PFS 8.3 mo) (*JCO* 2021;39(30):3391) or 2L+ **mobocertinib,** EGFR TKI (ORR 28%, PFS 7.3 mos) (*Cancer Discov* 2021;11(7):1688)
- ***ERBB2/HER2* mt:** Trastuzumab deruxtecan-nxki (T-DXd, ORR 55%, PFS 8.2 mos), trasuzumab emtansine (T-DM1, ORR 44%) (*JCO* 2018;36:2532)
- ***KRAS* G12C mt:** 2L+ **sotorasib** (ORR 37%, PFS 6.8 mos), adagrasib
- ***MET* exon 14 alteration: Capmatinib** (ORR 68% tx naïve, ORR 41% pretx) (*NEJM* 2020;383:944) or **tepotinib** (ORR 46%, PFS 8.5 mos); crizotinib. S/e: Peripheral edema
- ***MET* high amp** (GCN ≥10 or MET/CEP7 ≥4): Capmatinib (ORR 40% tx naïve, ORR 29% pre-treated.) (*NEJM* 2020;383:944), crizotinib (ORR 38%)
- ***BRAF* V600E: Dabrafenib + trametinib** (ORR 64%, PFS 10.9 mos) (*Lancet Onc* 2017;18:1307)
- ***ALK* fusion:**
  - Initial tx: **Alectinib** (ORR 83%, PFS 34.8 mos) (*NEJM* 2017;377:829), **brigatinib** (ORR 74%, PFS 24.0 mos), **ceritinib,** or **lorlatinib** (ORR 76%)
  - Subsequent tx: **Lorlatinib** if previously treated w/ alectinib or brigatinib; consider **alectinib, ceritinib,** or **brigatinib** if previously treated w/ crizotinib. Rebiopsy may guide agent choice based on resistance mts
- ***ROS1* fusion:**
  - Initial tx: **Entrectinib** (ORR 77%, PFS 19.0 mos) (*JCO* 2021;39:1253), **crizotinib,** or ceritinib. Tox: Fluid retention, visual Δs
  - Subsequent tx: Lorlatinib
- ***RET* fusion: Selpercatinib** (ORR 85% tx naïve, ORR 64% pretx) (*NEJM* 2020;383:813) or **pralsetinib** (ORR 79% tx naïve, ORR 62% pretx)
- ***NTRK1/2/3* fusion: Larotrectinib** (ORR 73%, PFS 35.0 mo) or **entrectinib** (ORR 69%, PFS 15.0 mos)

SMALL CELL LUNG CANCER

Epidemiology

- SCLC accounts for ~30k new lung CAs in the U.S. annually, majority w/ extensive stage at dx (60–70%). Seen almost exclusively in pts w/ smoking hx, related to both dur & intensity. Smoking cessation leads to better tolerance of therapy & longer life expectancy

Pathology

- Dx based primarily on light microscopy w/ confirmatory IHC
- IHC: +TTF1, +CD56, +chromogranin, +synaptophysin (75% w/ ≥1 NE marker)
- Rarely can coexist w/ SQCLC, ADCL, or other histologies

Pulmonary NETs (WHO Classification)	
Typical carcinoid	Carcinoid morphology, <2 mitoses/10 hpf, lacking necrosis
Atypical carcinoid	Carcinoid morphology, 2–10 mitoses/10 hpf or necrosis
Large cell	NE morphology, high mitotic rate (>10/10 hpf), necrosis, cytologic features of NSCLC (large cells, abundant cytoplasm), +IHC for 1 or more NE markers
Small cell	Small size, scant cytoplasm, nuclei w/ finely granular chromatin, absent nucleoli, high mitotic rate (>10/10 hpf), freq. necrosis

Clinical manifestations

- Often presents as large hilar mass w/ bulky mediastinal LAD
- Sx: Fatigue, cough, dyspnea, wt loss, hemoptysis
- Most common sites of distant mets: Adrenals, bone, & brain

Paraneoplastic Syndromes	
Endocrine	
Ectopic ACTH secretion	Cushing syn, causing muscle weakness, HTN, hirsutism, hypoglycemia, osteoporosis
Ectopic ADH secretion	SIADH, causing hyponatremia, seen in ~10% of pts w/ SCLC, causing cerebral edema, confusion, irritability, seizures
Ectopic PTHrP secretion	Tumor secretion of PTHrP, causing anorexia, vomiting, constipation, lethargy
Neurologic	
Lambert–Eaton	(Affects 3% of pts) p/w symmetrical proximal muscle weakness, also w/ autonomic dysfxn (dry mouth, impotence), dx made clinically, confirmed by EMG & presence of Ab to voltage-gated calcium channel. Treat by addressing underlying malignancy
Other	Cerebellar degeneration, opsoclonus myoclonus, encephalitis, neuropathy

Molecular biology

- Near universal inactivation of TP53 (75–90%) (*Oncogene* 1991;6:1775) & frequent RB1
- *Subtypes based on genomic profiling of transcription regulators:* SCLC-A – ASCL1, classic NE features, SCLC-N – NeuroD1, characterized by NOTCH1 & MYC pathway activation, SCLC-Y – YAP1, SCLC-P – POU (*Nat Rev Cancer* 2019;19:289)
- Other Mts: SOX2 Mts/amp (*Nat Genet* 2012;44:1111), FGFR1 amp (*Nat Genet* 2012;44:1104), inactivation of NOTCH (25%) (*Nature* 2015;524:47)
- Cyto: LOH at 9p, 10q (PTEN) (*Cancer Res* 1997;57:400), deletion 3p (*Cell* 1996;85:17), loss of Rb gene fxn (13q14) (*PNAS* 1997;94:6933)
- Expression: DLL3 (*Sci Transl Med* 2015;7:302), activation of telomerase, upregulation of c-kit (*Clin Cancer Res* 2004;10:8214), c-myc (*Oncogene* 2006;25:130), bcl-2

Workup, staging, prognosis

- After tissue dx w/u includes imaging of chest, liver/adrenals, & CNS

Staging		Median OS	1-y Survival	5-y Survival
Limited dz	Confined to ipsilateral hemithorax & w/in a single radiotherapy port	20 mos	60%	20%
Extensive dz	Met dz outside the ipsilateral hemithorax	10–13 mos	30%	1%

- Poor prognostic factors include poor PS, wt loss, continued smoking, M sex, presence of paraneoplastic syn, elevated LDH

Management—Limited stage (lung confined)

- In rare cases, surgical resection may be curative for clinical stage I dz (5-y survival 40–50% for path stage I–II dz) (*J Thorac Oncol* 2009;4:1049), nodes need to be confirmed neg prior to resection, pts require neoadj chemoRT
- 4 cycles of concurrent chemoRT w/ an OS benefit (*NEJM* 1992;327:1618), RR of 80–90%, 50–60% w/ CR
- Dose: 45 Gy twice QD better than ~45 Gy QD (*NEJM* 1999;340:265), survival benefit for adding RT w/ cycle 1 or 2 (*JCO* 1993;11:336)
- Plat/etoposide is chemo of choice, plat/etoposide = plat/irinotecan, although irinotecan seldom used in US, as ↑ tox (*JCO* 2009;27:2530), CIS = carbo (*JCO* 2012;30:1692)

Management—Extensive stage

- **Atezolizumab + carbo/etoposide** preferred 1st line based on Impower133 (OS 12.3 vs 10.3 mos in platinum–etoposide group) (*NEJM* 2018;379:2220)
- Durvalumab + platinum/etoposide also an option based on improved OS (13 vs 10.3 mos) in Caspian trial (*Lancet* 2019;394:1929)
- Pembro + platinum/etoposide showed improved PFS, however OS benefit not significant (*JCO* 2020;38:2369). Ipi + chemo did not prolong OS (*JCO* 2016;34:3740)
- Recommend 4–6 cycles of induction chemoimmunotherapy, followed by maintenance IO until POD or unacceptable tox
- Thoracic RT in pts w/ residual dz after systemic therapy, OS 13% vs. 3% at 2 y (*Lancet* 2015; 385:36). However, not yet evaluated after CIT
- Elderly pts: If PS adequate, proceed w/ standard CIT
- Trilaciclib (CDK 4/6 inhibitor) approved to decrease myelosuppression during therapy (*Clin Lung Cancer* 2021;22:449)

Prophylactic cranial irradiation (PCI)

- Significant rate (17–38%) of CNS "failure" despite systemic response, CNS failure rate ~80% over 2 y
- PCI w/in 4–8 wks after completion of chemo, MRI brain before proceeding
- *LS-SCLC:* After CR or significant regression to chemo ↓ brain mets, ↑ OS w/ PCI (*NEJM* 1999;34:476)
- *ES-SCLC:* If tumor response to chemo, ↓ brain mets, but conflicting OS data (*NEJM* 2007;357:664; *Lancet Oncol* 2017;18:663). PCI & MRI surveillance both acceptable options
- Total dose of 25–30 Gy, can abbreviate if not PR or in ES-SCLC
- Tox: Fatigue, alopecia, neurocognitive impairment

Management—Relapsed disease

- Median survival after relapse 2–6 mos
- Prognostic factors: PS, tumor extent, time to relapse
- *Sensitive dz:* Initial PR/CR to Rx, progression ≥3 mos after last d of initial tx, high likelihood of response to additional Rx
- *Refractory dz:* Progression after ≤3 mos or lack of response during initial Rx, chance of response to additional Rx <10%
- In late relapse (≥6 mos), significant responses w/ reinduction w/ 1st-line chemo
- Combination therapies w/ ↑ RR, ↑ tox w/o survival benefit
- In pts w/ adequate PS, 2nd-line chemo vs. best supportive care improves OS & QoL
- **Topotecan:** 2nd-line phase III data vs. cyclophosphamide, Adriamycin (doxorubicin), vincristine (CAV) (cyclophosphamide, doxorubicin, vincristine) w/ similar RR, PFS, OS but improved control of sx (*JCO* 1999;17:658), oral topotecan compared to BSC w/ improved QoL (*J Clin Oncol* 2006;24:5411)
- **Lurbinectidin:** Single-arm phase II trial w/o brain mets w/ ORR 35%, toxicities mostly hematologic. Approved for dz progression after ≥1 platinum-based chemo (*Lancet Oncol* 2020;21:645)
- Other agents: Based on smaller, single-arm, phase II studies, irinotecan, temozolomide (*CCR* 2012;18:1138), paclitaxel, docetaxel, vinorelbine, GEM

Targeted therapy

- No improvements in survival w/ standard Rx, no FDA-approved targeted agents
- Angiogenesis inhibitors tested w/o clear efficacy (thalidomide, Bev, sorafenib)
- Ongoing studies: DLL3 Ab drug conjugate, inhibitors of IGF-1R, PI3K/Akt/mTOR, Hedgehog, PARP, HDAC, Notch, Bcl-2, Aurora kinase

THYMOMA AND THYMIC CARCINOMA

Epidemiology

- Exact incidence unclear, estimated 1.5 cases/million annually in the United States (80% thymoma, 20% thymic carcinoma (TC)), most common malignancy in the anterior mediastinum, no known RFs
- Most pts present btw ages 40–60, slight female predominance, Asian, AA > Caucasians

Pathology/Histology

- Histologic heterogeneity is common, difficult to identify degree of invasion on small bx
- IHC: Epithelial cells: +Keratin, +Leu-7, thymic lymphocytes: +LCA, +CD1/3, +CD99
- TC: +CD5, **CD117 (C-kit)**
- Rare (5%) thymic NETs "carcinoids," 25% found in assoc w/ MEN

Pathology (WHO Classification)	
Type A	Bland spindle epithelial cells, few lymphocytes
Type AB	2 components: Type A & predominant lymphocytic infiltrate
Type B1	Epithelial cells w/ vesicular nuclei, small nucleoli, & abundant lymphocytic pop
Type B2	Predominant lymphocytic pop w/ scattered epithelial cells w/ vesicular nuclei
Type B3	Polygonal/round epithelial cells w/ mild atypia
TC	Highly atypical cells, fewer lymphocytes (B cell, mature T cell types), histopathologic subtypes: SCC, sarcomatoid, clear cell, basaloid, papillary

Etiology and clinical manifestations

- 40% asx at dx, found incidentally
- Sx: Shortness of breath, cough, CP, trouble swallowing, wt loss, facial swelling/venous distension of neck & CW (SVC syn)
- **Paraneoplastic syn:** Almost exclusively w/ thymoma (30–50%)
- **Myasthenia gravis (MG)** (25–40%) p/w muscle weakness (esp. eyes), dx made w/ presence of auto-Ab against acetylcholine receptor, tx of MG is thymectomy; other tx: Acetylcholinesterase inhibitor, IO, plasmapheresis
- **Red cell aplasia** (5%), dx made w/ low reticulocyte count, absent erythroid precursors in BM
- **Hypogammaglobulinemia** (5–10%) w/ typically spindle-cell thymoma (Good syn), rarely other AI dz incl. lupus, PM, UC, vitiligo
- **Morvan syn** (<5%) neuromyotonia, pain, hyperhidrosis, wt loss, severe insomnia, & hallucinations, diagnosed by serum abs to VGKC

Molecular biology

- TC: **KIT** overexpression by IHC (86%)
- Thymoma/TC: Lowest somatic mutational load among adult CAs copy-number variation common. *GTF2I* mutations in ~40%; *HRAS, TP53, NRAS* also seen (*Cancer Cell* 2018;33;244)

Workup and staging

- Diff. dx for mediastinal mass: lymphoma, germ cell, thymus hyperplasia, cyst, thyroid tissue
- More than 1 histologic subtype may be found in a given tumor, difficult to determine subtype on a small bx
- W/u: CT chest, CBC, b-HCG, AFP, thyroid studies as appropriate, optional PET, optional MRI chest/cardiac, PFTs

Staging (Masaoka Clinical Staging) (*Cancer* 1981;48:2485)	
Stage I	Macroscopically (Macro) completed encapsulated, no microscopic (Micro) capsular invasion
Stage II	Macro invasion into fat/pleura, Micro invasion into capsule
Stage III	Macro invasion into neighboring organs (pericardium, vessels, lung)
Stage IVA	Pleural or pericardial dissemination
Stage IVB	Lymphogenous or hematogenous met

- Masaoka staging most common, alternative is the TNM staging system proposed by International Thymic Malignancy Interest Group (ITMIG)

Staging (TNM) (*JTO* 2014;9:S65–S72)			
Stage	**Tumor**	**Node**	**Mets**
Stage I	**T1A** (Encapsulated or unencapsulated, w/ or w/o extension into mediastinal fat) **T1B** (extension into mediastinal pleura)	**N0**	**M0**
Stage II	**T2** (invasion into pericardium)	**N0**	**M0**
Stage IIIA	**T3** (invasion of lung, brachiocephalic vein, SVC, CW, phrenic nerve, hilar [extrapericardial] pulm vessels)	**N0**	**M0**
Stage IIIB	**T4** (invasion of aorta, arch vessels, main PA, myocardium, trachea, or esophagus)		
Stage IVA	**Any T** **Any T**	**N1** (anterior perithymic nodes) **N0,1**	**M0** **M1a** (separate pleural or pericardial nodule)
Stage IVB	**Any T** **Any T**	**N2** (deep intrathoracic or cervical nodes) **Any N**	**M0, 1a** **M1b** (pulm nodule or distant organ met)

Prognosis

- Outcomes w/ thymoma superior to TC
- Prognostic factors: Resectability, staging, histologic features, age, presence of MG
- Thymomas a/w ↑ risk for 2nd malignancies incl. NHL & sarcoma (*Int J Cancer* 2003;105:546)

Prognosis: OS at 5 y (%)			
Stage	Localized	Regional	Distant
	93%	79%	40%

Management: Localized disease—intrathoracic (thymoma and TC)

- **Complete surgical resection** is tx of choice
- If resectable, neoadj chemo w/ plat-based combinations preferred, **CAP** for thymoma (CIS, doxorubicin, cyclophosphamide), RR ~70%, resectability 36–70%, s/e: Fatigue, N/V, alopecia, myelosuppression; plat/taxane for TC
- If unresectable, concurrent CRT vs. chemo w/ or w/o RT
- **RT:** Adj. RT for incomplete resection, +margins may be used w/ stage II or III dz, dose 45–60 Gy, ↓ recurrence, s/e: Pulm fibrosis, pericarditis
- **Surveillance:** Annual chest CT to assess for recurrence (can recur many y later, long-term surveillance recommended)

Management: Metastatic disease (thymoma)

- **Metastasectomy** can be a/w good outcome, esp. w/ A, B1 histology (*J Surg Oncol* 2007;95:40)
- **CAP** w/ ORR 50%, CR 10%, OS 38 mos in thymoma (*JCO* 1994:12:1164)
- **Carbo/paclitaxel** w/ good results in thymoma & TC (in TC: ORR 22%, PFS 5 mos) (*JCO* 2011;29:2060)
- **Other active agents:** CIS/etoposide (*JCO* 1996;14:814), peme, GEM, paclitaxel, **Octreotide:** has activity in octreotide scan + thymoma, CR 5%, PR 25% (*JCO* 2004;22:293). Avoid checkpoint inhibitors in thymoma due to high incidence of irAEs (71%) (*JCO* 2019;37:2162)

Metastatic disease (TC)

- 1st-line **chemo: Preferred carbo (AUC 6)/paclitaxel (200 mg/m^2 q3wks)** or CAP, CIS/etoposide, etoposide/ICE/CIS
- 2nd-line therapies: **Pembro** (19–22% RR, 15% grade ≥ irAEs) (*JCO* 2019;37:2162; *Lancet Onc* 2018;19:347), **sunitinib** activity in TC (PR 65%) but not thymoma (*Lancet Oncol* 2015;16:177), **everolimus** activity in both thymoma & TC (PFS 10 mo) (*JCO* 2018;36:342), **lenvatinib (38% ORR, 64% grade 3 HTN)** (*Lancet Onc* 2020;21:843), chemo: 5-FU & leucovorin, GEM/CAP, paclitaxel, peme

MALIGNANT PLEURAL MESOTHELIOMA

Definition

- Malignant proliferation of mesothelial cells that make up lining of pleura
- Note: Mesothelioma can occur in lining of other sites (pleura most common 85% peritoneum 15%, pericardium & tunica vaginalis testis—rare <1%)

Epidemiology/Risk factors

- Rare; ~3,500 new cases dx annually in the United States. Commonly develops in 5th to 7th decade
- Men: women ratio 4:1 w/ a slow but steady decline in the rate in men
- ~80% potentially a/w asbestos exposures. Typically, occupational (steam fitters, insulators, shipbuilders, brake mechanics) or environmental. However, only 5–10% of people w/ classic asbestos exposure are dx w/ mesothelioma
- Develops decades after asbestos exposure, averaging 30–40 y
- Other assocs: Radiotherapy, erionite (common in Cappadocia region of Turkey & also found in gravel roads in regions such as N Dakota)
- Genetics: Germline Mts in ~10% regardless of asbestos. Most common is *BAP1;* familial CA syn includes risk of mesothelioma, uveal/cutaneous melanoma, clear cell renal CA
- Smoking does not ↑ the risk of mesothelioma, though it does markedly ↑ the risk of lung CA together w/ asbestos exposure

Pathology

- Histologic subtypes: Epithelioid (heterogeneous & most common—75%), biphasic or mixed, & sarcomatoid
- Multiple chromosomal alterations. Significantly mutated genes: *BAP1, NF2, TP53, DDX3X, SETD2, CDKN2A/B.* 40–60% have *BAP1* loss. Low Mt burden (*Nat Genet* 2016;48:407–416)
- PD-L1 expression >1% in 40–50% pts. High expression in 9%. More in sarcomatoid
- Useful IHC markers noted below; of note TTF-1 & CEA, which are neg in pleural mesothelioma, are typically positive in ADCL
- DDx: Reactive atypical mesothelial hyperplasia

IHC Markers	
Positive	Calretinin, WT-1, D2-40, CK 5/6
Neg	TTF-1, CEA

Clinical manifestations

- Most commonly p/w unilateral pleural effusion; other sx include dyspnea, cough, CP, CW mass, or other symptomatic 2° to local invasion
- Constitutional sx: Fever, wt loss, diaphoresis
- Distant mets to the contralateral lung, peritoneum, bone, or liver

Diagnostic evaluation

- Thoracentesis (note: Cytologic samples are typically nondiagnostic)
- Pleural bx (thoracoscopic bx preferred)
- Following confirmation of mesothelioma, w/u includes: CT CAP w/ contrast, PET-CT, mediastinoscopy or EBUS FNA of mediastinal LN, VATS, &/or laparoscopy if suspicion of contralateral or peritoneal dz

Staging (IASLC Mesothelioma Staging Group—TNM, 8th Edition)

Key Δs arising from the new staging:

- **T:** Collapse subclassification of T1A & T1B into a single category as the clinical detection of visceral pleural involvement is impossible
- **N:** Survival appears to be influenced more by extent of nodal involvement than by specific location of involved nodes
    1. N1 any ipsilateral, intrathoracic node
    2. N2 ipsilateral supraclavicular or contralateral nodes (previously N3)

TNM Staging

Stage	TNM Classification
IA	T1, N0, M0
IB	T2–T3, N0, M0
II	T1–T2, N1, M0
IIIA	T3, N1, M0
IIIB	T4, any N, M0, or T1–T3, N2, M0
IV	any T, any N, M1

Treatment

- **Trimodality tx** is goal (see figure); however, high proportion of pts unable to complete all 3 modalities. Given rarity, always consider clinical trials

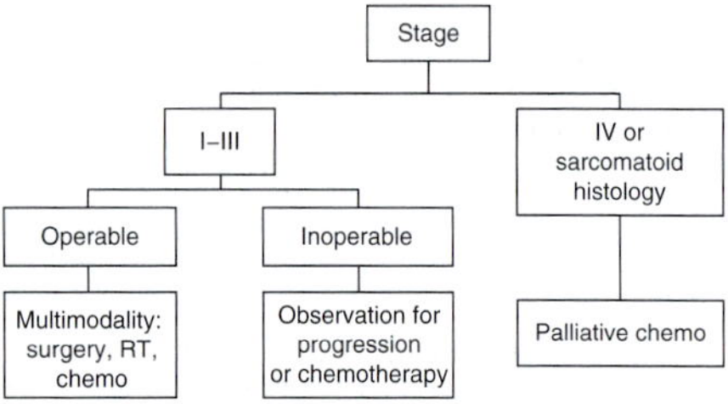

Surgery

- Pleurectomy/decortication (**P/D):** Complete removal of pleura & all gross tumor
- Extrapleural pneumonectomy (**EPP):** En bloc resection of the parietal & visceral pleura w/ the ipsilateral lung, diaphragm, & often pericardium
- For now, b/c met involvement of any LNs is a/w poor prog, surgeons should be encouraged to perform detailed node dissections for all pts undergoing a cytoreductive operation & to document precise location
- P/D & EPP are both choices; most prefer P/D. EPP is a/w significant morbidity & mortality; P/D may not offer complete resection (*J Thorac Cardiovasc Surg* 2008;135:620)
- Role of surgery in biphasic less clear than epithelioid; currently surgery for sarcomatoid histology not recommended (*J Surg Res* 2015;107:929–935)

RT

- Hemithoracic RT ↓ local recurrence after EPP (*J Thorac Cardiovasc Surg* 2001;122:788)
- Phase III trial of immediate prophylactic radiotherapy to prevent procedure-tract mets did not demonstrate superiority over deferred RT (*Lancet Oncol* 2016;17:1094)

Chemotherapy

- Phase III trial CIS/peme vs. CIS w/ OS 12.1 vs. 9.3 mos (*JCO* 2003;21:2636–2644)
- MAPS phase III trial: CIS/peme/Bev vs. CIS/peme up to 6 cycles. OS 18.8 vs. 16.1 mos; CIS/peme/Bev group w/ maintenance peme (*Lancet* 2016;387:1405)
- **1st line:** CIS 75 mg/m^2 + peme 500 mg/m^2 +/– Bev 15 mg/kg (combination IO preferred for nonepithelioid)
- Carbo may be substituted for CIS (*JCO* 2006;20:1443)
- Plat/peme only regimen w/ neoadj/adj. data regardless of histology
- 2nd-line chemo has unclear benefit. Active agents: GEM, anthracyclines, vinca alkaloids

Immunotherapy

- **1st line:** Ipi 1 mg/kg Q6wk + Nivo 360 mg Q3wks; preferred in nonepithelioid, also an option for epithelioid (Checkmate 743, *Lancet*; 2021;397:375). PD-L1 not fully validated as a biomarker. Nonepithelioid histology & age <75 seems important
- 2nd line: Pembrolizumab (KEYNOTE-02, *Lancet Oncol* 2017;18:623-630), Nivo (CONFIRM, IASLC WCLC 2020) & ipi+Nivo (MAPS2, *Lancet Oncol* 2019;20:239-253) (INITIATE, *Lancet Resp Med* 2019;7:260–270) options if no prior ICI

Clinical trials

- ***BAP1* mutant:** *BAP1* loss in mice incr. trimethylated histone H3 lysine 27 (H3K27me3) & dysregulated EZH2-dependent regulation, lineage commitment, & differentiation. Mesothelioma cells that lack BAP1 are sensitive to EZH2 (*Nat Med* 2015;21:1344–1349)
- **Neoadj/adj.:** Role of dual ICI & chemo/IO being evaluated
- **Combination chemo/IO:** CIS/peme/durvalumab 1st-line DREAM trial was positive (*Lancet Oncol* 2020;21:1213–1223); phase III trial underway (DREAM3R)
- Ongoing studies: Vaccine combinations (WT-1 vaccine), mesothelin specific CAR-T cells, mesothelin immunotoxin, VISTA abs, dendritic cell therapy

Prognosis

- Cure is rare; high risk of local & distant recurrence. Median survival: ~15 mos. Epithelioid subtype & women have a better outcome (*BJC* 2014;11:1860)
- The control arm in MAPS & Checkmate 743 trials (platinum/pemetrexed) lived ~50% longer than the same tx in prior platinum/pemetrexed phase III (*JCO* 2003;21:2636–44)
- Sarcomatoid subtype poor prog, rarely responds to chemo, but outlook may Δ w/ approval of 1st-line IO
- Screening not shown to ↓ mortality even in asbestos exposure

HEPATOCELLULAR CARCINOMA (HCC)

Epidemiology

- Primary liver CA—**6th most common CA worldwide** (905,000/y) & 3rd leading cause of worldwide CA mortality (830,000/y); ~80% is HCC
- >80% cases of HCC occur in sub-Saharan Africa, eastern & southeastern Asia; Europe & North America have intermediate incidence rates (*Globocan* 2020)
- **6th leading cause of CA mortality in US;** in recent years, decades-long ↑ in the incidence of HCC-related mortality in US has plateaued (*CA Cancer J Clin* 2020;70:7)

Risk factors

- **Viral hepatitis: HBV** & **HCV** are the **leading RFs** & account for **75% cases** worldwide; while HBV is the leading cause globally, HCV is the leading cause in North America
- **Metabolic d/os:** Metabolic syn, DM, **NAFLD;** overall prevalence of NAFLD is rising in US (32%) & NASH may overtake viral hepatitis as the leading cause of HCC
- **Acquired RFs:** Excessive EtOH → **alcoholic cirrhosis** (account for up to 1/3 of cases of HCC in US), environmental exposure to aflatoxin from Aspergillus fungus, tobacco
- Other RFs: AI hepatitis, hereditary hemochromatosis (muts in HFE gene), Wilson's dz & other rare metabolic d/os

Pathophysiology

- ~80% occurs in cirrhosis: acute or chronic injury to hepatocytes → repair/remodeling results in liver fibrosis/cirrhosis → stepwise accumulation of diverse genetic alterations & epigenetic modifications (*TERT*, p53, *CTNNB1*, etc.) → malignant transformation
- ~20% develops w/o underlying cirrhosis: HBV induces early genetic alterations through direct viral DNA insertion; HBV/HCV both induce early alterations through chronic inflammation/oxidative stress
- Histopathologic markers of HCC: For poorly differentiated cases, IHC markers (HepPar1, GPC-3, etc.) may be used for dx

Screening and prevention

- Screening w/ ultrasonography & AFP testing every 6 mos for **pts w/ established RFs for HCC;** these include pts w/ cirrhosis (HBV/HCV/alcohol/NASH/other causes), Hep B carriers w/o cirrhosis; early detection using cell-free DNA is currently under investigation (*Cell Res* 2021;31:589)
- Add'l imaging **(abd multiphasic CT or MRI)** in the setting of rising serum AFP or identification of liver mass (10 mm or greater) on U/S
- **HCV tx** w/ direct-acting antivirals (sofosbuvir, ledipasvir, etc.) is highly effective (cure rates >90%) & decreases HCC risk
- **HBV vaccination:** Decrease in HCC incidence is expected among cohorts born after 1960 (*JCO* 2016;34:1787)

Clinical manifestations

- **S/S:** No pathognomonic s/s for HCC. Abd pain may indicate rupture of a liver lesion & warrants immediate attention
- **Exam:** Usu unremarkable, hepatomegaly, ascites, jaundice, encephalopathy, & other s/s of adv cirrhosis
- **Lab findings:** Reflects level of liver dysfunction. ↑ Total bili., low albumin, & elevated INR in the setting of advanced cirrhosis

Diagnostic workup

- Includes imaging, pathologic confirmation of HCC, tumor markers, & LFTs
- **Imaging:** At least **3-phase contrast-enhanced CT scan** (arterial, portal venous, parenchymal phase), tumor enhances in arterial phase & becomes hypoattenuating in portal venous phase, or **gadolinium-enhanced MRI.** U/S primarily used as screening modality. PET/CT not adequate
- **Bx:** Dx can be made noninvasively by imaging w/o bx; bx may not be necessary for early curable stages when surgery or transplant are considered; bx should be strongly considered in pts in whom dx is in question & in pts w/o cirrhosis. LI-RADS helps standardize the reporting & data collection but does not confirm dx. **Core needle bx** rec for adv stages in view of the more sophisticated pathologic dx & genetic testing interest & value
- **Labs: LFTs, Hep B & C serologies** (it is critical to treat active Hep B even w/ the dx of CA)**, Serum AFP** (useful in conjunction w/ imaging for dx & monitoring tx response, but not sensitive or specific by itself)
- **Assessment of hepatic dysfunction: Child–Pugh classification**

The Child–Pugh Scoring System for Liver Cirrhosis			
	Points		
Parameter	**1**	**2**	**3**
Albumin	>3.5 g/dL	2.8–3.5 g/dL	<2.8 g/dL
Total bili.	<2 mg/dL	2–3 mg/dL	>3 mg/dL
INR	<1.7	1.7–2.3	>2.3
Clinical ascites	Absent	Mild	Moderate
Clinical encephalopathy	Absent	Grade 1–2	Grade 3–4

Staging

- No unified international staging system that accounts for CA & the assoc cirrhosis
- Most clinical trials are based on **AJCC**, which contains variables related to tumor stage (TNM), & **Child–Pugh** classification to assess cirrhosis
- **BCLC system** includes tumor stage, liver fxn, performance status, & serves as a road map to guide Rx; however, it has its limitations & has not been validated in the setting of adv dz (*JCO* 2010; 28:2889). BCLC B may need to be split into B1 & B2 based on up-to-7 criteria (*Dig Dis* 2015;33:751). BCLC C, eg, includes portal vein invasion, extra-hepatic mets, Child–Pugh score of A or B, & PS 1–2

Curative management

Surgical resection

- <25% of tumors are resectable; majority unresectable due to underlying liver dz, multifocal nature of dz, & late dx
- Generally, for pts w/ preserved liver fxn & low-volume dz, w/o major vessel involvement: **AJCC stage I–III A, Child–Pugh class A,** & **no evidence of portal HTN.** Highly selected cases of pts w/ Child–Pugh class B
- 5-y OS for resected pts >50%; tumor recurrence rates high, >70% at 5 y
- Ablation as alternative to surgery for small (<3 cm), properly located tumors (*Clin Radiol* 2017;72:1066); most common method is thermoablation (eg, RFA); percutaneous EtOH injection appears inferior to RFA (*Radiology* 2003;228:235)
- No role for adj. sorafenib (STORM, *Lancet Onc* 2015;16:1344)

Liver transplantation

- Potentially curative Rx for pts w/ early HCC, multinodular dz, &/or adv cirrhosis
- The **Milan Criteria** for eligibility of liver transplantation: A single solitary lesion ≤5 cm or up to 3 lesions each ≤3 cm, no macrovascular invasion or extrahepatic dz; for pts meeting the criteria, 4 y OS & RFS rates at 85 & 92%
- **HCC MELD exception:** MELD score as measure of liver fxn & pretransplant mortality, used to prioritize liver allocation; HCC pts w/ AFP ≤1,000 ng/mL & T2 tumors are eligible for a MELD exception. MELD = 3.8 [Ln serum bili. (mg/dL)] + 11.2 [Ln INR] + 9.6 [Ln serum Cr (mg/dL)] + 6.4)
- Bridge therapy (ie, therapies to control tumor prior to transplantation) is still debatable
- Transplantation can be considered for pts who did not meet the Milan Criteria initially but have undergone successful downstaging Rx

Palliative management

Locoregional therapies

- **Arterially directed therapies** (via hepatic artery branch that feeds tumor): **TAE** – arterial blockage → tumor ischemia/necrosis; **TACE** – arterial blockage + chemo; **TARE** – high dose β radiation from Y-90
- **RT:** EBRT or SBRT if ablation/embolization failed or is contraindicated

Systemic therapies

- 1st line: **Atezolizumab/bevacizumab** (C-P Class A only) improves OS vs. sorafenib (median OS 19.2 vs. 13.4 mos) (IMbrave150, *NEJM* 2020;382:1894; *JCO* 2021; 39(3_suppl):267); evaluate & treat esophageal varices before initiating tx; OS benefit was observed in antidrug ab (ADA) (–) pts but not ADA (+) pt (*Cancer Research* 2021;81(13_suppl): CT185). **Sorafenib** (C-P Class A only) improves OS vs. placebo (median OS 10.7 vs. 7.9 mos) (SHAPR, *NEJM* 2008;359:378; *Lancet Oncol* 2009;10:25); may be considered for C-P class B7. **Lenvatinib** (C-P Class A only) is noninferior to sorafenib (median OS 13.6 vs. 12.3 mos) (REFLECT, *Lancet* 2018:391:1163)
- Subsequent therapies: Regorafenib (*Lancet* 2017;389:56); cabozatinib (*NEJM* 2018:375:54); ramucirumab for AFP ≥400 ng/mL (*JCO* 2018;36:4003); sorafenib, lenvatinib if not previously used; nivolumab ± ipilimumab (CheckMate 040, *Lancet* 2017;389:2492; *JAMA Oncol* 2020;6(11):e204564); pembrolizumab (KEYNOTE-240, *JCO* 2021;39:268)
- **Best Supportive Care** for pts w/ adv dz & not candidates for other therapies or trials

CANCER OF THE BILIARY TREE

Definition

- Cholangiocarcinomas (CC), tumors of the bile duct (BD) epithelium, differentiated by anatomic site of origin. Further classified into intrahepatic & extrahepatic
  - *Intrahepatic CC* (10%): W/in the hepatic parenchyma
  - *Extrahepatic CC* (90%): W/in extrahepatic bile duct (incl. intrapancreatic duct)
    Hilar (40%), confluence of right/left hepatic duct **(Klatskin tumor)**
    Distal (50%), involve CBD/Ampulla of Vater
- Gallbladder carcinoma (GBC) is histologically = CC but ≠ epidemiology, staging system, & surgical Rx. Anatomic site of origin → fundus (60%), body (30%), neck (10%)

Epidemiology

- **Incidence:** ~11,900 new cases/y & ~4,300 deaths/y in the United States of CC & GBC; GBC is more common. Most cases are sporadic (*NEJM* 1999;341:1368), GWAS studies pending
- RFs: ↑ Risk w/ adv age, ↑ risk w/ **chronic inflammation**
- **CC** specific RFs: PSC, choledochal cysts, Asian liver flukes (*O. viverrini* & *C. sinensis*), chronic calculi of BD, HCV, HBV, cirrhosis, & M sex
- **GBC** specific RFs: Chronic cholelithiasis, GB calcification (ie, porcelain GB) & female

Pathophysiology

- Most common histologic subtype = adenoCA (90% CC, 80% GBC); less common: Small cell CA, SCC, sarcomas
- Underlying molecular biology & pathogenesis of GBC & CC is increasingly understood; new insights w/ genetic profiling; mut patterns vary by location, progenitor cell, pattern of growth: *P53, KRAS, BRAF, c-MET, PIK3CA, HER2/neu, EGFR* (*JCO* 2010;28:3531), *FGFR2, ROS1, ARID1A, IDH1/2* (*Oncotarget* 2016;7:46750)

Clinical manifestations

- **Sx** depend on location of lesion; include **painless jaundice,** pruritus, abd pain, biliary colic (esp in GBC), cholangitis, clay-colored stool, cola-colored urine, fever, anorexia, & wt loss. Intrahepatic CCA incidental finding in 25% cases
- **Exam:** Hepatomegaly, palpable GB due to obstruction of cystic duct (*Courvoisier sign*), jaundice, ascites
- **Labs & initial studies:** ↑ T. bili, ↑ AST/ALT, ↑ γ-GT, US ABD ± stones

Diagnostic evaluations

- **MRI/MRCP** w/ & w/o contrast or CT A/P (multiphase delayed contrast)
  Determines anatomy, location, & degree of obstruction
  Used to plan for bx, surgery, &/or stenting
- **ERCP or PTC:** Commonly employed but not required in all cases
  ERCP to stent/relieve obstruction, & for bx (cytology, brushings)
  If ERCP is nondiagnostic, consider EUS or CT-guided for FNA/core
- **In cases w/ suspicious lesion w/o biliary obstruction & distant dz** → surgery w/o bx
- **CA19-9** & CEA, CT chest

Staging and prognosis

- 4 unique AJCC TNM staging systems for CC (intrahepatic, hilar, distal, GBC)
- **Key differences for staging systems:** Intrahepatic T stage based on # of lesions & similar to HCC staging while hilar, distal, & GBC T staging reflects degree of invasion through BD epithelium
- **AJCC staging may not adequately predict surgical resectability** (specifically for hilar, consider Bismuth or Blumgart classification)
- OS in met setting is poor:
  GBC Stage IV → 5-y OS <1%, mOS ~6 mos; Stage III 5-y OS ~5%
  Intrahepatic CC Stage IV → 3-y OS ~10%, mOS ~13 mos

Surgical treatment

- **Early surgical consultation** is critical for CC & GBC
  R0 resection improves OS; **surgery is the only curative Rx, ~25% eligible**
  Avoid needless preoperative biliary stenting in resectable pt (*Ann Surg* 2002;236:17)
  Bx unnecessary if characteristic imaging, ↑ CA 19–9, nl IgG4, excl other CA
  Staging laparoscopy may be required in select cases; if high-risk disseminated dz
- **Intrahepatic CC resection**
  Requires hepatic lobectomy
  Contraindication to surgery: Multifocal tumor, extrahepatic extension, & N1 dz
  5-y OS s/p resection ~15–40%

- **Extrahepatic CC resection**
  Hilar → *en bloc* resection hepatic lobe + involved extrahepatic BD + periportal LND; if L main hepatic duct → caudate lobectomy
  Distal → Pancreaticoduodenectomy + extrahepatic BD to confluence (↑ surg morbidity & mortality)
  5-y OS s/p resection ~10–40%
- **GBC**
  Often laparoscopic surgery for suspected gallstones, incidental CA
  Only T1a (invades lamina propria) can be treated w/ simple cholecystectomy (CCY)
  Extended (radical) CCY → *en bloc* resection of GB, wedge resection of GB bed (segment IVB & V), regional LND
  If jaundiced at presentation, curative surgery unlikely
  5-y OS depends on T stage, approaches 100% T1, 0–40% T3/T4

Systemic and local regional treatment

Adj. Rx:

- Observation is rec for T1 GBC (long-term OS ~100%)
- Observation can be considered for R0 & N0 intra/extrahepatic CC
- In all other cases, adj. Rx is rec due to the high risk of locoregional & met recurrence
- For R1/R2 intrahepatic CC resections, consider reresection or radiation
- **BILCAP trial:** For resected biliary tract CA, **capecitabine** improves median RFS/OS vs. observational arm (24.4/51.1 mos vs. 17.5/36.4 mos) (*Lancet Oncol* 2019;20(5):663)
- Gem in BCAT study, gem/ox in PRODIGE-12 study failed to show benefit
- Ongoing studies: Cis/gem (ACTICCA-1 trial), liver transplantation for early-stage, unresectable, intrahepatic, & perihilar CC

Rx for unresectable & met dz

- Clinical trial preferred if candidate
- **ABC-02:** Randomized Phase III of GEM + CIS vs. GEM in 410 pts w/ adv GBC, CC, ampullary CA; **GEM + CIS superior** w/ median PFS/OS ~8 mos/12 mos vs. ~5 mos/8 mos in GEM arm (*NEJM* 2010;362:1273); GEM + CIS = standard of care
- Other combinations explored in first-line setting: Gem/cis + nab-paclitaxel (phase III pending results) or S1 (tegafur, gimeracil, oteracil), FOLFIRINOX, acelarin + cis vs. gem/cis
- ABC-06 showed benefit from second-line FOLFOX vs. active sx control after progression on gem/cis
- Concurrent chemoradiation (w/ 5-FU or capecitabine, not GEM) in select pts w/ unresectable locally adv dz
- Data for liver-directed therapies such as TACE in combination w/ systemic chemo pending
- Targeted therapies: **Pemigatinib & infigratinib** approved for *FGFR* fusions or rearrangements. Ivosidenib (IDH inhibitor) vs. placebo (in previously treated) w/ OS benefit in phase III Clar-IDHy Trial (*JAMA Oncol* 2021;7:1669)
- Ongoing: *ERBB2* targeting; specifically, in GB. Rare *NTRK, NRG1, ALK* fusions
- IO data (vaccines, CAR-T, checkpoint inhibitors) premature. MSI-H in dz-agnostic trials

Selected Chemotherapy for Unresectable and Metastatic Disease

Regimen[a]	Citation	ORR (%)	Median PFS (mos)	Median OS (mos)
GEM + CIS	*NEJM* 2010;362:1273	26	8	12
GEM + OX	*Ann Oncol* 2004;15:1339	22–36	~4–6	~8–15
GEM + Cape	*JCO* 2008;26:3702	25	~7	~13
Cap + OX[b]	*Br J Cancer* 2008;98:309	27	~7	~13
GEM	Multiple trials	0–30	NR	~5–12
5-FU or Cape	Multiple trials	10–32	NR	~5–7

[a]GEM, CIS, OX, Cape, 5-FU, NR; most trials, except for GEM + CIS, are phase II trials.
[b]Lower ORR for intrahepatic.

Surveillance and Rx of recurrence

- Serial exam, CT-CAP, CA19–9, CEA q6mos for 2 y then annually, if local recurrence → chemoRT (if none prior), ablation, reresection or chemo alone; if metastatic see above

PANCREATIC CANCER

Epidemiology

- **Incidence:** Estimated ~60,430 new cases/y & ~48,220 deaths/y in the United States (NCI SEER); increasing incidence, particularly early onset (<50 yo) (*Lancet* 2019;4(3):E137); 4th most common cause of CA deaths in U.S. men & women; estimated to be 2nd leading cause of CA-related mortality by 2030 (*Cancer Res* 2014;74:2913)
- **Acquired RFs:** Age (median: 70 yo), race, tobacco, EtOH, ↑ BMI, chronic pancreatitis, occupational exposure, DM
- **Hereditary RFs:** ↑ Risk w/ FHx, ~5–15% pts have genetic predisposition
  - Inherited susceptibility to pancreatic CA (*NEJM* 2008;359:2143)
    Familial atypical multiple-mole melanoma syn, *CDKN2A* (p16) (15% lifetime risk)
    Hereditary breast CA syn, *BRCA2* (5% lifetime risk) > *BRCA1* > *PALB2*
    Lynch syn, *MSH2*, & *MLH1*
    Peutz–Jeghers syn, *STK11* (30% lifetime risk)
    Ataxia–telangiectasia, *ATM*
    Hereditary chronic pancreatitis syn, germline muts in cationic trypsinogen (*PRSS1*) or secretory trypsin inhibitor (*SPINK1*) (40% lifetime risk)
  - Note FDRs of individuals w/ familial pancreatic CA → EUS + MRI (*Gut* 2013;62:339)

Pathophysiology

- Arises from acinar epithelial cells after acinar to ductal metaplasia, most common histology = adenoCA; 70% of tumor mass is nonneoplastic desmoplastic (stromal component) composed of numerous cell types
- Sequential progression from premalignant PanIN to invasive adenoCA
- PanIN ↑ in histologic grade (1A/B → 2 → 3) & genetic complexity (***KRAS* mut** overexpression → p16 loss → p53 & *BRCA2* loss)
- Likely slow evolution to invasive dz, over **decades** (*Nature* 2010;467:1114)

Clinical manifestations

- **Sx** dependent on location of lesion, **painless jaundice,** abd pain, anorexia, wt loss, **back pain** (RP involvement, predictor of unresectable tumor (*Surgery* 1997;122:53))
- New or worsening DM, acute pancreatitis, or malabsorption (steatorrhea)
- VTE or migratory thrombophlebitis (Trousseau sign)
- **Exam:** Most often nl; jaundice, hepatomegaly, ascites, abd mass, left supraclavicular LAD (Virchow node), periumbilical LAD (Sister Mary Joseph nodes)
- **Labs:** Hyperglycemia, ↑ AST/ALT, ↑ conjugated bili., ↑ amylase/lipase, anemia, prolonged PT/INR due to malabsorption of fat-soluble vitamins

Diagnostic evaluations and staging

- **Multiphase contrast-enhanced CT scan** or MRI/MRCP; CT Chest
  - If (+) pancreatic mass, stricture, dilated pancreatic duct → EUS FNA for bx; ERCP & metal stent if biliary stricture; if (+) cholangitis → temporary stent by ERCP + abx if (+) distal mets → bx
- **CA19-9** (↑ in biliary obstruction, not appropriate baseline until biliary decompression or surgery), LFTs
- **Universal germline/somatic NGS:** *KRAS* WT subset (~5%) enriched for potentially targetable drivers; targeted Rx a/w ↑ OS (*Lancet Oncol* 2020;12(4):508)

Staging of Exocrine Pancreas Cancer
(AJCC 8th ed. 2017 and NCCN Guidelines Pancreatic Adenocarcinoma v2.2021)

Stage (% at Resection)[a]	Tumor	Node (LN)	Mets	5-y OS (%)[b]
IA/B (17%)	Primary ≤4 cm	N0	None	*Local* ~42%
IIA (2%)	Primary >4 cm	N0	None	
IIB (42%)	Any size	1–3 regional (N1)	None	
III (39%)	Any size	≥4 regional (N2)	None	
	Involves celiac axis/SMA/CHA *See Resectable & Borderline Resectable definitions below*	NX	None	*Regional* ~14%
IV	Any size	NX	Distant mets	*Distant* ~3%

[a](*JAMA Surgery* 2018;153(12):e183617). Note, only 15% of patients undergo resection. >50% of patients present with metastatic disease. Staging is both clinical & pathologic.
[b]NCI SEER 18, 2011–2017; seer.cancer.gov, Accessed 2021, includes all patients; note, improved survival with resection. All stages = 10%.

Surgical treatment

- **Surgical resection** is delivered w/ curative intent; R0 resection optimal; 5-y OS resected pts = 20.2% (*JAMA Surgery*, 2018;153(12):e183617); High-volume surgical centers = ↓ morbidity & mortality
- **Definitions of resectability** (*Ann Surg Onc* 2009;16:1727; *Radiology* 2014;270(1):248)
  Resectable = clear fat planes around hepatic artery, celiac axis or SMA; no involvement or encasement of portal vein or SMV
  Borderline = abutment/limited involvement of PV, SMV, or hepatic artery. May abut SMA or CA by ≤180°
  Unresectable = CA/SMA encasement (>180°)
- **Type of resection** depends on size/location of tumor
  Head = pancreatoduodenectomy (Whipple procedure)
  Body or tail = distal or subtotal pancreatectomy ± splenectomy
  Multifocal = total pancreatectomy
- **Other surgical considerations:** Avoid extended lymphadenectomy (no improved OS); IP drains ↑ rate postop sepsis, fluid collections, & fistula (*Ann Surg* 2001;234:487); in resectable pts no benefit of preoperative biliary drainage unless other complicating issues (*NEJM* 2010;362:129)

GI 16-178

Radiotherapy and systemic treatment

- **Adj. Rx:** mFOLFIRINOX favored (ECOG 0–1), alternative: GEM/Cape
  - GITSG: 5-FU + RT vs. obs; chemoRT ↑ OS (20 vs. 11 mos) (*Arch Surg* 1985:120:899)
  - CONKO-001: GEM vs. observation; GEM ↑ DFS/OS (22.8 vs. 20.2 mos) (*JAMA* 2007;297:267)
  - ESPAC-1: Bolus 5-FU + RT vs. 5-FU only vs. 5-FU + RT → 5-FU vs. obs; ↑ DFS/OS for adj. 5-FU (20.1 vs. 15.5 mos); unclear benefit RT (*NEJM* 2004;350:1200)
    - ESPAC-3: GEM vs. 5-FU, no Δ DFS, OS, QoL (*JAMA* 2010;304:1073)
  - ESPAC-4: GEM/Cape vs. GEM; GEM/Cape ↑ OS (28.0 vs. 25.5 mos) (*JCO* 2016;34: no.18_suppl.LBA4006)
  - PRODIGE-24: mFOLFIRINOX vs. GEM; mFOLFIRINOX ↑ OS (54.4 vs. 35.0 mos) (*NEJM* 2018;379(25):2395)
- RT controversial—awaiting results of RTOG 0848
- **Neoadj/conversion Rx:** Limited prospective data, considered for borderline resectable tumors, restage prior to surgery
- **Surveillance & Rx of recurrence:** Serial exam, CT CAP, CA19-9 q3–6mos for 2–3 y then annually; if local recurrence consider systemic Rx &/or chemoRT (if none prior)

For unresectable & met dz

- Rx not curative, designed to ↑ survival & ↓ sx & maintain QoL
- **PS** dictates Rx
  Good PS (ECOG 0–1) → clinical trial, FOLFIRINOX or GEM + nab-paclitaxel
  Poor PS → GEM monoRx or best supportive care
  If locally adv dz w/ SD or better on chemo → consider chemoRT though no OS benefit (*JAMA* 2016;315:1844)
- ***gBRCA/PALB2:*** GEM + cis (*JCO* 2020;38(13):1378); if cis ineligible favor, other platinum-containing regimen
- ***gBRCA:*** If no POD on platinum, can consider olaparib maintenance (*NEJM* 2019;381:317)
- **2nd line:** 5-FU–based if prior GEM-based & vice versa; 5-FU/LV + liposomal irinotecan approved for previously treated w/ gem-containing regimen (*Lancet* 2016;387:545)

Selected Chemotherapy for Unresectable & Metastatic Disease

Regimen[a]	Citation	ORR (%)	Median PFS (mos)	Median OS (mos)
FOLFIRINOX	*NEJM* 2011;364:1817	32	6.4	11.1
GEM + ***nab*-P**	*NEJM* 2013;369:1691	23	5.5	8.5
GEMOX	*Br J Cancer* 2006;94:3778	23	4	6
GEM + **Cape**	*JCO* 2009; 27:5513	19	5	7
GEM	Multiple trials	10–15	2–3	5–7
CapeOX	*Cancer* 2008;113:2046	3	2.5	5.8

[a]FOLFIRINOX = 5-FU/LV, irinotecan, and OX; nab-P = nab-paclitaxel; w/ exception of CapeOX, all regimens were compared to GEM in randomized phase II or III studies.

- **Palliative & supportive measures:** Biliary or gastric outlet obstruction → stent; VTE → anticoagulation; pain → opioids, celiac plexus neurolysis, RT; malabsorption → pancreas enzyme replacement; psychosocial support, early GOC discussion

PANCREATIC AND GI NEUROENDOCRINE NEOPLASMS

Epidemiology

- Prevalence of neuroendocrine neoplasms (NENs) in US may exceed 170,000 (likely 2° to ↑ imaging & endoscopy surveillance) (*JAMA Oncol* 2017;3(10):1335)
- Pancreatic (panNENs) are 1–2% of pancreatic CA by incidence; 10% of pancreatic CA by prevalence
- Peak incidence of panNENs between ages 40–69

Classification

- **NENs:** Heterogeneous group of neoplasms composed of **neuroendocrine tumors (NETs**; mixed grades) **& carcinomas (NECs**; all high grade). NENs arise from enterochromaffin cells generally of the GI (2/3rds) & pulm tract but can also arise in the genitourinary & gynecologic systems. Rx is dependent on the site of origin & grade/differentiation
- The **WHO classification system** distinguishes well-differentiated & poorly differentiated neoplasms to prognostically stratify NENs. These are further classified by the European Neuroendocrine Tumor Society (ENETS) **TNM grading system**
- NEN pathology is defined by cell differentiation (ie, cell morphology, well vs. poor) & grading (**low, intermediate**, & **high grades** based on proliferative activity of the tumor, measured by Ki-67 proliferation index &/or mitotic rate)

Nomenclature and Classification of Neuroendocrine Neoplasms				
Differentiation & Grade	**Mitotic Rate (per mm²)**	**Ki-67 Proliferation Index (%)**	**Traditional Classification**	**ENETS/WHO Classification**
Well-Differentiated Neuroendocrine Tumors (NETs)				
Low grade (grade 1)	<2	≤2	Carcinoid, islet cell	NET, grade 1
Intermediate grade (grade 2)	2–20	3–20	Carcinoid, atypical carcinoid, islet cell	NET, grade 2
High grade (grade 3)	>20	>20	Carcinoid, islet cell	NET, grade 3
Poorly Differentiated Neuroendocrine Carcinomas (NECs)				
High grade (grade 3)	>20	>20	Small cell NEC[a], Large cell NEC[a]	NEC, grade 3, small cell

[a]High-grade small- and large-cell NECs generally have Ki-67 >50%.

Risk factors and genetics

- Majority of NENs are sporadic; RFs are poorly understood
- Rarely a/w **MEN type 1** (AD), w/ muts in the tumor suppressor gene *MEN1* that encodes the protein menin (tumors involving pancreas, pituitary, & parathyroid glands); **MEN type 2,** w/ muts in *RET* proto-oncogene (a/w medullary thyroid CA, pheochromocytoma, & HPT)
- Cases also a/w VHL dz, TSC, & neurofibromatosis; rare pancreatic CAs as part of Lynch syn also seen

Clinical presentation

- Frequently **asx (ie, nonfunctional tumors);** symptoms usu related to hormonal hypersecretion (ie, functional): Intermittent flushing, diarrhea, rarely tricuspid regurgitation/pulm stenosis in pts w/ **carcinoid syn,** & sx related to secretion of insulin, glucagon, gastrin, & other peptides in pts w/ panNETs

Diagnostic evaluation

- **Multiphasic CT** or **MRI** to assess extent of dz & possible 1° location
- **Gallium-68 DOTATATE PET-CT** (preferred) or **Octreotide scan** (radiolabeled somatostatin analog [^{111}In-DTPA]-octreotide may also be used given majority of NETs express somatostatin receptor (SSTR); SSTR-avid tumors on functional imaging have better prognosis
- Other imaging studies: EUS or EGD used for suspected duodenal & gastric NENs & panNENs; proctoscopic examination for rectal carcinoids; bronchoscopy as needed for thymic & bronchopulmonary carcinoids, TTE for carcinoid syn–related cardiac dz
- **Lab work:** R/o MEN1 syn in pts w/ suspected FHx. Hormone markers based on clinical sx (ie, 24-h 5-HIAA if suspected carcinoid syn)

Management: Resectable locoregional disease

- Depends on location of 1° site & tumor size; **Surgery** is mainstay Rx for resectable tumors for healthy pts

Management: Unresectable locoregional disease or metastatic disease

- Assess **grade/differentiation, goals of Rx** (stabilization/monitoring vs. shrinkage), & **extent of dz** (oligometastatic vs. disseminated). Slow growing tumors can undergo **active surveillance** to determine rate of dz growth

Regional therapies

- **Embolization** for liver dz. Bland, chemo, or radioembolization are options. Useful for reducing sx of tumor-assoc hormone production (in functional tumors) & a/w prolonged tumor regression. Observe for postembolization syn & allow recovery
- Debulking **cytoreductive surgery** can reduce burden & palliate hormone-producing sx

Systemic therapies

- **Octreotide** & **analogue Rx:** Used to control sx in hormonally active NETs. Analogues have tumorstatic rather than tumoricidal effect. Use of monthly **octreotide long-acting release (LAR),** compared to placebo, a/w delay in tumor progression (14.3 vs. 6 mos) in midgut NETs (PROMID, *JCO* 2009;27:4656). Use of monthly **lanreotide,** compared to placebo, a/w prolonged median PFS (not reached vs. 18 mos) in pancreatic, midgut, hindgut, or unknown origin NETs (CLARINET, *NEJM* 2014;371:224)
- **Radiolabeled octreotide Rx (peptide receptor radionuclide Rx [PRRT]):** Phase III study of ^{177}Lu-DOTA^{0}-Tyr^{3}-Octreotate (Lutathera) compared to high-dose octreotide LAR showed ↑ median PFS (not reached at 24 vs. 8.4 mos) in SSTR positive midgut NETs (NETTER-1, *NEJM* 2017;376:125); but no statistically significant ↑ OS (48.0 vs. 36.3 mos, p = 0.30) (*Lancet Onc* 2021;22(12):1752)
- **Cytotoxic chemo:** Consider in pts w/ heavy tumor burden, high-grade, & poorly differentiated/rapid growth
  - Temozolomide-based Rx in panNENs improves PFS & OS
  - Addition of capecitabine may ↑ median PFS
  - In panNETs, can consider streptozocin + doxorubicin (RR = 69%, OS = 2.2 y) (*NEJM* 1992;326:519), but tox is notable, & further studies suggest a MUCH lower degree of activity for this regimen (*Cancer* 1999;86:944)
  - Platinum-based combination Rx is also an option. Exceptional response to Rx can be managed w/ tx holidays
  - Chemo ineffective in midgut tumors, a/w variable response rates in other NEN types
- **Biologically targeted therapies**
  - **Sunitinib** (VEGF inhibitor): FDA-approved in panNETs. Phase III study in panNETs showed ↑ median PFS (5.5 to 11.4 mos, HR 0.42) compared to placebo (*NEJM* 2011;364:501)
  - **Everolimus** (mTOR inhibitor): FDA-approved for panNETs, well-differentiated GI or lung NET. Phase III study of everolimus in panNETs showed ↑ median PFS (4.6 to 11 mos, HR 0.35) compared to placebo (RADIANT-3, *NEJM* 2011;364:514). Phase III study of everolimus in lung or GI origin NETs showed ↑ median PFS (3.9 mos to 11 mos, HR 0.48) compared to placebo (RADIANT-4, *Lancet* 2016;387:968)

Epidemiology

- In the United States, ~19,000 new cases esophageal CA per y (*CA Cancer J Clin* 2021;71:7); worldwide 7th most common CA
- SCC most common in endemic regions of the world (South Africa, China, Iran, Russia); adenoCA more common in many Western European countries & North America; incidence rising

Risk factors

- **Squamous:** Tobacco & EtOH abuse, dietary factors, lye ingestion, achalasia, esophageal webs (Plummer–Vinson Syn), small subset a/w HPV in some endemic regions
- **Adenoca:** Tobacco, obesity ↑ BMI, 60% cases w/ evidence of **Barrett esophagus** (squamous epithelium replaced w/ intestinal columnar epithelium); found in 10–20% endoscopies evaluating GERD; w/ surveillance endoscopy, 0.1–0.2%/y risk of developing CA
- Age, male gender, long-standing GERD, hiatal hernia size, length of Barrett esophagus is a/w higher grades of dysplasia → 10%/y risk of developing CA (*Cancer* 2007;109:668)

Genetics

- Hereditary CA predisposition syns are rare; tylosis (focal nonepidermolytic palmoplantar keratoderma) is an AD d/o caused by germline mut in *RHBDF2* w/ lifetime risk esophageal SCC 90% by age 70
- AdenoCA enriched for chromosomal instability (CIN), frequent mut in *TP53*, RTK/RAS gene amp (ie, *ERBB2*, *EGFR*, *KRAS*), *VEGFA* amp (*Nature* 2017;541:169)

Pathology/Etiology

- **Squamous:** Preceded by squamous dysplasia; 60% in middle third of esophagus, 30% distal third, & 10% proximal third
- **AdenoCA:** Preceded by Barrett esophagus or incomplete intestinal metaplasia; low-grade → high-grade dysplasia → adenoCA; usu distal third of esophagus
- **Others:** Small cell (1%), SCC w/ sarcomatous features, adenoid cystic, & mucoepidermoid CA

Figure 16-1 Siewert classification.

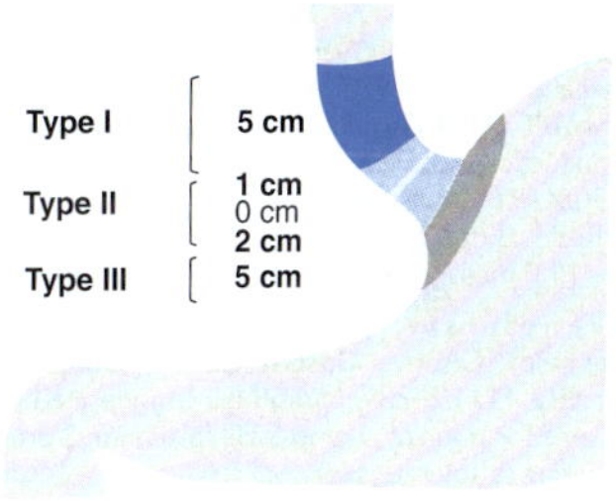

Siewert classification for GE junctions (*Br J Surg* 1998;85:1457)

- **Type 1:** Center of lesion 1–5 cm prox to GE jxn
- **Type 2:** 1 cm prox to, 2 cm distal to GE jxn
- **Type 3:** 2–5 cm distal to GE jxn**—**Treated like gastric CA** (AJCC 2017 8th ed.)

**Location defined by position of upper (proximal) edge of tumor.

Clinical manifestations

- Sx: Most commonly progressive dysphagia → solids then liquids → cachexia & substantial wt loss; odynophagia, GI bleeding

Screening and prevention

- In North America & Western Europe, no screening programs for early detection; at dx ~50% pts have locally adv CA

Staging and workup

- **PET/CT** has higher accuracy in preop, occult M1 dz dx'd in add'l ~10–15% pts, consider esp if CT w/ LN; also helps determine response to preop chemo
- **EUS** for assessing depth of tumor invasion & regional LN, limited depth, & visualization of transducer, suboptimal for distant LN
- Laparoscopy w/ peritoneal washings considered for cT3 or N+ tumors; M1 if positive
- T = depth of tumor invasion (staged by EUS) (T1a lamina propria, muscularis mucosae; T1b submucosa; T2 muscularis propria; T3 adventitia; T4a resectable invading pleura, pericardium, or diaphragm; T4b unresectable invading other adj. structures, such as aorta, vertebral body, trachea, etc.)
- N = # poss LNs in **regional** LN groups (N1 1–2 LN; N2 3–6 LN; N3 ≥7); nodes in nonregional areas (hepatoduodenal, portal, paraaortic etc.) = distant mets (M1)
- Separate staging (TNM + grade) for SCC & adenoCA, & postneoadj rx (AJCC 2017 8th ed.)

Early disease (stage I)

- **Esophagectomy;** consider endoscopic resection for Tis or T1a
- Most common surgical techniques: (1) Transhiatal esophagectomy (lower esophagus) & (2) Ivor Lewis resection, a transthoracic approach w/ thoracotomy + laparotomy

Locoregional disease (stage II–III)

- **Squamous:** Definitive chemoradiation (fluoropyrimidine- or taxane-based regimens), surgery reserved for bx proven residual dz only; chemoradiation alone vs. chemoradiation + surgery (for responders only) → no difference in median OS despite improved local control (*JCO* 2007;25:1160)
- **AdenoCA:** Preoperative chemo ±; radiotherapy → esophagectomy should be considered for all medically fit pts w/ resectable esophageal adenoCA (>5 cm from cricopharyngeus) b/c compared to squamous, adenoCA w/ lower rate of PCR after chemoradiation, 49% vs. 23% (CROSS, *NEJM* 2012;366:2074)
- **Neoadj Rx** improves outcomes (see below)
- T4b (unresectable) or cervical/cervicothoracic esophageal CA <**5 cm from cricopharyngeus:** Definitive chemoradiation

Neoadjuvant/Adjuvant therapy for locoregional disease

- **Periop ECF:** 13% ↑ 5-y OS rate, 36% vs. 23%, 26% pts had esophageal & GEJ CA, only 55% pts received postop Rx (MAGIC, *NEJM* 2006;355:11)
- **Periop FLOT:** ↑ median OS, 50 vs. 35 mos, FLOT vs. ECF/ECX; 56% pts had GEJ CA (FLOT4, *Lancet* 2019;393:1948)
- **Preop Carbo/Taxol w/ RT (41.4 Gy):** 13% ↑ 5-y OS rate, 47% vs. 34%, mOS 49.4 vs. 24 mos, ↑ R0 resection rates of 92% vs. 69% (CROSS, *NEJM* 2012;366:2074)
- **Preop FOLFOX w/ RT (50.4 Gy):** Preferred over carbo/taxol; pCR 38% in pts w/ adenoCA receiving induction FOLFOX & PET response (>35% decrease SUV) followed by concurrent FOLFOX/RT (CALGB 80803, *JCO* 2017;35:4_suppl,1-1)
- **Adj. nivolumab:** Residual dz after CRT & surgery, 11.4 mos ↑ mDFS w/ nivolumab vs. placebo, 22.4 vs. 11.0 mos (CheckMate 577, *NEJM* 2021;384:1191)

Advanced stage (IV) treatment

- Treated as adv stage gastric CA, (see **Gastric Cancer Chapter**)
- Biomarker testing: HER2, PD-L1, EBV, MMR/MSI, consider NGS
- Most pts are candidates for doublet chemo 5-FU/platinum; 3 drug (ie, FLOT or DCF) only in high-PS pts willing to tolerate s/e
- **Chemo + pembrolizumab:** ↑ Median OS vs. chemo alone, 12.4 vs. 9.8 mos (KEYNOTE-590, *Ann Oncol* 2020;31:S1192)
- **Chemo + nivolumab:** ↑ Median OS vs. chemo alone, 14.4 vs. 11.1 mos in pts w/ PD-L1 CPS ≥5 (CheckMate 649, *Ann Oncol* 2020;31:S1191)
- Second-line chemo: Fluoropyrimidines, platinums, taxanes, irinotecan

Immunotherapy and targeted therapy

- **Nivolumab:** SCC ↑ mOS w/ 2nd-line nivolumab vs. chemo 10.9 vs. 8.4 mos (ATTRACTION-3, *Lancet Oncol* 2019;20:1506)
- **Pembrolizumab:** ORR 15.5% w/ 3rd-line pembrolizumab in PD-L1-positive (CPS ≥1) gastric/GEJ CA (KEYNOTE-059, *JAMA Oncol* 2018;4:e180013) but no ↑ mOS in 2nd-line vs. paclitaxel (KEYNOTE-061, *Lancet* 2018;392:123); ↑ mOS w/ 2nd-line pembrolizumab vs. chemo, 10.3 vs. 6.7 mos, in PD-L1-positive (CPS ≥10) SCC (KEYNOTE-181, *JCO* 2020;38:4138)
- **See Gastric Cancer** for other targeted therapies incl. trastuzumab, trastuzumab deruxtecan, & ramucirumab for GEJ

GASTRIC CANCER

Epidemiology

- 5th most common CA in world, 3rd leading cause of CA death: Geographic variation, high incidence East Asia, South/Central America, Eastern Europe (*CA Cancer J Clin* 2018;68:394)
- United States: ~26,560 new cases for 2021, median age 68 y, 2x ↑ incidence in men, ↑ all groups except non-Hispanic whites (*SEER*Explorer*); ↑ early-onset gastric CA (*Surgery* 2019;166:547)
- Western countries: ↓ Intestinal-type distal stomach, ↑ diffuse-type proximal stomach

Risk factors

- *H. pylori* (*cagA*-positive), tobacco, EtOH (noncardia), obesity/high BMI, GERD, EBV, radiation, pernicious anemia, occupation exposure to coal/rubber
- Nutritional factors: ↑ salt/nitrate diet (synergistic w/ *H. pylori*), ↑ smoked or cured foods, poor-quality drinking water, diet low in vitamin A/C
- Precursor lesions: Adenomatous gastric polyps, dysplasia, chronic atrophic gastritis, & intestinal metaplasia

Genetics

- **Familial cases** account for up to 5–10% of all gastric CA
- **Lynch:** Germline muts of MMR genes (*MSH2, MLH1, MLH6, PMS2, EPCAM*)
- **Diffuse hereditary gastric CA:** Germline E-cadherin (*CDH1*) mut, AD, 60–80% penetrance, consider ppx gastrectomy (*NEJM* 2001;344:1904)
- **Others: FAP, Li–Fraumeni, juvenile polyposis, Peutz–Jeghers**

Pathology/biomarkers

- **Lauren's histologic classification**
  - **Intestinal:** Tumor cells arranged in tubular or glandular formations, spreads through gastric wall as part of a tumor mass
  - **Diffuse:** Defective intercellular adhesion molecules allow tumor cells to invade w/o formation of tubules or glands; spreads as discohesive cells throughout stomach wall; highly metastatic; signet-ring histology is a poor prognostic factor
- **WHO classification:** Tubular, papillary, mucinous, poorly cohesive incl. signet ring, adenosquamous, small cell, undifferentiated, squamous cell
- **The CA genome atlas** 4 subtypes: **EBV-positive** (w/ recurrent *PIK3CA* muts, higher prevalence of DNA hypermethylation), **microsatellite instability** (MSI), chromosomal instability (CIN) (↑ receptor tyrosine kinases incl. *VEGFR2*), **genomically stable** (GS)
- **Biomarkers w/ clinical implications**
  - **HER2 overexpression:** Determined by HER2 IHC (3+), IHC equivocal (2+), & FISH amp, or *HER2* gene amplification; 10–20% of gastric adenoCAs
  - **MMR:** Determined by IHC for MLH1, MSH2, MSH6, PMS2 proteins
  - **PD-L1:** Positive if combined positive score (CPS) ≥1; unclear utility as responses seen w/ checkpoint inhibition in PD-L1 (-) tumors & significant interobserver variability
  - **EBV:** Gold standard is EBV-encoded RNA in situ hybridization (EBER-ISH)
  - **NGS:** Tumor sequencing for other targets (eg, *NTRK*)

Clinical manifestations

- Sx: Wt loss, abd pain, early satiety, GI bleed, ascites; avg 6–9 mos from sx to dx
- Mets most common to liver, peritoneal surfaces, & nonregional LN

Screening and prevention

- Screening programs implemented only in Japan due to higher incidence

Workup and staging

- Upper endoscopy + bx (perform on any gastric ulcer); EUS can be used for T stage, suboptimal for LN staging; EUS-guided FNA is better
- **CT CAP** may detect occult M1 dz (bone, liver) in ~10% pts; consider esp if locally adv dz; consider **PET** if no evidence of M1 dz**; laparoscopy w/ peritoneal washings** detects M1 dz in ~20% pts

Locoregional disease (Stage I–III)

- Gastrectomy is potentially curative, >50% relapse; perioperative chemo if ≥T2 or N+
- **Resection:** Goal **R0** (Complete resection, clear margins [≥4 cm]); ~50% achieve R0 **R1:** Microscopic residual dz (+margins); **R2:** Gross (macroscopic) residual dz
- **LN dissection: D2** (standard of care)—includes D1 & removal of celiac, gastrohepatic, & splenic LN (15–30 LN for adequate staging); lower locoregional recurrence (12% vs. 22%) & CA-related mortality (37% vs. 48%) compared to D1 (*Lancet Oncol* 2010;11:439)
  D1: Gastrectomy w/ removal of greater & lesser omenta & associated LN
  D0: Incomplete resection of greater & lesser curvature LN
- **dMMR/MSI-H:** Always evaluate for mismatch repair deficiency prior to initiating periop Rx

AJCC TNM Pathologic Staging	
Stage	**TNM Criteria**
IA, IB	T1N0, T2N0
IIA	T1 N1–3, T2 N1–3, T3 N0
IIB	T1 N3a T3 N1 T2 N2 T4a N0
IIIA	T2 N3a T4a N1–2 T3 N2 T4b N0
IIIB	T1–2 N3b T4b N1–2 T3–4a N3a
IIIC	T3–4b N3b, T4b N3a
IV	Any T, Any N, M1

AJCC TNM Categories	
T = depth of tumor invasion	
T1	Lamina propria, muscularis mucosae, or submucosa
T2	Muscularis propria
T3	Subserosal connective tissue w/o invasion visceral peritoneum, adj. structure
T4	Serosa/visceral peritoneum (a) or adj. structures (b)
N = number positive *regional* LN	
N1–2	1–2 LN (N1) or 3–6 LN (N2)
N3	7–15 LN (a) or ≥16 LN (b)
M = metastases	
M1	Distant mets incl. nonregional LN

Perioperative therapy for locoregional disease

Perioperative Therapy for Resectable Gastric Cancer		
Study Name	**Regimen**	**Outcomes**
dMMR/MSI-H		
JCO 2021;39;suppl	**No periop chemo**	3-y OS 80% chemo vs. 86% no chemo
Perioperative Chemotherapy*†		
FLOT4 (*Lancet* 2019;393)	**Periop FLOT**	R0 resection rate 85% vs. 78% w/ periop ECF/ECX, pCR rate 15% vs. 6%, median OS 50 mos vs. 35 mos
Postoperative Chemotherapy		
NEJM 2007;357:1810	**Oral S-1**	3-y OS 80.1% vs. 70.1% surgery only; can use cape in US
CLASSIC (*Lancet* 2014;15:1389)	**CAPEOX**	3-y DFS 73% vs. 61% surgery only, 5-y OS rate 78% vs. 69%
Postoperative Chemoradiotherapy—*RT is only considered if <D2 or non-R0*		
INT-0116 (*NEJM* 2001;345:725)	**5-FU/LV + RT (45 Gy)**	Compared to surgery only, median OS 36 vs. 27 mos, but <50% D1 dissection & only local recurrence reduced
ARTIST (*JCO* 2012;30:268)	**Cape/Cis + RT (45 Gy)**	Compared to cape/cis, all D2 LN, no Δ in DFS/OS, subgroup w/ pathologic LN mets & intestinal type gastric CA may have ↑ DFS
ARTIST 2 (*Ann Oncol* 2021;32:3)	**Surgery + D2 → SOX → SOXRT**	Compared to SOX, no benefit w/ RT; SOX, & SOXRT prolonged DFS vs. S-1 alone; benefit for adj. oxaliplatin w/ S-1
CRITICS (*Lancet Oncol* 2018;19:616)	**mECF → surgery + D1 + LN → chemoRT**	No difference in median EFS or 5-y OS w/ chemo alone vs. chemoRT; no role for adj. chemoRT if preop chemo

*Ongoing study to evaluate role of RT: TOPGEAR (periop ECF ± preop chemoRT)
†Periop ECF is no longer used (MAGIC trial, *NEJM* 2006;355:11).

Systemic Therapy for Stage IV Gastric Cancer		
Subtype	**Regimen**	**Outcomes**
First-Line Therapy: Platinum (cis or oxaliplatin) + fluoropyrimidine backbone		
HER2 overexpression	**Fluoropyrimidine + oxaliplatin + trastuzumab ± pembrolizumab** (KEYNOTE-811, *JCO* 2020;38:TPS463)	ORR 74% in pembro arm vs. 52% in placebo arm, accelerated FDA approval
	Fluoropyrimidine + platinum + trastuzumab (TOGA, *Lancet* 2010;376:687)	Compared w/ chemo alone, ↑ median OS 13.8 vs. 11.1 mos, ↑ PFS & response, FDA approved
HER2 (–) & any PD-L1	**Fluoropyrimidine + platinum + nivolumab** (CheckMate-649, *Lancet* 2021)	Median OS 14.4 mos in pembro arm vs. 11.1 mos in placebo arm (HR 0.71)
	Fluoropyrimidine + platinum ± docetaxel (*JCO* 2006;24:4991)	Docetaxel: Improves RR & minimal OS benefit (OS 9.2 vs. 8.6 mos) but ↑ tox; only in fit pt
Second-Line or Subsequent Therapy: Irinotecan or paclitaxel ± ramucirumab or targeted therapy		
HER2 overexpression	**Fam-trastuzumab deruxtecan** (*NEJM* 2020;382:2419)	ORR 51% in trastuzumab deruxtecan arm vs. 14% in chemo arm; median OS 12.5 vs. 8.4 mos
HER2 (–)	**Paclitaxel + ramucirumab (VEGFR2 mAb)** (REGARD, *Lancet* 2014;383:31) (RAINBOW, *Lancet Oncol* 2014;15:1224)	Ram vs. BSC: ↑ Median OS 5.2 vs. 3.8 mos, ↑ PFS 2.1 vs. 1.3 mos (REGARD) Paclitaxel + Ram vs. paclitaxel alone: ↑ Median OS 9.6 vs. 7.4 mos, ↑ PFS 4.4 vs. 2.9 mos (RAINBOW)
	FOLFIRI ± ramucirumab	No median OS difference between irinotecan & paclitaxel (WJOG 4007, *JCO* 2013;31:4438)
***NTRK* fusion (+)**	**Entrectinib or Larotrectinib**	(*Lancet Oncol* 2019;21:271, *NEJM* 2018;378:731)
MSI-H or dMMR	**Pembrolizumab** (KEYNOTE-158, *JCO* 2020;38:1)	Objective response rate 34.3% in pretreated noncolorectal CA

Advanced stage (IV) treatment

Other targets

- No role of EGFR mAbs cetuximab or panitumumab (EXPAND *Lancet Oncol* 2013;14:490; REAL3 *Lancet Oncol* 2013;14:481)
- Ongoing targeted studies: Claudin 18.2 inhibitors; matrix metalloproteinase-9 inhibitors

APPENDIX AND SMALL BOWEL CARCINOMA

Appendiceal Carcinoma

Epidemiology and classification

- Found in 1% of appendectomy specimens, <1% of all intestinal neoplasms
- **Main histologic types:** Classification controversial; mucinous neoplasm, colorectal-type adenoCA, goblet-cell adenoCA, NEN
- **Mucinous neoplasms** most frequent & range from low-grade to high-grade mucinous, can develop into mucoceles, & recur → **pseudomyxoma peritonei**

Clinical presentation and prognosis

- **S/S:** Acute appendicitis, abd pain, ascites, abd mass
- **Prognosis:** Varies w/ histology & differentiation. Mucinous neoplasms & well-differentiated tumors = slow growing, 5-y survival >80%. Poorly diff & signet-ring features have poor survival (*Cancer* 2016;122(2):213). Mets often contained w/in peritoneal cavity

Management

- **Surgery:** R hemicolectomy for local dz. In select pts w/ met dz to peritoneum, cytoreductive surgery +/– intraperitoneal chemo can prolong OS
- **Systemic:** No direct data. Metastatic well-differentiated adenoCA have lower chemo response rates (*J Surg Oncol* 2019;120(3):446) & may be observable given slow growth. Chemo in unresectable metastatic dz based on extrapolation of metastatic colon CA (FOLFOX, FOLFIRI, FOLFOXIRI). Likely no benefit from anti-EGFR Rx in RAS wt tumors

Small Bowel Carcinoma

Epidemiology

- Rare; approximately 10,000 new cases & 1,500 deaths annually in the United States; accounts for approximately 2% of all GI tract CAs
- ↑ Incidence in last decade; ↑ in African–Americans, slight male predominance (male: female 1.5:1); mean age at dx = 66 y
- Types: AdenoCA (30–40%) & neuroendocrine (29%)

RFs & pathophysiology

- Majority in duodenum; most arise from adenomas; likely accumulation of somatic muts
- Small bowel: **Hereditary CA syn** (<10% cases): Lynch, FAP, Peutz–Jeghers syn; screening rec for all new dx
- Pts w/ colon adenoCA a/w ↑ risk of small bowel adenoCA
- Small bowel CA = ↑ of 2° CA of colon, rectum, ampulla of Vater, endometrium, & ovary
- Other RFs: **Chronic inflammation** (eg, Crohn) ↑ risk small-bowel adenoCA & lymphoma; diet (red meat, smoked foods, EtOH intake), tobacco, obesity

Clinical manifestations

- **S/S:** Nonspecific; abd pain, N/V, wt loss, anemia, GIB, obstruction (duodenal adenoCA can p/w **gastric outlet obstruction**). Vague s/s = adv stage by dx

Staging and prognosis

- # of LN evaluated prognostic w/ improved **5-y dz-specific survival** in pts w/ >8 LN evaluated: Stage I 95%, Stage II 83%, Stage III 56%
- 5-y survival w/ small-bowel adenoCA are usu worse than similarly staged colon CAs
- Poor prognostic indicators: Duodenal primary, + resection margins, LVI, T4 stage, extent of nodal dz, poorly differentiated

Management

Locoregional dz

- If resectable (65–75% at dx), manage w/ **wide segmental surgical resection** of 1° tumor & en bloc mesentery/LN. **Right colectomy** for tumors in distal ileum. Consider **pancreaticoduodenectomy** for tumors in 1st/2nd portion of duodenum
- **Adj. systemic Rx:** No direct data, typically treat along colon paradigm w/ 3–6 mos of CAPEOX or FOLFOX based on extrapolation from colon CA (MOSAIC, IDEA trials)

Unresectable or met dz

- Chemo based on extrapolation of metastatic colon CA (FOLFOX, FOLFIRI, FOLFOXIRI); palliative resection of 1° tumor/RT for local sx control
- Taxanes w/ modest efficacy in later line (*Ann Oncol* 2018;29:139; *Oncologist* 2019;24:e384); EGFR targeted Rx ineffective (*Oncologist* 2018;23:277); mgmt of dMMR/MSI tumors extrapolated from colon CA

COLON CANCER

Epidemiology

- ~149,500 estimated annual new cases of CRC in the United States in 2021: 104,270 colon, 45,230 rectal, accounting for 52,980 annual deaths (American Cancer Society)
- Highest incidence in Australia & New Zealand, Europe & North America
- Overall incidence has decreased but incidence has increased in adults 50 y or under

Risk factors

- **Age,** increasing incidence w/ age w/ relative rise starting at age 40–50
- **Familial syn** (FAP, Lynch, *MUTYH*-assoc polyposis, Peutz–Jeghers, Juvenile polyposis) (see **Lynch/FAP chapter**)
- **Personal or FHx** of CRC or adenomatous polyps
- **IBD:** UC > CD, increasing risk 8–10 y after initial dx
- **Other associations:** Consumptions of red or processed meats, EtOH, tobacco, obesity, diabetes: Adherence to healthy lifestyle (healthy weight, physical activity, nonsmoking, limited EtOH use, & healthy diet) can reduce the risk of CRC

Prevention

- **ASA & NSAIDs:** Potential protective effect of ASA & NSAIDs on development of colonic adenomas & CRC (*JAMA* 2005;294:914; *Lancet* 2010;376:1741)
- **Diet:** Potential protective benefit of avoidance of red meat, limited caloric intake
- **Vitamin D:** Although low vitamin D levels may be a/w higher incidence & increased mortality of CRC, supplementation has not yet shown any benefits

Pathophysiology

- **Adenoma-CA sequence:** Most common pathway, adenomas on avg take 10 y to develop (*Cell* 1990;61:759). Accumulation of genetic muts (*APC* → *TP53*, *KRAS*, *SMAD4*, etc.) leads to tumorigenesis; usu a/w chromosomal instability (CIN); risk of CRC ↑ w/ adenoma size, number, & histology (villous > tubular)
- **Serrated polyp pathway:** Alternative route for CRC development through serrated adenomas; *BRAF* mut & CpG Island Methylation Phenotype (CIMP); hypermethylation of promoters of MMR genes such as *MLH1* & tumor suppressors → gene silencing
- **Lynch:** Hereditary, 2° to muts in MMR genes *MLH1, MSH2, MSH6, PMS2, EPCAM*), MSI high, (–) CIN, (–) *BRAF* mutant

Molecular classification

- Consensus molecular subtypes of colon CA: **CMS1** (MSI Immune, hypermutated, immune infiltrated, *BRAF* V600E mut), **CMS2** (canonical/epithelial, MSS, CIN, Wnt/Myc activation, EGFR dependent), **CMS3** (metabolic, CIN–MSI mixed, metabolic dysregulation, *KRAS* mut), **CMS4** (mesenchymal, MSS, CIN, activated TGFb, & angiogenesis pathway, immune tolerant, worst prognosis)

Clinical presentation

- Sx are generally nonspecific & many pts are asx until adv dz
- **Distal colon:** Hematochezia, abd pain, obstruction, overflow diarrhea
- **Proximal colon:** Iron deficiency anemia, melena, hematochezia, obstruction (rare)
- **Met dz:** RUQ pain, ascites, wt loss, fatigue
- **Other sx:** Sx from local invasion (bladder, small bowel); may mimic diverticulitis; FUO; *S. bovis* bacteremia & *C. septicum* sepsis

Screening in average risk populations

- **Preferred by most guidelines:** Colonoscopy every 10 y starting at 45; 45–49 y—qualified recommendation given prevalence of large polyps in adults by age 50–54 y & rising incidence/mortality of CRC in younger pts; 50 y or older—strong recommendation, highest Se & Sp, ↓ mortality in RCT (*NEJM* 2012;366:687); 76–85 y—individualized by health status, life expectancy, & pt preference; 86 y or older—usu discouraged
- **Other options (less preferrable):** CT colonography q 5 y; flexible sigmoidoscopy q 5 y; FOBT annually; fecal immunochemical test (FIT) annually; stool DNA q 3 y
- See **Cancer Genetics** chapter for screening recommendations in increased risk pops (incl. Lynch/FAP)

Diagnostic evaluation

- Colonoscopy
- CT chest/abdomen/pelvis
- Hepatic fxn panel, CEA
- ***KRAS/NRAS/BRAF*** **mutant status &** ***HER2*** **amplification** only in pts w/ met dz
- **MSI testing** or **IHC for MMR proteins** for all pts

Staging and prognosis

- Right-sided tumors generally have a worse prognosis

Staging, Prognosis, & Treatment of Colorectal Cancer				
Stage	**T**	**N**	**M**	**Rx**
I	T1–2	N0		Surgery alone
IIA	T3	N0		Surgery ± adj. chemo[a]
IIB	T4a	N0		
IIC	T4b	N0		
IIIA	T1–2, N1/1c; T1, N2a			Surgery + adj. chemo
IIIB	T3–4a, N1/1c; T2–T3, N2a; T1–2, N2b			3–6 mos CAPEOX or FOLFOX[b] (MOSAIC, *NEJM* 2004;350:2343; IDEA, *Lancet Oncol* 2020;21:1620)
IIIC	T4a, N2a; T3–4a, N2b; T4b, N1/2			
IVA			M1a	Chemo ± surgery[c]
IVB			M1b	Chemo ± surgery[c]
IVC			M1c	Chemo

[a]High-risk features for recurrence (poorly differentiated, T4, LVI, PNI, inadequate LN sampling [<12], obstruction/perforation, etc.) may prompt consideration of chemo but data on the absolute benefit in stage II disease is mixed and the decision to observe or treat should be based on shared decision making between the clinician and pt. Adjuvant chemo is not recommended in MSI-H stage II.
[b]In low-risk stage III (T1-3, N1), 3 mos CAPEOX is noninferior to 6 mos in 5-y DFS and OS; in high-risk stage III (T4 or N2), noninferiority is not established but the difference in OS is less than 1%. For all stage III, 3 mos CAPEOX should be strongly considered as standard care given risk of neurotoxicity. For FOLFOX, noninferiority is not established for 3 mos vs. 6 mos. In low-risk stage III, the difference is small, and 3 mos FOLFOX should be discussed with pts. In high-risk stage III, 3 mos FOLFOX was inferior to 6 mos.
[c]Pts w/ limited hepatic or pulm mets may benefit from metastasectomy either preceded or followed by chemotherapy.

Surveillance after initial therapy

- Hx & physical & CEA every 6 mos for 5 y
- **CT chest/abd/pelvis** annually for 5 y—no role for PET scans
- **Colonoscopy** 1 y after surgery; if no adv adenoma repeat in 3 y, then every 5 y

Chemotherapy for advanced and metastatic disease

- **Definitions: FOLFOX:** Infusional 5-FU/LV + OX; **FOLFIRI:** Infusional 5-FU/LV + irinotecan; **FOLFOXIRI:** Infusional 5-FU/LV + OX + irinotecan; **CAPEOX:** Cape + OX
- **1st line:** FOLFOX (*JCO* 2004;22:23) ± Bevacizumab (*JCO* 2008;26:2013); CAPEOX; FOLFIRI (*JCO* 2004;22:229) ± Bev (*JCO* 2007;25:4779); FOLFOXIRI ± Bev (TRIBE, *NEJM* 2014;371:1609)
  - If pts not appropriate for intense Rx: Infusional 5-FU/LV; Cape
  - For pts w/ **L-sided CRC & wt *RAS/BRAF***: FOLFOX or FOLFIRI ± cetuximab/panitumumab (CRYSTAL, *NEJM* 2009;360:1408; PRIME, *JCO* 2010;28:4697)
- **2nd line:** FOLFIRI or irinotecan for pts who received prior FOLFOX; FOLFOX/CAPEOX for pts w/ prior FOLFIRI; FOLFOX/CAPEOX, or FOLFIRI for prior 5-FU/LV or Cape; all regimens ± Bev/ziv-aflibercept/ramucirumab (note that Bev is preferred over ziv-aflibercept/ramucirumab because of tox &/or cost); irinotecan-based regimens ±; cetuximab/panitumumab if not previously used
- **3rd line:** Irinotecan ± panitumumab/cetuximab (BOND, *NEJM* 2004;351:337) or single-agent panitumumab/cetuximab, or single-agent regorafenib or TAS-102; overall benefits of regorafenib or TAS-102 are modest w/ significant s/e
- **1st line for MSI-H/dMMR:** Pembrolizumab (KEYNOTE-177, *NEJM* 2020;383:2207) or nivolumab ± ipilimumab (CHECKMATE 142, *Lancet Oncol* 2017;18:1182)
- **Later line for *BRAF* V600E mut:** encorafenib + cetuximab/panitumumab (BEACON, *NEJM* 2019;381:1632); addition of binimetinib did not improve OS or ORR
- **Later line for *HER2* amplified & *RAS/BRAF* wildtype:** Trastuzumab + pertuzumab; trastuzumab + lapatinib; trastuzumab deruxtecan
- For FOLFOX, OX should be discontinued after first 3 mos of Rx till progression to reduce risk of severe neurotoxicity. Can be resumed at or after progression (OPTIMOX1, *JCO* 2006;24:394)
- Do not use concurrent anti-EGFR + anti-VEGF Rx (*CAIRO2, NEJM* 2009;360:563)
- **Do not use anti-EGFR Rx** in **RAS/BRAF mut or any R sided CRC** (*JCO* 2016;34(suppl, abstr 3504, 3505, 3506; *JAMA Oncol* 2017;3:211)
- For pts progressing on anti-EGFR, use of anti-EGFR is not rec in subsequent lines

RECTAL CANCER

Epidemiology
- See colon cancer

Risk factors
- See colon cancer

Genetics
- See colon cancer

Pathology
- See colon cancer

Screening
- See colon cancer

Clinical presentation
- See colon cancer. Sxs may include tenesmus, rectal pain, hematochezia, diminished caliber of stools

Figure 16-2 Anatomy of rectum.

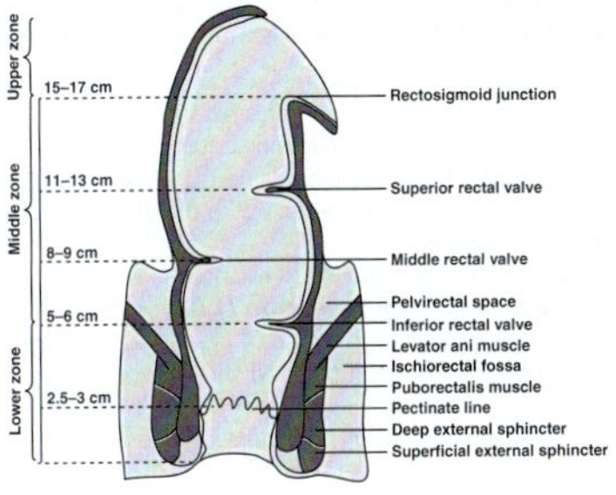

General diagnostic evaluation
- Colonoscopy, bx, & pathology review
- CT chest/abdomen (IV contrast), & pelvis MRI. PET scan is not indicated
- CBC, chemistry profile w/ LFTs, CEA
- Universal IHC for MMR proteins or MSI testing
- ***KRAS, NRAS, BRAF, & HER2* status** for pts w/ met dz. Consider NGS panel.

Diagnostic evaluation for localized staging
- **Pelvis MRI:** High degree of accuracy in predicting involvement of circumferential resection margin (CRM) (MERCURY, *BMJ* 2006;333:779), as well as T & N stage
- **TRUS:** Operator dependent. Inadequate for high or bulky tumors, evaluation of tumor deposits, vascular invasion or iliac adenopathies. May be considered if MRI is contraindicated
- **CT:** Helpful for evaluation of distant mets, limited for local tumor & nodal staging
- **PET:** Offers no add'l information & is not routinely indicated.

Clinical staging & treatment

Treatment of Rectal Cancer Based on Clinical Staging

Stage	T	N	M	Rx
I	cT1[a]	cN0		Surgery alone (transanal local excision)
I	cT2	cN0		TME[b]
IIA	cT3	cN0		Neoadj RT[c] followed by FOLFOX × 4 mos or CAPEOX × 3 mos (or chemo followed by RT [c]) followed by resection (or observation in pts w/ complete clinical response), OR Clear CRM: Neoadj RT[c] followed by resection & adj. FOLFOX or CAPEOX Involved CRM: Neoadj RT[c] followed by FOLFOX or CAPEOX & resection
IIB	cT4	cN0		
IIIA	cT1–2	cN1		
IIIB	cT3–4	cN1		
IIIC	cT1–4	cN2		
IV			M1	Systemic Rx ± local therapies[d]

[a]T1–2, N0 should be based on assessment by MRI (preferred) or TRUS. If pathologic staging indicates ≥T2 disease, positive LN, or high-risk features, chemoRT, or transabdominal resection ± adjuvant chemotherapy (FOLFOX or CAPEOX) is indicated. High-risk features: (+) margins, LVI, PNI, poor differentiation, or deep submucosal invasion

[b]Neoadjuvant chemoRT may be considered in patients with a distal cT2, cN0 tumor in attempt to convert an abdominoperineal resection (APR) into a low-anterior resection (LAR). Initial chemoRT can also be considered in poor surgical candidates or patients who refuse surgery. Patients who achieve a complete response after initial chemoRT may be observed

[c]RT can be long or short course. Long-course RT is given with concurrent capecitabine or 5-FU. Short course (500 cGy/d × 5 d) is given without concurrent chemo

[d]Pts w/ limited hepatic or pulm mets may benefit from metastasectomy (before or after chemotherapy)

Principles of surgical resection

- **TME:** Indicated for all pts (LAR or APR). Involves precise en bloc removal of the perirectal areolar tissue to include all margins of the mesorectal envelope, lymphatics, & tumor deposits. Improved local control & survival compared to blunt dissection (*Lancet* 1993;341:457)
- **Regional LND:** Dissection of mesorectum & regional LN (>12 LN)

Surgical procedures and criteria

- **Local excision:** Includes transanal local excision & transanal endoscopic microsurgery (TEM). Must meet the following criteria:
  - Selected T1, N0 tumors w/ no high-risk features (poorly differentiated, LVI, PNI)
  - Tumors <3 cm in diameter, <30% of rectal circumference, & w/in 8 cm of anal verge
  - Clear margins
  - Reliable postoperative surveillance
- **Sphincter-sparing resection (LAR w/ primary anastomosis):** Removes sigmoid & rectum to the level of clear distant margin. A temporary stoma may be considered for low tumors or if the pt received preop RT. Must meet the following criteria:
  - Stage cT2-4 (invasion beyond submucosa)
  - Neg distal margin can be achieved
    - Adequate presurgical sphincter fxn
- **APR:** Involves resection of the sigmoid colon, rectum, & anus w/ permanent colostomy. Indicated for pts w/ ≥1 of the following criteria:
  - Neg distal margin (1 cm) cannot be achieved w/ sphincter-sparing procedures
  - Low tumor involving the anal sphincter
  - Salvage procedure for locally recurrent low-rectal tumor
- **Nonoperative mgmt (total neoadj therapy or TNT)**
  Upfront chemo (CAPEOX or FOLFOX) & RT. Unclear whether it is better to start w/ chemo or RT. Upfront chemo provides faster relief if symptomatic. In pts who achieve a complete clinical response (by MRI, endoscopy, & DRE), close observation may be considered w/o surgery

Principles of radiation and chemoradiation

- Adj. RT reduces local recurrence, but has no OS benefit
- Adj. chemoRT is superior to adj. RT alone w/ OS benefit (*NEJM* 1994;331:502)
- Neoadj chemoRT is superior to adj. chemoRT w/ decreased local relapse rate & improved tolerance, but no OS benefit (*NEJM* 2004;351:1731)
- Neoadj chemoRT w/ infusional 5-FU is superior to RT alone w/ improved response rate & local control (*NEJM* 2006;355:1114)
- **No benefit w/ addition of oxaliplatin or irinotecan** to 5-FU during radiation
- ChemoRT w/ Cape is equivalent to chemoRT w/ 5-FU (*Lancet Oncol* 2012;13:579)
- **Current guidelines:** 45–50 Gy in 25–28 fractions to the pelvis. Short-course RT w/out concurrent chemo (25 Gy in 5 fractions) can also be considered

Principles of adjuvant chemotherapy in early-stage disease

- No direct evidence in favor of adj. chemo after preoperative chemoradiation, but FOLFOX/CAPEOX rec as extrapolation from colon CA data (MOSAIC, *NEJM* 2004;350:2343)
- Total duration of perioperative Rx, incl. chemo & chemoRT, should not exceed 6 mos

Surveillance after initial therapy

- Hx & physical & CEA every 6 mos for 5 y
- CT chest/abd/pelvis annually for 5 y
- Colonoscopy 1 y postsurgery; if no adv adenoma repeat in 3 y, then every 5 y

Chemotherapy in advanced and metastatic disease

- See **Colon Cancer** chapter

ANAL CANCER

Epidemiology

- Estimated 9,090 new cases & 1,430 deaths in 2021 (American Cancer Society)
- Increasing incidence (1.9-fold for men, 1.5 for women) from 1970s to 2000s
- **A/w HPV,** receptive anal intercourse, MSM, STD, cervical/vulvovaginal CA, immunosuppression (transplant or HIV), hematologic malignancy, AI d/os, smoking
- HPV (dsDNA nonenveloped virus) is the #1 causative agent; HPV DNA detected in 84% of specimens (commonly HPV-16, HPV-18)
- HPV prevalence is ↑ in MSM pop (detectable in 1/3 of HIV+ men & 1/8 of HIV– men)
- HAART ↑ HIV-assoc survival but does not impact progression of anal CA. This contributes to recent ↑ in anal CA incidence from 19 → 78/100k among HIV+ pts
- HPV vaccination likely to be effective (*NEJM* 2011;365:1576)
- High-grade squamous intraepithelial neoplasia (HSIL) can be a precursor lesion
- Evidence for screening & tx of HSIL (vs. observation) is limited

Clinical manifestations

- **Symptoms:** 45% rectal bleeding, 30% symptoms of mass incl. pain & tenesmus
- 50% of CAs are localized at presentation (80% 5-y OS); 29% have regional LN involvement (60% 5-y OS); 12% present w/ distant mets (31% 5-y OS)
- Stepwise model of premalignant LSIL → high-grade SIL → CA is less validated compared to cervical neoplasia & progression rates are slower (*Lancet Oncol* 2012;13:487)
- Anatomic zones separated by anorectal ring & anal verge: **Anal canal** → between anorectal ring & anal verge; **anal margin**→ includes anal verge & 6 cm radius of surrounding skin

Figure 16-3 *Devita, Hellman, and Rosenberg's Cancer: Principles and Practice of Oncology.* 9th edition. 2011.

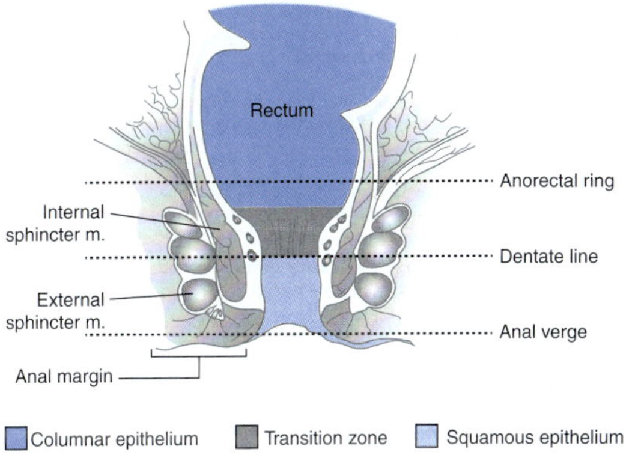

- **LN drainage:** Proximal to dentate line → anorectal, perirectal, & paravertebral LN, possibly internal iliac & inferior mesenteric if more proximal; distal to dentate line → superficial inguinal nodes
- **Met sites:** Liver, lung, extrapelvic LNs

Pathology and molecular biology

- **HPV E2** peptide: Attaches HPV DNA to chromatin, allowing steady viral production
- **HPV E6** peptide: Mediates degradation of **p53**, impeding cellular arrest, & apoptosis; also mediates degradation of **NFX1-91** telomerase repressor
- **HPV E7** peptide: Inactivates **pRB**, promoting cell-cycle progression
- Most anal CAs are of **SCC** histotype. Histologic variants (keratinizing, nonkeratinizing, basaloid) do not alter tx. Anal adenoCA & anal melanoma are treated according to rectal CA & melanoma guidelines, respectively

Workup and staging

- DRE, anoscopy, inguinal exam, CT, or MRI pelvis + CT chest/abdomen, HIV test, GYN exam, consider fertility-risk discussion. Consider PET/CT
- **Stage 0:** Tis (HSIL); **Stage I:** Tumor ≤2 cm (T1); **Stage IIA:** Tumor 2–5 cm (T2), N0; **Stage IIB:** >5 cm (T3), N0; **Stage IIIA:** T1–T2 (≤5 cm) & involved regional LN (N1); **Stage IIIB:** Any size but invading adjacent organs (T4), neg LN; **Stage IIIC:** T3–T4 & positive LN (N1); **Stage IV:** Distant mets (M1)
- Consider bx by FNA for clinically suspicious LN

Management: Nonmetastatic disease

- **1st line: Nigro Protocol** in 1970s established chemoRT as standard compared to APR; chemoRT is superior to RT (*JCO* 1997;15:2040)

Chemoradiotherapy Protocol Using RTOG 98-11 Schedule

Wk (d)	1 (1–4)	2–4 (5–28)	5 (29–32)	
Chemo	5-FU d1–4		5-FU d1–4	
	MMC d1		MMC d1	
RT	d1–5 fractions weekly, 45 Gy in total			Boost[a]: 10–14 Gy/5–7d

[a]N1, T3–T4, or T1–T2 w/ residual disease should receive boost (*JAMA* 2008;299:1914).
MMC, mitomycin-C.

- **Chemo: Capecitabine + MMC** or **infusional 5-FU + MMC.** Infusional 5-FU w/ bolus MMC as above (*JCO* 1996;14:2527). Capecitabine, Mon–Fri on days of RT, also widely used based on retrospective data (*Br J Cancer* 2014;111:1726) & other small studies. 5-FU + cis may be considered if MMC contraindicated
- **Radiation:** Dosing of ≤59 Gy is sufficient, w/ no additional benefit to high-dose RT or induction chemo (ACCORD-03, *JCO* 2009;27:4033); Rx breaks should be minimized, but may be necessary due to acute anoproctitis, perineal dermatitis, or cytopenia. Chronic adverse effects may include anal ulcers, stenosis, & necrosis
- **IMRT:** ↓ Tox & effective (*J Radiat Oncol* 2012;1:165); IMRT is acceptable only at experienced centers (must avoid "marginal-miss" ↓ in local control)
- 3-fold ↑ pelvic fracture risk in women s/p RT
- Women should be considered for vaginal dilator to reduce vaginal stenosis
- Post-Rx follow-up: DRE 8–12 weeks after Rx. If regression w/o CR, repeat DRE in 4 wks. Pts w/ persistent dz may be followed for up to 6 mos, provided there is no progression. If CR, repeat DRE, inguinal exam q3–6mos for 5 y, anoscopy every 6–12 mos for 3 y, annual CT C/A/P for 3 y
- HIV pts w/ adequate T4 counts & undetectable viral load should be treated w/ same protocols. Data suggests similar ORR & OS but ↑ skin tox & local relapse

Management: Perianal cancer

- **T1–T2 (select), N0, well or moderately differentiated, not involving the sphincter:** Surgical excision. If inadequate margins, re-excision preferred over RT ± chemo
- **Higher stage:** Treat w/ chemoRT (as above)

Management: Refractory/recurrent and metastatic disease

- **Confirm progression w/ bx** & restaging CT or MRI, consider PET
- If locally progressive, proceed to salvage APR (removal of anus, rectum, partial sigmoid, regional nodes) w/ colostomy (*Ann Surg Oncol* 2007;14:478)
- For unresectable or metastatic, 1st-line standard Rx includes carbo/paclitaxel (preferred), FOLFCIS, FOLFOX, 5-FU + cis, modified DCF. 2nd line includes nivolumab & pembrolizumab. Modification to dose & schedule may be necessary
- **No evidence exists to support metastasectomy in anal CA.** Regional Rx may be considered in select pts w/ limited dz
- Clinical trial preferred for subsequent Rx

CANCER OF UNKNOWN PRIMARY (CUP)

Overview

- **CUP: Histologically proven malignant tumors** w/o an identified 1° site
- About 2–5% of all malignant epithelial tumors
- Median survival of 7–10 mos; 2-y survival rates of 20–25% (*Semin Oncol* 2009;36:65; *Lancet* 2012;379:9824)
- 1° tumor site found in <30% of pts w/ CUP
- Multiple sites involved in >50% pts
- **Unfavorable features** include poor performance status, pathologic dx of adenoCA, mets involving multiple organs, presence of liver mets, elevated LDH

Initial diagnostic workup

- **Lab studies:** CBC, electrolytes, LFTs, U/A, occult blood-stool testing. In men, consider serum PSA. Common tumor markers (CEA, CA19-9, CA 15-3, CA 125) generally not useful for dx
- **Imaging:** CT chest & CT or MRI of the abdomen & pelvis used to determine extent of dz. In women, consider mammography & pelvic imaging. Consider EGD. PET/CT not rec for routine screening
- **Tissue bx:** Core-needle bx preferred over FNA. Detailed review of pathology findings & review of past biopsies or malignancies

Pathology

- **Classified into 5 major subtypes:** AdenoCA (60%), poorly differentiated carcinoma (30%), SCC (5%), neuroendocrine carcinoma (3%), other (2%)
- IHC useful in characterization of poorly differentiated or undifferentiated tumors but large marker panels not rec
- NGS can be considered to identify potential actionable genomic aberrations; TMB testing, MSI/MMR status, & *NTRK* fusion testing also rec
- Key screening markers for CUPs summarized below

Tumor-Specific IHC Markers

Marker	Malignancy
TTF-1	Lung, thyroid
Thyroglobulin	Thyroid
GCDFP-15	Breast
Uroplakin III	Urothelial
WT1	Epithelioid mesothelioma Ovarian serous carcinoma Desmoplastic small round cell
CDX2	Colorectal, duodenal
PSA, PAP	Prostate
ER/PR	Breast, ovary, endometrium
Hep Par-1	Hepatocellular
Melan-A	Adrenocortical, melanoma
Calretinin	Mesothelioma, sex-cord stromal, adrenocortical

Key Screening Antibodies for Undifferentiated Malignancy

Antibody	Malignancy
S-100	Melanoma, clear-cell carcinoma, glioma, malignant peripheral nerve sheath tumors
HMB45	Melanoma (highly specific)
LCA or CD45	Hematolymphoid malignancies (all) NHL (highly specific)
PLAP	Seminomas (also in some NSGCT, GI, genitourinary, & pulmonary carcinomas)

Patterns of Expression of CK7 & CK20 Keratins in Epithelial Malignancies	
CK7+ CK20+	Ovarian mucinous adenoCA (90%), transitional cell (65%), pancreatic adenoCA (65%), cholangiocarcinoma (65%), gastric adenoCA (40%)
CK7+ CK20–	Ovarian serous (100%), thyroid (all 3 types) (100%), breast (90%), NSCLC (90%), endometrial (85%), embryonal (80%), mesothelioma (65%), transitional cell (35%), pancreatic (30%)
CK7– CK20+	Colorectal (80%), Merkel cell (70%), gastric adenoCA (35%)
CK7– CK20–	Adrenal (100%), seminoma & yolk sac tumor (95%), prostate (85%), hepatocellular (80%), renal cell (80%), carcinoid GI & lung (80%), squamous carcinoma (70%)

Management

- Consider surgery &/or RT for localized dz & systemic therapies for met dz
- No specific chemo regimen considered standard of care
- Choice of chemo regimen based on histology & likely 1° site of dz
- Specific chemo regimens based on phase II/III trials include
  1. **AdenoCA or squamous cell CA of unknown 1°:** Platinum-based combinations w/ taxanes, gem, or 5-FU
  2. **Neuroendocrine carcinoma:** Well-differentiated, treated as carcinoid tumors; high-grade or small-cell carcinoma treated as small-cell lung CA w/ platinum & etoposide
  3. **dMMR/MSI-high or TMB-high (≥10 mut/Mb):** Consider pembrolizumab (*JCO* 2020;38:1; *Lancet Oncol* 2020;21:1353)
- No clear role for gene expression testing to evaluate for a potential primary site of dz (*Ann Oncol* 2019;30:V851; *JCO* 2019;37:7)
- Important role of psychosocial support & symptomatic mgmt, incl. palliative & hospice care

Treatment Recommendations for Specific Subsets of CUP

Histology	Clinical Feature	Tx Recommendation
AdenoCA	Women w/ isolated axillary LAN	Treat as stage II breast CA
	Men w/ elevated PSA or blastic bone mets	Treat as adv prostate CA
	Colon CA profile (CK20 + CDX2)	Treat as adv colon CA
	Peritoneal, serous papillary	Treat as primary peritoneal, Stage III ovarian CA
AdenoCA or poorly differentiated carcinoma	Single met lesion	Definitive local tx w/ surgical resection &/or radiotherapy
Poorly differentiated carcinoma	Young men w/ midline tumor or elevated hCG/AFP	Treat as extragonadal germ-cell tumor
	Other clinical presentations	Empiric platinum/taxol chemo
SCC	Cervical LAN	Treat as head & neck CA w/ involved LN
	Inguinal LAN	Inguinal LN dissection Consider postoperative radiation
Poorly differentiated NET	Varied clinical presentations	Treat w/ platinum/etoposide

BASAL AND SQUAMOUS CELL CARCINOMAS

Epidemiology

- Most common CA in the United States; collectively known as non-melanoma skin cancer (NMSC)
- BCC is at least twice as common as SCC
- Lifetime risk of BCC ≥20% overall (≥30% in white populations)
- BCC rarely metastasizes; however, can be locally aggressive & disfiguring; SCC w/ greater potential for metastases (3–7%)

Risk factors

- **Sunlight:** UVB 1° cause of carcinogenesis; fair-skinned individuals at greatest risk
- Ionizing radiation exposure, particularly at a young age
- Prolonged psoralen & ultraviolet A (PUVA) exposure
- Arsenic exposure
- Immunosuppression (organ transplant recipients (OTRs) have >100× risk of SCC)
- For SCC, other RFs include beta HPVs, chronic inflammation, voriconazole

Pathogenesis

- SCC arise from keratinocytes
- Most BCC arise from keratinocyte progenitor cells in the epidermis & hair bulb

Genetics

- BCC has highest mut burden of any human CA
- UV-signature mut (C → T, CC → TT) observed in NMSC
- Muts in BCC frequently involve the *PTCH1* gene or members of the sonic **hedgehog signaling pathway** → overexpression of transcription factor GLI1
- Most common muts in SCC tumor suppressor genes *TP53* & *CDKN2A*
- **Genetic syndromes** predisposing to BCC & SCC: Albinism, xeroderma pigmentosum, epidermolysis bullosa. BCC: Nevoid BCC, Rombo, Bazex–Dupré–Christol syndromes
- Nevoid BCC syn (aka basal cell nevus syn, Gorlin–Goltz syn)

Nevoid BCC syn	**AD;** mut in the *PTCH1* gene at 9q22.3 Multiple BCC, starting in childhood Palmoplantar pits, epidermoid cysts, lipomas Developmental anomalies: Odontogenic cysts of the maxilla & mandible, dental defects, bifid ribs, scoliosis, hypertelorism, frontal bossing **Assoc tumors:** Medulloblastoma, ovarian fibromas, cardiac fibromas, mesenteric lymphatic cysts

Clinical features

- **Most develop on head & neck (80%)** & are more likely to recur compared to lesions developing on the trunk or extremities
- SCC can arise on mucosal membranes, BCC do not
- SCC appear as hyperkeratotic papules or plaques often w/ crust or ulceration
- **SCC precursor lesions:** Actinic keratoses, cutaneous horn
- **Bowen dz:** SCC in situ on the skin
- **Basosquamous carcinomas:** Mixed histology of both BCC & SCC; classified under SCC & risk of met determined by the squamous component

Types of BCC	
Nodular BCC	Most common variant (50–80%) Pearly, telangiectatic dome-shaped nodule often w/ central ulceration, may also appear pigmented
Superficial BCC	Flat, tan/red patch or plaque, may also appear pigmented
Morpheaform BCC	Atrophic plaque, typically around nose or ears
Infiltrative BCC	Poorly defined plaque w/ white/yellow/pink color & ulceration
Ulcus terebrans	Extremely aggressive BCC, invades underlying structures, frequently fatal but rare

Diagnosis

- Complete skin examination including mucous membranes, dermoscopy
- LN evaluation (for SCC; FNA, or core bx if enlarged)
- Bx (should include deep reticular dermis)
- Imaging if extensive dz (bone, perineural, or lymphovascular invasion)

AJCC 8 Staging: BCC and SCC	
Stage 0	Carcinoma in situ
Stage I	Tumor size ≤2 cm
Stage II	Tumor size >2 cm but ≤4 cm
Stage III	Tumor size ≥4 cm or minor bone erosion or specified perineural invasion or deep invasion (>6 mm &/or beyond subcutaneous fat) OR tumor of any size & ipsilateral nodal involvement ≤3 cm
Stage IV	Ipsilateral nodal involvement ≥3 cm or <3 cm w/ ENE, bilateral or contralateral nodal involvement, multiple ipsilateral LN involvement, LN ≥6 cm, distant met
High-risk features: >2-mm thickness, Clark level IV, perineural invasion/neurologic sxs, 1° site on "mask areas" of face, genitalia, hands or feet, aggressive growth pattern (infiltrative, micronodular, morpheaform, basosquamous, sclerosing, or carcinosarcomatous in BCC), poorly differentiated (SCC), immunosuppression, site of prior RT, recurrent dz, poorly defined borders	

Treatment-localized disease: BCC, SCC

- **Surgical excision w/ histologic control of margins:** Excision w/ POMA, Mohs surgery for high risk (above features + ≥2-cm diameter [≥1-cm non "mask area" head & neck/pretibial]) or positive margins postexcision
- Consider electrodessication & curettage for select low-risk lesions, excluding terminal hair-bearing areas
- Cryotherapy for pre-SCC lesions & sBCC
  - Topical therapies for sBCC (5-FU, imiquimod, PDT) & pre-SCC (+ diclofenac, ingenol mebutate, tirbanibulin (*NEJM* 2021;384:512))
- LND if regional LN involvement
- Adj. RT for pts who have undergone LND; otherwise use of radiation Rx is controversial. Consider for positive margins, evidence of substantial perineural involvement. Consider 1° RT for nonsurgical candidates >60 y

Treatment-metastatic and locally advanced disease: BCC

- Mets exceptionally rare; however, systemic therapy is indicated
- **Vismodegib or sonidegib** (hedgehog pathway inhibitors, HHI) FDA-approved for residual or met dz, use limited by s/e (*NEJM* 2012;366:2171; *Lancet Onc* 2015;16:716)
- Platinum-based chemo regimens
- Cemiplimab approved in 2021 for locally adv/metastatic BCC after HHI or in pts for whom HHI therapy is not appropriate (Study 1620, *Lancet Onc* 2021;22(6):848)
- Consider clinical trials

Treatment-metastatic and locally advanced disease: SCC

- CIS-based regimens, checkpoint inhibitors: Cemiplimab (*NEJM* 2018;279(4):341), pembrolizumab (*Lancet Onc* 2020;21:294; *JCO* 2020;38:2916)
- Consider clinical trials
- If OTR on immunosuppressive Rx, consider adjusting dose of immunosuppressive Rx or using mTOR inhibitor if appropriate

Prognosis and follow-up

- Localized dz has good prog, poor prog for metastatic SCC
- Worse prog for SCC of the genitalia, mucous membranes, ears
- Perineural involvement increases the risk of recurrence for BCC & SCC & increases met risk for SCC
- Close surveillance for high-risk pts (immunosuppression, organ transplantation)
  - In OTR w/ multiple SCC, consider reducing immunosuppression, starting mTOR inhibitor or chemoprevention w/ acitretin
- Encourage sun protection strategies & self-skin checks
- Pts w/ h/o NMSC are likely to develop further skin CAs including melanoma; perform at least annual skin exams & consider LN evaluation
- Limited evidence that nicotinamide may reduce risk of further SCC

MELANOMA

Epidemiology

- **Incidence:** ~100,000 new cases/y & ~7,000 deaths/y in the United States
- Only a small % of all skin CA (<5%) but has the highest morbidity & mortality
- ↑ Incidence, affects younger individuals
- **RFs:** Higher number of moles, atypical nevi, h/o prior melanoma, 1st-degree relative w/ melanoma, prior NMSC, freckles, sunburns easily, UVA/UVB exposure (esp before age 15), h/o indoor tanning, red-hair, immunosuppression
- **Hereditary RFs:** Rarely inherited, some syndromes include: Familial atypical multiple mole melanoma syn (*CDKN2A*, p16), Xeroderma pigmentosum (muts in NER), Li–Fraumeni syn (*TP53*), *RB1*, *BRCA2*, Cowden syn (*PTEN*), Werner syn (*WRN*), *BAP1*

Pathology

- **Histologic subtypes**
  - **Cutaneous** (most common)
    - *Superficial spreading:* Most common, radial growth
    - *Nodular:* Vertical growth into dermis, worse prog
    - *Lentigo maligna:* Sun-damaged skin in elderly or middle-aged pts, usu on face
    - *Acral lentiginous:* Most common in Asian or African Americans, usu on palm/soles
    - *Desmoplastic/Neurotropic:* Locally invasive, less likely to metastasize, CN involvement
  - **Uveal:** Arise from melanocytes in iris, ciliary body, or choroid
  - **Mucosal:** Arise from melanocytes in mucosal surfaces (ie, nasopharynx, vagina)
- **Molecular subtypes**
  - Majority of melanomas are driven by overactivation of the MAPK pathway
    - *BRAF V600* (~50–60%): V600E > V600K, commonly observed in younger pts w/ nodular/superficial spreading melanoma of the trunk. Sensitive to targeted therapy w/ combined oral BRAF + MEK inhibitors
    - *NRAS* (15–20%): No specific targeted Rx available (MEK inhibitors studied versus darcarbazine but not approved based on minimal clinical benefit)
    - *KIT:* ↑ In mucosal, chronically sun-damaged skin, acral sites (~20%); similar muts as in GIST. Oral KIT inhibitors more effective in pts w/ Exon 11 or 13 muts
    - *GNAQ/GNA11:* Not observed in cutaneous melanomas, ↑ in uveal melanomas (>80%), activates heterotrimeric G-protein–coupled receptors → activates MAPK pathway
    - *Other muts: PIK3CA/AKT*, *PTEN* loss, *NF1*, & *BAP1*

Clinical manifestations

- **Sx:** Cutaneous: Most melanomas found by pt at early stage; adv dz → enlarged LN, skin nodules, sx related to lung, liver, bowel/mesenteric, or brain mets **Uveal:** Incidental finding or visual complaints. **Mucosal:** Mucosal bleeding
- **PEx:** Evaluate skin & mucosal surfaces; **ABCDEs: A**symmetry, **B**orders irregular, **C**olor variegated, **D**iameter >5 mm, **E**volution; check for LAN or subcutaneous met, sequela of widespread met dz, *melanosis* → rare, blackening of the skin & urine due to ↑ melanin production, poor prog
- **Labs:** Microcytic anemia, suspect chronic blood loss from bowel mets; ↑ LDH

Diagnostic evaluations and staging

- Punch bx preferred over shave bx; shave bx can transect the tumor & prevent proper depth assessment (T-staging)
- EOD w/ **CT-CAP** or **PET** (esp if 1° lesions is in the distal extremity), if distant dz, FNA or core bx
- Baseline MRI-brain w/ gadolinium for stage III dz or higher to r/o intracranial met
- Evaluation/staging/tx of uveal melanoma is different. In stage IV dz, staging based on size of largest met

Treatment of localized cutaneous melanoma (stages I–III)

- **Wide local excision of 1°:** Margin of 1 cm if tumor ≤1 mm deep, margin of 2 cm for all other lesions

Sentinel LN mapping & bx: Lymphoscintigraphy w/ Tc99 colloid, usu used for lesions >1 mm, if <1 mm consider if high-risk features

AJCC Staging of Locoregional Cutaneous Melanoma (CA Clin J 2017;67:472)				
Stage (~% at Dx)[1]	Tumor	Node	Mets	5-Year Recurrence-Free Survival[2]
IA/B	≤1 mm or 1.01–2 mm w/o ulceration	None	None	IA: 91% IB: 86%
IIA–C (I/II = 83%)	1.01–2 mm w/ ulceration, or any ≥2.01 mm	None	None	IIA: 75% IIB: 55% IIC: 27%
IIIA–D (9%)	Any T	+ LN or in-transit mets	None	IIIA: 56% IIIB: 43% IIIC: 14% IIID: 24%

[1]Based on SEER 18; 5% with unknown stage.
[2]*JNCI* 2020;112:921.

- **Completion LND:** SOC for clinically positive LNs; not indicated for positive sentinel LN bx. DeCOG-SLT RCT showed no ↑ OS (*Lancet Onc* 2016;17:757) but underpowered; MSLT-II showed ↑ regional dz control but no benefit of melanoma-specific survival (*NEJM* 2017;376:2211)
- **Neoadj Rx:** Not SOC, but some increasing adoption. Two doses of preop ipilimumab 1 mg/kg + nivolumab 3 mg/kg q3wk assoc w/ 77% pathologic complete response (*Lancet Onc* 2019;20:948)
- **Adj. Rx & surveillance:** For resected stage IIB–IV melanomas, observation (serial exam/imaging) vs. 1-year adj. nivolumab, pembrolizumab, or dabrafenib/trametinib (for *BRAF* V600E/K). ↑ RFS for LN+ dz, OS benefits unknown (*NEJM* 2017;377:1824; *NEJM* 2018;378:1789; *NEJM* 2020;383:1139). Only pembrolizumab currently approved for IIB–IIC dz (ESMO 2021, Abstr. LBA3_PR (Ann Oncol 2021;32_suppl5:S1283)). Radiotherapy to high-risk nodal basins can ↑ local control but no effect on OS. Increased lymphedema after groin RT

Treatment of metastatic cutaneous melanoma

- **Metastasectomy:** In properly selected pts, long-term OS 20–40%. M1a dz assoc w/ more favorable prog after surgery
- **Immunotherapy:**
  - **Nivolumab/Pembrolizumab (PD-1–blocking Abs):** RR ~30–40% & ↑ PFS/OS (*NEJM* 2015;372:320; *NEJM* 2015;372:2521); ~35% 5-y OS
  - **Nivolumab + Ipilimumab:** Superior RR (~60%); ↑ PFS & ↑ OS compared to ipi monotherapy (*NEJM* 2015;372:2006; *NEJM* 2015;373:23; *NEJM* 2017;377:1345). Higher rate of grade 3–4 irAEs compared to PD-1 or ipi monotherapy (~55%); intracranial clinical benefit 58% in pts w/ asx untreated brain mets (*NEJM* 2018;379:722)
  - **Nivolumab + Relatlimab (LAG-3 blocking ab):** ↑ PFS compared to nivolumab monotherapy; grade 3–4 irAEs appear less common than w/ combined ipi + nivolumab (ASCO 2021 abstr. 9503); not FDA-approved by December 2021
  - **Ipilimumab (CTLA-4 blocking ab):** ↑ OS in 2 RCT (*NEJM* 2010;363:711; *NEJM* 2011;364:2517), slow acting, monitor for immune-mediated tox (ie, colitis, dermatitis, hepatitis, etc.) (See **Toxicities of Immunotherapies** section)
  - **IL-2:** Given in ICU setting, 2–6% pts w/ durable dz control/cure
  - **Autologous ex vivo expanded TILs (lifileucel):** 36% RR in Phase II trial of pts previously treated w/ PD-1 blockade (ASCO 2020, Abstr. 10006); not FDA-approved at time of print
- **Targeted Rx:**
  - **RAF + MEK inhibitor (vem + cobimetinib, dab + trametinib, enco + binimetinib):** ↑ PFS/OS compared to BRAF monotherapy (*JCO* 2015;33:9020; *NEJM* 2012;367:107; *Lancet Onc* 2018;19:603); RR 63–68% w/ median PFS only ~11–14 mos
  - **KIT inhibitors (imatinib/dasatinib/nilotinib):** May be particularly effective for exon 11 & exon 13 mts
- **Chemo:** DTIC/Temozolomide, RR 7–19%; Combination chemo: CVT RR 30–40%, carbo/paclitaxel RR 11–20%, no OS advantage

Treatment of uveal melanoma

- **Locoregional dz:** Brachytherapy, particle beam RT, or enucleation
- **Metastatic dz:** OS benefit w/ bispecific TCR fusion protein tebentafusp in HLA-A*02:01 positive pts (*NEJM* 2021;385:1196), not FDA-approved at time of print

SOFT TISSUE SARCOMAS (STS)

Epidemiology and etiology

- Majority of soft tissue tumors are benign; STSs are rare dzs
- STS = 1% of adult malignancies, >50 histotypes; ~13,000 cases & 5,000 deaths annually
- A/w **radiation** (osteosarcoma, UPS, angiosarcoma), lymphedema (angiosarcoma), genetic syndromes (eg, **FAP** → desmoid; **NF-1** → MPNST; **Li–Fraumeni syn** → osteosarcoma, UPS, angiosarcoma, LMS; **Retinoblastoma** → 2° LMS)

Clinical manifestations

- Presents as mass of the extremities (43%), viscera (19%), RP (15%), trunk (10%), head & neck (9%); ± sx depending on location; rare constitutional sx
- At dx, 57% localized, 22% regional, & 15% w/ mets (3% LN, **80% lung**)

Workup and staging

- **Bx:** Incisional or core (w/ multiple specimens), ensuring resectability of bx tract, as well as hemostasis to minimize seeding
- **Path:** Histology (WHO Classification is standard), IHC, FISH & PCR for dx; NGS for identification of recurrent translocations or other alterations can be useful
- **Imaging:**
  - CT-CAP w/ contrast to evaluate truncal 1°, r/o mets in extremity 1°
  - Consider the following special cases: MRI or CT angio for nontruncal primaries; consider PET to assess chemo response in neoadj tx; CNS imaging (MRI) useful for alveolar soft part sarcoma, solitary fibrous tumor, PNET, angiosarcoma, left-sided cardiac sarcomas; MRI to assess cellularity in desmoid
- **Staging:** Controversial utility; consider AJCC 8th ed. 2017 (trunk/extremity shown)
  Stage IA: Tumor ≤5 cm (T1) + no nodes (N0), grade undetermined (X) or G1
  Stage IB: Tumor >5 cm (T2+) +N0, GX-1
  Stage II: T1N0 + G2–3
  Stage IIIA: T2 (5–10 cm) N0 + G2–3; *Stage IIIB:* T3 (>10 cm) N0 + G2–3
  Stage IV: Nodal involvement (N1) or distant met (M1)
  - Localized tumors should be designated as superficial (superficial fascia uninvolved) or deep
- **Prognostication:** For resected tumors, nomogram predicts 12-y sarcoma-specific death (*JCO* 2002;20:791). Risk ↑ w/ age, tumor size, grade; depth, location, & histology also incorporated. Available at: https://www.mskcc.org/nomograms/sarcoma

Most common types

- **Liposarcoma** (19%): Arise from adipocytes. Most commonly in extremities & RP
  1. Well-diff/de-differentiated—low metastatic potential; however frequent local recurrence problematic. ***MDM2 & CDK4* amp**
  2. Myxoid/round cell—local fat met to RP, spine > lung/liver. t(12;16)(q13;p11)
  3. Pleomorphic—high metastatic potential esp to lung/liver; *TP53* muts common
- **UPS** (formerly malignant fibrous histiocytoma, 16%): NOS dx
- **Leiomyosarcoma** (15%): Arise from smooth muscles; uterine vs. extrauterine sites
- **Synovial** (6%): Misnomer, unknown cell of origin. Most commonly a young adult extremity tumor. t(X;18)(p11;q11) common. IHC: Cytokeratin
- **MPNST** (3%): Arise from peripheral nerves. 50% in NF-1. Most commonly in trunk, extremities, head, & neck. IHC: S100
- **Fibrosarcoma** (2%): Fibroblastic morphology, commonly bone. IHC: Vimentin
- **Desmoid** (2%): Arise from mesenchymal progenitor cell. Most commonly in trunk/extremity, abdominal wall, & intra-abdominal (esp if FAP). No distant metastatic potential. IHC: Vimentin, SMA, nuclear beta-catenin
- **Angiosarcoma** (1%): Arise from endothelia. Most commonly breast, head, & neck, most a/w RT after 8–10 y. IHC: Factor VIII & CD31
- **Rhabdomyosarcoma:** Arise from mesenchyme w/ myogenic potential. 90% in age <25. Pleomorphic subtype tx as STS; others (alveolar, embryonal, spindle cell/sclerosing) have separate tx (below). IHC: Desmin, SMA, myogenin, myoD1

Localized disease: Management

- Malignant dz, if localized, is potentially curable; tx at sarcoma referral center is advised & clinical trials encouraged
- **Surgery:** R0 en bloc resection is mainstay
- **RT:** Meta-analysis shows perioperative RT decreases local recurrence risk at multiple anatomic locations (*Ann Surg Onc* 2018;25:754); *preop RT* smaller field, but doubles wound complication; *postop RT* ↑ fibrosis, edema, joint stiffness due to larger field

- **Adj. chemo:** Standard in GIST & some adult bone malignancies (see **GIST, Bone Sarcoma, & ESFT** chapters) but remains controversial in adult STS
  - Large meta-analysis found ↑ OS for doxorubicin/ifosfamide (OR 0.56) (*Cancer* 2008;113:573). Largest RCT (350 pts w/ STS) found no benefit to adj. Rx (*Lancet Onc* 2012;13:1045); however heterogeneous population & low ifosfamide dose. Indeed, ↑ OS in high-risk subgroup on post hoc analysis (*EJC* 2019;109:51)
  - Considered case-by-case: Eg, if unable to achieve R0 or high risk of recurrence
  - If using adj., combination doxorubicin & ifosfamide favored (*Cancer* 2008;113:573)
- **Neoadj chemo ± RT:** Consider to downstage unresectable lesions; intraoperative RT also employed. Histotype-tailored neoadj therapy does not improve outcomes over anthracycline/ifosfamide chemo (*Lancet Onc* 2017;18:812). Regional hyperthermia may have a role in high-risk extremity sarcomas (*JAMA Onc* 2018;4:483)
- **Surveillance:** PEx & imaging of chest & 1° interval depends on histotype
- **Oligometastatic dz:** Surgical resection & other localized therapies (RT, ablation) in selected pts yield long-term survival & possibility of cure

Metastatic/unresectable disease: management

- Observation may be considered in selected pts w/ low-grade asx dz
- Multiple classes of antineoplastics have activity in STS writ large, including anthracyclines, GEM, taxanes, alkylators, vinca alkaloids, multitargeted TKIs
- Classic 1st-line therapy is **doxorubicin**. Addition of **ifosfamide** ↑ PFS (7.4 vs. 4.6 mos) & ORR (60% vs. 31%) but not OS & ↑ tox (*Lancet Onc* 2014;15:415). Addition of olaratumab to doxorubicin did not ↑ OS in phase III trial (*JAMA* 2020;323:1266)
- **GEM/docetaxel** also considered in 1st line: no Δ PFS/OS vs. doxorubicin (GeDDiS *Lancet Onc* 2017;18:1397). **GEM/DTIC** also active (*JCO* 2011;29:2528)
- **Pazopanib** (TKI of VEGFR, PDGFR-α & -β, & c-Kit): 2nd line in anthracycline-experienced nonadipocytic STS based upon ↑ PFS (RR 6%, no Δ OS, PALETTE *Lancet* 2012;379:1879). s/e: Fatigue, diarrhea, nausea, vomiting, wt loss, HTN, anorexia, hair hyperpigmentation. Other multitargeted TKIs may have utility in adv sarcoma—eg, regorafenib (REGOSARC *Lancet Onc* 2016;17:1732)
- **Trabectedin** (complex mechanism including DNA binding): 2nd line for "L sarcomas" (LMS & liposarcoma) based upon ↑ PFS (RR 10%, no Δ OS), particularly effective in myxoid/round-cell liposarcoma (*JCO* 2015;34:786). May be active in translocation-driven dz more broadly. S/e: Nausea, vomiting, diarrhea, fatigue, transaminitis, cytopenias
- **Eribulin** (microtubule inhibitor): Approved 2nd line for liposarcoma based upon ↑ OS (RR 4%, no Δ PFS), (*Lancet* 2016;387:1629). S/e: Fatigue, GI, alopecia, pyrexia, & anemia

Additional Histotype-Specific Therapies to Consider	
UPS	Pembrolizumab (*Lancet Onc* 2017;18:1493)
Alveolar soft part sarcoma	Pembrolizumab +/– TKI (*Lancet Onc* 2019;20:837), TKIs
LMS	Doxorubicin + DTIC (*Cancer* 2020;126:2637)
Well-differentiated/dedifferentiated liposarcoma	CDK4/6 inhibitors (*JAMA Onc* 2016;2:937)
Angiosarcoma	Taxanes (ANGIOTAX *JCO* 2008;26:5269), VEGF inhib
Rhabdomyosarcoma (Nonpleomorphic)	VAC: Vincristine+dactinomycin+cyclophosphamide (*JCO* 2009;27:5128)
Epithelioid sarcoma	Tazometostat (*Lancet Onc* 2020;21:1423)
Solitary fibrous tumor	Temozolomide + bev (*Cancer* 2011;117:4939)
PEComa, epithelioid hemangioendothelioma	Sirolimus (*JCO* 2010;28:835 & *Cancer* 2021;127:569)
Tenosynovial giant cell tumor	Pexidartinib (ENLIVEN *Lancet* 2019;394:478)
Dermatofibrosarcoma protuberans	Imatinib (*JCO* 2010;28:1772)
Desmoid	NSAIDs, tamoxifen, sorafenib, liposomal doxorubicin, MTX, vinca alkaloids

Kaposi sarcoma: Management

- A/w immunodeficiency (HIV); classified & treated separately from other sarcomas
- In persons w/ HIV, co-mgmt of HIV, including HAART & OI ppx is critical
- **HAART:** CR in 80%; immune reconstitution inflammatory syn **(KS-IRIS)** occurs in <10% & be severe—glucocorticoids contraindicated, consider thalidomide
- **Localized tx:** Resection, RT, cryotherapy, intralesional vinblastine/bleomycin, topical alitretinoin, imiquimod
- **Systemic Tx:** 1st line → **liposomal doxorubicin;** paclitaxel is the favored alternative (*Cancer* 2010;116:3969); pomalidomide for KS refractory to the above (*JCO* 2016;34:4125)

GASTROINTESTINAL STROMAL TUMOR

Epidemiology

- **Incidence:** ~5,000 new cases/y in US, underreported for many years
- 1–3% all GI malignancies; most common gut mesenchymal tumor
- No clear RFs, median dx age ~60, more common in men
- Rare hereditary syndromes affecting RTK signaling or SDH
  Germline mt **c-*KIT*** or ***PDGDR*-α:** GIST, skin hyperpigmentation, urticaria pigmentosa
  Neurofibromatosis type 1 (germline *NF1* Mts): ↑ incidence GIST
  Carney–Stratakis syn (germline *SDH* Mts): GIST, paraganglioma

Pathology

- Cell of origin likely *interstitial cells of Cajal* (myenteric plexus, control-gut peristalsis)
- ***c-KIT*** oncogene encodes the cell-surface RTK, KIT (CD117)
  Nl pathway: Stem cell factor, the ligand for KIT → KIT dimerization & phosphorylation → activation of multiple signaling cascades, including MAPK-dependent stabilization of ETV1 → cell growth
- *c-KIT* is mutated & activated in ~80% of GISTs; particularly **exons 11** (intracellular juxtamembrane domain, ~70% cases), 9 (extracellular domain, up to 20% cases, ↑ intestinal GIST), 13 & 17 (tyrosine kinase domain, <5%)
- ~5–10% have somatic mts in *PDGFR-α* (exon 18, ↑ gastric) → MAPK activation
- Other MAPK-activating somatic muts seen, including *BRAF* & *NF1*
- RTK/MAPK wild-type GIST can have somatic *SDH* alteration (SDHB-neg on IHC)
  Carney's triad: GIST + paraganglioma + pulmonary chondroma, a/w somatic *SDHB,C,D* muts or epigenetic silencing
- **Anatomic sites:** Stomach (~60%), small intestine (~30%); less common sites include large bowel (rectum → aggressive), esophagus, & mesentery

Clinical manifestations

- **Sx:** Incidentally found or after the evaluation of nonspecific sx; abd pain, n/v, gastric outlet obstruction, early satiety, anorexia, wt loss, upper GIB (occult or acute hemorrhage), intraperitoneal hemorrhage
- Adv GIST disseminates in IP cavity, liver; less commonly lung, LN (*SDH* mts), bone
- **Exam:** Palpable abdominal mass
- **Labs:** Microcytic anemia, paraneoplastic hypothyroidism (*NEJM* 2014;370:1327)

Diagnostic evaluations and staging

- **Bx:** EGD or EUS w/ FNA to establish dx
- Friable tumor can hemorrhage, EUS–FNA is preferred to percutaneous bx by NCCN
- **Pathology review:**
  IHC CD117+, diagnostic molecular pathology for *c-KIT* or *PDGFR-α* mt
  DOG1, a receptor chloride channel, is expressed on both KIT ±; GISTs, can make dx in difficult cases; CD34+ also common
- **Imaging:**
  - EOD w/ CT-CAP +/– MRI
  - FDG–PET scan: Highly avid, early marker of response to TKIs
- **Prog** depends upon: Size of 1°, location of 1°, & mitotic index; **Gold Nomogram** (*Lancet Onc* 2009;10:1045) freely available: www.mskcc.org/nomograms/gastrointestinal
- Nonlinear modeling w/ add'l consideration of surgical tumor rupture may further refine prognostication (*Lancet Onc* 2012;13:265)

Treatment of resectable and locally advanced disease

- **1° tx modality is surgical resection**
  - Complete resection w/ neg margins is goal, possible in majority of cases
  - Lymphadenectomy usu not required except if LN enlarged (some SDH-deficient tumors)
  - Tumor is friable, forms pseudocapsule, surgery is optimized to prevent rupture → peritoneal dissemination
  - 1° resected GIST 5-y dz-specific survival ~50% (*Ann Surg* 2002;231:51)
  - Consider periodic endoscopic surveillance vs. resection in <2 cm, no high-risk features (eg, even when <2 cm, rectal GIST can be high risk)
- **Neoadj Rx:** Reserved for borderline resectable/unresectable dz as limits staging & prognostication. Prospective trials indicate safety of imatinib in preop setting; difficult to ascertain if preop Rx ↑ OS as most trials gave postresection Rx; preferred strategy in rectal GIST to improve surgical outcome

- **Adj. Rx:** Imatinib ↑ OS w/ longer duration of Rx in high-risk pts; key trials:
  - ACOSOG Z9001 (*Lancet* 2009;373:1097): Phase III RCT, localized GIST (>3 cm) s/p resection → 1 y of placebo vs. imatinib, ↑ **RFS, no Δ OS**. Subgroup analysis shows benefit for ***KIT* exon 11 deletion**, but not in *KIT* exon 11 insertion, point mut, *KIT* exon 9 mut or *PDGFRA* muts (*JCO* 2014;32:1563)
  - Scandinavian sarcoma group: Phase III RCT of 1-y vs. 3-y imatinib in high-risk GIST, ↑ **RFS/OS** w/ **3 y** of Rx. ~10% absolute ↑ in 5-y OS (*JAMA* 2012;307:1265)
  - PERSIST-5 (*JAMA Onc* 2018;4:e184060): Single arm phase II of 5 y imatinib for resected GIST >5-cm nongastric OR >2 cm any location w/ >5 mitoses/50 hpf; no pt w/ imatinib-sensitive dz recurred on tx, but only ~50% completed 5 y of therapy
  - Adj. KIT inhibition indefinitely may be reasonable for high-risk pts w/ imatinib-sensitive muts
- **Surveillance:** CT-CAP or MRI q3–6mos for 3–5 y; should continue if persisting on tx

Treatment of unresectable and metastatic disease

- Prior to TKI, GIST considered not sensitive to chemo
- **Imatinib Mesylate**
  - Inhibitor of KIT RTK; blocks ATP-binding
  - Multiple Phase II/III clinical trials shown benefit. Overall, KIT exon 11 > exon 9 > exon 13 or 17 mts. SDH deficient GIST is generally more resistant to TKIs
  - Key trials of imatinib dosing in adv/met GIST:
    - RCT of 400 mg QD vs. 600 mg QD imatinib; **ORR in all pts >50%,** no Δ PFS/OS (*NEJM* 2002;347:472)
    - RCT of 400 mg QD (low dose) vs. 400 mg BID (high dose) imatinib; ORR & OS equivalent; ↑ tox but ↑ PFS w/ high dose (*Lancet* 2004;364:1127)
    - RCT of low-dose vs. high-dose imatinib; **median OS 51–55 mos;** no Δ ORR/PFS/OS between groups; after POD, pts who cross over to high dose had 33% ORR or SD (*JCO* 2008;26:626)
  - *Standard therefore is imatinib 400 mg QD for adv/met GIST*; consider ↑ to high dose in exon 9 mts; *PDGFR-α* D842V insensitive to imatinib—consider avaprinitib (see below)
  - S/e: Fluid retention, fatigue, GI, myalgia, rash, cytopenias, rare transaminitis
- **Resistance to imatinib/POD:** 1° = POD <6 mos (more common in exon 9 mt), 2° = >6 mos (typically develop separate 2° resistance Mts in KIT)
- **Sunitinib**
  - Multitargeted TKI; second line tx after imatinib failure; good activity in exon 9, 13/14 Mts
  - RCT sunitinib vs. placebo in imatinib-resistant GIST, sunitinib ↑ PFS/OS, RR ~10% (*Lancet* 2006;368:1329)
- **Regorafenib**
  - Multitarget TKI; third line; activity in exon 17/18 acquired resistance Mts
  - GRID trial → Phase III RCT of GIST pts w/ failure to imatinib/sunitinib to regorafenib vs. placebo; regorafenib w/ ↑ PFS compared to placebo (~5 mos vs. 1 mo) (*Lancet* 2013;381:295)
- **Ripretinib**
  - Unique "switch control" mechanism extends the spectrum of susceptible muts to those targeted by both type I & type II kinase inhibitors (*Cancer Cell* 2019;35:738)
  - INVICTUS phase III RCT of ripretinib vs. placebo in 4th-line setting (*Lancet Onc* 2020;21:923) median PFS increased (6.3 vs. 1.0 mos); common s/e—alopecia, myalgia/arthralgia, fatigue, PPES, GI toxicities, cardiotoxicity
  - INTRIGUE trial will assess ripretinib vs. sunitinib in the 2nd-line setting (ongoing)
- **Avapritinib**
  - TKI w/ exceptional activity against PDGFR-α exon 18 muts, including D842V Mt pts on NAVIGATOR trial who had ORR of 88% (*Lancet Onc* 2020;21:935)
  - FDA approved in *PDGFRA* exon 18 Mts; NCCN recommends use in place of imatinib for these pts in the neoadj & 1st-line settings
  - Cognitive s/e can be problematic, monitor closely
- Other TKIs may have utility after failure of the above—eg, sorafenib, pazopanib, nilotinib, cabozantinib; dasatinib for PDGFR-α D842V after avapritinib
- May be a role for augmentation of TKIs w/ mTOR inhibition on progression
- Investigational: TKI + MEK inhibitor combinations
- Monitoring: CT-CAP/MRI q3mos, responses can correlate w/ Δ density, consider Choi criteria, which incorporates Hounsfield units as a measure of density (*JCO* 2007;25:1753)
- Consider metastasectomy or RT in cases of limited progression (*Ann Surg* 2006;244:176, *Cancer* 2006;107:2833)

BONE SARCOMAS

Epidemiology

- Estimated 3,600 cases, 1,700 deaths/y in US in 2020
- Common subtypes include chondrosarcoma (40%), osteosarcoma (28%), chordoma (10%), Ewing Sarcoma (ES) (8%, see **ESFT** chapter), UPS of bone (<5%), fibrosarcoma of bone (<2%), & giant cell tumor of bone

Osteosarcoma: Clinical manifestations and molecular biology

- Commonly presents as bone pain or swelling, particularly w/ activity
- Met spread is almost exclusively **hematogenous** → lung & bone; lymphatic involvement is rare (<10%) w/ poor prog; localized CAs likely have micrometastatic dz; likelihood of mets correlate w/ tumor size
  - *Skip mets*: Discontinuous tumor in same bone 2/2 sinusoidal or venous anastomotic embolization; frequent in high-grade lesions
- **RFs:** RT, Paget dz, fibrous dysplasia; no proven association w/ trauma
- **Assoc hereditary syndromes:** *LFS* (*TP53* Mt); hereditary *retinoblastoma* (*RB1* Mt, relative risk 30); *RECQ helicase syndromes*: Rothmund–Thomson, Bloom, Werner, & RAPADILINO syndromes; Diamond Blackfan Anemia
- **Rb pathway:** Loss of heterozygosity in >50% osteosarcoma; **p16^{INK4a}** in add'l 15%
- **HER2:** Overexpressed in 42%; worse prog; no proven benefit w/ trastuzumab

Common Osteosarcoma Subtypes	
Low/Intermediate Grade	
Low-grade intramedullary	Occurs in same sites as classic intramedullary; rare (<2%)
Parosteal (5%)	Older individuals, F > M; site: Cortical bone, ↑ distal femur; ↑ late mets; can transform to high grade
Periosteal	Intermediate grade, commonly affecting femur & tibial, "scooped-out" Codman triangle
High Grade	
"Classic" high-grade intramedullary (~80%)	Subclassified into osteoblastic (50%), chondroblastic (25%), or fibroblastic (25%). Mgmt same among all types
Small cell	Requires IHC, cytogenetics, molecular studies to distinguish between other similar histologies
Telangiectatic	Vascular tumors w/ lytic appearance on radiographs
Multifocal	Unclear synchrony, but poor prog
High-grade surface	Median age 13.5 y; mostly diaphysis of bone; high met rate

Chondrosarcoma: Clinical manifestations and molecular biology

- Commonly presents as dull, achy pain often at night; long latency between onset of sx & dx
- **Conventional chondrosarcoma of bone (~90%):**
  - **Central chondrosarcomas:** *IDH1/IDH2* Mt is early genetic event in 65%. Median age 50; M > F; proximal femur, humerus, pelvis; enchondromas are precursor lesions
    - **Ollier dz/Maffucci syn:** Somatic mosaic *IDH1/IDH2* Mt leading to precursor enchondromas → transformation to central chondrosarcoma in ~50%; Maffucci also p/w soft-tissue hemangiomas
  - **Peripheral chondrosarcomas:** Osteochondromas are precursor lesions. EXT1 loss in osteochondroma creates niche for development of chondrosarcoma (*Oncogene* 2012;31:1095). Young median age; pelvis, shoulder, long bones
    - **Hereditary multiple exostoses:** AD *EXT1/EXT2* Mt leading to precursor osteochondroma lesions → transformation to peripheral chondrosarcoma in ~5%

Rare Chondrosarcoma Subtypes (Orthopedic Onc 2014;162:117)	
Periosteal	Median age 20–30; M > F; metaphysis of long bone (femur); ↑ prog despite ↑ grade
Dedifferentiated	Median age 50–60; medullary bone (pelvis, femur, humerus); ↓ prog w/ 21% mets at dx; high-grade noncartilaginous tumor arising from (subclone of) low-grade cartilaginous lesion
Mesenchymal	Median age 25; skeletal (axial) but many extraskeletal (meninges); ↓ prog w/ 20% mets at dx
Clear cell	3:1 M:F; humerus/femur epiphyses; low grade but ↑ late mets
Skeletal myxoid	Poorly understood entity; tx as int/high-grade chondrosarcoma; hip location

Workup and staging

- Referral to multidisciplinary referral center strongly preferred
- Painful bone lesions in pts <40 y should be worked up as a malignant 1°; in >40 y, must r/o met carcinoma or myeloma
- Bone should be evaluated & treated for impending **pathologic fracture**
- **Bx:** Open bx most sensitive, but core needle bx w/ multiple cores sufficient if adequate sample. Bx tract resected & meticulous hemostasis achieved to prevent seeding
- **Imaging:** Plain image to start; MRI most accurate. Staging depends on tumor type; CT chest, CT/MR of 1° PET or bone scan useful for bony mets; PET/CT useful for monitoring response in osteosarcoma, whole-body MRI sensitive for skeletal mets; CT/MR angiography useful for surgical planning
- **Staging: MSTS (Enneking)** staging used for osteosarcoma
  Stage IA: Low grade (G1), intracompartmental (T1, confined by cortex), M0
  Stage IB: G1 + extracompartmental (T2, beyond cortex) + M0
  Stage IIA: High grade (G2) + T1M0
  Stage IIB: G2T2M0
  Stage III: Met (M1)
- AJCC 8th ed. 2018 staging (TNM) also referenced for osteosarcoma (see **EFTS** section)
- Staging of limited utility in chondrosarcoma
- **Labs:** LDH & alk phos should be obtained, trended as tumor marker (also prognostic)
- Fertility consultation prior to chemo, including possible need for sperm banking/egg harvesting; pain mgmt, physical/occupational rehab, sexual counseling, psychotherapeutic counseling postoperatively; **AYA programs** where available

Osteosarcoma and UPS of bone: Management

- **Initial mgmt** of localized dz is surgery +/– chemo
  - **Low–intermediate grade dz:** Wide excision w/ neg margins; perioperative chemo may be considered for periosteal type, but not proven
  - **High-grade dz:** Wide excision w/ perioperative chemo; preop chemo may ↑ likelihood of limb-sparing surgery, allow for assessment of tx response, but intensifying chemo for poor response not effective (EURAMOS-1 *Lancet Onc* 2016;17:1396)
  - **HEENT osteosarcoma:** Generally low grade; tx w/ wide local excision; consider adj. CIS-based chemo RT if unable to obtain neg margins; consider adj. CIS-based chemo if >5 cm or high grade
  - **Chemo:** CIS + doxorubicin (*Lancet* 1997;350:911), MAP are favored. Addition of ifosfamide to MAP can be considered but did not improve outcomes in peds (*JCO* 2008;26:633)
  - **Mifamurtide (MTP):** Immune stimulant**;** addition of MTP to MAP chemo ↑ OS (HR 0.71); however, not FDA approved (*JCO* 2008;26:633)
  - **Surveillance:** Imaging of 1° site & chest, bone scan/PET scan, & exam q3mos y 1–2, q4mos y 3, q6mos y 3–5, & q12mos subsequently. Consider survivorship clinic
- **Relapsed/met dz:** Resection if possible ± systemic Rx; original chemo may be rechallenged if initial response >1 y; ↑ prog if lung-only
- **2nd-line chemo:** Clinical trial if available; GEM ± docetaxel; cyclophosphamide + etoposide or topotecan; ifosfamide + etoposide ± carbo or high-dose MTX
  - **TKIs:** Regorafenib, cabozantinib, sorafenib have activity in relapsed/refractory
- **Samarium-153:** Bone-seeking beta-emitter for pain palliation (*JCO* 2002;20:189)

Chondrosarcoma: Management

- **Dedifferentiated histotype:** Technically a low-grade chondrosarcoma admixed w/ high-grade sarcoma component; tx as high-grade osteosarcoma (see above)
- **Mesenchymal histotype:** Tx as Ewing Sarcoma (see **EFTS** section)
- **Low-grade, nonpelvic intracompartmental lesions:** Consider intralesional excision w/ adj. cryosurgery, or wide local excision
- All other histotypes are managed surgically w/ wide excision; margins should extend 3 cm beyond abnl bone on imaging; (+) margins portend poor prog (10-y OS 61% vs. 17%); limb-sparing surgery contraindicated if neurovascular involvement
- Classical cytotoxic chemo of no proven benefit; **Dasatinib & pazopanib** may have activity though
- ***IDH1* mutated:** Consider **ivosidenib**. Median PFS 5.6 mos. Durable dz control in subgroup w/ conventional histology & no additional drivers (*JCO* 2020;38:1693)

EWING SARCOMA FAMILY (ESFT)

Epidemiology

- Annual incidence in the United States: 300–400 cases
- 70% in <20 y, incidence 2.9/million among <20 y; 9:1 White:Black
- 65–90% p/w localized dz (55% 5-y OS); 10–35% p/w mets (22% OS) (EICESS *JCO* 2000;18:3108)

The Ewing Sarcoma Family and Select-Related Small Round-Cell Tumors	
Osseous ES	Long bones, pelvis, & ribs; frequently in diaphysis; **"onion skinning"** XR periosteal rxn
Extraosseous Ewing	Paravertebral & CW masses, also in lower extremities
PNET	Cerebrum, pineal gland, or peripheral; PNETs of cerebellum are classified as **medulloblastomas** & are clinically/pathologically distinct from supratentorial CNS PNET
Askin tumor "CW PNET"	CW soft tissue mass ±; pleura/rib; frequent mets to bone, sympathetic chain
Esthesioneuroblastoma	Tumor of nasal vault probably developing from olfactory placode
Peripheral neuroepithelioma	Extremities (buttock, upper thigh, shoulder, upper arm); Homer–Wright rosettes (small cells arranged w/ neurofibrillar center)
Desmoplastic small round-cell tumor	Abdominal mass most common; frequent in males aged 18–21; canonical *EWS-WT1* translocation

Etiology and clinical manifestations

- ESFTs are **small round-cell** neoplasms thought to originate from **neural crest** cells w/ shared genetic alterations
- Bone pain/swelling, constitutional sx, leukocytosis
- Met sites: Lungs, bones, BM
- Poor prognostic factors: Mets, pelvic bone, & vertebral involvement, adult age, large tumor
- Favorable prognostic factors: Distal 1°, nl LDH, localized dz, tx response

Molecular biology

- Characterized by **canonical translocations** & varying degrees of neuroectodermal differentiation
  - ***EWS-ETS* t(11;22):** Prototypical Ewing translocations fuse the *EWS* gene (22q12, potent transcriptional activator) w/ members of the *ETS* family of genes
    ETS family: *FLI1* most frequent fusion partner for *EWS* (85% of ESFTs), others include *ERG, ETV1, ETV4,* or *FEV*
  - ***EWS-WT1:*** Diagnostic of desmoplastic small round-cell tumor
  - ***FUS-ETS:*** Rare ESFTs will exhibit fusion of *FUS-ETS* fusions instead of *EWS-ETS*
  - ***CIC-DUX4:*** Identified in some *EWS*-neg primitive round-cell tumors, poor prog
  - ***BCOR-CCNB3:*** Male predominance occurring in Ewing-like & undifferentiated sarcomas
- Other sites of recurrent genomic alterations include *STAG2, TP53, CDKN2A*
- **MIC2(CD99):** Glycoprotein strongly expressed in many ESFTs; can be used to histologically support dx

Workup and staging

- **Bx:** Core needle or open, send for cytogenetic/FISH analysis, avoid FNA; bx tract must be resected at time of surgery given high risk of seeding
- **Imaging/Staging:** CT chest; MR +/– CT of 1°; Whole-body PET or bone scan (whole-body MRI may be of utility in pediatric pts); consider bone marrow bx
- Staging systems are not often clinically utilized given poor prognostic performance & high likelihood of subclinical metastatic dz but can consider use of AJCC staging
- AJCC 8th ed. TNM 2017 staging for nonspine, nonpelvis 1°s (separate T staging)
  Stage IA: Tumor ≤8 cm (T1) + N0 + GX/G1
  Stage IB: Tumor >8 cm (T2) or discontinuous tumors (T3) + N0 + GX/G1
  Stage IIA: T1N0 + G2–3
  Stage IIB: T2N0 + G2–3
  Stage III: T3N0 + G2–3
  Stage IV: Distant mets &/or nodal involvement
- Fertility consultation should be offered prior to chemo

Management: Localized disease

- *Accepted paradigm: Neoadj chemo followed by restaging, local tx(surgery +/– RT), & then adj. chemo*
- **Neoadj multiagent chemo:** Downstages tumor (↑ probability of complete resection), treats micrometastatic dz, allows for assessment of response prior to local Rx
- **Neoadj regimens:** 12–24 wks tx, w/ G-CSF support
  - **VDC/IE:** Vincristine + doxorubicin + cyclophosphamide alternating w/ ifosfamide + etoposide q3wks (q2wks if <18 yo) (*NEJM* 2003;348:694)
  - **VIDE:** Vincristine + ifosfamide + doxorubicin + etoposide
  - **VAI:** Vincristine + D-actinomycin + ifosfamide
  - Note: **VDC/IE now preferred;** superior to European standard of VIDE → VAI or VAC (HR EFS 0.70, HR OS 0.64; Euro Ewing 2012 (*JCO* 2020;38(suppl_15):abstr 11500)
- Interval-compressed tx (q2wks chemo) may improve efficacy, subgroup analysis suggests benefit limited to pts <18 y (*JCO* 2012;30:4148)
- **Restaging:** MR of 1° & CXR, or PET/bone scan. If stable or response → proceed to local Rx & adj. chemo; if no response → RT ± surgery followed by 2nd-line chemo (below)
- **Local Rx:** Either preop RT + surgery, surgery + postop RT (if positive margin), or definitive RT. Consider hemithorax RT or DP-IMRT for 1° or infiltrative pleural dz
- **Surgery:** Limb-sparing resection preferred if limb functionality can be retained, alternative is amputation. Physiatry consultation rec
- **Adj. Chemo:** 28–49 wks add'l chemo (same regimens as above; drop anthracycline at lifetime max, can consider substituting D-actinomycin)
- **Surveillance:** PE, chest imaging, & 1° site imaging q3mos, ↑ interval after 24 mos, annually after 5 y; monitor for tx-related malignancies

Management: Primary metastatic disease

- **Multiagent chemo:** Preferred regimen is **VDC** (*JCO* 2004;22:2873)
- Neoadj regimens (above) are accepted alternatives
- If clinical response, consider surgical resection/RT of residual dz

Management: Relapsed and primary refractory disease

- 30–40% pts recur; portends poor prog (50% 5-y OS if local recurrence; 14% if distant recurrence)
- **Late relapse (≥2 y):** 50% 5-y OS, retreat w/ original regimen, resection if possible
- **Early relapse (<2 y):** 8% 5-y OS, clinical trial preferred, or 2nd-line chemo
- **2nd-line chemo:** Cyclophosphamide + topotecan; temozolomide + irinotecan; ifosfamide + etoposide ± carbo; docetaxel + GEM (vincristine may be added to any of these regimens)
- **Cabozantinib** (VEGFR2 & MET TKI) can be considered. In single arm study ORR 25% at 6 mos, median OS 10 mos, median PFS 4.4 mos (CABONE *Lancet Onc* 2020;21:446)
- Isolated pulmonary mets: ↑ Prog; tx w/ serial resection + chemo ± RT (whole lung RT in pediatrics; controversial in adults)

Management: CNS PNET

- Very rare dzs w/ poor prog & heterogeneous pathobiology (*Cell* 2016;164:1060) complicates unifying mgmt recommendations
- Paradigm is surgical resection followed by adj. RT then chemo
- **Surgery:** Maximal surgical resection if possible, otherwise a partial resection at referral center. 2nd-look surgery may be necessary to remove residual tumors. Consider neoadj chemo to downstage
- **Adj. tx:** Radiation benefit is dose dependent & stereotactic techniques are being investigated to reduce tox; enrollment in adj. clinical trial is preferred for chemo (multiple regimens are utilized)
- Craniospinal axis radiation is used for pts w/ spinal dissemination

HEAD & NECK SQUAMOUS CELL CANCER

Epidemiology

- **H&N CA:** 66K cases/y, 14.6K deaths/y in the United States projected in 2021, ↑ due to HPV surge. >90% = SCC (SCCHN)
- **M:F:** 3:1
- **RF:** Tobacco, EtOH, HPV, betel nut chewing
- **Genetic syns:** Overall rare; Fanconi most common. Others: Bloom, Li–Fraumeni, xeroderma pigmentosa
- **Risk of 2nd 1° CA:** 3–7% /y for lung & aerodigestive tracts due to "field cancerization" by tobacco/EtOH (not HPV). Solitary lung mass → r/o 2nd 1°

Anatomic divisions of H&N cancer

- **Oral cavity:** Buccal mucosa, alveolar ridges, floor of mouth, retromolar trigone, hard palate, anterior 2/3 tongue
- **Oropharynx:** Tongue base (posterior 1/3), tonsils, glossotonsilar sulcus, inferior surface of soft palate, vallecula, posterior pharyngeal wall to level of hyoid
- **Nasopharynx:** Superior to soft palate posterior to nasal cavity
- **Hypopharynx:** Hyoid bone to cricoid cartilage
- **Larynx:** Divided into supraglottic, glottic, subglottic (rare)

Molecular pathogenesis

- **HPV:** E6, E7 viral protein → inhibit p53, Rb, other tumor suppressors
- **p16:** Tumor suppressor overexpressed in HPV-assoc CAs (E7 protein inhibits Rb fxn, leading to compensatory p16 upregulation), frequently inactivated in tobacco-assoc SCCHN
- **EGFR:** Overexpressed in >80% SCCHN; ↑ correlates w/ poorer prog (*Mol Can Ther* 2019;18:1909)
- ***TP53*:** Inactivated in >50% SCCHN, more common in tobacco/EtOH-associated tumors
- ***CCND1* (cyclin D1):** ↑ cell-cycle progression
- **Others:** *PI3K/AKT/mTOR* (primarily in HPV+), *HRAS*, & *PTEN*

Pathology

- **Precursor lesions:** Hyperplasia → dysplasia → carcinoma in situ → invasive CA
  - Leukoplakia—fixed white plaques, hyperparakeratosis w/ hyperplasia
  - Erythroplakia—red patches, often a/w epithelial dysplasia
- **Molecular studies**
  - **p16 (+)** by IHC in HPV-associated tumors due to inactivated Rb
  - **RNA in situ hybridization high-risk HPV** gold standard

HPV-associated SCCHN

- **Serotypes:** Most commonly a/w **HPV-16 (>90%), HPV-18** (*NEJM* 2001;344:1125)
- **Dx:** p16+ IHC (more sensitive), HPV in situ hybridization (more specific), HPV DNA PCR
- **Location:** Most commonly **oropharyngeal**, infrequently other sites
- **Demographics:** Younger pt w/o smoking/EtOH hx & few comorbidities, typically p/w nodal dz → w/u locates small oropharyngeal 1° tumor
- **Prog:** Dramatically better than stage-matched HPV-neg tumors, therefore, separate staging system (*NEJM* 2010;363:24; *JCO* 2015;33:836-845)
- **Prevention:** Although not proven, preventative HPV vaccine likely decreases risk of HPV-associated SCCHN

Initial workup

- **Sx:** Dysphagia, poor PO, voice changes, trismus/pain, wt loss, neck mass (enlarged cervical LNs)
- **H&P:** EtOH, tobacco. Detailed H&N exam w/ mirror exam &/or direct visualization
- **Imaging:** CT/MRI of neck, chest imaging = CXR at minimum. Consider CT chest or PET/CT if N2 or N3 dz
- **Bx:** After imaging if possible to avoid false (+), esp PET/CT; FNA of involved neck node well tolerated, convenient; tissue HPV testing if oropharynx
- **Multidisciplinary care:** Rad onc, surgery, med onc; nutrition (consider PEG at baseline only if +malnutrition); dental, speech/swallow; smoking/EtOH cessation

Staging (TNM, AJCC 8th ed.)

- T stage is variable by site; N & M stages are more uniform
- **HPV+ oropharyngeal CA: stage I** = T0–T2, N0–N1; **stage II** = N2 or T3 (>4 cm or extending to epiglottis) N0–2; **stage III** = T0–T3N3 or T4N0–3; **stage IV** = M1 dz

- **Non–HPV-assoc SCCHN: Stage I** = T1N0; **stage II** = T2N0; **stage III** = T3N0 or T1-3N1 (single ipsilateral LN ≤3 cm); **stage IV** = still potentially curable:
  - IVA = "moderately advanced local dz," T4a or T1–T3N2 (LN <3 cm + ENE, 1 LN 3–6 cm, or 2+ LNs <6 cm)
  - IVB = "very advanced local dz" T4b or N3 (any LN >6 cm or >3 cm + ENE)
  - IVC = M1 dz = considered incurable
- Depth of invasion (DOI) is part of T staging for oral cavity CA & is an independent prognostic factor: (T1: DOI ≤5 mm; T2: DOI ≤10 mm; T3: >10 mm)
- Nasopharyngeal staging system differs from other upper aerodigestive CA

Treatment–curative intent (stage I–IVB)

- **Early-stage:** Surgery or RT alone
- **Locally advanced:** Surgery followed by adj. RT (± chemo for high-risk features) or upfront concurrent CRT (see CRT below) with surgery reserved for salvage
- No OS benefit to adj. chemo alone (MACH-NC, *Radiother Oncol* 2009;92:4)
- RT—when surgery is not technically feasible or undesirable (eg, larynx preservation). SEs of RT—both short- & long-term fatigue, mucositis, xerostomia, dermatitis, rarely 2° malignancies (sarcomas). IMRT standard 66–70-Gy, 2-Gy fractions to 1° tumor &/or side of neck with LNs. "Hyperfractionation" = potential higher cumulative doses in smaller fractions

Role of chemoradiation (CRT)

- **Concurrent CRT:** Used as alternative to surgery for organ preservation or for unresectable dz
- CRT for locally advanced dz: CIS CRT ↑ OS but also ↑ tox (cytopenias, renal, n/v) (*JCO* 2003;21:92). Carbo + 5-FU CRT ↑ OS in oropharyngeal (*JCO* 2004;22:69); cetuximab CRT ↓ OS & ↓ locoregional control in HPV+ locally advanced dz compared to CIS RT (RTOG 1016, *Lancet* 2019; 393:40; *Lancet* 2019;393:51)
- Cumulative dose of CIS >200 mg/m^2 is rec regardless of bolus or weekly dosing
- Larynx preservation improved w/ concurrent CIS + RT (RTOG 91, *JCO* 2013;31:845)
- **Postop adj. CRT w/ CIS for high-risk features of (+) margins or ENE** in LN (*Head Neck* 2005;27:843): ↑ DFS (*NEJM* 2004;350:1937) & OS (*NEJM* 2004;350:1945)

Role of induction chemotherapy

- Rationale: ↓ sxs a/w 1° tumor size, organ preservation, ↓ risk of distant mets; controversial as ↑ duration of tx, potential ↑ tox risk, no trials have yet shown OS advantage of induction + CRT vs. CRT alone
- If induction chosen, docetaxel, CIS, 5-FU standard (EORTC 24971/TAX 323 *NEJM* 2007;357:1695)

Treatment: Palliative intent

- For distant mets or recurrent dz s/p RT that is unresectable or ineligible for more RT
- 1st-line preferred: Platinum-doublet (CIS/carbo + 5-FU) with pembrolizumab or pembrolizumab monotherapy in PD-L1 (+) tumors with CPS ≥1. Both regimens demonstrated OS advantage over EXTREME; no PFS advantage (KEYNOTE-048, *Lancet* 2019;349;1915)
- Historically & alternatively: EXTREME (CIS/carbo + 5-FU with cetuximab) was the 1st-line regimen due to improved efficacy with addition of cetuximab to platinum doublet (EXTREME, *NEJM* 2008;359:1116)
- Cetuximab tox: Acneiform rash (correlates w/ response), GI complaints, hypersensitivity rxn
- 2nd-line (if not previously used): Nivolumab & pembrolizumab following progression on or after platinum therapy

Posttherapy surveillance

- H&P q1–3 mos × 1 y, then gradually lengthen interval until yearly >5 y
- New baseline imaging w/in 6 mos of tx
- Surveillance for 2° CA, complications of RT (eg, thyroid dysfunction)

NASOPHARYNGEAL CARCINOMA

Epidemiology/risk factors

- Uncommon in the United States & Western Europe
- **Endemic to southern China;** high risk in Southeast Asia, Mediterranean basin (North Africa, Middle East, Southeast Europe)
- >90% a/w **EBV**
- Environmental factors: High intake of salt-preserved foods

Molecular pathogenesis

- **EBV** → LMP1, other viral proteins → ↑ cell replication

Diagnosis/workup

- **Sx:** Nasal obstruction/epistaxis, HA, enlarged cervical LN, otitis media (eustachian tube obstruction), diplopia, facial numbness/paresthesias (invasion of cavernous sinus—CN III, IV, V1–3, VI)
- **H&P:** W/ nasopharyngeal exam; mirror & fiberoptic exam
- **Imaging:** MRI ± CT w/ contrast of nasopharynx, base of skull to clavicles. Body contrast CT or PET-CT when advanced neck dz is present
- **Bx:** Nasopharyngeal bx
- **Multidisciplinary care:** Dental evaluation, nutrition, speech, & swallow evaluation, audiogram before starting plat-based chemo

Pathology

WHO type I	SCC	Behaves more like other head & neck CA
WHO type II	Nonkeratinizing CA	Endemic areas; >90% a/w EBV
WHO type III	Undifferentiated CA	

- Basaloid squamous CA: Rare subtype
- Neuroendocrine & SNUC may arise in the nasopharynx but are distinct clinical entities

Staging (TMN, AJCC 8th ed.)

T0	No tumor identified, but EBV-positive cervical LN
T1	Confined to NP or extends to OP &/or nasal cavity w/o posterolateral infiltration
T2	Parapharyngeal extension &/or involvement of prevertebral muscles
T3	Bony involvement of skull base, cervical vertebra, &/or paranasal sinuses
T4	Intracranial extension &/or involvement of CN, hypopharynx, orbit, parotid gland, or w/ extension to the infratemporal fossa/masticator space
N0	No LN mets
N1	Unilateral cervical LN ≤6 cm &/or unilateral or bilateral retropharyngeal LN ≤6 cm above caudal border of cricoid cartilage
N2	Bilateral cervical LN ≤6 cm, above caudal border of cricoid cartilage
N3	(a) LN >6 cm (b) extension below caudal border of cricoid cartilage
M0	No distant met
M1	Distant met

- **Stage I:** T1 N0; **stage II:** T0–1 N1 or T2 N0–1; **stage III:** T0–2 N2 or T3 N0–3; **stage IVA: T4** N0–N2, M0 or Any T & N3, M0; **stage IVB:** Any T, any N, **M1**

Treatment

- Due to the base of skull location, tx for nasopharyngeal carcinomas is radiation based
- **Stage I:** RT alone
- **Stage II, III, & IVA:** Concurrent CRT w/ CIS (INT 0099, *JCO* 1998;16:1310)
- Adj. CIS & 5-FU after concurrent CRT, trend toward benefit without meeting statistical significance (*Lancet Oncol* 2012:13:163). Ongoing trial evaluating adj. chemo based on EBV DNA level (NCT02135042)
- Induction therapy with GEM/CIS often used for pts with T4 or N3 lesions based, although trial data mixed on OS benefit (*NEJM* 2019;381:1124; *Lancet Oncol* 2016;17:1509; *European J Cancer* 2019;119:87; *Ann Oncol* 2018;29:1972)
- Concurrent carbo–RT may replace CIS–RT if CIS contraindicated (*EJC* 2007;43:1399)
- Salvage surgery for small local recurrences & residual dz in neck after CRT
- **Met dz/stage IVB:** Initial tx platinum doublet. GEM + CIS > 5-FU + CIS (*Lancet* 2016;388:1883). The addition of anti-PD1 therapy to platinum-GEM is under investigation

SALIVARY GLAND TUMORS

Definition

- **Major salivary glands:**
  - Parotid (80% of salivary gland tumors, 20% malignant)
  - Submandibular (10% of salivary gland tumors, 50% malignant)
  - Sublingual (<1% of salivary gland tumors, 80% malignant)
- **Minor salivary glands** (throughout upper aerodigestive tract, trachea, breast)

Epidemiology

- 5% of head & neck CAs, 0.5% of all malignancies. 2,000–2,500 cases/y in US

Pathology

- WHO classification into 24 distinct histologic subtypes; heterogeneous tumors that vary in molecular drivers, behaviors, & responses to therapy
- MEC, adenoid cystic carcinoma, adenoCA comprise 75% of salivary gland CAs

Histologic Subtypes

Histologic Subtype	Parotid Gland (%)	Submandibular Gland (%)	Minor Salivary Glands (%)
Adenoid cystic carcinoma	15	45	45
AdenoCA	15	15	20
MEC	40	10	30
Other subtypes	30	30	5

Molecular features

- **Adenoid cystic carcinoma:** t(6;9): *MYB-NFIB* fusion leads to overexpression of c-Myb target genes; high c-kit expression
- **MEC:** t(11;19): *MECT1-MAML2* fusion
- **SDC:** High AR expression, HER2 overexpression
- **Mammary analog secretary tumors:** *ETV6-NTRK3* fusion

General staging

- **Stage I:** ≤2 cm w/o extraparenchymal extension**; stage II:** 2–4 cm w/o extraparenchymal extension**; stage III:** >4 cm &/or extraparenchymal extension &/or + LN <6 cm
- **Stage IV:** Invades skin, mandible, ear canal, facial nerve, skull base, encases carotid artery, &/or LN >6 cm, &/or distant met dz (stage IVC)

Localized disease (stage I–IVB) management

- **Complete surgical resection** if feasible
- **Adj. radiation** if advanced T stage, high-grade, +margins, +locoregional LN

Locoregional recurrence management

- If resectable → salvage surgery; if not resectable → RT for selected pts
- If dz is not amenable to surgery or RT: treat w/ systemic therapy

Metastatic disease (stage IVC) management

- Limited clinical trials to guide systemic therapy
- **Adenoid cystic carcinoma:** Wide natural hx spectrum; indolent, asx dz (especially pulmonary-only mets) is observed; progressive/symptomatic dz is treated
  - **Chemo:** Active agents include CIS, vinorelbine, anthracycline combination tx can result in ↑ ORR, but unclear advantage over monotherapy; Tx includes CIS/doxorubicin/cyclophosphamide (CAP) & CIS/vinorelbine (*Lancet Oncol* 2011;12:815)
  - **VEGFR TKI:** Phase II trial of lenvatinib w/ ↑ ORR/PFS compared to historical studies of other TKIs (*JCO* 2019;37:1529). Phase III trial of axitinib vs observation w/ ↑ PFS benefit (*JCO* 2020;38:no15_suppl:6503)
- **MEC/SDC:**
  - Chemo: Single-agent paclitaxel & CIS-based combination regimens (CAP, CAP-5-FU, CIS/doxorubicin/5-FU, & CIS/methotrexate/bleomycin) have activity, but benefit of triplet over doublet therapy unknown (*JCO* 2006;24:2673)
  - **HER2 overexpression:** 1st line: Trastuzumab/docetaxel with high ORR in phase II (*JCO* 2019;37:125–134). 2nd line: T-DM1 (*JCO* 2019;37:15)
- **AR+ SDC, adenoCA NOS:** Combined androgen blockade (*Ann Oncol* 2018;29:979)
- **Mammary analog secretory tumors:** TRK TKI for *NTRK(+)* fusion (*NEJM* 2018;378:731–739)
- **Histology-agnostic approaches:** IO for TMB high/MMR-deficient tumors

THYROID CANCER

Epidemiology

- Incidence: 2.3% of all CA cases. **Incidence doubled** over the last 20 y, in part due to ↑ detection of small papillary CA; incidence of anaplastic thyroid CA declining
- Mortality: **Mortality rate stable;** 0.4% of all CA deaths, accounts for 95% of endocrine malignancies, but 66% of endocrine CA death
- **Subtypes:**
  Follicular derived:
  - Differentiated: Papillary (80–85% of all thyroid CAs), follicular, Hürthle cell
  - Poorly differentiated & Anaplastic (4–6%)

  C-cell derived (produce calcitonin): Medullary (3–6%)
- Median age at dx 51 y for papillary, late 60s for follicular; 70–80 y for anaplastic

Risk Factors	
Papillary Follicular Anaplastic	• **Radiation** exposure to thyroid gland (esp younger age w/ latency period at least 3–5 y, **linear relationship to exposure dose,** nuclear fallout events including Chernobyl) • Age • Female sex • **FHx** (4–10× ↑ risk in 1st-degree family of papillary/follicular CA pts) • 5% differentiated thyroid CA are a/w FAP, Gardner syn, Cowden syn, Carney complex • No clear causal a/w iodine ingestion • Papillary may have ***RET* fusions**
Medullary	• **20–25%** familial MTC syn (**FMTC), a subtype of MEN2** involves *RET* mt • 75–80% sporadic/nonfamilial involving ***RET* mt**

Biology

- ***MAPK*-signaling pathway:** Mts in 1 of 3 driver genes that do not co-occur in same papillary CA: *BRAF* (~60%), *RAS* (10–15%) & *RET/PTC* (rearrangement in 7%)
- ***RAS* mt & *PAX8-PPAR*** in 35% follicular carcinomas

Clinical presentation and diagnosis

- **Commonly p/w incidental solitary thyroid nodules:** Median tumor size 2–3 cm; 5–10% malignant; higher percentage if radiation exposure; majority nonfunctional; presence of microcalcifications, irregular margins, taller than wide, intranodular hypervascularity are suggestive of malignancy
- U/S: For FNA, to assess number & sonographic characteristics of nodules
- **FNA:** Accuracy of dx 70–97%; varies w/ sample quality, cytopathologist skill; ~70% benign, 4% malignant, 15% suspicious/indeterminate; 10% insufficient sample ***Molecular testing*** can be done on FNA to improve accuracy
- **Medullary:** Familial often detected by genetic screening, test for calcium & plasma metanephrines presurgically; sporadic by asx thyroid mass; **secretory diarrhea if bulky dz with high calcitonin**
- **Anaplastic:** Often prior or concurrent dx of well-diff thyroid CA or benign nodular thyroid dz; **rapidly ↑ palpable neck mass** (median tumor size 8–9 cm); **invasion into airways & recurrent laryngeal nerve (RLN) leads to obstructive sx, hemoptysis, dysphagia, hoarseness;** 20–50% have **distant mets** at dx in lung > bone, liver
- Familial tumors tend to be more aggressive than nonfamilial
- Young pts tend to have bilateral cervical LN mets

Natural history and prognosis

- **Natural hx:** 2/3 pts w/ papillary carcinomas have dz limited to thyroid at dx
- **Prog:** Papillary: 90–95% long-term survival; follicular: 70–80% long-term survival; distant mets strong neg prognostic indicator; anaplastic: Median survival 6–12 mos
- **Poor prognostic factors for well-diff thyroid CA:** Age >55 y, male sex, poorly differentiated histology, tumor size, macroscopic extrathyroidal extension at dx; nodal involvement does not confer ↓ survival in younger pts
- **Several prognostic scoring strategies:** EORTC, AMES (age, mets, extent, & size), & AGES (age, tumor grade, extent, & size)

Staging (AJCC 8 predicts mortality; ATA risk stratification predicts recurrence & mortality)

- **Papillary/follicular, under age 55:** Stage I: M0; stage II: M1
- **Papillary/follicular, 55+:** Stage I: T1–T2 (<4 cm confined to thyroid ± minor ETE); stage II: T1–T2 + N1a/N1b (any size tumor plus LNs) or T3 regardless of LN; stage III: Macro extension to subcutaneous tissues, trachea, esophagus, RLN; stage IVa: Macro extension to prevertebral fascia, major vessels; stage IVb: M1
- **Medullary:** Stage I: T1, node neg; stage II: T2–T3, node neg; stage III: T1–T3, central compartment nodal involvement (N1a); stage IVa: T1–3 + lateral LN involvement (N1b), T4a (macro extension to subcutaneous tissues, trachea, esophagus, RLN); stage IVb: Macro extension to prevertebral fascia, major vessels; stage IVc: M1
- **Anaplastic:** Stage IVa: Intrathyroidal dz; stage IVb: Gross extrathyroidal extension or LN mets; stage IVc: Distant mets

Pathology

- **Cell derivation:** Papillary, follicular, Hürthle cell, anaplastic arise from follicular cells that produce thyroid hormones; tumors usu stain for PAX8, TTF1, Tg positive

Pathology	
Papillary	Papillae; follicular variant has no papillary areas; enlarged, ovoid nuclei that frequently overlap; **propensity to invade lymphatic spaces so high incidence of regional node involvement;** microcarcinoma <1 cm
Follicular	True follicular carcinoma rare (5–10% of nonendemic goiter area thyroid malignancies); unifocal, thickly encapsulated, **invasion of capsule/vessels frequent**
NIFT-P	Noninvasive follicular papillary-like nuclear features (NIFT-P): Premalignant tumor composed of papillae, follicular variant, completely encapsulated, no capsular or vascular invasion. Should not recur or metastasize
Intermediately differentiated tumors	**More aggressive.** 10–15% tumors w/in papillary (tall cell, columnar cell, & diffuse sclerosing variants, insular carcinoma) & follicular subtypes (Hürthle cell [oncocytic, oxyphilic] carcinomas)
Poorly differentiated tumors	Have increased mitoses & necrosis. Follow Turin diagnostic criteria of poorly differentiated thyroid carcinomas. Aggressive locally & with distant mets. Poor survival in the elderly
Medullary	Arises **from calcitonin-producing parafollicular C-cells,** w/c are embryologically from neural crest
Anaplastic	**"Giant cell"** variant, possibly a/w de-differentiation of previously well-diff tumor, rapidly growing, invasive

Treatment

- **Surgery:** Mainstay of tx for all subtypes but rarely possible w/ anaplastic; **complications of total thyroidectomy include recurrent laryngeal nerve injury & hypocalcemia 2/2 hypoparathyroidism**
- **Follicular cell–derived differentiated thyroid CA:** Levothyroxine **suppression of TSH** (a growth factor for thyroid tissue), **RAI administration** to ablate any nl thyroid remnant & as adj. therapy
  - **Met dz:** RAI; external-beam radiotherapy for locally invasive or progressing met; observe indolent, asx metastatic dz; for RAI-refractory dz that is progressive &/or symptomatic: Attempt at redifferentiation with vemurafenib/dabrafenib + RAI for *BRAF* mt tumors; Trametinib + RAI for *RAS* mt tumors. Systemic tx w/ **TKIs, sorafenib** (*JCO* 2008;26:4714) & **lenvatinib** (*NEJM* 2015;372:621). **Selpercatinib** (*Ann Oncol* 2018;29:1869) & **pralsetinib** (*Cancer Disc* 2018;8:836) for *RET* fusion + dz
- **Medullary:** Total thyroidectomy w/ b/l central-compartment node dissection & at least unilateral lateral neck dissection; often resistant to radiation & chemo; targeted therapies **vandetanib** (*JCO* 2012;30:134) & **cabozantinib** (*JCO* 2011;29:2660), **Selpercatinib** & **pralsetinib** for tx of met *RET* mt dz; treat local recurrences surgically; **screen** for germline *RET* gene mt, as total thyroidectomy is preventive in young at-risk family members.
- **Anaplastic thyroid CA: May require urgent tracheostomy;** test for *BRAF* 1st: if positive, start **dabrafenib/trametinib** (*JCO* 2018; 36:7); if unresectable at dx, radiation-based tx, often w/ chemo for sensitization; **RAI not useful**
- **Tumor markers for surveillance: Thyroglobulin** (highly sensitive & specific in the absence of nl thyroid tissue) for follicular-cell origin, differentiated CA; surveillance w/ **CEA & calcitonin** for medullary

SELLAR TUMORS

Sellar masses

Presentation

- Neuro sx: HA (expansion of sella), diplopia (oculomotor nerve compression), visual field deficits (optic chiasm), pituitary apoplexy (sudden hemorrhage into mass), CSF rhinorrhea (inferior extension of mass)
- Hormonal abnormalities (hyper- or hyposecretion; see below)
- Incidental finding on MRI ("incidentaloma")

Causes

- **Pituitary adenomas** = most common cause; ~85% of sellar masses, a/w MEN1
- Also: Physiologic pituitary hyperplasia (pregnancy, 1° hypothyroidism); cyst; abscess; AV fistula of cavernous sinus; hypophysitis (after ICI tx [anti-CTLA4 > anti-PD1/PDL-1] = most common, lymphocytic in postpartum); benign tumors (craniopharyngioma, meningioma); 1° malignant tumors (germ cell, chordoma, 1° CNS lymphoma, sarcoma, pituitary carcinoma—rare); met dz (breast/lung 1° most common); other autoimmune (sarcoidosis, histiocytosis)

Evaluation

- **Sellar MRI w/ & w/o gadolinium:** Best imaging modality
- **Evaluation of pituitary & end organ hormonal fxn:**
  - If <1 cm & asx, prolactin (PRL) screening alone may be the most cost-effective approach (*J Clin Endocrinol Metab* 1997;82:3625)
  - Hormonal *hyper*secretion is caused only by pituitary adenomas (obtain PRL, IGF-1, ACTH, cortisol, 24-h UFC)
  - Hormonal *hypo*secretion can be caused by any hypothalamic or pituitary lesion (2° adrenal insuff, hypothyroidism, hypogonadism, GH def); exception is central DI which indicates a lesion of hypothalamus or stalk
  - Visual field testing if lesion abuts optic chiasm

Pituitary adenoma

Classification: By size & cell of origin

- Size: <1 cm = microadenoma; >1 cm = macroadenoma
- Cell type: Arise from any anterior pituitary cell type; can ↑ secretion of hormone(s) made by that cell &/or ↓ secretion of other hormones due to compression of the nl gland
  - **Gonadotroph:** Usu clinically nonfunctional
  - **Corticotroph:** Cushing w/ nl or ↑ ACTH, defined by elevated 24-h UFC, late night salivary cortisol, & dexamethasone-suppressed serum cortisol
  - **Lactotroph:** ↑ PRL → hypogonadism (M/F)
  - **Thyrotroph:** Can be clinically nonfunctional (secreting only α or TSH-β subunits, or can cause hyperthyroidism from ↑ secretion of intact TSH)
  - **Somatotroph:** ↑ GH/IGF-1 → acromegaly
  - **Lactotroph/somatotroph** combinations also occur, leading to sx of both

Tx

- **Nonfunctioning adenomas:** If neuro sx, TSS is 1st line. If asx but w/ extrasellar extension (ie, optic chiasm contact), discuss TSS (preferred) vs. monitor w/ q3–6 mos exam/MRI. Postop steroid taper, monitor for hormone deficiency, f/u w/ MRI; consider repeat surgery or RT if growth of residual tumor
- **Corticotroph:** 1st r/o other sources for Cushing then TSS is 1st line. If persistence/recurrence: Repeat surgery, medical Rx (adrenal enzyme inhibitors: Ketoconazole, metyrapone, osilodrostat; somatostatin receptor ligand: Pasireotide; dopamine agonist: Cabergoline; cortisol receptor antagonist: Mifepristone), RT if needed for tumor control, or b/l adrenalectomy
- **Lactotroph:** Tx if existing/impending neuro sx due to size, hypogonadism, or other sx due to inc PRL; DA agonist (cabergoline, bromocriptine) is 1st line regardless of tumor size. Pts w /nl PRL & no visible adenoma on MR while on low-dose DA agonist for at least 2 y, can taper down/off w/ monitoring. If drugs ineffective (ie, substantial tumor remains or sx due to ↑ PRL persist), or if fertility is desired, consider TSS. If persistent dz after surgery, consider RT or DA agonist tx
- **Thyrotroph:** Octreotide till euthyroid then TSS is 1st line; many need additional tx (DA agonist/octreotide/RT). βB can ↓ s/s of hyperthyroidism
- **Somatotroph:** TSS is 1st line. If unresectable or if IGF-1 still high following surgery, consider medical tx w/ somatostatin receptor ligand; cabergoline; &/or pegvisomant. If still not successful, RT (for tumor control) or repeat operation

Craniopharyngioma

- Slow growing benign solid & cystic tumors from Rathke's pouch remnants, bimodal age distribution
- **Workup:** MRI or CT (typically a cystic calcified parasellar lesion), endocrine testing
- **Tx:** Surgical resection; if incomplete resection, early postop RT. If recurring *BRAF* V600E-mt papillary craniopharyngioma, consider BRAF +/− MEK inhibitor (*Cancer* 2019;125:2910). If cyst recurs, intracavitary irradiation or chemo w/ bleomycin (*Cancer* 2007;109:2124)

Rathke cleft cyst

- Benign noncancerous cystic remnant from Rathke's pouch, may be asx or cause neuro sx due to local compression
- **Tx:** If neuro sx, TSS is 1st line. If no sx, f/u w/ serial MRI, 15% will ↓ in size, ~30% ↑ in size, & >50% will remain stable (*J Clin Endocrinol Metab* 2015;100:3943)

Primary malignant tumors

Aggressive & malignant pituitary tumors

- Rapidly growing (aggressive) &/or locally invasive. Malignancy defined by presence of noncontiguous mets
- More commonly in males, functional, & with higher Ki-67 index
- **Tx:** Will require multiple surgeries & RT; temozolomide after other tx have failed (*Eur J Endocrinol* 2018;178:G1)

Intracranial GCTs

- Usu occur in children & through 3rd decade of life (up to 40% in young adults; M > F)
- Intracranial GCTs make up ~0.5–3% of pediatric CNS tumors in the United States (more frequent in Asian countries) (*Oncologist* 2008;13:690)
- Sx: Pineal—HA, n/v, lethargy, diplopia, pyramidal tract signs, & ataxia (from ↑ ICP/hydrocephalus), paralysis of upward gaze; suprasellar—hypopituitarism, DI
- **Intracranial GCTs** = germinomas & NGGCTs; the latter includes embryonal carcinoma, endodermal sinus tumor/yolk sac tumor, choriocarcinoma, teratoma (immature & mature), mixed tumors consisting of a combination of these types
  - **Characteristic genetic mts:** *KIT*, *RAS*, & isochromosome 12p in germinomas; *TNFRSF8* in embryonal carcinoma; *ERBB4* in yolk sac tumor (*Commun Biol* 2020;3:544)
  - **Workup:** CSF & serum levels of tumor markers (see below) eval of pituitary fxn, CSF cytology, MRI brain/spine for staging as 10–15% will have leptomeningeal spread at time of dx (*Oncologist* 2000;5:312), bx

Risk Category	Tumor Type	βhCG	AFP	PLAP	c-Kit
Low-risk	Pure germinoma	−	−	+/−	+
	Mature teratoma	−	−	−	−
Intermediate-risk	Immature teratoma	+/−	+/−	−	+/−
	Mixed NGGCTs w/ tumor types from multiple-risk groups	+/−	+/−	+/−	+/−
High-risk	Choriocarcinoma	+	−	+/−	−
	Yolk sac tumor	−	+	+/−	−
	Embryonal carcinoma	−	−	+	−
	Mixed NGGCTs composed mainly of high-risk histologies	+/−	+/−	+/−	+/−

Tx:

- **Localized pure germinoma:** Whole-ventricular RT (21–24 Gy) w/ boost to 1° tumor (total dose 40–45 Gy) (*Int J Radiat Oncol Biol Phys* 2003;56:511) or neoadj chemo w/ 2 courses of carboplatin & etoposide, alternating w/etoposide & ifosfamide followed by ↓ dose RT (*Neuro Oncol* 2013;15;788). Note: Treat bifocal tumors (pineal & suprasellar components) as localized tumors if MRI spine & CSF cytology are neg (*Int J Radiat Oncol Biol Phys* 82:1341)
- **Disseminated germinoma** (identified by MRI &/or CSF cytology): Craniospinal RT (24 Gy) w/ boost to 1° tumor (total dose 40 Gy) (*Neuro Oncol* 2013;15:788)
- **NGGCT:** Neoadj plat & etoposide (*Cancer* 2003;98:369) +/− ifosfamide or cyclophosphamide (*JCO* 2015;33;2464)) followed by craniospinal RT w/ tumor boost (*Neuropediatrics* 2005;36:71). If residual tumor, "second-look" surgery with total resection (*J Neurosurg Pediatr* 2010;6:125)
- **Mature teratoma:** Surgical resection (do not respond to chemo/RT)

Chordomas

- Rare (~300 cases in the United States annually), slow growing, locally aggressive neoplasms of bone that arise from embryonic remnants of notochord; can arise in the clivus
- **Common sx:** HA, diplopia, facial numbness, & cranial neuropathies

- **Histologic subtypes:** Conventional (most common, cartilaginous, or other mesenchymal components absent), chondroid (chordomatous & chondromatous features); sarcomatous transformation (2–8% of chordomas; poorer prog)
- **Workup:** MRI w/ contrast, IHC w/ + CK; + EMA >80% of cases; other stains variable
- **Tx:** Surgical resection followed by RT (proton preferred) (*Surg Neurol Int* 2019;10:96). If advanced dx, imatinib (*Eur J Cancer* 2015;51:2609) vs. targeted tx (against PDFGR, EGFR, VEGFR, or mTOR)

Primary CNS lymphoma involving the pituitary

- Very rare ~0.1–0.3% of pituitary tumors
- **Common sx:** HA & visual/oculomotor impairment &/or deficiencies of anterior pituitary hormones & ADH/DI
- **Workup:** Contrast-enhanced MRI = sellar mass w/ variable extrasellar extension
- **Tx:** Remains controversial—some treat as a systemic lymphoma; some w/ CNS lymphoma regimens; some w/ a combination of both (see Primary CNS Lymphoma)

Metastases to the pituitary gland

- Mets to the hypothalamus & pituitary gland = ~1–2% of sellar masses. Most common w/ breast & lung CA but also occurs in other CA (renal cell, hepatocellular, prostate, colon)
- **Presentation** (sx occur in ~60%): DI (most common), panhypopituitarism, visual field deficits, retroorbital pain, ophthalmoplegia
- **Tx:** Local surgery or RT for sx mets; systemic Rx is dictated by 1° tumor type
- **OS** very poor (between 6–22 mos) (*Neurosurg Focus* 2004;16:E8)

PHEOCHROMOCYTOMA/PARAGANGLIOMA

Epidemiology & biology

- Catecholamine (norepi, epi, dopamine) secreting tumor arising from chromaffin cells in adrenal medulla (pheochromocytoma) or sympathetic ganglia (paraganglioma)
- Sporadic cases present at 40–50 y, no gender predilection
- **40% hereditary:** >30 genes assoc, most commonly *VHL* mt (1/3 of cases), MEN2 (*RET* mt), *NF1* mt, often detected earlier in childhood due to biochemical surveillance
- SDHA/SDHB/SDHC/SDHD: Familial pheochromocytoma/paraganglioma syn. *SDHB* mts—assoc with malignant potential, shorter survival, GIST, RCC
- **10% rule:** 10% bilateral, 10% extraadrenal, 10% metastatic/malignant
- 60% dx'd in presympatomatic phase due to incidental adrenal mass on imaging

Clinical presentation & diagnosis

- **Classic sx triad:** HA, diaphoresis, tachycardia; refractory or paroxysmal HTN/ "spells"; other = palpitations, tremor, pallor, dyspnea
- More commonly assoc with systolic & diastolic HTN, 15% have nl BP
- Initial testing: **24-h urine-fractionated metanephrines** + **catecholamines** (98% sens, 98% spec); if high suspicion (family hx, genetic syn, prior pheo, adrenal mass with imaging characteristics of pheo), **plasma fract metanephrines** (~100% sens, 85% spec). If nl, no further testing. If ↑, obtain CT AP or MRI
- CT/MRI findings: Hounsfield unit (HU) >10 on noncon CT, contrast enhancement with delayed washout (<50% at 10 min), high signal intensity on T2-weighted MR, cystic & hemorrhagic changes, bilaterality, or large size (>4 cm)
- If neg CT/MRI & high suspicion, consider MIBG (norepi analog), FDG-PET, DOTATE-PET, octreotide scan (useful in detecting dedifferentiated pheos)

Treatment

- **Surgery:** Preop management w/ BP control, HTN crisis prevention, volume expansion
  - Avoid unopposed β-blockade, glucagon, histamine, metoclopramide, & high dose corticosteroids as these can provoke pheochromocytoma paroxysm
  - **α-adrenergic blockade** with phenoxybenzamine (preferred) or selective α-1-adrenergic blockers (prazosin, terazosin, doxazosin) 7–14-d preop to control BP/ expand contracted blood volume, then **low-dose β-blockade** 2–3-d preop
  - **High sodium diet** (>5 g/day) after 2–3 d of α-blockade to counteract volume contraction & orthostasis (may be contraindicated in CHF/renal insuff)
  - **Ca channel blockers** (nicardipine, amlodipine) to supplement BP control as needed or as alternative if **α-blockers** not tolerated
  - **Metyrosine** (inhibits catecholamine synthesis) alternative agent when α/β-blockade is ineffective or contraindicated, or if plans for RFA or cryoablation of mets
  - Sporadic adrenal pheo requires complete adrenalectomy (laparoscopic vs. retroperitoneal approach); familial pheo (ie, *MEN2, VHL*) can consider partial cortical-sparing adrenalectomy to prevent adrenal insufficiency given ↑ incidence of bilateral tumors. If bilateral adrenalectomy, administer stress-dose steroids
  - Intraoperative phentolamine drip. For HTN crisis tx: Nitroprusside, phentolamine or nicardipine
  - Given risk of recurrence, monitor with annual biochemical screening after surgery. Genetic testing rec for all pts for malignant risk stratification
- **Metastatic pheo (10%):** Histologically/biochemically identical to benign; dx by local invasion (LN, kidney, liver) or distant mets. Paragangliomas 20% malignant
  - **No curative tx.** Surgical resection of 1° tumor & mets to decrease hormone secretion & sx, improve response to subsequent tx. No improved survival.
  - Local therapy: EBRT, RFA, cryoablation, percutaneous EtOH injection, transarterial chemoembolization of liver mets, all demonstrate local tumor burden control & symptomatic relief; can induce catecholamine secretion/HTN crisis
  - Systemic therapy: Goal is sx palliation & tumor stabilization/regression
    - **MIBG/I-131** effective in 60% of tumors that take up MIBG, most effective if low dz burden & soft tissue (not bone) mets, ineffective after EBRT
    - **Radiolabeled somatostatin analogs** if tumor expresses somatostatin receptors (DOTATE PET uptake), currently investigational use only (Lutetium)
    - **Octreotide**—unclear benefit, trial if not a candidate for other systemic therapy

- **Chemo—**if unresectable, rapidly progressive, high tumor burden, significant bone mets. Regimens include cyclophosphamide, dacarbazine, vincristine, doxorubicin. Temozolomide may be useful if *SDHB* mt (case reports only)
- **TKIs—**sunitinib may be useful in small open-label trial. Other TKIs in clinical trials
- Additional trials of everolimus & HIF2A inhibitors are ongoing

MEN1

- **Autosomal dominant** mt in *MEN1* gene, **3 Ps**: Parathyroid, anterior pituitary, enteropancreatic cell tumors

Clinical presentation

- **1° hyperPTH/multiple parathyroid adenomas:** Often 1st manifestation, almost 100% penetrance by 40–50 y. Usu asx, ↑ Ca^{2+} & inappropriately ↑ serum PTH. High risk of recurrence even after adenoma resection. Multiple gland involvement more common in MEN1 than sporadic hyperPTH
- **Pituitary adenomas:** 15–20% penetrance. Prolactinoma most common; lower frequency of somatotroph, corticotroph, cosecreting, nonfunctional tumors; macroadenomas & hormonal hypersecretion after tx more common in pts w/ MEN
- **Pancreatic islet cell/GI tumors:** 30% penetrance. Zollinger–Ellison most common (gastrin); also insulinoma, somatostatinoma, glucagonoma, VIPoma, clinically nonfunctioning tumors
- **Other tumors:** Carcinoid, cutaneous tumors, adrenal tumors, pheo, ependymoma

Diagnosis and treatment

- **Dx: 2 of 3 main MEN-assoc tumors** (1 of 3 in family members of MEN1 pt). Genetic testing rec in all index cases & 1st -degree relatives
- **Tx: Subtotal parathyroidectomy** or complete parathyroidectomy with autotransplantation of parathyroid tissue for pts with symptomatic hyperCA; pituitary adenomas tx similar to sporadic cases (see Pituitary Adenomas under Sellar Tumors); **PPI** for gastrinoma, unclear role of surgical resection given often multifocal & small; **surgery** for insulinoma (local excision of tumor in pancreatic head + distal subtotal pancreatectomy)
- **Screening:** Established MEN1 pts, known carriers, at-risk family members monitor **sx of MEN1-assoc tumors** (nephrolithiasis, amenorrhea, galactorrhea, erectile dysfunction, peptic ulcers, diarrhea, hypoglycemia); annual serum Ca^{2+}, PTH, & prolactin

MEN2

- Autosomal dominant mt in *RET* proto-oncogene; predisposition to thyroid, parathyroid, & adrenal tumors

Clinical presentation

MEN2A	- MTC (100%), pheo (50%), 1° hyperparathyroidism (HPT) (25%) - Penetrance of MTC nearly 100% but variability in other manifestations - Regular evaluation for pheo & hyperPTH is rec - Further subclassified into classic, cutaneous lichen amyloidosis (CLA), Hirschsprung dz (HD), & familial MTC (FMTC) - FMTC has strong predisposition to MTC w/o other CAs; difficult to distinguish in small families
MEN2B	- MTC (earlier, more aggressive phenotype than MEN2A), pheo, mucosal neuromas, intestinal ganglioneuromas, marfanoid habitus; no hyperPTH

Diagnosis and treatment

- Suspect dx in any pt with MTC or pheochromocytoma, especially if dx <35 y
- Index pt with 1–2 classical clinical features should be genotyped to identify **germline *RET* mt**. 1st & 2nd-degree family members should be genotyped as early dx & specific *RET* allele predicts age of onset, aggressiveness of MTC, & incidence of other endocrine neoplasms
- For family members of MEN2 pts who refuse genetic testing, **pentagastrin** or **Ca stimulation test** can be used to screen for MTC
- All pts require **prophylactic thyroidectomy** (timing depends on specific *RET* mt [M918T most aggressive]), & annual screening for pheo & hyperPTH
- **Initial management of MTC** in suspected MEN2 pts:
  - **Screen for pheo** prior to thyroidectomy. If found, resect pheo 1st (note freq bilateral)

- **Limited local dz/local mets:** Total thyroidectomy & central neck dissection; if lateral neck LNs & no/limited distant mets, proceed with lateral neck dissection; if adv local/distant dz, consider limited neck surgery
- **Postoperative monitoring** for recurrent MTC

Undetectable postop calcitonin	- Check calcitonin/CEA q6–12 mos - Neck U/S 6–12 mos postop
Detectable postop calcitonin <150 pg/mL	- Neck U/S ± baseline CT/MRI
Postop calcitonin >150 pg/mL	- CT or MRI of CAP + bone scan or bone MRI to r/o distant metastatic dz

- **Persistent/metastatic MTC: RT** to neck/upper mediastinum in pts with extrathyroidal dz/nodal mets (if curative dissection impossible)
- **Systemic tx for progressive met dz:** Oral TKIs (vandetanib, cabozantinib preferred over sorafenib or sunitinib); dacarbazine-based chemo if dz progresses despite multiple TKIs; immunotherapy & radiolabeled octreotide (investigational)
  - ***RET*-mt:** FDA-approved RET inhibitors: Selpercatinib, pralsetinib

TUMORS OF THE ADRENAL CORTEX

Epidemiology

- **Adrenal "incidentalomas"** are adrenal nodules identified on imaging performed for other reasons. Prevalence is 4% on abdominal imaging. Most are benign & nonfunctional
- **ACC** are extremely rare (incidence 1–2 per million), bimodal age distribution (1st & 5th decade); female to male ratio is ~2:1

Etiology and genetics of ACC

- RF are not understood due to rarity; possibly smoking & contraceptive use in women
- Majority are **sporadic**. Can be a/w **hereditary syn:** Li–Fraumeni, Beckwith–Wiedemann, MEN1, Lynch, FAP, NF-1. High incidence in Southern Brazilian children, distinct germline *TP53* mt identified (R337H)
- Susceptibility genes: Sporadic tumors have been a/w *TP53* mt

Clinical manifestation

- Vast majority are unilateral (90–98%)
- Most met at dx; most common to periadrenal tissue, LN, lungs, liver, bone
- Nonfunctional tumors (30%) p/w fever, abdominal/back pain, early satiety, wt loss
- **40–60% ACC are hormone secreting** & p/w signs & sx of hormone excess (see table)

Hormone Secretion	Presentation	Functional Evaluation
Cortisol (Cushing syn, also known as ACTH-independent Cushing)—30–40%	Wt gain, proximal weakness, hirsutism, psychiatric disturbances, HTN, osteoporosis, edema, hypokalemia, central obesity, purple striae, hyperglycemia	ACTH, cortisol levels → overnight dexamethasone suppression test w/ AM cortisol testing OR × 3 midnight salivary cortisol OR 24-h urine cortisol w/ suppressed ACTH
Androgen-secreting tumor—20–30%	Hirsutism, male pattern baldness, deepening of voice, oligo/amenorrhea	DHEAS, testosterone
Estrogen-secreting tumor—10%	Gynecomastia & testicular atrophy	Estradiol
Aldosterone-secreting tumor—<5%	HTN, hypokalemia, alkalosis	Screening test: Serum aldosterone: Renin ratio >30 w/ an aldosterone >15 If screen is +, need to do either salt, saline, or captopril suppression testing to confirm

Workup and evaluation of adrenal nodule/mass

- Structural evaluation: CT scan or MRI abdomen to determine size, heterogeneity, lipid content (MRI), Hounsfield Units (HU), margin characteristics
- **Imaging characteristics of adenomas vs. carcinomas**
  - **Adenomas:** Often <4 cm, HU <10 precontrast, >50% HU washout 15 min post-IV contrast, signal drop off on MRI chemical shift (*Radiology* 2002;222:629)
  - **ACC:** Ave size: 10–13 cm, only 3% are less than 4 cm; w/ heterogeneous, irregular margins; local invasion w/ evidence of necrosis on CT
- FNA bx will not distinguish adenoma from ACC but can help distinguish ACC vs. met
- Is there a h/o prior malignancy? → met adrenal masses are common in pts w/ active 1° dz; it is typically not the 1st presentation of 1° CA elsewhere
- Most common potential primaries of met dz are lung, breast, melanoma, RCC, lymphoma, leukemia, pancreatic, colonic, ovarian
- **Must r/o pheochromocytoma prior to bx or surgery.** Otherwise, risk of hypertensive crisis w/o α-adrenergic blockade. Sporadic pheochromocytomas can be found in adrenal cortex. Pheo typically have high HU on CT (>30 sec) & bright on T2 MRI. Exclude pheo w/ fractionated plasma &/or 24-h urine metanephrines
- Surgical pathology confirms dx w/ ≥3 Weiss criteria: Capsule/vessel invasion, changes in growth patterns, tumor necrosis, increased mitotic rates, & atypical mitotic figures

Staging

- Multiple staging systems exist: ENSAT, most common AJCC/UICC for adults:
  - Stage I: Tumor ≤5 cm (T1N0M0)

- Stage II: Tumor >5 cm, no extraadrenal invasion (T2N0M0)
- Stage III: Any regional LN spread (T1–2N1M0) or local invasion (T3–T4N0M0)
- Stage IV: Distant mets (T1–3, N0–1, M1)

Management: Localized adrenal carcinoma

- **Surgery:** Complete surgical resection is the only potentially curative tx for adrenal carcinoma. Open adrenalectomy w/ lymphadenectomy should be performed at specialized referral center. Complete resection may require removal of adjacent structures (liver, kidney, pancreas, spleen). ↑ risk for local recurrence & peritoneal spread when done laparoscopically. Retrospective data of locoregional LN dissection showed reduced recurrence & dz-related death (*Ann Surg* 2012;255:363)
- **Adj. chemo:** Adj. mitotane to be considered, esp in high-risk pts (eg, incomplete resection, Ki67 >10%, >20 mitotic figures per 50 hpf, tumor spillage, or vascular/capsular invasion). Improved DFS vs. observation alone in retrospective study (*NEJM* 2007;356:2372); however, data are scarce. Optimal duration of tx also unknown
- **Adj. radiation:** Controversial; consider external beam RT to tumor bed, esp if close margins or tumor spillage. Small retrospective analyses show ↓ local recurrence but no DFS or OS benefit (*J Clin Endocrinol Metab* 2006;91:4501; *Int J Radiat Oncol Biol Phys* 2015;92:252)
- **Surveillance:** Imaging & hormone testing every 3–6 mos until 5 y

Management: Metastatic adrenal carcinoma

- Clinical trials should be considered for all eligible pts
  - **Low-grade tumor:** Consider resection of 1° tumor & mets if >90% removable, particularly if functional. ↓ tumor burden, sx
  - **Metastatic/unresectable:**

    Mitotane monotherapy—only FDA-approved drug, RR <25% (*JCEM* 2006;91(6):2027). No standard optimal dose of mitotane; has narrow therapeutic index. Some institutions recommend target serum levels of 14–20 μg/mL if tolerated. Studies suggest such levels are needed to achieve benefit. Mitotane is adrenolytic → pts should receive hydrocortisone empirically to prevent the development of adrenal insufficiency; can also cause aldosterone deficiency, hypothyroidism, hyperlipidemia

    EDP (etoposide, doxorubicin, cisplatin) + mitotane: ↑ RR (23% vs. 9.2%), PFS (5 mos vs. 2.1 mos) but no OS benefit vs. streptozocin + mitotane. Significant tox 58% AEs (FIRM-ACT, *NEJM* 2012;366:2189)

    Consider **RT** or **RFA** for palliative local control

    Newer agents in clinical trials–PD-1 inhibitors, proteasome inhibitors, [^{131}I]IMTO radionuclide therapy

Medical management for hormonal control

- Hypercortisolism: Mitotane, mifepristone, metyrapone, ketoconazole
- Hyperandrogenemia: Spironolactone
- Hyperestrogenism: Aromatase inhibitors & SERMS
- Hyperaldosteronism: Spironolactone or eplerenone

Prognosis

- Overall prog remains very poor
- 5-y survival at MSKCC in 1999 reported at 37% (median survival 38 mos), which had a strong association w/ completeness of resection (*Ann Surg Oncol* 1999;6:719). Median OS 17 mos (*J Clin Med Res* 2018;10:636)
- Even stage I, II, & III dz have a 27%, 46%, 63% 2-y risk of distant met, respectively (*J Clin Endocrinol Metab* 2006;91:2650)
- Stage, completeness of resection, pathologic grade are most important prognostic factors

MSKCC Poor Prognostic Factors
1. Stage; presence of distant met at presentation
2. Venous, capsular, or adjacent organ invasion
3. Presence of tumor necrosis
4. Mitotic figures >5/50 hpf
5. Presence of atypical mitoses
6. Mdm2 overexpression (staining of target gene of p53)

(*JCO* 2002;20:941)

Figure 19-1 Survival by number of prognostic factors.

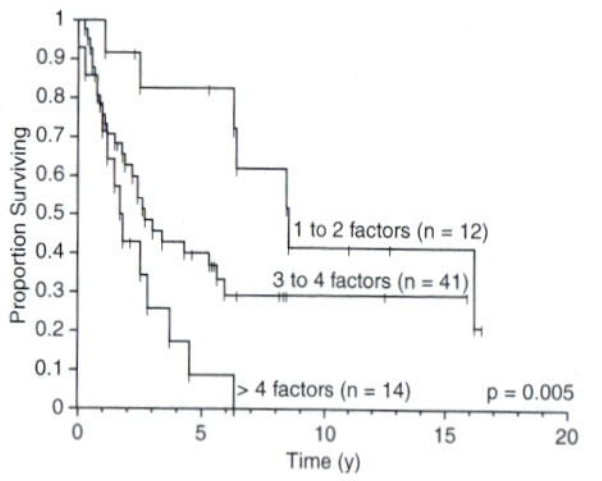

OVARIAN CANCER

Epidemiology

- Ovarian CA is the leading cause of death from gyn CA in the United States
- 5th most common cause of CA mortality in ♀ in the United States, ~21,500 new cases/y
- Median age at dx is 63 y; >70% present w/ adv dz
- Fallopian tube & 1° peritoneal CA: Similar entities to Ovarian CA

Risk factors

- Advancing age, early menarche, late menopause, obesity, PCOS, nulliparity, infertility, older age at 1st birth (>35 y)
- Conversely, a 30–60% ↓ risk of CA a/w younger age at pregnancy & 1st birth (≤25 y), OCPs, salpingectomy, &/or breast-feeding
- Up to 24% of ♀ w/ ovarian CA have a germline CA-predisposition gene mt (*PNAS* 2011;108:18032)

Etiology

- HGS may originate in fallopian tube fimbria as STIC (*J Clin Oncol* 2008;26:4160)
- Low-grade serous & serous borderline a/w *KRAS/BRAF* muts
- Clear cell & endometrioid histologies a/w endometriosis (*ARID1A/MMR*)

Germline genetics (see Principles of Hereditary Cancer Syndromes and Hereditary Breast and Ovarian Cancers chapter)

- All pts w/ EOC should be referred for genetic risk evaluation & potential opportunity for cascade testing
- ***BRCA1* or 2 mt:** AD inheritance. ~12–15% of women w/ ovarian CA. Most definable cause of hereditary ovarian CA, esp in AJ population. *BRCA1:* By age 70, risk of ovarian CA 40%. *BRCA2*: By age 70, risk of ovarian CA 10–20%. Possible better progs: ↑ sensitivity to platinum-based chemo (*JCO* 2012;30:2654) & PARP inhibitors (see below)
- **DDR mt:** *BRIP1* (RRSO 45–50 y), *RAD51C/D* > *PALB2*, *ATM* > *NBN* consider management of the latter 3 based on FHx; a/w ~3–8% hereditary ovarian CA
- **Lynch syn:** AD inheritance. Germline mt of MMR genes (*MLH1, MSH2, MLH6, PMS2*). Lifetime risk of ovarian CA 5–15%, ↑ risk CRC, uterine CA, stomach CA

Pathology subtypes

- **Epithelial (EOC)** (90%): 5 main types—HGS (most common ~75%, WT1+ &/or PAX8+), endometrioid, clear cell, low-grade serous, mucinous, transitional cell
- **Germ cell** (See Ovarian Germ Cell Tumor chapter)
- **Sex cord-stromal** (<2%) heterogeneous, often early stage, can produce androgens, estrogen: Granulosa (inhibin B as tumor marker, 5–10% a/w early-stage uterine CA), theca, Sertoli–Leydig (*DICER1*). Surgery ± chemo (BEP or taxane/carbo [T/C]). Consider RT if pelvic recurrence. Consider hormone manipulation

Screening and prevention

- Asx ♀ at average risk should NOT undergo ovarian CA screening
- UKCTOCS trial: Screening w/ annual TVUS vs. CA 125 vs. no screening × 16.3 y did not ↓ ovarian CA mortality (*Lancet* 2021;397:2182)
- In high-risk ♀ (hereditary syn, *BRCA1/2+*) can consider multimodality screening (TVUS & CA 125 every 6 mos starting at age 30–35 or 5–10 y earlier than earliest age of 1st ovarian CA in family), but RRSO is most effective way to ↓ risk of ovarian/fallopian tube CA. RRSO is rec post childbearing or by age 35–40 y. In premenopausal *BRCA*+ ♀ can also ↓ breast CA risk
- OCP use in *BRCA*+ ♀ a/w ↓ ovarian CA risk (~5%/y of OCP use)

Clinical manifestations/diagnosis

- 70% EOC tumors have spread beyond true pelvis (≥ stage III) at dx
- Persistent, nonspecific sxs: abd/pelvic pain/mass/bloating, urinary urgency or frequency, constipation, early satiety, dyspnea, VTE (↑ in clear cell), torsion (germ cell), rarely vaginal bleeding or paraneoplastic syn: Cerebellar degeneration, polyneuritis, DM, ↑ Ca^{2+} (small cell)
- ↑ CA 125 in 20% early & 80% adv-stage EOC; CA 125: CEA >25 = müllerian 1° likely
- CT CAP to determine if complete gross resection feasible

Surgical management EOC

- **Presumed early stage:** Hysterectomy/BSO w/ comprehensive staging (inspection of all peritoneal surfaces, bx of suspicious areas/adhesions, omentectomy, pelvic, & paraaortic LND) is 1° procedure to establish dx/accurate dz extent, & for maximal cytoreduction

- **Presumed adv stage:** Diagnostic laparoscopy to determine resectability if appropriate. If resectable, proceed to primary debulking (PDS). If not resectable, consider neoadj therapy followed by interval debulking surgery (IDS)
- Mucinous tumors: + Appendectomy & explore upper & lower GI tract
- **Optimal debulking (opt)** → residual tumor <1 cm max diameter or thickness
- Ideally performed by gyn oncologist & goal is complete gross resection

Stage	Definition	5-y Survival (%)[a]
Stage I	Confined to ovary or ovaries. A: 1 ovary; B: Both ovaries; C: Surgical spill, capsule rupture before surgery or surface involvement, or malig cells in peritoneal washings or ascites	85–95 (90–95 for IA or IB)
Stage II	Pelvic extension. A: Implants/extension on uterus, fallopian tubes or ovaries; B: Extension to other pelvic tissues	70–80
Stage III	Spread into but confined to abdomen. A: Abd mets microscopic or + RP LNs; B: Abd mets macroscopic but ≤2 cm; C: Abd mets >2 cm	25–50
Stage IV	Spread outside abd &/or parenchymal mets	5–19

[a]Prognosis also depends on age, extent of residual disease, and histology.

Early-stage adjuvant treatment of EOC

- **Low-grade serous or endometrioid:** No role for adj. chemo in select pts
- **HGS or endometrioid:** Grade 3+ stage IA/IB or any grade stage IC → adj. tx w/ IV T/C × 3–6 cycles; ↑ DFS & OS
- **Less common histologies:** Tx depends on histology

Advanced-stage (II–IV) treatment

- 6 cycles taxane/platinum chemo; consider Bev if suboptimal debulking, ascites, stage IV
- **Maintenance:** If *BRCA* mut → olaparib (SOLO-1, *NEJM* 2018;379:2495) OR niraparib (PRIMA, *NEJM* 2019;381:2391). If *BRCA*1/2 neg (germline or somatic), perform HRD testing. If HRD+ consider niraparib (PRIMA) OR Bev + olaparib (PAOLA-1); if HRD test (–) observe or continue Bev maintenance
- **Stage II & stage III optimally debulked (<1 cm):** IV/IP paclitaxel & IP CIS vs. IV alone as IP more toxic. In stage III opt debulked pts, median PFS ↑ 6 mos (23.8 vs. 18), median OS ↑ 16 mos (65.6 vs. 49.7) compared w/ q3wk IV dosing. ↑ Tox w/ IP: Fatigue, pain, neuropathy, renal, IP port complications (GOG 172, *NEJM* 1996;354:34). Bev ↑ PFS 1.7–4 mos but not OS (*NEJM* 2011;365:2473; *NEJM* 2011;365:2484)
- **Residual dz >1 cm, stage IV, not IP candidate:** Q3wk dosing vs. consider dose-dense IV T/C (weekly paclitaxel) esp Japanese pts. In stage II–IV (opt & subop) dose-dense IV T/C vs. q3wk T/C: ↑ PFS 11 mos (28 vs. 17) & ↑ 3-y OS by 7% (72% vs. 65%) (*Lancet* 2009;374:1331). In stage III & IV (subop), dose-dense IV T/C vs. q3wk T/C, ± Bev: ↑ PFS (14.2 vs. 10.3 mos) w/ dose dense in pts who did not receive Bev (*NEJM* 2016;374:738)
- **Unresectable bulky dz or poor PS:** Obtain bx for dx. Neoadj T/C chemo × 3–6 cycles → interval tumor debulking → postop chemo (EORTC-GCG/NCIC 55971 *NEJM* 2010;363:943-53); MRC CHORUS trial (*Lancet* 2015;386:249-57) also showed neoadj chemo → interval debulking surgery (IDS) not inferior to primary debulking surgery (PDS). Complete gross resection strongest predictor of OS
- **HIPEC:** Stage III dz: Neoadj → IDS + HIPEC ↑ RFS 3.5 mos, ↑ OS 12 mos (*NEJM* 2018;378:230)

Recurrent disease

- Majority of adv-stage recur. Platinum-refractory if progression on or <1 mo from 1° platinum. Platinum-resistant if recurrence 1–6 mos after completing platinum
- **Platinum-resistant:** Single-agent lipo dox, gem, topo, taxane + Bev ↑ PFS by ~3 mos (AURELIA *JCO* 2014;32:1302)
- **Platinum-sensitive (recurrence ≥6 mos):** Platinum-based doublet (carbo+gem/liposomal dox/paclitaxel) ± 2° cytoreduction. 1st recurrence → +Bev ↑ PFS 4 mos (12.4 vs. 8.4) (OCEANS *JCO* 2012;30:2039); serial relapse/remission w/ chemo until platinum-resistant
- **PARPi** (See section on Pharmacology): Olaparib approved for germline *BRCA* 1/2+ s/p ≥3 lines of chemo, RR 31% (*J Clin Oncol* 2015;33:244); rucaparib approved for germline or somatic *BRCA*1/2+ s/p ≥2 lines of chemo, RR 42% (ARIEL2 *Lancet Oncol.* 2017;18(1):75); niraparib approved for platinum-sensitive HRD+ s/p ≥4 lines of chemo, RR 29% (QUADRA *Lancet Oncol* 2019;20:636).
  - **Maintenance:** All 3 PARPi approved as maintenance in phase III studies of PARPi post response to platinum retreatment w/ ↑ PFS (SOLO2 *Lancet Oncol* 2017;18(9):1274; ARIEL3 *Lancet* 2017;390(10106):1949; NOVA *NEJM* 2016;375:2154)
  - **Tox:** PARPi a/w ~2% ↑ MDS/leukemia, among other AEs

OVARIAN GERM CELL TUMORS

Epidemiology

- 0.41 per 100,000 in the United States; 2–3% of all ovarian malignancies; 11% of CAs in adolescents
- 20% of all benign ovarian tumors; usu present at **early stage** in **young women** median age 16–20 y (range 6–60 y) (*IJGC* 2020;30:879)
- ↑ rate in Asian/Pacific islanders/Hispanic population > Caucasians
- Risk factor: Gonadal dysgenesis (developmental anomaly) (*IJGC* 2014;24:S48)
- Tumors tend to be large at dx (median size = 16 cm)

Benign Tumors
Mature cystic teratoma: 5–25% of OGCTs; 10–20% bilateral; 1–2% malignant degeneration; often present w/ thickened area from which hair & teeth can arise (Rokitansky protuberance)
Malignant OGCT (MOGCT)
• **Dysgerminoma (35–50%):** Most common MOGCT; ovarian counterpart of testicular seminoma; 75% of pts are adolescents & young adults (avg age = 19); can produce estrogen, testosterone, β-hCG, & LDH; can cause menstrual abnormalities; usu diagnosed at stage IA; spreads via lymphatics; highly radiosensitive; 10–15% bilateral; histology w/ fried egg appearance; better prog than nondysgerminomas • **Yolk sac/endodermal sinus tumors (14–20%):** Usu present in adolescents (median age = 19); spreads intraperitoneally & hematogenously, usu produces AFP & LDH; histology w/ Schiller–Duval bodies • **Embryonal carcinoma (4%):** Most aggressive OGCT; usu produce hCG ±; AFP; spreads intraperitoneally; mean age <30 y; histology w/ sheets & ribbons • **Polyembryoma:** Rare, treated like nondysgerminomas • **Nongestational choriocarcinoma (2.1%):** Aggressive; mean age 20; produces β-hCG if arise from ovary; can cause precocious puberty; relatively chemoresistant • **Mixed germ cell tumor: (10–15%):** Treated like nondysgerminomas; 5–10% bilateral
Malignant Teratoma
• **Immature teratoma (~20%):** Graded from well-diff to poorly differentiated based on portion of tissue in histologic section containing immature neural elements; 75% present in 1st, 2nd decades of life; 12–15% bilateral; 60–70% stage I; rarely produce tumor markers • **Monodermal teratoma:** Teratoma composed predominantly of 1 tissue element; most common **"struma ovarii":** Mature thyroid tissue which can cause hyperthyroidism; can be benign. Other types: **Carcinoid** (1/3 present w/ carcinoid syn), **melanoma, sarcoma, sebaceous tumor, pituitary type, etc.;** chemo directed at transformed component

Risk factors and clinical manifestations

- **Risk factors for poor prog:** Advanced FIGO stage, age >45 y, nondysgerminoma or grade 2/3 immature teratoma, incomplete surgical resection/residual dz, elevation of both hCG & AFP tumor markers preoperatively (*JCO* 2006;24:4862; *IJGC*, 2014;24:S48)
- **Sx:** Abd pain & palpable pelvic abd mass (85%), distension (35%), fever (10-25%), vaginal bleeding from β-hCG/estrogen production (10%), precocious puberty 2/2 to β-hCG production (rare), NMDA receptor encephalitis (rare), hyperthyroidism (2/2 struma ovarii)
- **Growing teratoma syn:** Rare complication of immature teratomas 2/2 enlarging teratoma that becomes mature during chemo; needs prompt surgery

Serum Tumor Markers in MOGCTs

Histology	AFP	β-hCG	LDH
Dysgerminoma	–	±	+
Yolk sac/endodermal sinus tumor	+	–	+
Immature teratoma	±	–	±
Mixed germ cell tumor	±	±	±
Choriocarcinoma	–	+	±
Embryonal carcinoma	±	+	±
Polyembryoma	±	+	±

Staging and workup

- **Laparotomy w/ TAH/BSO w/ comprehensive staging** (for all ovarian CAs, establish stage, & max cytoreduction) + serum tumor markers: AFP, LDH, β-hCG, CA 125; CXR, pelvic U/S or MRI/CT abd/pelvis. Karyotype if gonadal dygenesis suspected. Use tumor markers to monitor response to tx & recurrence. R/O pregnancy if β-hCG ↑ if malignancy suspected in young pt. Tumor markers (AFP, LDH, β-hCG) should be measured *preoperatively* to determine if these are good markers to follow
- **Fertility preservation:** Fertility-sparing surgery (unilateral salpingo-oophorectomy, removal of abnl lesions) for pt w/ apparent early-stage & good-risk tumor; for children or adolescents, comprehensive staging may be omitted (based on tumor type, imaging/markers). Discuss embryo cryopreservation. If not feasible, cryopreservation of oocytes or ovarian tissue are options (experimental)
- **Stage I:** Confined to ovaries or fallopian tubes (FT) (**IA:** Single ovary/FT; **IB:** Both ovaries or FTs; **IC:** Ovarian/FT involvement w/: ***IC1*** surgical spill; ***IC2*** surface involvement or preop capsule rupture; ***IC3*** positive peritoneal/ascitic washings)
- **Stage II:** Extension to other pelvic tissues or **1**° peritoneal (**IIA:** Extension to uterus/FT; **IIB:** Extension to other pelvic intraperitoneal tissues
- **Stage III:** Dz spread beyond pelvis or to LN but remains in abd (**IIIA: IIIA1** dz in RP LNs; **IIIA1i** LN ≤10 mm; **IIIA1ii** >10 mm. **IIIA2:** Microscopic abd mets; **IIIB:** macroscopic abd mets [≤2 cm] ± RP LNs; **IIIC:** abd mets >2 cm ± LNs; includes tumor extension in spleen/liver capsule w/o parenchymal involvement)
- **Stage IV:** Distant mets excluding peritoneal mets (**IVA:** Pleural effusion w/ + cytology, **IVB** parenchymal met, extraabdominal mets including inguinal or extraabdominal LNs)

Management low-risk disease (benign OGCT; stage IA, grade 1 immature teratoma and stage IA dysgerminoma)

- **Definitive surgery:** Completed w/ comprehensive staging laparotomy; if fertility-sparing surgery done, should include U/S w/ monitoring
- **Surveillance:** Physical exam & tumor markers q2–4mos × 2 y, q6mos × 5 y, thereafter yearly exam. Imaging if clinically indicated (*Am J Obstet Gynecol* 2011;204:466; *NCCN Ovarian Cancer* v1.2021)

Management: All other MOGCT

- **1° Surgery:** Perform before chemo, pts w/ completely resected dz have improved outcomes, although data inconclusive. May be more critical for nondysgerminomas
- **Adj. chemo for adults:** Standard of care w/ 3–4 cycles of BEP. Ideally give 7–10 d after surgery; do NOT dose reduce even w/ myelosuppression (*NEJM* 1987;316:1435; *JCO* 1994;12:701; *NCCN Ovarian Cancer* v1.2021)
- For select pts w/ IB–III resected dysgerminoma, can consider 3 cycles etoposide/carbo if minimizing tox is critical
- All pts getting bleomycin need PFTs before & during tx

Residual disease

- **Residual dz:** After adj. chemo, nl markers: Surgical resection; persistently elevated markers: TIP (paclitaxel, ifosfamide, CIS) (*NCCN Ovarian Cancer v1.2021*)
- Surgery can prevent growing teratoma syn & dedifferentiation of teratoma into active CA (*Gynecol Oncol* 1994;55:217)

Recurrent MOGCT

- If they recur, 90% recur w/in 2 y after chemo completion; if recurs after 2 y, usu slow growing & chemo resistant. Tx is resection
- **Salvage chemo:** If no prior chemo: BEP; if prior chemo: TIP, VIP (etoposide, ifosfamide, CIS), VeIP (vinblastine, ifosfamide, CIS). Palliative options: Paclitaxel, GEM ± CIS, epirubicin + CIS
- **HDC w/ stem-cell rescue:** Consider for persistent, refractory, or platinum-resistant dz. Strongly rec referral to tertiary-care center (*JCO* 2000;18:1173)

Long-term side effects of BEP chemotherapy

- Renal insufficiency, gonadal dysfunction, neurotoxicity, cardiovascular tox 2/2 CIS, 2° malignancies 2/2 etoposide (solid tumors, leukemias), & pulm fibrosis 2/2 bleomycin. >80% pts preserve menstrual fxn after fertility-sparing surgery/platinum-based chemo (*Obstet Gyn* 2003;101:251, *Gynecol Oncol* 158(2):467).

Prognosis, MOGCT

- 5-y OS 95% for stage I dz; 73% for adv stage dz
- Age >45 & tx not at a referral center are independent RFs for recurrence; stage >I & yolk sac histology are independent poor prognostic indicators (*IJGC* 2011;21(8):1414)
- Modified IGCCC is prognostic for ovarian GCT & identifies poor-risk groups that may benefit from high-intensity 1st-line chemo (*Gynecol Oncol* 2015;138:566)

ENDOMETRIAL CARCINOMA

Epidemiology

- Most common gyn CA in developed countries; 2nd most common in developing countries
- Approx 62,000 new cases w/ 12,000 deaths annually in the United States
- Median age at dx is 62y
- Nearly 80% p/w early-stage, uterine-confined dz
- AA women: ↑ mortality, p/w more advanced dz & higher incidence of aggressive histology

Pathology	
Preinvasive lesions	Type I: Estrogen-related → simple hyperplasia (low risk) → complex hyperplasia → endometrial intraepithelial neoplasm (EIN) (25–33% risk) → endometrioid CA Type II: Nonestrogen-related→ atrophy → EIN → serous CA
Invasive lesions	Type I: **Endometrioid adenoCA (85%):** Usu well-to-moderately differentiated (FIGO grade 1–2) w/ minimal myometrial invasion, estrogen responsive; *PTEN* mut common; favorable prog Type II: **Nonendometrioid histology (15%):** Usu poorly differentiated (FIGO grade 3), w/ myometrial invasion, not a/w hormone exposure, ER/PR neg, *TP53* > *PTEN*, spread intra-abdominally, poor prog • **Papillary serous (5–10%):** Poorly differentiated, aggressive, older women • **Clear cell (<5%):** Aggressive, hobnail appearance on histology • **Rare subtypes:** Endometrial stromal sarcoma, uterine leiomyosarcoma, carcinosarcoma, adenosarcoma
Molecular classification	Active area of research. TCGA (*Nature* 2013,497:67–73) divided endometrial CA into 4 molecular subgroups w/ prognostic value demonstrated in PORTEC3 cohort (*JCO* 2020,38(29):3388–3397) (5 y OS = 98% [POLE], 91% [MSI-H], 54% [CN-H], 89% [CN-L]): 1) **POLE:** <10%, ultramutated, *POLE* mut, endometrioid—favorable prog 2) **MSI-H:** ~25–30%, MMRd, endometrioid/clear cell—intermediate prog 3) **CN-H:** ~25%, "serous-like", *TP53* mut, endometrioid/serous—poor prog 4) **CN-L:** ~50%, *TP53* wildtype, endometrioid/clear cell—intermediate prog Refer to genetics if <50 y or FHx of uterine/CRC or known Lynch syndrome. Consider prophylactic TAH/BSO after completion of childbearing (*NEJM* 2006;354:261)

Etiology, risk factors, and clinical manifestations

- **Unopposed estrogen:** Exogenous (tamoxifen, HRT w/o progestins) or endogenous (obesity, PCOS, early menarche, late menopause, nulliparity, chronic anovulation)
- Tamoxifen: ↑ risk of high-grade, poor-risk histology (*Gynecol Oncol.* 2013;129:277)
  No difference in incidence between raloxifene & tamoxifen (STAR *JAMA* 2006;295:2727)
- ↑ risk w/ age, HTN, DM, metabolic syn; ↑ BMI a/w type I tumors; combined oral contraceptives may ↓ risk
- **Lynch** carries 40–60% of lifetime risk of developing endometrial CA
- **Sx:** Postmenopausal vaginal bleeding (75–80%), abdominal/pelvic pain, cough, wt loss

Screening and prevention

- **Screening:** ACS recommends annual screening w/ EMBX at 35 y for women w/ Lynch even in absence of sx. If using tamoxifen, need to evaluate all abnl bleeding, although no clinical data justifies routine screening. All postmenopausal vaginal bleeding needs to be evaluated w/ endometrial sampling as 15% have endometrial carcinoma

Workup and staging

- **Workup:** TVUS & EMBX. Hysteroscopy if high suspicion & EMBX neg; CXR, CT scan of abd/pelvis; surgical staging required if medically fit. **Standard surgical staging** w/ TAH, BSO, washings, abdominal cavity eval, & SLN mapping
- **FIGO 2009 staging:**
  Stage I (80%): Tumor limited to the corpus uteri; **IA** w/ <50% myometrial invasion, **IB** w/ >50% myometrial invasion; **stage II (11%):** Uterine cervical-stromal invasion; **stage III (6%): IIIA** w/ uterine serosa &/or adnexae, **IIIB** w/ vaginal or parametrial involvement, **IIIC** w/ pelvic (IIIC1) &/or paraaortic LN (IIIC2);

stage IV (2%): IVA tumor invading bladder/bowel mucosa; **IVB** w/ distant mets (including inguinal LN, intraperitoneal dz, lung, liver, or bone). Washings/cytology not used in staging

Management and risk stratification

Surgery: TAH/BSO w/ complete surgical staging. Adj. Rx depends on stage, grade, & histologic subtype. Molecular subtype may become important factor

Risk Stratification	
Low risk	Grade 1/2, stage IA, no LVSI, endometrioid adenoCA histology
Intermediate risk	Stage IB–stage II
High risk	Stage III–IVA OR nonendometrioid histology OR age + risk features: • >70 y w/ 1 risk feature • 50–69 y w/ 2 risk features • >18y w/ 3 risk features Risk features = grade 2/3, LVSI, outer 1/3 myometrial invasion

Management: Stage IA disease, low risk

- **No adj. tx necessary** (PORTEC-1, *Lancet* 2000;355:1404)
- **Radiation:** Consider as primary tx for nonsurgical candidates
- **Endocrine therapy:** Progestin-based therapy w/ endometrial sampling q3–6mos. Acceptable for some pts who want to preserve fertility. Surgical staging after childbearing or POD

Management: Stage IB–stage II disease, intermediate risk

- **Adj. radiation:** Vaginal ± pelvic RT (consider EBRT if high grade, deep invasion)
  - GOG 99: Radiation ↓ rate of local recurrence but = OS (GOG 99 *Gynecol Oncol* 2004;92:740)
  - PORTEC-2: Intravaginal brachytherapy has = recurrence rates, PFS, & OS vs. whole pelvic radiation, & has ↓ tox & superior QoL (PORTEC-2 *Lancet* 2010;375:816)
  - PORTEC-3: No 5-y OS difference w/ chemo but significant ↑ 5y FFS. Worse tox w/ chemo-RT. Molecular subtypes may determine benefit for adj. therapy
- **Adj. chemo:** Unclear role but consider for high-grade/high-risk histology. GOG 249: Intermediate risk stage I–II dz (including serous/clear cell), PFS same in adj. paclitaxel/carbo plus intravaginal brachytherapy vs. whole pelvic radiation w/ optional vaginal brachytherapy (*Gynecol Oncol.* 2014;134:438)
- **Nonendometrioid:** Prospective data lacking but overall higher risk. Consider/discuss adj. therapy: Stage IA (w/o myometrial invasion) → vaginal brachytherapy; stage IA (w/ myometrial invasion &/or + pelvic wash)–II → brachytherapy or pelvic RT ± chemo

Management: Stage III/IVa disease, high risk

- **Multimodality therapy:** Optimal adj. therapy yet to be defined
- **Adj. chemo:** Platinum-based chemo should be considered for pts w/ residual dz <2 cm. **Carbo/paclitaxel noninferior to TAP, considered 1st-line therapy** (GOG 209 *Gynecol Oncol.* 2012;125:771)
- **Adj. radiation:** Tumor volume–directed RT, pelvic ± vaginal RT, depends on risk of locoregional/metastatic dz
- **Adj. CRT:** Concurrent CIS + RT followed by carbo/paclitaxel (preferred for stage III, consider for stage IVA [PORTEC-3])

Management: Stage IV metastatic and recurrent disease

- **Debulking surgery:** Consider for recurrent abdominopelvic dz in highly selected pts
- **Chemo: Carbo/paclitaxel considered 1st-line Rx,** as noninferior to CIS/dox/paclitaxel in PFS & OS, (GOG 209 *Gynecol Oncol* 2012;125:771). If recurrence <6 mos after receiving prior platinum-based regimen, lenvatinib/pembro ORR 32% (SGO, 2021), but ↑ tox (HTN, diarrhea) > single-agent doxorubicin or paclitaxel
- **Endocrine therapy:** 10–30% RR. FIGO grade 1–2, endometrioid, long dz-free interval, & ER/PR receptor positivity ↑ probability of response. Use in minimally symptomatic dz. If progression, should switch to chemo
- **IO:** Pembrolizumab (TMB-H/MSI-H): ORR 57% (*J Clin Oncol* 2020;38(1):1–10); lenvatinib/pembrolizumab: ORR wk24 36% MSS (*J Clin Oncol* 2020;38(26):2981–2992); nivolumab; dostarlimab-gxly
- **Targeted Rx:** Bevacizumab (VEGF): 40% PFS at 6 mos (*J Clin Oncol* 2011;29:2259); temsirolimus (mTOR inhibitor): RR 14% (*J Clin Oncol* 2011;29:3278); larotrectinib or entrectinib (*NTRK* gene fusion positive)

Prognosis: OS at 5 y (%)				
Stage	**I**	**II**	**III**	**IV**
	80–90%	60–75%	40–50%	10–30%

GESTATIONAL TROPHOBLASTIC DISEASE

Definition

- **Gestational trophoblastic disease (GTD):** Includes both benign & malignant pathological disorders arising from the placental trophoblast
- **Gestational trophoblastic neoplasm (GTN):** Persistent GTD, includes invasive mole (partial & complete), choriocarcinoma, PSTT & ETT

Epidemiology

- Complete & partial hydatidiform moles comprise 80% of GTD cases, invasive moles ~15%, choriocarcinoma ~5%
  - Incidence of GTD ~ 1 in 1,000 pregnancies in the US

Risk factors

- Extremes of maternal age (>40 y w/ 5–10× greater risk), h/o previous GTD, cigarette smoking, nulliparity, h/o infertility, use of oral contraceptives. Incidence increased in East Asia (unknown if genetic or environmental)

Clinical subtypes

- **Hydatidiform mole (complete or partial)**
  - **Partial hydatidiform mole:** Triploid karyotype, generally dispermic, arising from fertilization of an egg by 2 sperm, only type of GTD a/w a fetus, embryo survives until 8th wk of gestation, presents as missed abortion, less likely to become malignant
  - **Complete hydatidiform mole:** Extremes of reproductive age <20 & >40 y, diploid but androgenic, usu arise by fertilization of an enucleate egg by a single sperm that duplicates (46XX, most common) or by 2 sperm (46XY)
    - Early presentation: Absence of p57 (KIP2), immunostaining (paternally imprinted)
    - Late presentation: Uterus large for date, U/S (hydropic changes, no embryo), vaginal bleeding, theca lutein cysts, preeclampsia, hyperemesis, hyperthyroidism
    - **Tx:** Both partial & complete hydatidiform moles are treated w/ surgical evacuation & weekly β-hCG monitoring until normalized
- **GTN**
  - **Persistent/invasive GTN:** Malignant transformation of a molar pregnancy (~15% of complete moles s/p evacuation & 0.5% of partial moles s/p complete evacuation). Most common sx is vaginal bleeding. Persistent hCG elevation after evacuation. **Risk factors:** Large theca lutein cysts (≥6 cm), age >40 y, previous GTD, initial hCG >100,000 mIU/mL, excessively enlarged uterus for date. Always r/o new IUP
  - **Choriocarcinoma:** Most aggressive GTN, arise from villous trophoblasts, early vascular invasion, widespread mets (including brain), often present as late postpartum bleeding, malignant transformation of molar tissues or *de novo* lesion arising spontaneously
    - Surgical evacuation: D&C, hysterectomy
    - Close monitoring of postevacuation hCG levels (baseline w/in 48 h of evacuation, weekly until nl)
- **PSTT:** Rare (<0.2% of GTD), slow-growing malignant tumors, arise from intermediate cytotrophoblast cells in the placenta (*Lancet* 2009;374:48). More resistant to chemo compared to other GTN, hCG may be low, early-stage dz mandates hysterectomy
- **ETT:** Rare, similar behavior to PSTT. More resistant to chemo compared to other GTN, early-stage dz mandates hysterectomy

Diagnosis

- Obtain an hCG level & if elevated order pelvic U/S
- **Caution w/ bx as GTN are highly vascular**
- Always send a urine pregnancy test & confirm hCG reliability w/ serial dilutions
  - False (+) hCG may occur due to heterophile ab or nonspecific protein interference
- Criteria for dx of GTN (1 of the following):
  - 4 values or more of plateau of hCG over at least 3 wks
  - Rise of hCG of 10% or greater for 3 values or longer over at least 2 wks
  - Persistence of hCG 6 mos after mole evacuation (*Lancet* 2012;379:130)
  - Presence of histologic choriocarcinoma, PSTT, or ETT

FIGO anatomic staging

Based on extent of GTN

- **Stage I:** Tumor confined to the uterus
- **Stage II:** Tumor extension outside the uterus but confined to the pelvis
- **Stage III:** Tumor extension to the lungs
- **Stage IV:** All other met sites

Prognostic scoring system (GOG)

International Federation of Gynecology & Obstetrics (2000) scoring system for GTN, by WHO prognostic factor

	0	**1**	**2**	**4**
Age (y)	<40	≥40	—	—
Antecedent pregnancy	Mole	Abortion	Term	—
Interval from antecedent pregnancy to chemo-tx (mos)	<4	4–6	7–12	>12
hCG conc. (IU/L)	<1,000	1,000–10,000	10,000–100,000	>100,000
Number of mets	0	1–4	5–8	>8
Site of mets	Lung	Spleen, kidney	GI tract	Brain, liver
Largest tumor mass diameter (cm)	<3	3–5	≥5	—
Previous chemo-tx	—	—	Monotherapy	Combined Rx

- CXR (not CT) used to count number of mets. PSTT/ETT: Allot anatomic stage only (risk score is not applicable)
- **Low-risk:** Score of ≤6, tend to respond well to chemo: Typically treated w/ single-agent chemo
- **High-risk:** Score of >7, tend to respond less well to chemo: Typically treated w/ multiagent chemo

Management

- Early referral to trophoblastic dz center
- Curettage/hysterectomy depending on risk factors & fertility preferences
- **Single-agent tx**
  - MTX is the rec tx
  - Dactinomycin more severe SE profile; RCT comparing MTX vs. dactinomycin as 1st-line ongoing. Has activity in pts w/ low-risk GTN who develop MTX resistance & whose hCG is low (*J Clin Oncol* 2002;20:1838)
- **Combination chemo**
  - EMA-CO: Etoposide/MTX/actinomycin + cyclophosphamide/vincristine (*J Clin Oncol* 2013;31:280)
  - If resistance to EMA-CO develops, consider EMA-EP: Etoposide/MTX/actinomycin + etoposide/cis
  - Brain mets require MTX (1 g/m^2) w/ leucovorin rescue
  - For very high-risk pts, consider induction w/ etoposide/cis 1–2 cycles for gradual reduction in tumor volume prior to EMA-CO to reduce the risk of hemorrhage in critical organs (*J Clin Oncol* 2013:31:280)
- **PSTT/ETT:** (NCCN 2021, v2.2021)
  - Stage 1 (nonmetastatic): Surgery w/ hysterectomy, salpingectomy, & pelvic LN bx. Consider systemic therapy for deep invasion, necrosis, mitotic count >5/10 hpf, or antecedent pregnancy ≥2 y
  - Stage 2 (metastatic): Surgery as per stage 1 & platinum/etoposide containing regimen such as EMA-EP
- Avelumab for single-agent chemo resistant GTN (*J Clin Oncol* 2020;3129–3137)
- Monitor hCG until normalized, continue to monitor 6–12 mos or longer depending on risk factors. Note, hCG can initially spike 2/2 tumor lysis
- Strongly encourage reliable contraception during period of monitoring

CERVICAL CANCER

Epidemiology

- 4th most common CA & 4th most frequent cause of CA death in women worldwide; 14,000 cases w/ 4,000 death in the United States per y. Rates ↓ in the United States due to early detection w/ pap smears; still prevalent in pts w/ low socioeconomic status & poor access to medical care. Mean age of dx = 50 y

Pathology	
Preinvasive lesions	CIN, precursor to squamous carcinoma, characterized by dysplastic changes in the epithelium (low-grade: CIN1 vs. high-grade: CIN2 & 3). Lesions usu found in squamocolumnar jxn in the transition zone AIS, precursor to HPV-assoc adenoCA. Usu originates in the squamocolumnar jxn, may originate w/in endocervical canal, possible skip lesions
Invasive lesions	• **SCC:** Most common histology, 80% • **AdenoCA (including adenosquamous):** 15–20% • Rare histology: **Neuroendocrine/small cell carcinoma; rhabdomyosarcoma** (usu seen in adolescent/young women); 1° **cervical lymphoma; cervical sarcoma.** Tx based on histology

Etiology and clinical manifestations

- **RF:** Persistent HPV infection: High risk in pts w/ early age at coitarche, multiple sexual partners, high-risk sexual partners, h/o STIs (including genital warts), ↑ parity, smokers, OCP users, chronic immunosuppression (eg, HIV, organ transplant), low socioeconomic status (2/2 low rate of screening)
- **Sx:** Often asx & found at screening. Can cause abnl vaginal bleeding (postmenopausal, intermenstrual, postcoital), pelvic pain, bowel/urinary sx, or vaginal discharge w/ advanced stage

Molecular biology

- HPV genes E6 & E7 incorporate into genome of cervical cells & produce viral proteins capable of binding to & inactivating tumor suppressor proteins P53 & RB1. 15 subtypes of HPV considered high risk; HPV 16/18 most prevalent (70% of cervical CA cases); other high-risk subtypes: 31, 33, 35, 39, 45, 51, 52, 56, 58, 59, 68, 73, 82

Screening and prevention

- Cervical CA rate has ↓ by 70–90% in well-screened populations. Screening starts no younger than age 21. Vaccination does not alter screening guidelines

Cervical Cancer Screening Guidelines			
	ACS 2020	**USPSTF 2018**	**ACOG 2016**
Age to start	25	21	21
21–29 y of age	HPV test alone q5y (preferred) or Cotesting q5y or Pap q3y	Pap q3y	Pap q3y
30–65 y of age		HrHPV q5y or Cotesting q5y or Pap q3 y	Cotesting q5y (preferred) or Pap q3 y
All recommend that women who have been adequately screened in the previous 10 y and no precancerous lesions in previous 20 y can discontinue screening at age >65			

- **High-risk pts** (hx of CIN2/CIN3, HIV, diethylstilbestrol exposure in utero): q1 y
- **S/p hysterectomy:** Stop if no h/o CIN2/CIN3/CA. If h/o CIN2/CIN3, continue for 20 y

Prevention

- HPV vaccination ↓ incidence of premalignant lesion development; 9vHPV (Gardasil 9) given to females/males at 11 or 12 y (can be given as early as age 9, rec up to age 26, covered up to age 45) (ideally before HPV exposure)

Workup and staging

- **Workup:** If lesion seen during cervical exam: Perform cervical punch bx or endocervical curettage; for abnl Pap smear w/o visible lesion follow ASCCP guidelines (*J Low Genit Tract Dis* 2020;24:102–131)
- For invasive dz stage 1A: CXR. For ≥ stage IB: CXR w/ MRI or CT of chest/abd/pelvis vs. PET/CT (preferred). Cystoscopy & proctoscopy if concern for bladder/rectal involvement

- **Clinical FIGO 2018 staging: Stage 0:** Carcinoma in situ; **stage I:** Tumor limited to the cervix; **stage IA:** Tumor dx'd only by microscopy**; stage IB:** Clinical visible tumor confined to the cervix; **stage IB1:** <2 cm, **stage IB2:** 2–4 cm, **stage IB3:** >4 cm (bulky); **stage II:** Tumor invading beyond uterus into upper 2/3rd of vagina &/or parametria but not to pelvic side wall; **stage III:** Tumor involves lower 1/3rd of vagina &/or extends to pelvic wall (+/– hydronephrosis) &/or involves LNs; **stage IVa:** Tumor invades mucosa of adjacent organs (bladder/rectum); **stage IVb:** Tumor extends beyond true pelvis (no longer curable)

Management: Premalignant lesions

- CIN 1: Observe as 60% of lesions will resolve w/o intervention
- CIN 2/3: Excisional procedure w/ LEEP or cervical conization to r/o invasive carcinoma
- AIS: Excisional procedure w/ LEEP or cervical conization to r/o invasive CA followed by hysterectomy (consider close surveillance if fertility sparing desired)

Management of stage IA disease w/o lymphovascular space invasion (LVSI)

- **Surgery:** Simple hysterectomy alone
  Fertility preservation options: CKC w/ neg margins

Management of early-invasive disease (stage IA disease with LVSI or nonbulky <4 cm stage IB1/stage IB2/IIA1 disease)

- **Surgery:** Radical hysterectomy & pelvic LN dissection ± para-aortic LN sampling (consider SLN mapping)
  Fertility preservation options: CKC or Trachelectomy w/ LN assessment can be considered in pts w/ stage IA1 w/ LVSI or Stage IA2. Trachelectomy w/ LN assessment for stage IB1/IB2
- **Adj. radiation:** For pts at intermediate/high risk for relapse (2+ RF: Outer 1/3 cervical stromal invasion, LVSI, or tumor >4 cm), ↑ RFS (Sedlis Criteria, GOG 92, *Gynecol Oncol* 1999;73:177)
- **Adj. CRT:** For pts w/ + LNs, + margins, or microscopic parametrial extension—CIS-based CRT ↑ PFS/5-y OS compared to RT alone (Peter Criteria, GOG 109, *JCO* 2000;18:1606)
- **1° RT** ± **chemo:** Brachytherapy + pelvic RT for inoperable pts. Yields comparable 5-y OS to surgery

Management of local regionally advanced disease (bulky >4-cm stage IB3/IIA2–stage IVA)

- **CRT: Preferred tx** for extensive, bulky local dz; 1° whole pelvic radiation or extended-field radiation (for + para-aortic LN) w/ chemo followed by brachytherapy. Chemo options include platinum or platinum/5-FU; weekly CIS (40 mg/m^2, max dose 70 mg) w/ RT is preferred regimen (Keys Trial, *GOG 123, NEJM* 1999;340:1154)
- **Adj. hysterectomy:** Benefit unclear

Management of metastatic IVB disease/recurrent disease

- **Chemo:** CIS, carbo, paclitaxel, docetaxel, topotecan, vinorelbine, GEM, & ifosfamide all have activity, but duration of response is generally <4 mos. CIS/paclitaxel ↑ RR & PFS compared to single-agent CIS but approx = OS (*JCO* 2004;22:3113). CIS/topotecan combination ↑ RR, PFS, & OS compared to single-agent CIS (GOG 179 *JCO* 2005;23:4626); CIS doublets (CIS + paclitaxel OR vinorelbine OR GEM OR topotecan) = OS. However, trend in RR, PFS, & OS favors **CIS + paclitaxel** (*JCO* 2009;27:4649). Addition of **bevacizumab to CIS + paclitaxel ↑ OS by 4 mos** (*NEJM* 2014;370:734). Standard of care is **CIS/Taxol/Bev**
- **IO: Pembrolizumab** had 14.3% overall RR w/ a 2.6% complete RR & an 11.7% partial RR in 77 pts w/ PD-L1 + tumors who had received ≥ 1 prior chemo (KEYNOTE-158; see: *J Clin Oncol* 2019;37:1470). FDA Approval (2018) w/ PD-L1 staining companion diagnostic. Mostly used as 2nd-line therapy for pts w/ PD-L1 + tumors defined as having a CPS ≥1
  Cemiplimab had 16.4% ORR, ↑ OS compared to chemo in pts w/ ≥1 prior platinum-based chemo tx (HR 0.69, $P < 0.001$), regardless of PD-L1 status (RCT EMPOWER-Cervical1/GOG-3016/ENGOT-CX9, ESMO 2021)
- **Palliative radiation:** Consider for symptomatic relief for pt w/ extensive prior pelvic RT
- **Pelvic exenteration:** Consider in selected pts who have isolated pelvic recurrence w/in previous radiation field

Prognosis based on stage

- Prog depends on stage. For FIGO 2018, 5 y OS: Stage I—85.6%; II—56.1%, III—39.3%, IVA—24.0%, IVB—14.7% (*Obstet Gynecol* 2019;134:49)

VULVAR CANCER

Epidemiology

- Estimated 6,100 new cases dx'd & 1,500 deaths in US in 2021
- Occurs most frequently in **postmenopausal women** (mean age at dx 65), but age at dx is ↓, possibly due to ↑ HPV-related CA in younger women (women <45 y w/ vulvar CA more likely to have assoc condyloma, $p < 0.001$) (*Obstet Gynecol* 1995;86:51)
- **RF:** Tobacco use, vulvar dystrophy, vulvar or CIN, HPV, immunodeficiency, cervical CA

Clinical manifestations and diagnosis

- Plaque, ulcer, or mass usu on labia majora; in 10%, lesion too extensive to determine site of origin; in up to 22%, synchronous 2nd malignancy (most often cervical), is found commonly in HPV+ (*Am J Obstet Gynecol* 1971;109:446)
- Typically solitary mass in HPV– vs. multifocal in HPV+
- Vulvar bleeding, dysuria, groin LAN suggest advanced dz
- Dx: Made by vulvar bx; also need Pap & colposcopy to r/o synchronous vaginal/cervical lesions; CT, PET/CT, &/or MRI to determine extent of dz & for surgical planning

Histologic subtypes

- **SCC** (over 90% of 1° vulvar neoplasms)
  - Keratinizing/differentiated/simplex → most common: Older pts, a/w lichen sclerosus & chronic venereal granulomatous dz, NOT HPV assoc
  - Classic/warty/Bowenoid type → younger pts, assoc w/ HPV 16, 18, & 33; early age at 1st intercourse; multiple sexual partners; HIV; smoking
  - Verrucous carcinoma: SCC variant; grows slowly, rare LN mets, locally destructive
- **Melanoma** (5–10%): Usu pigmented but can be amelanotic
- **BCC** (2%): Postmenopausal White women, locally invasive (usu nonmetastasizing); high incidence of antecedent/concomitant malignancy
- **Sarcoma** (1–2%): Poor prog
- **Extramammary Paget dz** (<1%): Older White women; pruritus in 70%; eczematoid appearance. Evaluate for synchronous neoplasms (20–30%)
- **Bartholin gland adenoCA** (<1%): Solid, deeply infiltrating, often metastasize

Staging (FIGO 2009)

- Staging & 1° surgical tx performed simultaneously; **inguinofemoral LN (IFLN) status** most important predictor of overall prog (70–93% 5 y survival if neg, 25–41% if positive [*Crit Rev Oncol Hematol* 2006;60:227])

Stage I	Tumor confined to the vulva & perineum w/o LN mets (IA: ≤ 2 cm in greatest dimension & ≤1-mm stromal invasion, IB: >2 cm OR >1-mm stromal invasion)
Stage II	Tumor of any size w/ extension to adjacent perineal structures w/o LN mets (lower 1/3 urethra, lower 1/3 vagina, anal involvement)
Stage III	Regional nodes: **IIIA:** ≤2 LN mets ≤5 mm or 1 LN met ≥5 mm; **IIIB:** ≥3 LN mets <5 mm or ≥2 LN mets ≥5 mm; **IIIC:** Extracapsular spread of LN met
Stage IVA	Tumor w/ extension to upper 2/3 urethra, upper 2/3 vagina, bladder or rectal mucosa, fixed to pelvic bone, &/or fixed/ulcerated regional LN mets
Stage IVB	Any distant mets (including pelvic LNs)

Staging/treatment

- **Initial tx based on clinical size/extent of 1° tumor:**
  - **Stage IA (<1 mm invasion)**: Wide local excision/simple partial vulvectomy w/ a goal of ≥1 cm clinical intraop tumor-free margin (no LND assessment)
  - **Early stage (IB & tumor ≤4 cm):** Surgery (radical local excision, partial vulvectomy, radical vulvectomy)—use most conservative procedure allowing a ≥1 cm clinical intraoperative tumor-free margin w/ SLNB or IFND

    → SNLB is alternative to IFND in select Stage IB or II: No palpable LN, unifocal, <4 cm, no prior surgery, SNLB performed by experienced surgeon (*Gynecol Onc* 2015;137:351)

    If <u>neg margins</u> → observe

    If <u>positive margins</u>→ re-excision (adj. EBRT if re-exicision not feasible w/o extent)

    If <u>margins±</u> for invasive dz after re-excision→ adj. EBRT

    If <u>margins-</u> after reresection, consider EBRT if high-risk features (LVI, close margins, tumor size, diffuse 1°, & depth)

Adj. for nodal dz: If + SNLB ≤2 mm → EBRT ± concurrent chemo (CIS, CIS/5-FU, mitomycin/5-FU). If + SLNB >2 mm → Complete IFND w/ adj. EBRT ± chemo. Positive 1° IFND → EBRT ± chemo

- **Locally adv (>4-cm tumor &/or stage IVA based on tumor extent):**
  → With node neg by imaging/palpation: IFND
  → With node positive by imaging/palpation: IFND vs. FNA
  Adj.: If node neg by path: EBRT to 1° tumor (± groin nodes) + chemo; if node positive by path → EBRT to 1° tumor/groin/pelvic LN + chemo
- **Metastatic (stage IVB):** Pelvic LN mets only: EBRT to 1° tumor/groin/pelvic LN + chemo; distant mets: EBRT for local control &/or chemo (no evidence for best regimen—1st line: CIS doublet; 2nd line: Single agent [see cervical CA chapter]) or supportive care
- **Recurrent dz:** >50% recurrences are perineal & tx = re-excision ± RT if not given prior; inguinal/pelvic recurrence tx = RT + surgery if no prior RT; groin recurrence tx = RT only if unresectable, otherwise systemic tx ± resection; distant = salvage chemo
- **IO:** Investigational, possible role for pembrolizumab (KEYNOTE 158, *J Clin Oncol* 2020;38:1) & nivolumab (CHECKMATE 358, *J Clin Oncol* 2019;37:2825)
- **Vulvar melanoma:** Excise locoregional. Little data in met dz; although a type of mucosal dz, can use principles of cutaneous melanoma tx (*Int J Gynecol Cancer* 2014;24:S117)

Vaginal Cancer

Epidemiology
- ~ 8,000 new cases & 1,500 deaths in the United States in 2021; up to half have hx prior gyn malignancy
- **RF:** Similar to cervical SCC: HPV (75%), ↑ sexual partners, smoking, early coitarche

Clinical presentation and diagnosis
- **Sx:** Postcoital or postmenopausal vaginal bleeding, vaginal mass, urinary frequency or dysuria, tenesmus, constipation, melena, pelvic pain. 20% asx at time of dx
- Posterior wall of upper 1/3 of vagina = most common site
- **Dx:** Mass, plaque, or ulcer on exam; + Pap or colposcopy; definitive test = vaginal bx & absence of h/o other gyn malignancy that could be recurrent in the vagina

Histologic subtypes
- **SCC** (~84%): Incidence ↑ w/ age (mean age at dx = 60 y); a/w HPV. Verrucous carcinoma: Fungating, rare, well-diff; locally aggressive but mets rare
- **AdenoCA** (~10%): Predominant in pts <20 y; clear-cell variant a/w diethylstilbestrol exposure in utero. Polypoid masses often on ant. vaginal wall; 70% stage I at dx; improved outcome compared to nondiethylstilbestrol-assoc vaginal adenoCA; median age at dx = 19 y
- **Sarcoma** (~2.5%): Most vaginal sarcomas are embryonal rhabdomyosarcomas. Mostly young children (mean age 3 y), "bunch of grapes"
- **Melanoma** (~2.5%): Mean age 60, p/w vaginal bleed & blue-black/black-brown mass (or nonpigmented), plaque, ulceration of distal 1/3 ant. vaginal wall. 5 y OS <20%

Staging (FIGO)
- Staging is clinical (pelvic exam, cystoscopy, imaging) + any available pathology
- Stage I = confined to vagina, II = invades paravaginal tissues but not to pelvic wall, III = extends to pelvic wall, or pelvic or inguinal LN mets, IVA = invades bladder or rectum &/or extends beyond true pelvis, IVB = distant mets

Tx and prognosis
- Paucity of clinical trials to define optimal therapy
- **Stage I:** Surgery if neg margin is attainable (radical hysterectomy, upper vaginectomy, bilateral pelvic lymphadenectomy) or EBRT followed by brachytherapy
- **Stage II–IVA:** Poor prog w/ RT alone; 5-FU or CIS often used concurrently w/ RT for high-risk dz = tumor >4 cm or stage III/IVA dz (*Int J Radiat Oncol Biol Phys* 2005;62:138); pelvic exenteration a consideration in stage IVA dz
  Potential role for neoadj paclitaxel/CIS in stage II dz (*Gynecol Oncol* 2008;111:307)
  Complications of tx (10–15%): Rectovaginal, vesicovaginal fistulas; radiation cystitis, proctitis; rectal/vaginal strictures; rarely vaginal necrosis, radiation-induced premature menopause. Vaginal dilator use rec following RT
- **Stage IVB:** Systemic therapy (evidence lacking for specific regimens). 1st line: Usu CIS doublet; 2nd line: Single agent (see Cervical CA chapter)
- **Recurrent dz:** Pelvic exenteration w/ or w/o vaginal reconstruction. Chemo if no options for local tx
- **IO:** Same as vulvar CA—investigational, possible role for pembrolizumab (KEYNOTE 158) & nivolumab (CHECKMATE 358)
- 5 y OS: 77.6% stage I, 52.2% stage II, 42.5% stage III, 20.5% stage IVA, 12.9% stage IVB (*Int J Gynaecol Obstet* 2006;95:S29)

BREAST CANCER: INTRODUCTION

Epidemiology

- Most common CA affecting women & 2nd most common cause of CA death in the United States
- In the United States, approx 286,000 new cases in 2019 & 42,000 deaths. Approx 2.2 million new cases dx'd worldwide in 2020
- ↑ incidence, but ↓ mortality in past decades (↑ screening, ↑ therapeutic options)

Risk factors

- **Strongest:** Female gender, ↑ age
- **↑ Estrogen:** Early menarche, late menopause, late/nulliparity (*NEJM* 2006;354:270); prolonged HRT (*JAMA* 2003;289:3243); no increased risk w/ OCP
- **Certain benign conditions ↑ risk:** Proliferative features (ductal hyperplasia, papilloma, radial scars, sclerosing adenosis); atypia (atypical ductal or lobular hyperplasia); dense breast tissue (decreased mammographic sensitivity)
- **No ↑ risk from:** Cysts, fibroadenoma, columnar Δs (*NEJM* 2005;353:229)
- **Other:** BMI, FHx, smoking, EtOH, prior thoracic irradiation
- **Modified Gail model:** (www.cancer.gov/bcrisktool). Provides 5 y & lifetime risk. Average risk is <15%. **Do not use Gail model if prior Dx of breast CA, DCIS, LCIS, or inherited breast CA**

Genetics (see Cancer Genetics Section)

- **BRCA1/2 mt:** 56–84% lifetime risk of breast CA
- **Other familial/hereditary breast CA:** *CDH1* (lobular), *CHEK2* (ER+), *TP53, PALB2, PTEN, ATM, NF1, STK11*

Screening (for women with average risk)

	NCCN (2016)	ACS (2015)	USPSTF (2016)	ACOG (2017)
Ages rec	40+	≥45	50–74	≥40
Ages for individualized decision	–	40–44	40–49	–
Interval	1 y	1 y (45–54), 2 y (55+)	2 y	1–2 y
Exam	Clinical exam, MMG	MMG alone	MMG alone	Clinical exam, MMG

- **Mammography:** 20–30% ↓ breast CA mortality (smaller absolute benefit for women <50 y) (*Lancet* 2001;358:1340; 2002;359:909; *Ann Intern Med* 2002;137:347; *Lancet* 2012;380:1778)

Screening (for women with greater than average risk)

- ***BRCA1/2*:** CBE q6–12mos beginning age 25, **annual MMG + annual breast MRI** beginning age 25 or younger based on earliest onset in affected family member; consider U/S as adjunct to mammography for women w/ dense breasts due to decreased Se, though questionable utility if performing MRI
- **Consider MRI for mut in:** *ATM, CDH1, CHK2, NF1, PALB2*
- **≥20% lifetime risk (but not *BRCA*), as calculated by predictive models (Gail model):** CBE q6–12mos beginning age 25, annual MMG, & consider annual breast MRI
- **Hx of thoracic RT:** CBE q6–12mos starting 8–10 y after RT exposure, annual MMG + annual MRI starting 8–10 y after RT or age 40, whichever comes 1st
- **Hx of LCIS or ALH/ADH:** CBE q6–12 mos & annual MMG

Prevention

- **Tamoxifen (TAM):** Risk–benefit: 43% 7-y RR of invasive breast CA but ↑ DVT/PE, ↑ endometrial CA (NSABP P-1 (BCPT) *JNCI* 1998;90:1371; *Lancet* 2002;360:817)
- **Raloxifene:** 76% as effective as tam for RR also ↓ vertebral fractures, ↑ risk of stroke, DVT/PE, cataracts but < tam (RUTH, *NEJM* 2006;355:125), trend toward ↓ uterine CA (NSABP P-2 (STAR), *JAMA* 2006;295:2727), FDA approved in postmenopausal women
- **AIs:** Exemestane & anastrozole are not FDA approved for chemoprevention, no prospective data on AIs vs. tam or raloxifene. 65% 3-y RR of invasive breast CA w/ exemestane (MAP.3, *NEJM* 2011;364:2381) & 50% 7-y RR of invasive breast CA w/ anastrozole in postmenopausal women vs. placebo (IBIS-2, *Lancet* 2014;383:1041)
- **Prophylactic bilateral mastectomy:** 90% breast CA risk reduction for women at high risk (ie, *BRCA1/2, TP53*) (*JAMA* 2010;304:967)

- **Prophylactic bilateral salpingoophorectomy:** ↓ ovarian CA risk by 85–90% & breast CA risk by approx 50% & decrease in all-cause + CA-specific mortality in high-risk women (*BRCA 1/2*) (*JAMA* 2010;304:967)

Staging

- Isolated tumor cells (≤0.2 mm or <200 cells) in nodes by H&E are N0(I+)
- **Stage 0:** Carcinoma in situ; **stage IA:** T1 (tumor ≤2 cm), N0; **stage IB:** T1N1mi (micromet to LN >0.2 mm but ≤2 mm); **stage IIA:** T2 (tumor 2–5 cm), N0 or T1N1 (1–3 axillary nodes); **stage IIB:** T2N1 or T3 (tumor >5 cm), N0; **stage IIIA:** N2 (4–9 axillary nodes) or T3N1; **stage IIIB:** T4 (direct extension to CW &/or skin or inflammatory); **stage IIIC:** N3 (≥10 axillary nodes or any infraclavicular or ipsilateral supraclavicular nodes); **stage IV:** Distant mets

DCIS/LCIS

- **DCIS:** ~15–50% will progress to invasive breast CA if untreated
- Tx: Active surveillance, lumpectomy w/o SLN bx + RT, mastectomy ± SLN bx. ER+ DCIS: Tam (premenopausal), tam or AI (postmenopausal), no ↑ survival but reduces risk of ipsi- & contralateral recurrence (*Cochrane* 2012; *Lancet* 2016;387:849)
- **LCIS:** 10–20% will progress to invasive breast CA if untreated
- Tx: No surgical tx for classical LCIS, chemoprevention rec

Histology

- **Ductal:** Invasive ductal carcinoma (IDC) comprises 75% of all breast CAs
- **Lobular (ILC):** 10% of breast CAs, a/w germline or somatic *CDH1* mts. Difficult to detect on MMG. Increased frequency of multifocal & bilateral dz, equivalent prog to IDC
- **Mucinous, medullary, papillary, adenocystic:** Favorable prog
- **Metaplastic:** Extremely unfav. prog
- **Phyllodes tumor:** Composed of stromal & epithelial elements; tx is surgery w/ margins > 1 cm; ALND; adj. RT, or adj. chemo not indicated
- **TILs:** A/w improved prog (*J Clin Oncol* 2013;31:860)

Molecular pathology

- **ER+:** >1% **PR+:** > 1%
- **Other IHC markers:** Mammaglobin, AR, CK5, CK6, CK17
- **HER2 testing:** *HER2/neu* gene amplification observed in 20–30% of invasive breast CA. Assoc w/ worse prog (↑ risk of dz progression, ↓ OS) if untreated
- **IHC:** 3+ = HER2+; 0–1+ = HER2–; 2+ = equivocal → refer for **FISH**
- **FISH:** Positive if HER2/CEP17 ratio ≥2 & copy number/cell ≥4. If discordant, see ASCO/CAP 2018 guidelines (*J Clin Oncol* 2018;36:2105)

Molecular & Receptor Classification (*JCO* 2010;28:1684)

	ER/PR	HER2	Outcomes
Luminal A	+	–	Favorable
Luminal B	+	–	Intermediate
Luminal-HER2	+	+	Intermediate
HER2 enriched	–	+	Poor
Basal-like/TNBC	–	–	Poor

Inflammatory breast cancer

- **Epidemiology & dx:** ~2% of breast CA; worse prog. Clinical dx of skin erythema, *peau d'orange*, & breast pain & enlargement; T4 dz
- **Pathology:** Dermal lymphatic involvement by tumor emboli often found, but is neither necessary nor sufficient for dx
- **Tx:** Neoadj chemo → mastectomy w/ ALND → adj. radiation → adj. endocrine therapy if indicated

Male breast cancer

- **Epidemiology:** ~1% of breast CA, usu dx'd at later stage vs. females, ↑ risk w/ *BRCA1/2* mt
- **Pathology:** Most hormone-receptor positive (85–95%)
- **Local control:** Same tx paradigm as women
- **Systemic control:** Tam is the preferred endocrine agent; little data on AIs, LHRH agonists, fulvestrant, or CDK4/6 inhibitors

Local management with surgery and radiation

- Mastectomy = lumpectomy + RT in OS (*NEJM* 2002;347:1227)
- **SLNB** for (1) clinically neg axillary exam or (2) after NAC in cN1 converted to cN0 (ACOSOG Z1071, *JAMA* 2013;310(14):1455–1461)
- **ALND** for (1) ≥3 positive SLN; no OS benefit if <3 SLN (Z0011, *JAMA* 2011;305:569) (2) cN1–3 or positive axillary bx if surgery upfront, (3) clinically evident nodes or SLN+ (any) after NAC
- **RT:** No OS for RT after BCS for pts >70 yo, ER+, & node (–) (CALGB 9343, *JCO* 2013;31:2382)
  - Post mastectomy RT (PMRT): ↓ locoregional recurrence & ↑ survival. Recommend for ≥4 pos. LNs (if 1–3 pos. LNs, recommend rad onc referral for discussion), tumor >5 cm, higher stage (III), or pos. surgical margins (*Lancet* 2005;366:2087)
  - Consider addition of regional nodal irradiation to whole-breast irradiation after BCS if pos. LN (*NEJM* 2015;373:307; *NEJM* 2015;373:317)

General (neo)adjuvant principles

- **Aims:** ↓ recurrence risk & ↑ survival, NAC ~ adj. (*JCO* 2008;26:778)
- Additional aims of NAC: (1) Downstaging for cT > 2 cm, cN1+
  (2) sparing ALND (↓ lymphedema), mastectomy → lumpectomy
  (3) if no pCR → alter postsurgical tx in TNBC, HER2+ (as below)
- **Recurrence:** TNBC, HER2+ mostly in 1st 3–5 y. ER+ steady risk 0–14 y
- **Isolated local recurrence:** Tx decision case-by-case; chemo benefit limited to ER-neg dz (CALOR, *Lancet Onc* 2014;15:156)

Chemotherapy regimens for (neo)adjuvant use in HR+ and TNBC

- 3 most common regimens: **CMF** (cyclophosphamide, MTX, 5-FU), **TC** (docetaxel, cyclophosphamide), & **dd** (dose-dense) **AC → T** (doxorubicin + cyclophosphamide ×4, followed by paclitaxel ×4 or weekly paclitaxel ×12)
- Dose dense schedule (q2w) + G-CSF > 3 wk regimen → ↓ of 10-y risk of recurrence or death (*Lancet* 2019;393:1440–1452)
- Anthracycline (Anthra) & taxane-based tx > TC if HER2(–) & high-risk (ABC, *JCO* 2017;35(23): 2647–2655). If low-risk, TC not < ACT (PlanB, *JCO* 2019;37(10):799–808)
- CMF: ↑ OS at 30-y follow-up (RR of death = 0.79) vs. no chemo after surgery (*BMJ* 2005;330:217); not rec for high-risk dz
- ↑ DFS & OS w/ anthra containing tx > CMF (EBCTCG, *Lancet* 2005;365:1687)
- ↑ DFS w/ anthra & T-containing tx > TC × 6 for HER2(–) high-risk pts (ABC, *JCO* 2016;34:1000)
- ↑ DFS & OS when taxane added to anthra-based regimens (EBCTCG *Lancet* 2012;379:432; NSABP B-28, *JCO* 2005;23:3686)

Hormone positive disease—adjuvant endocrine treatment

- **ER &/or PR positive** (IHC > 10%): Always needs endocrine tx. Use of chemo depends on node status & molecular assays
- **ER &/or PR low** (IHC < 10%): Consider endocrine tx
- **Premenopausal:** If high risk (age < 35 y +/– any high-risk factor, eg, node +) → OFS+TAM or OFS+AI (based on distant relapse & OS ↑). Note: OFS+AI > OFS + TAM (based on recurrence risk), no OS benefit. (SOFT/TEXT, *NEJM* 2018;379:122–137; *NEJM* 2014;371:107–118; *JCO* 2016;34:1689)
  - OFS: Achieve w/ LHRH analogues vs. b/l oophorectomy
  - **Tox:** ↑ menopausal sxs (Grade 3,4 ~ 30%) & ↓ bone density
  - **Low risk:** TAM alone, ↓ breast CA mortality (*Lancet* 1998;351:1451–1467)
  - **Extended TAM:** ↓ breast CA mortality Δ 2.8% vs. 5-y tx, slight ↑ DVT/PE & endometrial CA (ATLAS, *Lancet* 2012;381:805; aTTom *JCO* 2013;13:(suppl; abstr 5))
  - **TAM tox:** DVT, endometrial CA, hot flashes
- **Postmenopausal:** AI either upfront or sequentially after 5 y of TAM.
  - Extended AI (10 y): ↓ Contralateral breast CA, w/ absolute benefit of 4%. No OS benefit. (MA.17R, *NEJM* 2016;375:209; NSABP-B42, SABC, 2019).
  - **AI types:** (1) Nonsteroidal: Anastrozole, letrozole (2) Steroidal: Exemestane
  - **AI tox:** Arthralgias, ↓ bone density, vaginal dryness
- **Additional strategies:** Zometa OR denosumab (60 mg q6mos) ↓ skeletal related events & ↑ DFS for pts on AI, independent of BMD (*Lancet* 2015;386:433; ABCSG, SABC, 2015)
  - CDK4/6 inhibitors + AI currently under investigation (monarchE, PALLAS, NATALEE, PENELOPE B)

Hormone-positive disease—adjuvant chemotherapy

- **Oncotype DX:** 21-gene signature RT-PCR assay to calculate Risk Score (RS)—predicts 9-y distant recurrence rate: Low (**RS ≤11**); Intermediate (**RS 12–25**); High (**RS ≥26**)
  - Any pT ≥5 mm, pN0, & **RS 0–11:** ET alone. **RS 12–25:** ET alone, but consider chemo if <50 & high clinical risk. **RS ≥26:** Chemo then ET (TAILORx trial: *NEJM* 2015;373:2005; *NEJM* 2018;379:111–121, *NEJM* 2019;380:2395–2405)
  - pN1 (1–3 N+), postmenopausal pt, & **RS ≤25:** ET only (IDFS ET alone ~ chemo + ET); **RS >25:** Chemo then ET. If premenopausal, chemo always indicated regardless of RS (RxPONDER, *NEJM* 2021;385:2336–2347)

Hormone-positive disease—prognostic models

- **MammaPrint:** 70-gene signature to categorize into 2 groups—good vs. poor prog irrespective of ER status; if high clinical risk, including 1–3 LN, but good prog on genetic risk, may be able to avoid chemo in postmenopausal pts (MINDACT, *Lancet* 2005;365:671; updated *NEJM* 2016;375:717, SABCS 2020)

Hormone-positive disease—neoadjuvant therapy

- **Chemo:** Consider for downstaging breast &/or axillary nodes for BCS & to spare ALND in inoperable or cN1 pts. ddACT preferred in this instance. Chances of pCR ~20%, but pCR not strongly assoc w/ survival outcome
- **Neoadj endocrine therapy (NET):** Preferred regimen: AI for at least 6 mos. NET may have equal BCS rates & clinical response as combination chemo (*JAMA Oncol* 2016;2:1477). pCR rate: NET < NAC
  - All AIs equal (*JCO* 2011;29:2342) & AI > tam (*Lancet Oncol*, 13:345–352)
  - Adding CDK4/6 not rec—no clear benefit in pCR rate vs. AI alone & vs. chemo. New biomarkers under investigation (*Ann Oncol* 2018;29:2334–2340: *summarizes results of NeoPalAna, neoMONARCH, NeoPAL trials*)
  - Premenopausal pts w/ cN1 → Chemo preferred (RxPONDER: *NEJM* 2021;385:2336–2347)

Triple negative disease

- **Stage I:** pT1aN0: No chemo; pT1b/c: Discuss w/ pt; pT2: Recommend chemo
- **Clinical Stage II–III:** NAC rec for T ≥ 2 cm. Preferred regimens: ddACT, CMF or TC if anthracycline contraindicated
- Adding **carbo** to NAC ↑ pCR, independent of *BRCA* status, but conflicting data on DFS impact (↑ in GeparSixto, [*Lancet Onc* 2014;15:747]; no effect in CALGB 40603 [*JCO* 2014;33:13])
- Addition of **ICI:** Remains under investigation
- **After NAC:** If pCR → observation. If nonpCR → capecitabine (cape) for 6–8 cycles (recurrence & survival benefit) (CREATE-X, *NEJM* 2017;376:2147–2159)
- **Pathologic stage II–III:** Adj. chemo is rec (anthra & taxane-based regimens as above. CMF or TC if anthra contraindicated)

HER2-positive disease

- **Anti-HER2 agents** approved in (neo) adj. setting
  - **Trastuzumab (Herceptin, H):** Recombinant, humanized mAb binds to extracellular HER2 domain
  - **Pertuzumab (P):** MAb, inhibits HER2 dimerization
  - **T-DM1:** Antibody–drug conjugate of trastuzumab + antimicrotubule agent
  - **Duration:** 6 mos of H not noninferior to 12 (PHARE, *Lancet Oncol* 2013;14:741, PERSPHONE trial. *Lancet* 2019;393:2599–2612); 24 mos = 12 mos (HERA, *Lancet* 2013;382:1021)
  - **Toxicities:** Cardiac, NYHA III–IV or G3–4 cardiac events <4%. Risk ↑ if pretreated w/ anthracycline. Addition of P: No further ↑ in risk
  - Echo/MUGA at baseline, postanthracycline, & serially every 3 mos. If symptomatic ↓ in EF or asx ↓ EF ≥ 10% below LLN or ≥ 16%, hold H
- **Stage I:** TH followed by H in T1b/c, consider for T1a
- **cStage II–III:** NAC is rec. ddACT-THP or TCbHP (taxane/carbo + HP)
- Addition of P: ↑ pCR (46% v. 29%) (NeoSphere, *Lancet Onc* 2012;13:25)
- pCR ~ 60% w/ HP + anthra & T, no ↑ cardiotox (TRYPHAENA, *Ann Oncol* 2013;24:2278; BERENICE, ESMO Breast 2021)
- Anthracycline-free regimen: TCbHP every 3 wks × 9 cycles. pCR rate & 3 y EFS of TCbHP ≈ FEC – TCbHP (TRAIN2, *JAMA Onc* 2021;7:978–984)
- **If non-PCR:** T-DM1 for 14 cycles (KATHERINE, *NEJM* 2019;380:617–628)
- **pStage II–III:** After surgery → adj. AC-THP (APHINITY, *NEJM* 2017;377:122–131)

Considerations for young patients

- Addition of OFS during chemo ↓ ovarian failure & early menopause & ↑ DFS &OS (POEMS, *NEJM* 2015;372:923)

Workup

- H&P: Including KPS, dz-related sxs
- Labs: CBC, CMP, consider baseline tumor markers (CEA, CA15-3, CA 27.29)
- Imaging: PET-CT vs. CT C/A/P & Bone Scan (BS), additional imaging for specific concerns (fracture → X-ray, brain met → MRI, equivocal staging → PET)
- Bx: Strongly consider for the 1st met/recurrence to document met & ER/PR/HER2 status & obtain NGS. Can have discordance in receptor status between 1° & met (due to sampling bias, Δ in tumor biology, proliferation of different clone, or lab error)

General management principles

- Goal of tx: ↑ survival, ↓ sxs, ↑ QoL
- Systemic therapy (prioritizing nonchemo options 1st, per ER/HER2); local intervention (eg, surgery/RT) for symptomatic control & imminent organ threat (eg, bone pain, cord compression, brain met)

Hormone-receptor positive (HER2 negative) disease

- Tx paradigm: Serial endocrine therapy ± targeted agents until failure → chemo (start w/ chemo if visceral crisis or rapid POD)
- **Endocrine therapy**
  - **1st line:** ET + CDK4/6i (AI + palbociclib, abemaciclib, ribociclib all w/ similar PFS benefit (HR 0.48 to 0.55), OS maturing. See Table below for tox (PALOMA-2, *NEJM* 2016;375:1925; MONALEESA-2, *Ann Oncol* 2018;29:1541; MONARCH 3, *JCO* 2019;5:5)
    - If premenopausal, OFS + AI + CDK4/6. Ribociclib vs. placebo + ET (tam/AI+OFS) showed ↑ PFS, OS (MONALEESA-7, *Lancet* 2018;19:904)
    - Fulvestrant + ribociclib (MONALEESA-3, *NEJM* 2020;382:514) (especially if met <12 mos on adj. AI) vs. fulvestrant + AI vs. single agent ET
  - **2nd line or later:** Fulvestrant + CDK4/6i (if not received 1st line) (PALOMA-3, *NEJM* 2018;379:1926; MONALEESA-3, *NEJM* 2020;382:514; 29:1541; MONARCH 2, *JAMA Onc* 2019;6:116)
  - If *PIK3CA* mut: Fulvestrant + alpelisib—↑ PFS (SOLAR1, *NEJM* 2019;380:1929)
    - Requires monitoring for hyperglycemia, stomatitis, rash, diarrhea
  - Everolimus + exemestane: ↑ PFS (BOLERO-2, *NEJM* 2012;366:520)
  - Abemaciclib single agent: Clinical benefit rate of 42% (MONARCH-1, *CCR* 2017;23:5218)
  - Single agent ET in case of elderly or poor KPS pts
- **Chemo** (same paradigm as in TNBC section below), but favor cape if gradual pace of progression
- **Therapies under development:** Oral SERD (multiple in development), PI3K delta-selective inhibitors, AKTi, CDK2/4/6 inhibitor

Differential Toxicities of CDK4/6 Inhibitor Therapy

	Palbociclib		Abemaciclib		Ribociclib	
Dosing	125 mg qD (3 wks on, 1 wk off)		200 mg BID (continuously)		600 mg qD (3 wks on, 1 wk off)	
CNS penetration	No		Yes		No	
Common AE (%)	**All**	**Gr. 3/4**	**All**	**Gr. 3/4**	**All**	**Gr. 3/4**
Neutropenia	95	54	88	27	46	29
Diarrhea	16	0	90	20	22	3
Cr increase	NR	NR	98.5	0.8	NR	NR
QTc increase	NR	NR	NR	NR	8	0

HER2 positive disease

- **1st line: Dual anti-HER2 agents: ↑ PFS & ↑ OS**
  - Docetaxel/trastuzumab/pertuzumab (DHP) vs. DH (CLEOPATRA, *NEJM* 2012;366:109); or can use weekly paclitaxel—↑ tolerability **(T)+HP** (*JCO* 2015;33:442)
  - Aim for combination chemo + HP for 6 mos; consider switch to vinorelbine or gem if taxane not tolerate (VELVET2, *Oncologist* 2017;22:1160)
- **2nd line**
  - T-DM1 > lapatinib (L) + cape: ↑ PFS & ↑ OS (EMILIA, *NEJM* 2012;367:1783)
  - Tucatinib + cape + H: ↑ PFS overall, ↑ PFS, & OS in pts w/ brain mets; included pts w/ active/untreated brain mets (HER2CLIMB, *NEJM* 2020;382:597)

- **3rd line & beyond**
  - Trastuzumab–Deruxtecan (T-DXd)—ORR 60%, PFS 12.7-NR (DESTINY-01, *NEJM* 2020;382:610)
  - Margetuximab + chemo—↑ PFS but Δ of 0.9 mos (SOPHIA, *JAMA Onc* 2021;7(4):573)
  - May continue H + other options (ie, chemo or hormone (NCCN 2021, *JCO* 2018;36:2736)
  - Other TKIs: **L + Cape** (*NEJM* 2006;355:2733); neratinib + Cape (*JCO* 2010;28:1124)
- **Therapies under development:** T-DXd for HER2 "low" (IHC 1–2+), combination anti-HER2, & IO, further development of ADCs
- **ER+/PR+/HER2+:** Distinct biologic & clinical subtype
  - Recommend 1st-line THP given OS benefit, but AI + HP may be appropriate in pts unable to tolerate chemo (PERTAIN, *JCO* 2018;36:2826)

Triple negative disease

- Initial work-up: PD-L1 IHC, NGS, germline genetic testing
- **Targeted/ IO:**
  - If **PD-L1** > = 1%: Atezo + nab-paclitaxel (IMpassion130, *NEJM* 2018;379:2108)
  - If **CPS** > = 10, pembro + chemo (nab-paclitaxel, paclitaxel, gem + carbo) (KEYNOTE-355 *Lancet* 2020;396;1817). PFS benefit for both
  - If ***BRCA1/2* germline positive,** consider olaparib/talazoparib: ↑ PFS (OlympiAD, *NEJM* 380;985; EMBARCA, *NEJM* 2018;379:753)—note: ORR & PFS benefit for olaparib seen in somatic *BRCA1/2*, germline *PALB2* as well in phase II setting (TBCRC 048, *JCO* 2020;36:4274)
  - For **3rd line:** Sacituzumab–govitecan (ADC to Trop2)—demonstrated ↑ PFS & ↑ OS benefit (ASCENT, *NEJM* 2021;384;1529)
    - Monitor for pancytopenia
  - ***NTRK* fusion** → laro/entrectinib
- **Chemo**
  - Sequential single-agent chemo preferred over combination, but combo could be considered if significant burden of dz & rapid progression (no OS benefit of combo AT vs. A –>T but ↑ RR w/ combo)
  - Combo docetaxel/cape ↑ OS vs. doce alone (*JCO* 2002;20:2812) & paclitaxel/gem ↑ OS vs. paclitaxel alone but incl. tox & never tested vs. sequential Rx (*JCO* 2008;26:3950)
  - No standard sequence of agents, although weekly paclitaxel is typically 1st-line (CALGB 40502) → cape & eribulin 2nd/3rd
  - **Taxanes:** Paclitaxel, docetaxel, & albumin-bound paclitaxel; paclitaxel weekly > q3wks (↑ OS) (*JCO* 2008;26:1642) & paclitaxel = albumin-bound paclitaxel but cheaper
  - **Other antimicrotubule agents:** Eribulin & vinorelbine; eribulin > "Physician's choice" (↑ OS) for 3rd-line & beyond (EMBRACE, *Lancet* 2011;277:914)
  - **Anthracyclines:** Doxorubicin, epirubicin, & pegylated liposomal doxorubicin; consider addition of dexrazoxane if >300 mg/m^2 of lifetime doxorubicin exposure (*JCO* 1999;17:3333); pegylated liposomal doxorubicin is less cardiotoxic
  - **Antimetabolite:** Cape & gemcitabine
  - **Less commonly used:** Infusional 5-FU, ixabepilone, vinblastine, etoposide, cis, cyclophosphamide, mitoxantrone, irinotecan
  - **Combinations:** Gem/carbo, CAF, FEC, AC, EC, AT, CMF, doce/cape, gem/taxol, cape/ixabepilone

Bone metastasis

- Treat w/ bone-strengthening agent if CrCl > 30 to ↓ skeletal-related events; denosumab > zoledronic acid (*JCO* 2010;28:5132)
  - **Bisphosphonates:** Zoledronic acid (4 mg IV q12wks)
  - **Anti-RANK ligand ab:** Denosumab (120 mg SQ q4wks)
  - Recommend preventive dentistry to avoid ONJ, Ca^{2+} monitoring (risk of hypocalcemia, esp w/ denosumab), & creatinine monitoring (esp w/ bisphosphonates)

Monitoring

- H&P, labs (CBC, CMP, ± consider tumor markers), optional imaging (CT C/A/P w/ bone scan or PET/CT) every 2–4 cycles on chemo or as clinically indicated

LOW-GRADE GLIOMA

Epidemiology/risk factors

- Gliomas are classified under a grading system: Grade 1 (typically benign), grade 2 (low grade), grade 3 (anaplastic), & grade 4 (GBM)
- Incidence 5.1 & 2.5 per 1,000,000 in the United States for low-grade astrocytoma & oligodendroglioma, respectively (*Neuro Oncol* 2019;21:v1–v100)
- 6.4% of all CNS tumors
- Peak incidence in 4th decade of life
- Risk factors: Remote hx of ionizing radiation (IR), familial tumor predisposition syns (NF1, LS, Li–Fraumeni)

Clinical manifestations and features

- Presentation is determined by the area of parenchymal involvement but includes seizure (most common), headache, weakness, sensory changes, vision changes, or aphasia
- Uncommon to p/w change in mental status or elevated ICP

Grading classification/pathology

- **WHO classification:**
  The 2016 WHO classification for CNS tumors incorporates **both histologic & molecular** findings in the dx of CNS tumors. WHO grade determinations are still based on histologic criteria alone
- **Molecular genetics:**
  ***IDH1* mut:** Stronger predictor of survival than grade
  - *IDH1* & *IDH2* are mutated in >75% of LGGs
  - Approx 90% of muts result in an amino acid substitution at arginine 132 (R132) w/in the enzyme's active site
  - Testing can be done through IHC for IDH1 R132H (most common mt) or through genetic sequencing. Only if sequencing is neg should a tumor be called *IDH* wt. If sequencing cannot be performed, the dx should be NOS

  ***IDH*wt:** Uncommon in LGG, but if present behaves like HGG w/ poor prog
  1p19q codeletion: Requirement for the dx of oligodendroglioma. A/w response to tx & increased OS
  Other molecular alterations: Astrocytomas: *ATRX* mt, *TP53* mt; Oligodendrogliomas: *ATRX* wt, *TP53* wt
- **Pathologic classification**
  The new pathologic criteria separate the astrocytomas into 2 major groups: The well-circumscribed lesions vs. the diffuse gliomas
  Diffuse gliomas:
  - **Diffuse astrocytoma, (WHO grade II):** Well-diff fibrillary or gemistocytic neoplastic astrocytes on a loose matrix w/ only ↑ cellularity, often *IDH* mut, absent 1p/19q codeletion
  - **Oligodendroglioma (WHO grade II):** Characteristic histology "fried egg" appearance seen on paraffin but not frozen, *IDH* mut, 1p/19q codeleted required
  - **Oligoastrocytoma:** No longer a WHO classification. If on histopathology the specimen has oligodendrocytes & astrocytes, then classification is determined by *IDH*, *ATRX*, & 1p19q molecular status (see above)

  Circumscribed astrocytomas:
  - **Pilocytic astrocytoma (WHO grade I):** Lack *IDH* mts & frequently have *BRAF* alterations. Typically benign. Rarely transform to a higher grade, often resectable. Usu cured by surgery alone & if incomplete resection, can be treated w/ RT
  - **SEGA (WHO grade I):** A/w *TSC1*/*TSC2* mts
  - **Pleomorphic xanthoastrocytoma (PXA) (WHO grade II):** Highly a/w *BRAF* mts, supratentorial, mural nodule, capable of malignant transformation

Diagnostic evaluation

- **MRI brain w/ & w/o contrast:**
  Astrocytomas: Typically nonenhancing, low-attenuation lesions on CT & MRI; T2-weighted or FLAIR MRI preferred (Figure 22-1)
  Oligodendroglioma: Typically T2 hyperintense w/o contrast enhancement. On CT, these tumors appear as low-density masses & can have calcifications that are suggestive but not specific for oligodendrogliomas
  2HG MR spectroscopy: IDH1 (R132H) mt results in excess production of the 2-HG metabolite. Detection of 2HG spike on MR spectroscopy suggests *IDH* mt. Used in initial dx & recurrence when dx is unclear
- **Bx/resection:**
  Utilized to make a definitive dx & for tx in the case of resections
  Histology & molecular genetics of the tumor will guide tx

Poor Prognostic Features in Low-Grade Gliomas
Age ≥40 y
Tumor ≥6 cm
Tumor crossing midline
Preoperative neurologic deficit present
Astrocytoma histology

(*J Clin Oncol* 2002;20:2076)

Initial treatment: (NCCN Clinical Practice Guidelines 2020)

Low-grade infiltrative supratentorial astrocytoma or oligodendroglioma: Traditionally considered low risk & avoided intervention until neurologic sxs became unmanageable. However, recent studies show continuous growth & improved outcomes w/ upfront maximal safe resection (cat 2A)

- Maximal safe resection → postop MRI w/in 48 h to assess extent of resection
- Low risk = ≤40 yo & GTR
  - → Observe **or** clinical trial
  - → Fractionated EBRT or chemo alone can be considered (cat 2B)
- High risk = >40 yo & subtotal resection
  - → RT (54 Gy given in 30 fractions) + adj. PCV chemo **or** RT + adj. TMZ **or** RT + concurrent & adj. TMZ **or** observe (*NEJM* 2016;374:1344)
  - → *IDH* wt often considered in this group, treat w/ RT + concurrent & adj. TMZ

Other low-grade astrocytomas

- Pilocytic astrocytoma: Surgery typically curative
- SEGA: Surgery is often curative. mTOR inhibitors (everolimus & sirolimus)
- PXA: BRAF/MEK inhibitors (dabrafenib/trametinib, vemurafenib/cobimetinib)

Surveillance after treatment

- Diffuse LGG will recur & often transform into HGG
- Surveillance MRI every 3–6 mos for 5 y & then every 6–12 mos thereafter
- RANO guidelines (replaced Macdonald criteria): Progression determined by 25% increase in product of perpendicular diameters
- 2HG MR spectroscopy, MR perfusion, & PET imaging can help determine tumor recurrence vs tx effect

Management of recurrent or progressive disease

- **No prior RT:** Surgery (if resectable) followed by chemo &/or RT or best supportive care
- **Prior RT:** Surgery (if resectable) followed by chemo or best supportive care
- Bx should be considered for unresectable dz to confirm recurrence
- Reirradiation to be considered if recurrence >2 y after prior RT, new lesion outside of prior RT field or small lesion
- Chemo: Active agents include TMZ, nitrosourea, PCV, platinum-based drugs (cis, carbo)

Prognosis

- WHO Grade II Astrocytoma, *IDH* mut: Median OS 10–12 y
- WHO Grade II Astrocytoma, *IDH* wt: Median OS 1.5–3 y (*NEJM* 2015;372(26):2481)
- WHO Grade II Oligodendroglioma, *IDH* mut, 1p/19q codeleted: Median OS 10 y (*Neuro Oncol* 2017;19:suppl5:v1-v88)

HIGH-GRADE GLIOMA

Epidemiology/risk factors

- GBM is the most common malignant 1° brain tumor; >80% of all gliomas
- HGG are 1° (de novo) or 2° (developing from LGG) in origin
- Incidence (per 100,000 persons): GBM 3.23, anaplastic astrocytoma 0.42, anaplastic oligodendroglioma 0.11 (*Neuro Oncol* 2020;22:iv1)
- Median age at dx: GBM 65 y, anaplastic astrocytoma 53 y, anaplastic oligodendroglioma 49 y (*Neuro Oncol* 2020;22:iv1)
- Risk factors: ionizing radiation & rarely familial CA predisposition syns

Clinical manifestations

- Sx related to mass effect, parenchymal infiltration, hydrocephalus, tissue destruction
- Headache, seizures, focal neurologic deficits; progressive over d to wks

Grading classification/pathology

- **WHO classification:** Incorporates **both histologic & molecular** findings in the dx of CNS tumors. Grade determinations are based on histologic criteria alone
  - **Anaplastic oligodendroglioma, WHO grade III:** Anaplastic histology w/ *IDH* mut & 1p/19q-codeletion
  - **Anaplastic astrocytoma, WHO grade III:** Anaplastic histology usu w/ *IDH* mut, absent 1p/19q-codeletion
  - **Glioblastoma, WHO grade IV:** ↑ cellularity, endothelial proliferation, pseudopalisading necrosis
- **Molecular findings:**
  - ***IDH* mut:** *IDH* muts are present in ~12% of GBMs & ~80% of anaplastic astrocytomas. Essential for dx & prognostication. Astrocytic tumors are classified as *IDH* mut or wt. A designation of NOS (eg, glioblastoma NOS) is used when sequencing cannot be performed. *IDH* mut a/w prolonged survival
  - ***MGMT* methylation:** Present in ~40% of GBM; a/w response to alkylating therapy & prolonged survival
  - **1p19q codeletion:** Requirement for the dx of oligodendroglioma; favorable prog

Diagnostic evaluation

- **MRI brain w/ & w/o contrast:**
  - Anaplastic glioma: Often a/w contrast enhancement, but may also appear as nonenhancing expansile T2 hyperintense mass indistinguishable from LGG
  - GBM: Typical appearance is a ring-enhancing mass w/ central necrosis surrounded by T2-hyperintense vasogenic edema (Figure 22-2)
- **Surgical bx or resection** required when possible to distinguish from other CNS masses

Treatment principles

- **Surgery:** In all diffuse gliomas, the goal is maximal resection to reduce mass effect & obtain histologic & molecular dx, while preserving neurologic fxn. Postop MRI should be obtained w/in 24–72 h to document extent of dz following surgery
- **RT:** EBRT w/ partial brain radiation is standard; as effective as WBRT while preserving nl brain tissue & reducing late neurotoxic effects
  - Complications: Radionecrosis (presents as a focal mass lesion w/ contrast enhancement & mass effect); cognitive decline; radiation-induced leukoencephalopathy (mos to y after, MRI shows diffuse ↑ T2/FLAIR signal abnormality & atrophy)

Chemotherapy

- Limited benefit; used in combination w/ surgery & radiation
- TMZ is the most commonly used agent for astrocytic tumors; *MGMT* methylation predicts better response
- PCV is often used for oligodendroglial tumors, both TMZ & PCV are active against oligodendroglioma but have not been directly compared
- Initial therapy w/ combination lomustine & TMZ may improve survival but has greater tox in *MGMT* methylated glioblastoma (*Lancet* 2019;393:678)

Alternating electric field therapy: Prolonged survival when added to RT + TMZ for supratentorial GBM. Device carried & worn ≥18 h daily on a shaved scalp; may result in significant burden (*JAMA* 2017;318:2306)

Initial treatment (NCCN Clinical Practice Guidelines 2020)

Anaplastic glioma: Maximal safe resection followed by:

- Anaplastic oligodendroglioma: RT + neoadj or adj. PCV **or** RT + concurrent & adj. TMZ **or** RT + adj. TMZ (*JCO* 2013;31:344; *JCO* 2013;31:337)
- Anaplastic astrocytoma: RT + adj. TMZ **or** RT + concurrent & adj. TMZ **or** RT + adj. PCV (*Neuro Oncol* 2006;8:253; *Lancet* 2017;390:1645)
- Anaplastic glioma w/ poor functional status (KPS <60): RT (hypofractionated [preferred] or standard) **or** TMZ **or** palliative/BSC

Glioblastoma: Maximal safe resection followed by:

- *MGMT* methylated: RT w/ concurrent & adj. TMZ, consider addition of either alternating electric field therapy or lomustine (*JAMA* 2005;352:987)
- Unmethylated: RT w/ concurrent & adj. TMZ ± alternating electric field therapy **or** RT alone (*JAMA* 2005;352:987)
- Age >70 y, KPS >60: Consider hypofractionated RT rather than standard RT (*JCO* 2004;22:1583)
- KPS <60: Hypofractionated RT (age <70 y: ± concurrent or adj. TMZ) **or** TMZ **or** palliative/BSC

Surveillance

- Surveillance MRI 2–8 wks after RT, then every 2–4 mos for 3y, then every 3–6 mos
- Pseudoprogression: Lesions may increase in size particularly following RT w/ similar appearance to dz progression. More likely ≤3 mos after RT, *MGMT* methylated tumors. MR perfusion, MR spectroscopy, PET/CT, or bx may help diagnose

Recurrent or progressive disease

- There is no established optimal therapy, tx plans are individualized, & clinical trial participation is encouraged
- **Surgical resection:** Esp focal recurrent lesions where GTR is possible. Best candidates are young, ↑ KPS, ↑ interval between initial resection & recurrence
- **Reirradiation:** Esp if recurrent lesion is small or outside initial radiation field. Best candidates are young, ↑ KPS, ↑ interval between initial RT & recurrence
- **Alkylating therapy:** TMZ, PCV, nitrosoureas (carmustine, lomustine), platinum-based therapies. Esp w/ recurrence during tx-free observation, *MGMT* methylation
- **Bev** monotherapy is FDA approved; also used in combination therapy as steroid-sparing agent. Esp w/ enhancing dz & steroid-refractory cerebral edema (*JCO* 2009;27:740; *JCO* 2009;27:4733)
- **Regorafenib:** Oral multikinase inhibitor; ↑ OS in phase II trial in GBM (*Lancet Onc* 2019;20:110)
- **Alternating electric field therapy:** FDA approved; similar efficacy to best-choice chemo in phase III study in GBM (*Eur J Cancer* 2012;48:2192)
- **Palliative/BSC**

Prognosis

- HGG are fast growing & generally considered incurable w/ recurrence inevitable
- Median OS: GBM = 16.7 mos; anaplastic astrocytoma = *IDH* mut 9.7 y, *IDH* wt 1.6 y; anaplastic oligodendroglioma = 14.7 y (*NEJM* 2014;370:709; *JCO* 2019;37:no15_suppl:2000; *JCO* 2013;31:337)

Figure 22-1 Low-grade Astrocytoma T2 FLAIR MSKCC. Courtesy of Dr. T. Kaley.

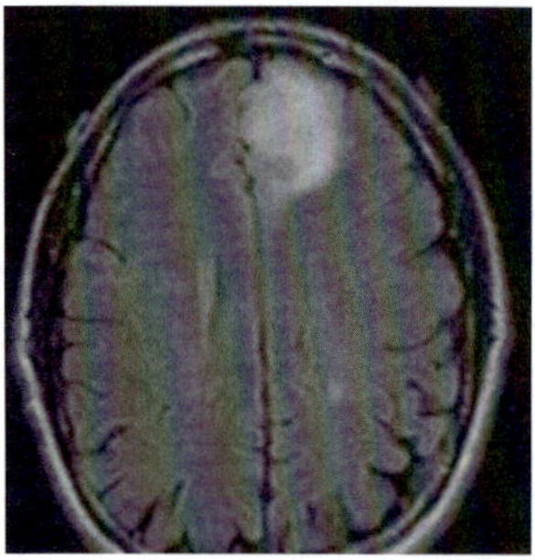

Figure 22-2 GBM T1 postcontrast MRI MSKCC. Courtesy of Dr. T. Kaley.

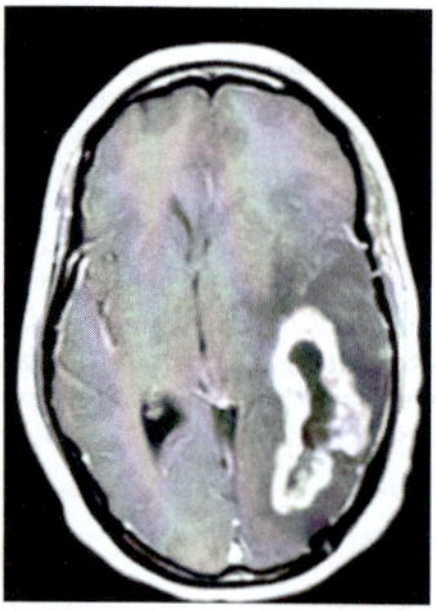

CNS METASTATIC DISEASE

Epidemiology

- CNS mets occur in **20–40%** of adult pts w/ CA (*J Neuro Onc* 2005;75:5)
- Most commonly a/w lung (20%), melanoma (7%), renal (7%), breast (5%), colorectal (2%), but any CA can spread to CNS (*JCO* 2004;22:2865)
- Estimated incidence of brain mets in pts newly dx'd w/ CA is 23,598 annually in the United States (*Neuro Oncol* 2017;19:1511)

Clinical manifestations and diagnosis

- **80% cerebral hemispheres,** 15% cerebellum, 5% brainstem
- **Hematogenous spread** to gray–white jxn where narrow blood vessels trap tumor emboli
- Headache, neurologic deficit (weakness, numbness, tingling), seizures, AMS, ataxia
- **MRI is the most important diagnostic tool & more sensitive than CT.** Can visualize solitary met vs. multiple vs. leptomeningeal dz w/ contrast-enhanced T1-weighted images
- Other imaging modalities: MR spectroscopy (measure metabolites), MR perfusion (measure cerebral blood flow), brain FDG-PET (measure radiolabeled tracer) may help differentiate radiation necrosis from active tumor
- Size, number, & location of lesions, along w/ amount of edema, PS, & status of systemic illness guide decision to resect vs. stereotactic radiation

Prognosis

- RTOG retrospective recursive partitioning analysis:
  - **RPA class I:** <65 y, KPS >70%, controlled 1°, no extracranial met → median survival 7.1 mos
  - **RPA class II:** KPS >70% but >65 y; not controlled 1° or extracranial met → median survival 4.2 mos
  - **RPA class III:** KPS <70% → median survival 2.3 mos (*Int J Radiat Oncol Biol Phys* 2000;47:1001)

Risk of Death and Median Survival by Treatment and Diagnosis (HR/Median Survival) (*JCO* 2012;30:419)

	NSCLC	SCLC	Melanoma	Breast	GI
WBRT	HR = 1 3.5 mos	HR = 1 4.2 mos	HR = 1 2.9 mos	HR = 1 7.4 mos	HR = 1 3 mos
SRS	HR = 0.6 10 mos				
WBRT + SRS	HR = 0.5 12.7 mos	HR = 0.2 15.3 mos			
Surg + SRS	HR = 0.5 11.9 mos				
Surg + WBRT	HR = 0.5 11.6 mos	HR = 0.4 14.7 mos	HR = 0.6 11 mos		HR = 0.3 10.7 mos
Surg + WBRT + SRS	HR = 0.4 12 mos		HR = 0.5 13 mos	HR = 0.5 29.5 mos	HR = 0.4 7.9 mos

Management

Sx control

- **Corticosteroids:** Lowest dose for shortest time. Consider starting at dexa 4–8 mg q12h. Extensive mass effect should be premedicated w/ steroids for 24 h prior to RT
- **AEDs:** For pts who have not experienced a seizure, routine prophylactic use of anticonvulsants is not rec. Recommend use of non-CYP450 inducing AED (levetiracetam, lacosamide, valproic acid, clobazam) in pts w/ seizures. Inducers of CYP450 medications (phenytoin, phenobarbital) may be indicated if status epilepticus or AED-refractory. If surgical resection, short-term prophylactic AED w/ rapid tapering off w/ in 1st wk postop
- **Anticoagulation:** Can be administered in pts w/ brain mets for VTE prophylaxis & tx. Frequent CBC monitoring is indicated among pts w/ thrombocytopenia-inducing chemotherapeutic agents

Treatment of brain metastases (*JCO* 2015;33:3475)

- **Surgical resection:** May be indicated for symptomatic pts or if dx in question. 1–2 mets, esp w/ extensive cerebral edema, critical location. Trend towards postop SRS to resection cavity instead of WBRT
- **SRS:** Few (1–3) or multiple mets; smaller mets (≤3 cm in diameter); local relapse after resolution of single met; or for more radioresistant tumors, such as melanoma. Allows tx of medically or surgically inoperable pts &/or multiple lesions, eliminating need for craniotomy. Limited by lack of tissue dx, risk of radiation necrosis, inability to acutely reduce cerebral edema (*Radiat Oncol Biol Phys* 2000;47:291)
- **WBRT:** Multiple (>3–10) mets; large (>3 cm) met not amenable to SRS; concomitant leptomeningeal mets; postsurgical resection of a dominant met w/ multiple (>3–10) remaining. Rec dose is 30 Gy in 10 daily fractions. A/w delayed, progressive, irreversible cognitive dysfunction (*Lancet* 2004;363:1665)
- **Targeted therapy:** CNS-penetrant agents for select CA (ie, osimertinib for *EGFR*-mut lung CA, lorlatinib for *ALK*-mutated lung CA, lapatinib/tucatinib for HER2+ breast CA, dabrafenib/trametinib for *BRAF*-mutated melanoma); requires molecular confirmation via bx of 1° or metastatic site
- **IO:** Alone or in combination w/ chemo (ie, ipilimumab/nivolumab for melanoma, pembrolizumab for NSCLC, & high PD-1). Risk of CNS pseudoprogression (*NEJM* 2018;379:722; *NEJM* 2018;378:2078; *JCO* 2017;35:2439)
- **Chemo:** W/ highly chemo-sensitive tumor, in combination w/ targeted/immune therapies, or after 1st-line txs fail (ie, capecitabine for breast CA, cis-pemetrexed for NSCLC, high-dose MTX for lymphoma) (*Eur J Cancer* 2003;39:2114)

Follow-up: MRI q2–3mos for 1 y, then as clinically indicated

Salvage Rx

- Prev tx w/ surgery: Surgery, SRS, WBRT, or systemic therapy
- Prev tx w/ WBRT or SRS: Surgery if large or symptomatic; consider additional RT depending upon prior dose & location

Leptomeningeal metastasis

- Multifocal seeding of leptomeninges w/ tumor by hematogenous dissemination, lymphatic spread, or direct extension
- 5% of pts w/ CA
- Most commonly a/w breast (35%), lung (25%), lymphoma (11%), leukemia (8%), GI (6%), melanoma (5%) (*Neurology* 2010;74:1449)
- Median overall survival is 2–5 mos. High KPS & available targeted therapies are positive prognostic factors (*Ann Onc* 2016;27:1138, *Neuro Oncol* 2020;22:675; *Am J Cancer Res* 2013;3:117)

Clinical manifestation & Dx

- **Local injury** to nerves traveling through spinal fluid—peripheral nerve palsies, weakness, paresthesias, pain, bowel or bladder dysfunction
- **Direct invasion** into brain or spinal cord—focal findings, seizures
- **Obstruction of nl CSF flow**—HA & n/v, often worse when supine or w/ position change; hydrocephalus; ↑ ICP on LP
- **Cognitive dysfunction**—encephalopathy
- **CSF cytology** 50% positive w/ malignant cells, 90% w/ repeated CSF but 10% persistently neg CSF. CSF circulating tumor cell quantification may be more sensitive, but only available in specialized centers. LP contraindicated in pts w/ coagulopathy, thrombocytopenia, bulky intracranial dz. CSF pleocytosis, ↑ protein, ↓ glc
- MRI w/ diffuse &/or **nodular enhancement of leptomeninges or hydrocephalus** w/o mass lesion

Tx

- **Systemic therapy:** Chemo or targeted therapy using drugs w/ adequate CNS penetration
- **Intrathecal chemo:** Requires nl CSF flow dynamics; Ommaya reservoir improves ease of administration
- **Radiation:** Palliative tx that may improve sxs; focal RT to bulky/sx sites in spine or WBRT in brain
- **Surgery:** May benefit from palliative VP shunt to alleviate sxs of elevated ICP

PARANEOPLASTIC SYNDROMES

Paraneoplastic syndromes

- Clinical disorders a/w malignancy unrelated to physical effects of 1° or metastatic tumor
- Sxs typically begin acutely or subacutely, progress over wks to mos. Can precede CA dx by mos to y
- Mediated by hormones/cytokines excreted by tumor or an autoimmune resp to the tumor
- Tx of malignancy may improve the paraneoplastic syn

Endocrine

- Ectopic ACTH/**Cushing syn:** Classic Cushing syn often manifests w/ proximal muscle myopathy, truncal obesity, purple striae, HTN, ↓ K, ↑ glc, & fatigue. Classic Cushing signs/sx may be absent given rapid tumor progression. Assoc CA: **SCLC + bronchial carcinoid (50–60%),** mesothelioma, bladder, endometrial, prostate, Ewing sarcoma, thymoma, lymphoma, GI, breast
- **SIADH:** HypoNa mediated by ADH-induced water retention w/ ensuing volume expansion activating natriuresis & restoration of euvolemia. Assoc CA: **SCLC (10–45%),** neuroendocrine lung CA, thymoma, med thyroid, GI, pancreatic, adrenal, ovarian
- HyperCA: 10% pts w/ CA, confers poor prog. Mechanism: **PTHrP secretion 80%,** osteolytic activity 20%, vit D secretion, PTH secretion. Assoc CA: MM, breast, SCC esp lung, RCC, HTLV lymphoma, gyn
- **Carcinoid syn:** Flushing, diarrhea, from serotonin or vasoactive peptides, typically w/ carcinoids; also in medullary thyroid CA, RCC, & others. **Harlequin** syn is unilateral flushing, diaphoresis from ciliary ganglion destruction
- Nonislet cell tumor–induced hypoglycemia: Tumor production of IGF-2 or insulin (rare). Assoc CA: Mesenchymal & hepatic carcinomas, GIST, adrenal
- Oncogenic osteomalacia: Osteomalacia w/ ↓ PO4, ↓ vit D1,25 w/ bone pain, urine PO4 loss; possibly from ↑ FGF23. Assoc CA: Lung, MM, prostate

Acute Management of Endocrine Paraneoplastic Syndromes

	Dx	Tx
SIADH (*NEJM* 2007;356:2064)	↓ Na, ↑ UOsm	Fluid restrict <1 L/d, demeclocycline 300–600 mg BID, 3% saline
HyperCA	↑ Ca	NS 200–500 mL/h, intranasal calcitonin (acutely); IV bisphosphonates (acute & chronic tx), denosumab, steroids (in lymphoma/MM), dialysis
Ectopic ACTH causing **Cushing syn** (*Pituitary* 2002;5:77)	1-mg overnight dexa suppression test w/ nonsuppressed AM cortisol & ACTH; ↑ 24-h Ucortisol, ↑ midnight salivary cortisol, ↓ K	Ketoconazole 600–1,200 mg/d, metyrapone 1–4.5 g/d, mifepristone 300 mg daily (for ↑ glc 2/2 Cushing); spironolactone 25–100 mg daily, K supplements; bilat adrenalectomy if cannot reverse sx

Skin

- **Acanthosis nigricans:** Gray–brown symmetric velvety plaques on flexor, anogenital regions w/ malignant form progressing more rapidly. Assoc CA: AdenoCAs (95%), commonly gastric
- **Sweet syn:** Acute onset fever; neutrophilia; erythematous, painful, raised cutaneous plaques w/ dense dermal infiltrates of well-diff neutrophils on path. 20% a/w malignancy; AML, MDS, various carcinomas
- **Pyoderma gangrenosum:** Painful, purulent, nonhealing neutrophilic ulcers. Assoc CA: MGUS, MM, NHL. Superficial pyoderma gangrenosum w/ bullous changes most often a/w AML
- **Paraneoplastic pemphigus:** Painful stomatitis, conjunctival ulcers, erosive skin lesions, resp failure w/ 30% mortality. AutoAb cross react w/ epidermal proteins. Assoc CA: NHL, CLL, Castleman dz, sarcoma, WM. Antiepiligrin variant of cicatricial pemphigoid characterized by ab to epidermal basement membrane
- **Dermatomyositis:** Heliotrope rash, Gottron papules, shawl sign. 10–30% adults w/ dermatomyositis w/ malignancy. Strongest a/w ovarian CA. ("Paraneoplastic Syndromes", Devita, *Cancer: Principles & Practice of Oncology* 2019;2004–2005; *Ca Cancer J Clin* 2009;59:73)

Neurologic

- Sx (often preceding CA dx) a/w ab against neural Ag: Intracellular (classic/oncogenic ab: Almost always paraneoplastic) or cell surface (can be autoimmune)
- Ab can be detected in CSF± serum in some cases; not clearly pathogenic
- If involving the CNS, can be a/w transient CSF pleocytosis & an elevated IgG
- MRI is often nl; may show medial temporal FLAIR hyperintensity in limbic encephalitis, cerebellar atrophy in cerebellar degeneration (*Ca Cancer J Clin* 2009;59:73, *Mayo Clin Proc* 2010;85:838)

Neurologic Paraneoplastic Syndromes

	Sx	Assoc CA	Dx	Ab
Limbic Encephalitis	Mood Δ, seizures, hallucinations, memory loss, hypothalamic sx over days to months (less common)	SCLC (40–50%), testicular germ cell CA (20%), breast (8%), thymoma, teratoma, HL	Temporal Δs: Epileptic foci (EEG), hypermetabolism (PET), abnl FLAIR CSF: Pleocytosis, ↑ protein, ↑ IgG, oligoclonal bands	Anti-Hu (SCLC), anti-Ma2 (testicular), NMDAR (ovarian teratoma), anti-VGKC, anti-AMPAR, anti-CRMP5
Paraneoplastic Cerebellar Degeneration	Ataxia, diplopia, dysphagia, dysarthria, prodrome dizziness, n/v	SCLC, gyn CA, HL, breast	PET brain: Early stage ↑ FDG → late stage ↓ FDG in cerebellum; cerebellar atrophy	Anti-Yo, anti-Hu, anti-CRMP5, anti-Ma, anti-Tr, anti-Ri, anti-VGCC, anti-mGluR1
Lambert–Eaton Myasthenic Syn (LEMS)	LE prox muscle weakness (improves w/ exercise), fatigue, autonomic sx (ptosis, impotence, dry mouth)	3% of pts w/ SCLC; prostate, cervical, lymphoma, adenoCA	EMG w/ repetitive nerve stim: Low-rate stim: ↓ response High-rate stim: ↑ response	Anti-VGCC
MG	Fatigable weakness of ocular, bulbar, limb & respiratory muscles	Thymoma (15%)	EMG w/ ↓ response to repetitive nerve stim	Anti-AChR
Autonomic Neuropathy	Subacute onset of panautonomic dysfunction: Dry mouth, orthostatic hypotension, gastroparesis/chronic pseudo-obstruction, cardiac arrhythmia	SCLC, thymoma	Abd studies: CT/barium w/ GI dilation, slowing, no mech obs. Esophageal studies: Achalasia/spasms	Anti-Hu, anti-CRMP5, anti-nAChR, anti-amphiphysin
Subacute Sensory Neuropathy	Sensory ataxia, ↓ reflexes, paresthesia	SCLC (70–80%), breast, ovarian, sarcoma, HL, MGUS (10%)	Nerve conduction w/ ↓ sensory nerve potential	Anti-Hu, anti-CRMP5, anti-amphiphysin, anti-MAG
Opsoclonus–Myoclonus	Rapid, arrhythmic involuntary eye movements, muscle twitching, ataxia	neuroblastoma (children), breast + SCLC (adults)	Clinical	Anti-Ri (adults), anti-Hu, anti-neurofilament
CA-assoc Retinopathy	Night blindness, blurry vision from photoreceptor degeneration	SCLC (most common), melanoma	Clinical	Anti-recoverin
Stiff Person Syn	Progressive stiffness, rigidity, & spasms, typically truncal	Breast, SCLC	+ antibody titers in serum & CSF, EMG: Involuntary motor unity firing	Anti-amphiphysin, anti-GAD, anti-Ri

Mayo Clin Proc 2010;85:838.

Treatment of neurologic paraneoplastic syndromes

- Treat underlying CA: Chemo, radiation, or surgical resection
- Immunosuppression: Steroids, IVIG (0.4 g/kg/d for 5 d), plasmapheresis; if ineffective (or if onconeural ab), cyclophosphamide, rituximab (IV 375 mg/m^2 weekly for 4 doses)

HODGKIN LYMPHOMA

Epidemiology

- Represents ~10–12% of lymphomas, ~8–9K cases annually in United States, ~1,000 deaths
- Bimodal age distribution, younger pts (20s–30s), 2nd peak in older adults (>55)

Biology/Pathology

- 2 major types: **Classical HL (cHL, 95%) & nodular lymphocyte-predominant (NLPHL, 5%)**
- cHL characterized pathologically by the **Reed–Sternberg cell:** Large, multinucleated cell w/ classic **"owl's eyes"** appearance, **CD15+/CD30+;** 40% of cases EBV-assoc
- **Subtypes** of cHL include **nodular sclerosis, lymphocyte rich, mixed cellularity, & lymphocyte depleted.** Tx does not differ among these subtypes
- **9p24.1** gene **amp** is one of the most common genetic alterations (contains *PD-L1, PD-L2, JAK2*; muts in **beta-2 microglobulin** can lead to loss of MHC I, assoc w/ improved PFS/OS (*Blood* 2010;116:3268, *Blood* 2015;125:1061)
- **NLPHL** is more indolent, characterized by the **lymphocyte-predominant (LP) cells** which are **CD15–/CD30–/CD20+**

Workup

- H&P: B sx, EtOH intolerance, pruritus. Labs: CBC, **ESR**, LDH. **Excisional bx** preferred for initial dx; core-needle bx may be adequate, **FNA inadequate**
- Cross-sectional imaging w/ **PET/CT**
- **BMBx** no longer required (unless unexplained cytopenias)
- **TTE** if anthracycline to be used, **PFTs** if bleomycin to be used
- Fertility counseling (ABVD assoc w/ low risk of infertility)

Staging

- **Lugano classification** (modification of the Ann Arbor/Cotswalds modification)

Stage	Description (*JCO* 1989;7:1630; *JCO* 2014;32(27):3059)
I	Single LN or nodal group
II	2 or more nodal groups on the same side of the diaphragm
III	LN groups on both sides of the diaphragm
IV	Disseminated EN dz
Modifier	**Description**
B	"B" sx: Unexplained fever, wt loss (≥10% of wt), or drenching night sweats
A	Absence of "B" sx
X	No longer used; instead record largest tumor size by CT scan
E	EN extension: Limited involvement of an extralymphatic organ contiguous w/ nodal site
S	Spleen involvement

Risk factors

- Early stage: Different criteria exist, in general unfav criteria include age ≥50, ESR >50 or >30 if +B sx, bulky dz (>10 cm or >1/3 width of mediastinum), 3+ nodal regions involved
- Adv stage: **IPS** includes 7 RFs for adverse outcome (*NEJM* 1998;339:1506):

Serum albumin <4 g/dL	Hb <10.5 g/dL	Male sex
WBC ≥15K	Age ≥45	Stage IV

Lymphocyte count <600/mm^3 or <8% of WBC

Nodular lymphocyte predominant Hodgkin lymphoma

- Indolent, relapsing neoplasm w/ different natural hx & tx paradigm than classical HL
- Most commonly early stage; better prog than classical HL
- **RT alone,** or in combination w/ chemo effective in early stage
- **Rituximab** containing chemo (eg, R-CHOP) effective in adv stage

Management: Treatment considerations

- For ABVD, risk of infection low even in neutropenic pts not receiving G-CSF: **Tx delays should be avoided**. Neutropenia does not necessitate a dose delay or reduction
- For BV+AVD, G-CSF is **required**
- End-of-tx PET: If positive, confirm w/ bx. If bx positive proceed to salvage therapy

Management: Early-stage disease

Stage	Treatment	Notes
I–II, favorable	ABVD ×2 + ISRT 20 Gy	Combined modality therapy vs. chemo alone: ↓ risk of recurrence, no difference in OS
	ABVD ×3 → obs if PET (–)	RAPID: If PET (+) after ABVD ×3 → ABVD ×1 + ISRT 30 Gy (*NEJM* 2015;372:1598)
	ABVD ×2 + AVD ×4 if PET-2 neg	RATHL (*NEJM* 2016;374:2419)
I–II, unfav, nonbulky	ABVD ×2 followed by PET-2 w/ PET-adapted approach (see right)	If PET-2 (–), options include AVD ×4 (as per RATHL, see above), ABVD ×2 (CALGB 50604) or ABVD ×2 + ISRT 30 Gy (*JCO* 2017;35:1786) If PET-2 (+), confirm w/ re-bx; use escBEACOPP, other salvage therapy
I–II, bulky	ABVD ×4 + ISRT 30 Gy	7 cm or larger likely requires ISRT (*Haematologica* 2016;101:1237)
	A(B)VD ×6 w/o RT	AVD for cycles 3–6 if PET-2 (–) (as per RATHL) No RT if PET-2 & PET-6 neg (*JCO* 2020;38:3905)

Management: Advanced-stage disease

Stage	Treatment	Notes
IIBX, IIII, IV	A(B)VD ×6 w/ PET after 2 cycles	AVD for cycles 3–6 if PET-2 (–) Escalation to escBEACOPP if PET-2 (+) may increase cure rate (*NEJM* 2016;374:2419)
	BV + AVD (A+AVD)	Consider if bleomycin contraindicated, no neuropathy (*NEJM* 2018;378:331)
	escBEACOPP ×6 w/ PET after 2 cycles	Reserve for pts w/ high-risk (IPS ≥ 4) dz Consider de-escalating to ABVD if PET-2 (–) (*Blood* 2015;126:577)

Note: PET-#: refers to PET after # cycles of therapy.

Management: Relapsed/refractory classical Hodgkin lymphoma

- Salvage nonoverlapping chemo **(ICE, DHAP, GVD)**, novel regimens incorporate PD-1 blockade (BV-nivolumab, pembrolizumab + GVD) (*Blood* 2018;131:1183; *JCO* 2021;39:3109), consolidate w/ **ASCT** if responsive
- Most important pre-SCT predictor of outcomes is achievement of **PET-neg CR** (*Blood* 2012;119:1665)
- Consolidative RT to sites involved w/ dz at relapse is typically administered to pts w/ **early-stage dz at relapse who were not previously IRR**
- RFs for adverse outcome postrelapse: Remission duration <12 mos, B sx, EN dz (*Blood* 2001;97:616)
- In high-risk pts, maintenance BV after ASCT 12 mos ↑ PFS (*Lancet* 2015;385:1853)
- In pts relapsing after ASCT: **BV** has 75% RR post-ASCT, long-term remission in ~20% achieving a CR (*Blood* 2016;128:1562); nivolumab or pembrolizumab has a 65–70% RR post-ASCT, long-term remission in ~40% (*Lancet Oncol* 2016;17:1283; *JCO* 2016;34:2698)
- Role of allo transplant is unclear, particularly for pts receiving PD-1 blockade given the increased-risk GVHD (*Blood* 2020;135(24):2182)

Toxicity

- Monitor pulmonary tox w/ clinical surveillance ± routine PFTs (↓ DLCO)
  - Bleomycin, carmustine, radiotherapy, BV, & anti–PD-1 therapy all cause **pneumonitis**
- Note: Anti–PD-1-related pneumonitis can **often appear like pseudoprogression w/ nonclassical radiographic presentations** → consider bx

Survivorship

- **2° malignancies** overtake HL as the greatest risk of mortality (*JCO* 2014;32:163)
- **Annual breast screening** should begin 8–10 y (no later than age 40) in women who received RT to chest; MRI together w/ mammography between ages 10 & 30 is the standard screening for women at high risk for breast CA
- **TSH** annually in pts who received RT to the neck

FOLLICULAR LYMPHOMA

Epidemiology

- Most common indolent lymphoma & 2nd most common lymphoma overall, representing ~25% of NHLs. More prevalent among Caucasians, incidence ↑ w/ age, equal incidence between men & women

Biology/Pathology

- Composed primarily of small, cleaved lymphocytes that grow in a follicular pattern resembling that of nl 2° lymphoid tissue
- Variable numbers of larger centroblasts, w/ ↑ number indicating higher grade
- **Grade I, II, & IIIA** share the tx paradigm outlined below. **Grade IIIB is treated as DLBCL**
- Immunophenotypically, FL cells classically express the B-cell Ags **CD19 & CD20**, the follicular center Ags **CD10 & BCL-6**, & the antiapoptotic protein **BCL-2**. Does not express T-cell Ags, including CD3 or CD5 (latter is typically expressed in CLL/SLL or MCL)
- Overexpression of **BCL-2**, an antiapoptotic protein, is mediated by the **t(14:18)** w/c juxtaposes the *BCL-2* gene to the Ig heavy chain locus in a large majority of cases. Translocation not sufficient to diagnose FL
- As w/ other lymphomas, incisional or excisional bx is preferred for initial dx
- The term "follicular center cell lymphoma" is nonspecific & may refer to FL or DLBCL
- Testicular FL, duodenal-type FL, pediatric FL, & 1° cutaneous follicle center lymphoma are rare, distinct dzs & are managed differently than classic FL

Staging and workup

- Lugano staging (*JCO* 2014;27:3059)
- Staging primarily consists of cross-sectional imaging w/ either a **CT scan** of chest/abdomen/pelvis (preferred) ± neck or a **PET scan**
- PET particularly useful if there is concern for **transformed** dz or to confirm limited distribution in early stage & for response monitoring
- Peripheral nodal areas evaluated w/ physical exam
- **BMBx** needed to complete staging, but can be deferred if observation or standard tx for adv dz is planned
- CBC, comprehensive profile, LDH, HIV, & hepatitis B & C serologies

Risk Factors		
FLIPI	**FLIPI2**	**PRIMA-PI**
Stage ≥III	+ BM	+ BM
↑ LDH	β2M > ULN	β2M >3 mg/L
Age >60 y	Age >60 y	
Hb <12	Hb <12	
>4 nodal areas involved	Node >6 cm	

Prognostic models

- As w/ other lymphomas, stage alone confers limited prognostic info
- **FLIPI** (*Blood* 2004;104:1258) predictive of OS; **FLIPI2** (*JCO* 2009;27:4555) & **PRIMA-PI** predictive of PFS (*Blood* 2018;132:49)

Outcomes						
Risk	**FLIPI**	**5-y OS (%)**	**FLIPI2**	**5-y PFS (%)**	**PRIMA-PI**	**5-y PFS (%)**
Low	0–1	90.6	0	79.5	β2M < 3, BM–	69
Int	2	77.6	1–2	51.2	β2M < 3, BM+	55
High	3–5	52.5	3–5	18.8	β2M > 3	37

- Response duration following upfront CIT is prognostic for OS. POD w/in 24 mos is a/w 50% 5-y OS (*JCO* 2015;33:2516). However, significant proportion of early POD may be transformed high-grade dz, & true FL POD has better OS

Management: Stages I–II

- Stage I & contiguous stage II: ISRT alone can be curative. 10-y RFS of ~40%, w/ Stage I pts faring better than stage II (*JCO* 1996;14:1282)
- Standard RT dose 24 Gy; better local control, similar 5-y OS vs. 4 Gy (*Lancet Onc* 2021;22:332)
- Observation in selected cases where ISRT may result in significant morbidity w/ systemic being employed when indicated by NCCN/GELF criteria, as for stages III–IV

Management: Asymptomatic stages III–IV (or intra-abdominal stage II)

- **Observation** is rec for asx pts: Serial clinical exams & periodic CT (PET if suspicion for **transformation**). Optimal timing of scans not determined, tailored to individual pt characteristics
- In observed pts, median time to initiation of tx is ~3.5 y. ~20% never require tx
- No OS advantage has been demonstrated w/ early initiation of tx (either alkylator or rituximab)

Frontline management: Symptomatic stages III–IV (or bulky stage II)

- Enrollment in clinical trial should be encouraged
- Commonly accepted **indications for tx** include: Sx, any node >7 cm or 3 nodes >3 cm, cytopenias, fluid collections (ascites, pleural effusions), organ impairment, & leukemic phase of dz (*JCO* 1997;15:1110; NCCN: B-Cell Lymphomas [version 3.2021])
- **Multiple frontline therapeutic options:** Choice of tx is based on pt & dz characteristics including volume & distribution of dz, age & functional status of the pt, potential need for rapid response, or concern for transformed dz (see below)
  - **Rituximab (CD20 mab) monotherapy** (4 weekly doses) is used 1° in pts w/ **low-volume** dz. ORR ~70–75%, CR ~40–45% in untreated pts (*JCO* 2005;23:1103)
  - **Rituximab plus chemo** is more often used. Standard regimens include **R-CHOP, R-bendamustine, R-CVP.** Addition of rituximab to chemo improves RR, PFS, & OS over chemo alone. No single regimen is preferred, & individual pt factors guide choice
  - **Obinutuzumab plus chemo +/– obinutuzumab maintenance** could also be considered. Obinutuzumab-chemo → obinutuzumab maintenance improves PFS (but not OS) compared to R-chemo → rituximab maintenance (*NEJM* 2017;377:1331)

Maintenance and consolidation therapy

- **Rituximab maintenance** after completing initial tx ↑ PFS, not OS (*JNCI* 2011;103:1799)
- No trials have directly evaluated the role of maintenance obinutuzumab. If maintenance therapy is rec, **obinutuzumab-chemo → obinutuzumab maintenance** is superior to R-chemo → R maintenance (*NEJM* 2017;377:1331)

Relapsed or refractory disease

- Consider transformed dz at progression; eval w/ PET & bx when feasible. PET may be useful in determining a site for bx. SUV values >10–13 suggest transformation (*Ann Oncol* 2009;20:508)
- Asx relapsed pts can be observed, as w/ untreated pts
- Choice of 2nd-line Rx influenced by quality & duration of response to initial tx
- **If rituximab-sensitive (PFS >6 mos after last rituximab): Rituximab ± chemo** remains effective in relapsed pts. Rituximab monotherapy ORR is ~45%, but is more commonly combined w/ chemo in relapsed pts
- **Rituximab-refractory: Obinutuzumab-Benda → Obinu maintenance** improves PFS & OS c/w bendamustine monotherapy (*GADOLIN Study, Lancet Onc* 2016;17:1081)
- **Lenalidomide plus rituximab (R2):** Improved PFS vs. R alone in R/R FL w/ 1 prior line therapy in rituximab-sensitive dz (median PFS 39 vs. 14 mos) (*AUGMENT Study, JCO* 2019;37:1188)
- **PI3K Inhibitors** (idelalisib, duvelisib, copanlisib, umbralisib) approved in dz refractory to rituximab & alkylating agents, ORR 42–66% in single-arm studies
- **Tazemetostat** (EZH2 inhibitor): Approved in R/R FL; ORR 69% in EZH2-mut FL; ORR 35% in EZH2 nonmut FL (*Lancet Onc* 2020;21:1433)
- **CAR T-cell therapy:** Axicabtagene ciloleucel approved in R/R FL after ≥2 lines tx; ORR 94%, 12-mo PFS 78% (*Blood* 2020;136[Suppl 1]:40)
- Choice of **autologous** or **allo** transplant is made individually; usu based on such factors as pt age & comorbidity, availability of a suitable donor, & the biology & behavior of the lymphoma
- **Very low-dose RT** (400 cGy) provides excellent local control & palliation in 70% of R/R pts

Histologic transformation

- There is a ~**3% /y** risk of transformation from FL to DLBCL, usu characterized by rapid nodal enlargement & rising LDH, ± systemic sxs
- **Transformation to DLBCL** in a previously untreated pt treated similar to **de novo DLBCL**
- If histologic transformation occurs after prior chemo, consider consolidation w/ **HDT/ASCR** in chemosensitive dz

MARGINAL ZONE LYMPHOMA (MZL)

Definition and epidemiology

- Indolent neoplasm of mature, nongerminal center B lymphocytes arising from the marginal zone of lymphoid follicles
- **3 subtypes: Extranodal MZL** (**ENMZL** including **MALT** lymphoma), **splenic**, **nodal**
- Comprises approx 5–10% of all NHLs

Pathogenesis

- Some subtypes arise from **chronic Ag stimulation** due to infectious pathogens or other inflammatory states, such as AI disorders
- Multistep pathogenesis involving in some cases a variety of chromosomal translocations resulting in Ag-independent activation of **NF-κB pathway** (key signal for B-cell survival)

Suspected Antigen or Inflammatory Associations in MZL

Type	Disease Site	Associated Ag
ENMZL/MALT lymphoma	Gastric (most common)	*Helicobacter pylori*
	Intestine	*Campylobacter jejuni*
	Orbital/ocular	*Chlamydia psittaci*
	Salivary/lacrimal gland	Sjögren syn
	Thyroid	Hashimoto thyroiditis
	Joint/synovial tissue	Relapsing polychondritis
	Cutaneous	*Borrelia* species
	Lung	*Achromobacter xylosoxidans*
Splenic MZL	Spleen	HCV

Clinical presentation

- MZL can affect **diverse anatomical sites** & presentation varies accordingly
- Localized sx: Epigastric pain/GERD (gastric), abd pain/obstruction/malabsorption (intestine), orbital mass/eye redness/tearing (ocular), salivary gland mass, thyroid mass, skin nodules or rash (cutaneous), cough (bronchial), abd distension/early satiety/cytopenias (splenic MZL), painless LAN (nodal MZL)
- Systemic sx: B sx uncommon (~15%, **consider histologic transformation to DLBCL**)

Diagnostic evaluation

- **Bx** required: Either excisional/incisional or core. Splenic MZL may be d'xd on splenic bx or splenectomy & indirectly if splenomegaly w/ low FDG PET & characteristic immunophenotype on blood &/or BMBx
- **Histology:** Polymorphous **infiltrate of small lymphocytes,** centrocyte-like B cells, & plasma cells; reactive follicles; **lymphoepithelial lesions** (epithelial tissues) in MALT
  - **Splenic MZL** sometimes w/ characteristic **villous lymphocytes** on peripheral smear
- Immunophenotype: **CD5–, CD10–**, CD19+, **CD20+,** CD23–/+, CD43–/+, **CD103–**, CCND1-, BCL2-, κ or λ restricted, surface Ig+, often cytoplasmic Ig+. Variants can be CD5+. CLL markers such as CD200 absent
- Cytogenetics/FISH: **t(11;18) (BIRC3:MALT1)** (*H. pylori*-neg gastric, bronchial), t(1;14) (gastric, bronchial, skin), t(14;18) (note this is IgH:MALT1) (liver, skin, ocular, salivary), t(3;14) (thyroid, ocular, skin); del13q; del7q; cytogenetics may have prognostic value (*Lancet* 2001;357:39)
- Molecular diagnostics for clonal IgH rearrangement (proves malignancy), ***MYD88*** status to differentiate WM vs. MZL if plasmacytic differentiation though can be + especially in SMZL, ***NOTCH2,*** & ***KLF2*** can differentiate from other B-cell lymphoma subtypes
- Lab evaluation: CBC w/ diff, CMP, LDH, HBsAg/cAb, **HCV Ab,** HIV, SPEP/IFE (paraprotein often present, esp IgM), quantitative Igs & FLC
- BM aspirate & core bx: Useful in certain circumstances, such as to evaluate cytopenias
- Imaging: CT CAP w/ contrast; may need MRI orbits (ocular) or neck (salivary); FDG PET (w/ neck) if ISRT or to r/o areas to be biopsied for suspected transformation to DLBCL
- Special considerations for gastric ENMZL:
  - **Endoscopy** ± EUS w/ core bx required, **stain specimen for *H. pylori***
  - if *H. pylori* neg by histopath, then perform *H. pylori* stool Ag test, urea breath test, or *H. pylori* blood Ab test. *H. pylori* MALT treated w/ abx (see below)

Staging

- **Lugano modification of ann arbor staging** (for nodal, splenic, & nongastric ENMZL): **Stage I** = single LN region or single EN site (IE), **stage II** = ≥2 nodal groups on one side of diaphragm, **stage III** = nodes on both sides of diaphragm, **stage IV** = LN plus noncontiguous extralymphatic involvement

- **Lugano staging system for GI lymphomas** (for gastric ENMZL) (*Ann Oncol* 1994;5:397): **Stage I** = confined to GI tract (I_1 = mucosa, submucosa, I_2 = muscularis, serosa), **stage II** = local LN (II_1), distant regional LN (II_2), or adjacent organ involvement (IIE), no stage III, **stage IV** = disseminated EN or supradiaphragmatic LN involvement

Principles of treatment

- In some cases, **tx of underlying etiology can result in MZL regression**
  - *H. pylori* eradication w/ abx for gastric ENMZL (not effective if **t(11;18)** present or if there is muscularis or perigastric LN involvement), HCV for splenic MZL, doxycycline for ocular or cutaneous Borrelia-assoc ENMZL
- Localized dz common, can be tx curatively irrespective of sx often w/ limited RT
- Adv stage MZL is a chronic condition (typically incurable). Surveillance vs. tx is based on presence of ≥1 **GELF, NCCN or similar criteria** (like follicular lymphoma)
- **Transformation:** 5–10% transform to aggressive large-cell lymphoma often signaled by rapid ↑ LN, new B sx, or ↑ LDH. Consider FDG PET directed bx, tx like DLBCL

Upfront Treatment Approaches

Subtype	Stage	Status	Treatment
Gastric ENMZL (no stage III)	Lugano I1/2 or II1	*H. pylori*+, t(11;18) neg/unknown	*H. pylori* eradication
		H. pylori+, t(11;18) positive	*H. pylori* eradication + ISRT
		H. pylori-	ISRT
	Lugano II2/E or IV	GELF–	Observe
		GELF+	BR, R-CHOP, R-CVP, rituximab
Nongastric ENMZL	Ann Arbor I or II	NA	ISRT (preferred), consider resection, rituximab, observation in select cases
	Ann Arbor III or IV	GELF–	Observe
		GELF+	BR, R-CHOP, R-CVP, rituximab
Splenic MZL	Ann Arbor IV (always)	HCV+	Treat HCV (even w/o sxs)
		No sxs or cytopenias	Observe (even if splenomegaly)
		Sx or cytopenias	Rituximab (preferred) or splenectomy usu beyond 1st line
Nodal MZL	Ann Arbor I or II	Contiguous	ISRT
		Bulky or noncontiguous	Consider observation or BR, R-CHOP, R-CVP, rituximab
	Ann Arbor III or IV	GELF–	Observe
		GELF+	BR, R-CHOP, R-CVP, rituximab

Note: BR was superior to R-CHOP in terms of PFS in all indolent subtypes except MZL (StiL trial, *Lancet* 2013;381:1203), though was noninferior to R-CHOP/R-CVP in the phase III BRIGHT study (*Blood* 2014;123:2944). Rituximab + lenalidomide was superior to rituximab in AUGMENT, but the MZL subset was small and results may be inferior (*JCO* 2019;37:1188).

Relapsed disease

- **General approach:** Treat w/ nonoverlapping combination regimens + anti-CD20 (if >6 mos since last exposure) (benda + R/obinituzumab, R-CHOP, R-CVP, len + R) or BTKi
- **Ibrutinib** (BTKi) w/ **ORR 48%, PFS 14.2** mos in phase II trial, likely due to MZL dependence on B-cell receptor signaling (*Blood* 2017;129:2224; *Blood Adv* 2020;4:5773)
- **PI3K inhibitors:** Copanlisib, duvelisib, idelalisib, umbralisib (dual PI3K∂/CK1ε). Umbralisib is FDA approved for MZL (*ASH* 2020;Abs 623)

Supportive care and surveillance

- **Endoscopy:** Consider surveillance EGD w/ biopsies for pts w/ gastric ENMZL treated by *H. pylori* eradication or ISRT
- **Vaccines:** *H. influenzae*, pneumococcal, & meningococcal A/B 2 wk **prior to splenectomy**

MANTLE CELL LYMPHOMA

Epidemiology
- Represents ~6% of all lymphomas
- ↑ Incidence w/ ↑ age, male sex (~3:1 ratio), Caucasians

Biology/Pathology
- Derived from a naïve (IGHV unmutated, most common) or postgerminal center B cell. Most often appears histologically as an infiltrate of small lymphocytes w/ notched nuclei
- Variants include the **blastoid & pleomorphic variants,** which carry poor prog
- Typically expresses B-cell antigens (CD19 & CD20) &, aberrantly, the T-cell antigen **CD5** (also seen in CLL/SLL), but **not CD10** (FL), **CD23** (CLL), or **CD200** (CLL)
- **Hallmark cytogenetic abnormality** is **t(11;14)(q13;q32):** Juxtaposes **Cyclin D1** gene (*CCDN1*) w/ the Ig heavy chain locus; detectable by **FISH, karyotype, SNP Array,** or **IHC (= BCL1 stain)**
- Rare CCND1(–) cases are SOX11(+) & have Cyclin D2 or D3 lesions. Must be distinguished from CD23(–) CLL & CD5(+) MZL
- Clinical behavior is variable but generally aggressive
- Prognostic factors: **Proliferative index** (Ki-67) ≥30% vs. <30% (*Ann Oncol* 2010;21:133), **p53 abnormalities** (del17p or *TP53* mutn) are powerful in MCL & predict for aggressive dz & chemo responsiveness (*Blood* 2017;130:1903)
- Nonnodal leukemic MCL: Cases w/ **leukemic presentation** (spleen + BM) may display **indolent** clinical behavior, typically **SOX11–, IGHV hypermutated**

Staging and workup
- Lugano staging; most pts stage IV
- Excisional or core bx preferred for initial dx
- Staging: **FDG PET/CT (preferred)** or **CT scan** of chest/abdomen/pelvis ± neck
- **BMBx** needed to complete staging. Marrow involvement ± leukemic phase are common
- Evolving rationale for FISH evaluation of deletion 17p (TP53) in addition to t(11;14) given prognostic importance
- Sequencing of *TP53* gene to evaluate for hotspot mut a/w poor prog
- LP to evaluate for CNS involvement in pts w/ blastic morphology &/or +CNS sx

Treatment: Localized disease
- **Localized MCL is rare** (<5–10%). Endoscopic evaluation of GI tract (EGD & colonoscopy w/ blind biopsies), BMBx, & PET/CT needed to definitively r/o adv stage dz
- Mgmt options include **IFRT alone** or **combined modality tx**

Treatment: Asymptomatic patients
- **Observation** appears to be safe in asx pts w/ low tumor burden (*JCO* 2009;27:1209)
- Pattern of distribution (either **spleen/leukemic/BM** or **GI only**), low proliferative index by **Ki-67 staining** (<10%) & absence of **SOX11** possible markers of indolent course

Initial treatment: Transplant-eligible patients
- **Clinical trial enrollment encouraged**
- In pts who require tx & are eligible, an **upfront HDT/ASCR**-directed approach is favored by most (*Blood* 2005;105:2677)
  - Pts typically receive alternating or sequential schedules of multiagent chemo plus rituximab (*JCO* 2005;23:7013; *Blood* 2008;112:2687; *Blood* 2013;121:48; *Ann Oncol* 2010;21:133, *Bone Marrow Transplant* 2021;56(7):1700)
  - Inclusion of **high-dose cytarabine** (alone or in combination) w/ initial chemo improves outcomes (*Lancet* 2016;388:565)
  - R-CHOP alone is insufficient
  - **Rituximab maintenance** ↑ PFS & OS after R-DHAP → HDT/ASCR (*NEJM* 2017;377:1250)

Initial treatment: Transplant-ineligible patients
- R-Bendamustine achieves at least equivalent, possibly longer PFS w/ less tox compared to R-CHOP (*BRIGHT Study, Blood* 2014;123:2944 & *STIL Study, Lancet* 2013;381:1184)
- Multiple active regimens include rituximab in combination w/ CHOP, bendamustine, CVP or lenalidomide
- **Maintenance rituximab** ↑ OS after response to R-CHOP but may not after BR (*NEJM* 2012;367:520; *JCO* 2016;no.15suppl:7503)

Initial treatment: Patients with TP53-altered MCL

- *TP53* alterations (deletion, mut, or both) assoc w/ inferior outcomes w/ upfront immunochemotherapy followed by HDT/ASCR approach (*Blood* 2017;130:1903); clinical trial enrollment encouraged for these pts, incorporating novel agents

Relapsed disease

- No generally accepted SOC; clinical trial enrollment encouraged; care is highly individualized based on response/tolerability to prior tx, fitness, GOC, EOD
- The above-described initial Rx regimens are typically also active in the relapsed setting if not already used
- Other options:
  - **Ibrutinib** (*NEJM* 2013;369:507), can consider addition of rituximab (*Lancet Oncol* 2015;17:48)
  - Emerging data for **later-generation BTKi** (zanubrutinib, acalabrutinib) w/ potential for less tox (*Blood* 2020;136:2038)
  - **Lenalidomide plus rituximab** (*Lancet Oncol* 2012;13:716)
  - **Venetoclax** (*JCO* 2016;70:4320)
  - **Bortezomib** (± rituximab) approved for salvage tx based on a single-agent ORR of 33% w/ 8% CR (*JCO* 2006;24:4867)
  - Long-term dz control can be achieved w/ **alloSCT** in select cases. Compared to HDT/ASCR, alloSCT is a/w ↑ tox but also ↑ dz control
  - Emerging promising data for **CD19-directed CAR-T cell therapies** (brexucabtagene autoleucel (*NEJM* 2020;382:1331), lisocabtagene maraleucel (*ASH* 2020;Abs 118); longer follow-up needed to assess durability

Prognosis

- Considered incurable w/ standard therapies, although long-term remissions have been observed w/ upfront HDT/ASCR & potential for long-term cure w/ alloSCT
- The **MIPI** (age, performance status, LDH, WBC) & **MIPI-Biologic** (MIPI + Ki-67) are prognostic for OS (*Blood* 2008;111:558)

DIFFUSE LARGE B-CELL LYMPHOMA

Definition

- A heterogeneous group of neoplasms arising from mature B-cells, characterized pathologically by large, atypical lymphocytes w/ a diffuse growth pattern

Epidemiology

- Most common lymphoma type: ~30% of lymphomas, ~24K cases/y
- ↑ Incidence w/ age, ↑ incidence in Caucasians, slight male predominance

Clinicopathologic subtypes clinical and pathologic subtypes

- Many different subtypes including 1° mediastinal (PMBL), 1° CNS (PCNSL), testicular, high-grade B-cell lymphoma w/ *MYC* & *BCL2* &/or *BCL6* translocations (HGBCL), transformed lymphoma, etc. (2016 WHO classification, *Blood* 2016;127:2375)

Genetics and molecular subtypes

- Gene expression profiling (GEP) identifies three distinct subtypes: Germinal-center B-cell type (GCB), activated B-cell type (ABC), & unclassifiable (*NEJM* 2002;346:1937; *Nature* 2000;403:503). ABC phenotype a/w older age, worse prog
- **Immunohistochemical algorithms** can be used in lieu of GEP classifying cases into GCB & non-GCB (w/o unclassifiable; Figure 23-1) (*Blood* 2004;103:275)

Figure 23-1 Immunohistochemical algorithm.

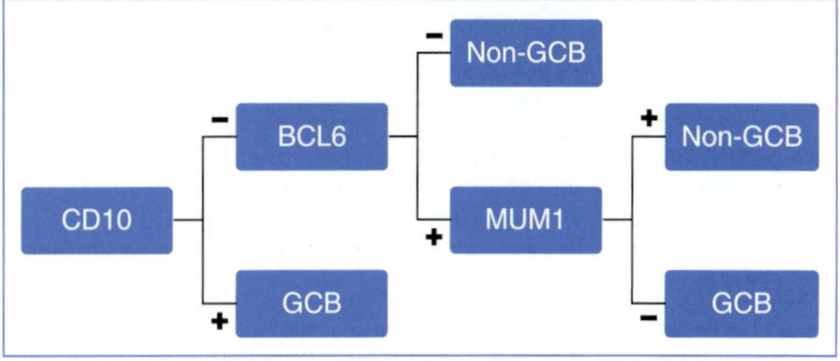

- High-grade B-cell lymphoma w/ *MYC* & *BCL2* &/or *BCL6* translocations by FISH (formerly "double-hit") represent ~8% of all DLBCL & have poorer prog. Almost always **GCB**. IHC detected "double expressors" (MYC >40% BCL2 >70%) may be assoc w/ ↓ prog (*JCO* 2012;30:3460). Burkitt typically BCL-2(–) vs. DLBCL nearly always BCL2(+)
- t(14:18) occurs in ~30% of DLBCLs (common in follicular lymphoma); juxtaposes *BCL-2* gene to the *IgH* gene. BCL-2+ IHC may be seen w/ or w/o this translocation

Staging

- Lugano classification (*JCO* 2014;32:3059). **Limited: Stage I** (one node or group of adjacent nodes), **stage II** (two or more nodal groups). **Adv: Stage III** (nodes on both sides of the diaphragm), **stage IV** (noncontiguous EN dz). Modifier 'X' (bulky ≥10 cm) & E (contiguous EN only w/ stage I/II). BMBx only for suspected discordant dz

Prognostic model

- IPI includes 5 adverse RFs: (APPLES) Age >60, ECOG PS ≥2, LDH>ULN, >1 EN site & stages III–IV (*NEJM* 1993;329:987)
- Outcomes w/ rituximab containing regimens (*Blood* 2020;135:2041):

# of Factors	Risk	5-y PFS	5-y OS
0–1	Low	81%	88%
2	Low–intermediate	67%	76%
3	High–intermediate	58%	67%
4–5	High	46%	54%

Management

- DLBCL is **curable** w/ chemo, even in adv stage
- **Rituximab + CHOP** is SOC for adv stage dz (cyclophosphamide, doxorubicin, vincristine, & prednisone): q3 wk for 6 cycles (*NEJM* 2002;346:235)
- Elderly frail pts can be treated w/ **R-mini-CHOP** or **R-GCVP**
- Check HBsAg & HBcAb > HBV PCR > entecavir ppx; age ≥60 GCSF support
- **LV fxn** is screened w/ MUGA or TTE before doxorubicin due to risk of cardiotox; incidence of clinical & subclinical CHF after R-CHOP is ~5% & risk is increased w/ >6 cycles (*Lancet Haem* 2020;7:e295). Cardiac tox ↓ w/ the infusional regimen **dose-adjusted EPOCH** (etoposide, prednisone, vincristine, cyclophosphamide & doxorubicin) **or liposomal doxorubicin**
- **Interim restaging by CT or PET** after 2–4 cycles. Consider bx prior to tx change if < PR due to high rate of false-positive PET. Later interim time points more predictive; emerging data on Δ SUV_{max} to discriminate responders (*Blood Adv* 2021;5:2375)
- **High risk of CNS** involvement or relapse (testis involvement, kidney/adrenal involvement; 2 EN sites w/ elevated LDH, high-risk IPI, HGBCL) (*JCO* 2016;34:3150). Role of prophylactic HD-MTX or IT-MTX is questionable (*ASH* 2020; Abs 477)
- Restage w/ PET after completion of tx (done 4–6 wk post tx to determine remission)
- **Surveillance:** CT CAP no more than every 6 mos for 2 y (some agencies recommend no further imaging); post-CR no tx required

Management: Limited stage disease

- ~1/3 of DLBCL pts have stage I–II dz that can be contained w/in a limited radiation field
- In nonbulky dz (<7.5 cm), R-CHOP (3 cycles) & 40 Gy IFRT results in 4-y PFS of 88% & OS of 92% (*JCO* 2008;26:2258)
- Tx w/ R-CHOP (4 cycles) + R (2 cycles) is noninferior to R-CHOP (6 cycles) in IPI < 1 dz & results in 3-y PFS of 96% & OS of 99% (*Lancet* 2019;394:2271)
- Tx w/ R-CHOP (4–6 cycles) equivalent to R-CHOP (4–6 cycles) + RT (5-y PFS 89% & OS 92%); RT used for consolidation of incomplete response (*Blood* 2018;131:174)
- In bulky dz (≥7.5 cm), consider R-CHOP (6 cycles) +/– ISRT

Management: Primary mediastinal BCL (PMBL)

- Aggressive lymphoma arising from thymic medullary B cells. Occurs in 30–40s, F > M
- Usu bulky but localized. Pts may p/w SVC syn
- Preferred tx is **(da)R-EPOCH** w/ 97% 5-y OS achieved (*NEJM* 2013;368:1408) but R-CHOP may have similar results. Residual dz can often be controlled w/ RT
- In relapsed/refractory dz, consider checkpoint blockade: **Pembrolizumab** (*JCO* 2019;37:3291) or **nivolumab + brentuximab vedotin** (*JCO* 2019;37:3081)

Management: High-grade B-cell lymphoma (HGBCL)

- Pts often p/w poor prognostic features, including CNS involvement & high IPI
- Optimal tx unknown but preferred is **(da)R-EPOCH** (*Lancet Haem* 2018;5:e609). Other options: R-hyperCVAD & R-CODOX-M/R-IVAC. Strongly consider clinical trials
- R-CHOP is assoc w/ inferior outcomes (*JCO* 2012;30:3452)
- ASCT in 1st remission does not ↑ OS, does ↑ morbidity (*Blood* 2014;124:2354)

Relapsed/refractory disease: Transplant eligible

- Pts **w/ chemosensitive** dz as demonstrated by PET CR to 2nd-line chemo such as **R-ICE** or **R-DHAP** are consolidated w/ BEAM ASCT (*JCO* 2010;28:4184)
- Pts w/ SD or PD to frontline chemo unlikely to respond to 2nd-line standard R-chemo (consider treating as transplant-ineligible)
- Consider pretransplant IFRT to sites of residual dz

Relapsed/refractory disease: Transplant ineligible

- No curative option available. Strongly consider clinical trials
- 2nd line & later options include **R-GemOx; BR + polatuzumab vedotin** (CD79b antibody-drug conjugate) (*JCO* 2020;38:155); **lenalidomide + tafasitamab** (antiCD19 antibody) (*Lancet Oncol* 2020;21:978); **loncastuximab tesirine** (antiCD19 ADC) (*EHA* 2020;Abs S233); **mosunetuzumab** (CD3–CD20 BiTE) (*ASH* 2020;Abs 401) all providing 25–45% CR rates w/ subsequent long-term remissions
- If ≤ PR after 2nd line, consider **anti-CD19 CAR-T-cell therapy**, axicabtagene ciloleucel (*NEJM* 2017:377:2531), tisagenlecleucel (*NEJM* 2019:380:45), or lisocabtagene maraleucel (*Lancet* 2020;396:839). All ~50% CR rate & subsequent long-term remission. Significant AEs include CRS (4–23%), ICANS (15–30%), & prolonged cytopenia (15%)

BURKITT LYMPHOMA

Definition and pathogenesis

- **Highly aggressive** B-cell NHL characterized by ***MYC* translocation** (**t[8;14]**[q24;q32] in 85% or light chain variants), *MYC* encodes a pleiotropic transcriptional regulator; absent for *bcl-2* translocation
- Cell of origin = **germinal center** B cell; immune: CD10+
- MYC overexpression occurs via translocations that place MYC expression under control of Ig gene enhancers → constitutive expression; other mechanisms include muts in regulatory regions, & decreased protein degradation (*JCO* 2000;18:3707)
- Whole genome sequencing studies identified recurrent somatic muts in *TCF3* (E2A), *ID3*, & *CCND3* (cyclinD3) (*Nature* 2012;490:116)
- EBV important in subset, likely stimulates B-cell expansion, once BL emerges likely minimal role in tumor maintenance

Epidemiology

- 3 distinct clinical forms: Endemic, sporadic (nonendemic), immunodeficiency-assoc
- **Endemic:** Primarily in equatorial **Africa** & New Guinea, 30–50% of childhood CA (peak age 4–7) male:female 2:1, strongly a/w **EBV** infection
- **Sporadic** (nonendemic): USA, Western Europe, 30% of pediatric lymphoma (peak age 11), <1% of adult NHL (peak age 30), male:female 4:1
- **Immunodeficiency-assoc: HIV+** pts, usu CD4 count >200, incidence not impacted by HAART, also in those w/ congenital immunodeficiency & after HCT
- EBV-driven cases share **common genetic pathway** irrespective of clinical subtype (*Blood* 2019;133:1313)

Clinical presentation

- **Rapidly growing mass, sometimes doubling time <24 h, B sx, spontaneous TLS**
- Typical site: **Endemic → jaw, sporadic → abdomen, HIV → LN + EN**
- Common involvement of **EN sites** including GI tract, CNS, pharynx, bone, testis, ovary, kidney, breast, nasopharynx, orbit, effusions

Diagnostic evaluation

- Excisional/incisional bx → histology shows sheets of medium-sized atypical lymphoid cells, extensive necrosis, frequent mitosis **(Ki-67 near 100%),** classic **"starry sky"** appearance, prominent **cytoplasmic vacuoles**
- Immunophenotype: **CD10+, CD19+, CD20+, BCL2–, BCL6+, TdT–**, κ/λ restricted (κ > λ), surface IgM+
- Karyotype, cytogenetics, FISH: Classically, simple karyotype w/ *MYC* gene rearrangement as sole abnormality, most common **t(8;14) = (MYC:IgHV)** >80% of cases, <20% t(2;8) = (κ light chain:MYC), t(8;22) = (Myc:λ light chain). FISH is current method of choice 2/2 rapidity
- FISH w/ break-apart probe or long-segment PCR more reliable for t(8;14) detection
- Other mature lymphomas acting clinically similar to BL w/o *MYC* considered as 2017 WHO provisional entry "BL w/ *11q* aberration," usu treated as BL though different gene expression profiles (*Mod Pathol* 2018;31:732)
- Lab evaluation: CBC w/ diff, CMP, phos, UA, LDH, **HIV testing**, HBsAg/cAb
- **BMBx:** BM involvement in ~70% of cases, **LP:** To r/o CNS involvement including cell markers even in the absence of pleocytosis ("occult positives")
- CT CAP w/ contrast &/or PET to determine EOD
- Fertility preservation: **Sperm banking** for men, women often have few options given rapid dz progression

Staging and risk stratification

- **Ann Arbor Staging**
  - Stage I = single LN region or single EN site (IE)
  - Stage II = multiple LN on one side of diaphragm
  - Stage III = multiple LN on both sides of diaphragm
  - Stage IV = LN plus EN sites or multiple EN sites
- **Risk stratification**
  - Low risk = nl LDH or stage I + completely resected abd lesion or single extra-abd mass <10 cm (need neg peripheral blood-cell markers)
  - High risk = any non–low-risk presentation (ie, stage I & abd mass or extra-abd mass >10 cm or stage II–IV), any peripheral blood, marrow, or CNS involvement

Principles of treatment

- BL is **curable w/ intensive multiagent chemo,** 2-y OS > 80–90% w/ modern tx regimens (see below), survival in older adults (age >60) worse in series other than R-EPOCH. No published randomized trials
- **Tx should be initiated ASAP,** often w/in 48 h
- Tx consists of intensive regimens, requiring inpt monitoring (limited exceptions), avoid dose reductions if at all possible
- **CHOP is not adequate therapy** & will result in frequent relapse. 2-y OS 39% in Danish registry (*Ann Oncol* 2013;24:1879)
- Addition of **rituximab** improves survival (*Blood* 2014;124:3870)
- Almost all BL regimens include **CNS ppx** in the absence of overt CNS dz
  - CNS penetrating systemic drugs = HD-MTX & cytarabine
  - IT-MTX & cytarabine alone = CNS PPX
  - Known leptomeningeal dz (even cell marker only) requires intensification of IT therapy, typically delivered via Ommaya reservoir
- **TLS ppx is mandatory:** IVF + allopurinol ± rasburicase
- No role for RT (unless palliative) or surgery unless for dx

Sample Treatment Regimens (most common in the United States, others exist)

Risk	Regimen	Drugs
Low	R-CODOX-M × 3 cycles	cyclosphosphamide, doxorubicin, vincristine + rituximab + IT-MTX & cytarabine + HD MTX
	R-HyperCVAD	hyperfractionated cyclophosphamide, vincristine, doxorubicin, dexamethasone + rituximab + IT-MTX & cytarabine + HD-MTX
	DA-R-EPOCH × 3 cycles (if PET + after cycle 2 → convert to high risk)	DA-etoposide, vincristine, doxorubicin, cyclophosphamide, prednisone + rituximab + IT-MTX (eliminated if first LP neg)
High	R-CODOX-M/IVAC × 2 cycles each	cyclosphosphamide, doxorubicin, vincristine/ ifosfamide, etoposide, cytarabine + rituximab + IT-MTX & cytarabine + HD-MTX
	R-HyperCVAD	hyperfractionated cyclophosphamide, vincristine, doxorubicin, dexamethasone + rituximab + IT-MTX & cytarabine + HD-MTX
	DA-EPOCH × 6 cycles	DA-etoposide, vincristine, doxorubicin, cyclophosphamide, prednisone + Rituximab + IT-MTX & Ara-C

DA = Dose-adjusted based on previous cycle with interim CBCs 2 per week 3 days apart.

Consolidation and surveillance

- No standard role for consolidation therapy or HDT/ASCR in CR1
- Relapses usu occur w/in the first 2 y & are symptomatic (rarely identified on imaging alone)
- No lymphoma-directed surveillance 2 y post-tx completion

Refractory disease

- **Clinical trial** is preferable, ideal tx is undefined
- Off-protocol tx includes regimen above (not previously received) or DLBCL-type salvage regimen followed by HDT/ASCR or allo transplant if BM involved
- **Survivors are rare** (*Am J Hematol* 2017;92:E114; *Blood* 2020;135:1124)

Supportive care

- Transfusions, growth factor support, infectious ppx all required, continue compatible HAART in HIV+ pts

PERIPHERAL T-CELL LYMPHOMA

Definition

- Heterogeneous group of often **aggressive** neoplasms arising from mature T lymphocytes & NK cells w/ 1° involvement of sites other than skin (eg, LN, blood, visceral organs)
- Precursor T-lymphoblastic lymphoma is a separate entity that is treated like T-cell ALL

Epidemiology

- Comprise approx 10% of all NHL, male > female

Clinical presentation

- **S/s:** Prominent B sx (wt loss, fevers, sweats), pruritus, generalized LAN, HSM, rash
- Relatively high rate of 2° hemophagocytosis
- Common **EN involvement (often subtype-specific):** BM, blood, skin, liver, GI tract, nasopharynx, testes, CNS

Type	Disease Features
Peripheral T-cell lymphoma, NOS (PTCL, NOS)	Clinical: **Most common** subtype of PTCL, genetically heterogeneous
	Path: Unfav markers include **CD8+, GATA3+**
ALCL	Clinical: **ALK+** (favorable) or **ALK–** (less favorable, frequent JAK/STAT activation. (*Cancer Cell* 2015;27:516)
	Path: **Strong CD30+, large cells,** often **t(2:5)**
Angioimmunoblastic T-cell lymphoma (AITL), PTCL-T-follicular helper phenotype, follicular T-cell lymphoma	Clinical: Fevers, rash, pruritus, arthritis, HSM, AI phenomena, +Coombs, ↑ eos, ↑ Ig
	Path: Follicular helper T-cell origin (**CD10+, Bcl6+, CXCL13+, PD1+**) heterogeneous immune infiltrate, **EBV+ B cells** (rarely coexisting EBV+ DLBCL) Frequent alterations in ***IDH2, DNMT3A, TET2, RHOA*** (*Nat Genet.* 2014;46:371)
EN NK/T-cell lymphoma, nasal type	Clinical: More common in Asia**, midline sinus/palate mass,** assoc w/ **EBV** (can have EBV-assoc HLH)
	Path: **CD56+,** perforin+, granzyme+, **EBER ISH+**
Adult T-cell leukemia/lymphoma (ATL)	Clinical: Caused by HTLV-1 = endemic to Caribbean & Japan (among others), ↑ **Ca, lytic bone lesions;** indolent & aggressive subtypes
	Path: **CD25+, FoxP3+, "clover leaf" or "flower"** cells
Enteropathy-type T-cell lymphoma (EATL)	Clinical: A/w **celiac** dz, HLA DQ1*0501 or DQB1&*0201, **intestinal involvement,** bowel perfs
	Path: **CD103+,** amp 9q34
Monomorphic epitheliotropic intestinal T-cell lymphoma (MEITL, prev. Type II EATL)	Clinical: NOT assoc w/ celiac dz; incr. risk in Asian/Hispanic populations
	Path: CD3, CD8, & CD56; γ/δ in 80% cases
Hepatosplenic T-cell lymphoma (HSTCL)	Clinical: **Young men, highly aggressive,** assoc w/ **IBD**
	Path: **CD4–/CD8–, CD16+, TCR expression** $\gamma/\delta > \alpha/\beta$, **sinusoidal infiltrate** in liver/spleen/BM, cyto: i7q

Lymphomas ordered most → least freq.
ALK, anaplastic lymphoma kinase.
Blood 2006;107:1255; *JCO* 2008;26:4124.

Diagnostic evaluation

- **Bx:** Excisional or incisional LN bx; skin or GI tract bx if involved
- Immunophenotype: **Variable expression of T-cell markers**; in general T-cell markers CD #s generally <10: CD2, CD3, CD4, CD5, CD7, CD8, CD25, CD30, CD56, granzyme, perforin, TCR expression $\alpha/\beta >> \gamma/\delta$, EBER ISH
- Cytogenetics/FISH**: t(2:5) (ALK:NPM);** other less common cytogenetic abnormalities
- Molecular evaluations: Clonal **TCR** β & γ **rearrangement;** consider **targeted genome sequencing** for all pts
- Lab evaluation: CBC w/ diff (often ↑ **eos**), CMP, LDH, quantitative Ig, Coombs, HBV/HCV serologies, HIV, **HTLV-1 serology (ATL), serum EBV PCR (AITL, NK/T)**
- BM aspirate & core bx: Hemophagocytosis may be seen
- LP: If CNS involvement suspected clinically or by imaging
- Imaging: FDG PET generally preferred; TTE prior to anthracycline
- Fertility preservation prior to tx if possible

Staging and risk stratification

- **Ann Arbor staging:** See **Burkitt Lymphoma** chapter for staging details; **most pts p/w stage III or IV**
- **IPI: "L-A-P-S-E"** acronym; **most pts w/ PTCL have high–int or high IPI;** 5-y OS after chemo, 74% (low), 49% (low-int), 21% (high-int), 6% (high), respectively (*Br J Haem* 2005;129:366)

Principles of treatment

- **Clinical trial preferred** if appropriate trial available
- **Induction chemo: Age <60 CHOEP** (*Blood* 2010;116:3418), **Age >60 CHOP vs. CHOEP, BV-CHP if CD30 >10%, especially for ALCL**
- Other options: DaEPOCH (ATL), ICE (HSTCL, MEITL), hyperCVAD
- **High-dose therapy + autologous rescue:** Consolidation w/ HDT/ASCR in 1st remission for fit pts should be considered/discussed (see "Special Tx Scenarios" for exceptions)
- **RT:** Curative intent as consolidation after induction chemo for localized dz; **essential component of care for localized NK/T-cell lymphoma**
- **Relapsed/refractory** dz: Clinical trial preferred, otherwise **combination vs. single-agent chemo** (see Table below)
- **AlloSCT:** Rec for selected pts w/ relapsed/refractory dz; upfront in select scenarios
- **Special tx scenarios/Subtype-specific regimens:**
  - ALK + ALCL = favorable outcome w/ BV-CHP alone
  - Localized (stage I/II) PTCL w/ low/low–intermediate IPI = favorable outcome w/ CHO(E)P (*Br J Haem* 2005;129:366)
  - Leukemic ATL: Zidovudine & IFNα can be used; for aggressive dz, combination chemo → **allo in 1st remission** (*NEJM* 1995;332:1749; *JCO* 2011;29:4696)
  - HSTCL = non-CHOP regimens (eg, ICE); consider allo in 1st remission
  - MEITL = CHOEP or non-CHOP regimens consider auto vs. allo in 1st remission
  - Localized EN NK/T-cell lymphoma, nasal type (stage IE/IIE) = sequential vs. concurrent CRT (*JCO* 2009;27:6027)
  - Adv-stage EN NK/T-cell lymphoma (stage IV) = SMILE regimen (*JCO* 2011;29:4410); allo vs. HDT/ASCR in first remission case-by-case
  - EATL = CHOEP followed by HDT/ASCR or Newcastle regimen IVE/MTX followed by HDT/ASCR (*Blood* 2010;115:3664)

Other Active Agents/Treatments

Class	Drug(s)	Notes
M abs	Alemtuzumab (anti-CD52)	Generally used as bridge to alloSCT; high risk of infections
Ab-drug conjugates	Brentuximab vedotin	For ALCL, CD30+ PTCL
Antimetabolites	Pralatrexate	Generally not used for AITL; vitamin B12/folate ppx essential
Histone deacetylase inhibitors	Romidepsin Belinostat	Active across all PTCL subtypes
Hypomethylating agents	Azacitidine, CC-486	Noteworthy activity in AITL
Immunosuppressants	Cyclosporine	Some single-agent activity in AITL, also used in SPTCL
Immunomodulatory agents (ImiDs)	Lenalidomide	Promote cereblon-mediated degradation of Ikaros transcription factors; especially active in ATLL
Steroids	Prednisone	Some single-agent activity in AITL
PI3K inhibitors	Duvelisib, tenalisib	Potential for colitis & other AI side effects
Proteasome inhibitor	Bortezomib	Potential for sensory neuropathy
ALK inhibitors	Crizotinib, ceritinib	High response rates in limited data; only given in R/R setting
Combination chemo	ICE, GemOx, DHAP, ESHAP, GDP	Usu as bridge to alloSCT
Single-agent chemo	Bendamustine, GEM	Responses are generally not durable

NCCN Guidelines; *NEJM* 1995;332:1749; 2010;363:1812; 2011;364:775; *JCO* 2009;27:abstract 8561;2012;30:2190; 2013;31:104.

Supportive care

- **CNS PPX:** Consider intrathecal MTX/cytarabine for high-risk dz involving paranasal sinuses, testes, epidural sites

CUTANEOUS T-CELL LYMPHOMA

Definition
- Neoplasms arising from mature T lymphocytes w/ 1° **involvement of skin** but also potential involvement of blood, BM, LNs, visceral organs
- "CTCL" most often refers to mycosis fungoides (MF) or SS but can signify any of the cutaneous lymphoma entities listed below

Epidemiology
- Comprise ~4–5% of all NHL, male > female

Clinical presentation
- **Patch** = any size skin lesion w/o significant elevation or induration (may have hypo- or hyperpigmentation, scaling, crusting, poikiloderma)
- **Plaque** = any size skin lesion that is elevated or indurated (may have ulceration)
- **Tumor** = >1 cm diameter solid or nodular lesion w/ depth &/or vertical growth
- **Erythroderma** = erythema of nearly the entire cutaneous surface
- **Systemic s/s** = pruritus; alopecia; LAN; HSM; B sx (wt loss >10%, fevers, sweats)

Type	Disease Features
MF	Clinical: Primarily involves **skin;** usu **indolent** but rarely can transform to aggressive large cell; most common CTCL (accounts for 50–70%)
	Path: **Epidermotropic** lymphoid infiltrate; **Pautrier** microabscesses; **haloed** lymphocytes
SS	Clinical: **Aggressive, erythrodermic,** often considered **leukemic form of MF**
	Path: **Circulating malignant cells** in blood w/ **"cerebriform"** nuclei
Subcutaneous panniculitis like T-cell lymphoma (SPTCL)	Clinical: Nodules or plaques w/o ulceration; female > male; often pre-existing AI d/o
	Path: **TCR** α/β+, **CD8+,** perforin+, granzyme+, **involves fat lobules,** spares dermis/epidermis
1° cutaneous γ-δ T cell lymphoma	Clinical: May presents like SPTCL but ulceration common; worse prog; **hemophagocytic syn common**
	Path: **TCR** γ/δ+, **CD56+,** involves dermis/epidermis
1° cutaneous ALCL (PCALCL)	Clinical: Firm, large **nodule(s),** often ulcerating; **indolent; relapsing/remitting** course; **rarely disseminates outside skin**
	Path: **CD30+; IRF4/MUM1** gene rearrangement; ***ALK–*** (no *ALK* gene rearrangement)
Lymphomatoid papulosis	Clinical: **Recurrent eruption of papules & nodules w/ spont remissions;** may be a/w PCALCL, MF, or other NHL
	Path: Can mimic ALCL, **CD30+,** no IRF4/MUM1 or ALK gene rearrangements **(ALK–)**

NEJM 2004;350:1978; *Blood* 2005;105:3768; *Blood* 2011;117:5019.

Diagnostic evaluation
- Physical: **Complete skin examination** w/ estimation of **% BSA involved**
- Bx: **Skin** bx, LN bx if present
- Immunophenotype (IHC or flow): **T-cell markers,** CD2, CD3, CD4, CD5, CD7, CD8, CD25, CD26, CD30, CD45RO, CD56, granzyme, perforin, TCR α/β/γ/δ
- Cytogenetics/FISH: **Not necessary for dx;** IRF4/MUM1 rearrangement present in PCALCL, *ALK* translocations not present [t(2;var)]
- Molecular diagnostics for **clonal TCR** β **or** γ **rearrangement**
- Lab evaluation: CBC w/ diff, peripheral smear, CMP, LDH, HBV sAg/cAb, HCV Ab, HIV, HTLV-1/2, **peripheral blood flow cytometry**
- BM aspirate & core bx: Not routinely necessary for MF/SS, but should be done if unexplained cytopenias
- Imaging in ≥ stage IB **CT CAP or FDG PET** often **required** to r/o systemic dz

Staging and risk stratification
- **TNMB staging system for MF/SS** (*Blood* 2007;110:1713)
  T = skin, N = nodes, M = visceral, B = blood; T1 = patches, plaques, or flat lesions on <10% of skin; T2 = >10% of skin; T3 = tumors; T4 = erythroderma >80% of body
  N0 = no nodal involvement; N1–N3 = clinically abnl LN
  M0 = no visceral organ involvement; M1 = visceral organ involvement

B0 = no significant blood involvement (<5% Sézary cells); B1 = low-blood tumor burden (>5% Sézary cells); B2 = high-blood tumor burden (>1,000/μL Sézary cells)
Adv stages (IIB–IVB) include T3, T4, B2, N3, & M1, respectively

- **Poor-risk features for MF/SS: T3, T4, any degree of blood involvement, ↑ LDH, large-cell transformation, folliculotropic pattern** (*JCO* 2010;28:4730)
- Other cutaneous lymphomas use Ann Arbor staging system or alternative TNM system (*Blood* 2007;110:479)

Principles of treatment

- **Skin-directed topical therapies for limited superficial dz:** Usu cared for by dermatologist alone or oncologist in collaboration w/ dermatologist
- **Systemic therapies reserved for adv stage or refractory cutaneous dz**
- AlloSCT: Only curative modality, limited evidence, reserved for R/R w/ significant systemic involvement.

Skin-Directed Therapies		
Class	**Drug**	**Notes**
Chemo	Nitrogen mustard	Topical alkylator agent
Electron beam Rx	TSEBT	Local fields for single or small number of lesions; total skin reserved for significant skin involvement (≥ T2)
Immune-modifying agents	Imiquimod	Topical TLR7 agonist that promotes Th1 immune response
Phototherapy	NB-UVB	Used for patches/thin plaques
	PUVA	Used after failure of NB-UVB
Retinoids	Bexarotene Isotretinoin	Vitamin A derivatives that modify response of skin to inflammation. **Monitor thyroid & triglycerides**
Steroids	Various	High-potency topical formulations

TSEBT, total skin electron beam therapy; TLR7, toll-like receptor 7; NB-UVB, narrowband ultraviolet B; PUVA, psoralen plus ultraviolet A.
NCCN guidelines; *NEJM* 1989;321:1784.

Systemic Therapies		
Class	**Drug**	**Notes**
Abs	Alemtuzumab Mogamulizumab	anti-CD52 (common lymph Ag) anti-CCR4 (for R/R dz, *Lancet Oncol* 2018;19:1192)
Ab drug conjugates	Brentuximab vedotin	For CD30+ dz only
Antimetabolites	Pralatrexate MTX	Inhibit folate metabolism; pralatrexate typically at low dose (*JCO* 2011;29:1182)
Chemo	Liposomal doxorubicin	Anthracycline
	GEM	Nucleoside analog
	Etoposide	Topoisomerase inhibitor
	Cyclophosphamide	Alkylating agent
Cytokines	Interferon α	Highly active immune modulator
Cytokine-toxin conjugates	Denileukin diftitox	IL-2 fused to diphtheria toxin (*JCO* 2010;28:1870)
Epigenetic modifiers	Romidepsin Vorinostat	HDAC inhibitors (*JCO* 2007;25:3109)
IO	Pembrolizumab	Phase II, potential flare reaction (*JCO* 2020;38:20)
Photopheresis	Extracorporeal photopheresis	WBC removed from body→ treated w/ photoactivated chemotherapeutic → reinfused
Retinoids	Bexarotene	Systemic formulation

Supportive care

- **Dermatology:** Aggressive dermatologic care for CTCL pts; sometimes **burn wound care** needed for pts w/ extensive desquamation
- **Skin CA screening:** UV light tx → may ↑ risk of **nonmelanoma skin** CA w/ long-term use
- **Prophylactic abx:** Prevent infection in pts w/ extensive skin involvement
- **Pruritus:** Moisturizers, topical steroids, antihistamines, SSRI, pregabalin, light therapy, etc.

PRIMARY CNS LYMPHOMA

Definition

- NHL involving the CNS, including the brain, leptomeninges, CSF, spinal cord, eye
- PCNSL solely involves the CNS & is the focus of this section
- **2° CNS lymphoma** is defined as systemic NHL w/ 2° spread to the CNS, w/c be seen at dx or more commonly at time of relapse. Mgmt involves both systemic & CNS-directed therapy

Epidemiology

- Rare subtype of NHL (1% of cases)
- Rare subtype of 1° CNS tumors (4% of cases)
- Age-adjusted incidence 0.47/100,000 person-y; 3/100,000 person-y in age >70
- In immunocompetent pts, median age at dx 60 y

Risk factors

- **Congenital immunosuppression:** Ataxia-telangiectasia, Wiskott–Aldrich syn & severe common & combined variable immunodeficiencies
- **HIV infection:** CD4 count <500 cells/μL
- **Iatrogenic immune suppression:** Solid organ transplant or SCT
- **AI disorder:** RA, SLE, Sjögren syn, MG, sarcoidosis, vasculitis

Pathogenesis

- Pathogenesis is incompletely understood
- **EBV** is a causal link, but only in immunodeficient individuals

Histopathology

- 95% of PCNSLs are **DLBCL**
- Angiocentric neoplasm, typically w/ perivascular distribution
- **Immunophenotype:** Positive B-cell markers (CD19, CD20). Majority positive for BCL-6, MUM1, & BCL-2 while neg for CD10; >80% nongerminal center subtype
- T-cell PCNSL approx 2% of cases
- **Molecular testing:** Positive for Ig heavy chain gene rearrangement; recurrent muts in the B-cell receptor pathway are common, particularly **MYD88** & **CD79b**

Clinical subtypes

- **Overlap between subtypes w/ multifocal dz in >50% of cases:**
  - **Intracranial parenchymal lesion:** Solitary or multiple (>90% of cases)
  - **Leptomeningeal or periventricular lesions:** Either w/ adjacent parenchymal dz or diffuse (30%)
  - **Ocular:** Infiltration of vitreous humor, retina, choroid, optic nerve (10–20%)
  - **Intradural spinal cord lesion:** Lower cervical & upper thoracic most common sites (rare)
  - **Neurolymphomatosis:** Invasion of peripheral nerves, cranial nerves, spinal nerves, or ganglia (rare; think 2° CNS lymphoma)

Clinical presentation

- **Presenting S/S may vary depending on site of dz:** Focal neurologic deficits (70%), mental status changes (43%), signs of elevated ICP (33%), seizures (14%), & visual sx (4%) (*J Neurosurg* 2000;92:261)

Diagnosis and initial evaluation

- **Contrast-enhanced brain MRI:** Lesions are isointense to hypointense on T1-weighted images & frequently enhancing. PCNSL presents as solitary intracranial lesion in 60–70% of cases, often located in deep structures (basal ganglia, corpus callosum, & periventricular regions)
- **Contrast-enhanced head CT if MRI contraindicated**
- **Definitive pathologic dx required:** Stereotactic needle bx of the brain indicated in most cases. In select cases, vitreous bx or CSF analysis may secure dx. W/ isolated neurolymphomatosis, nerve bx required
- **Withhold steroids if possible until pathologic dx confirmed:** PCNSL responds rapidly to steroid tx & lesions can regress on radiographs, making bx more difficult. Unless evidence of mass effect/impending herniation, hold initial steroids until bx performed
- **Initial evaluation:** Bilateral slit lamp eye examination, LP & CSF fluid analysis (if safe w/o evidence of elevated ICP), HIV testing, & PET/CT CAP. In select cases, MRI spine if spinal sx, BMBx or testicular ultrasound

Poor prognostic factors

- MSKCC prognostic score: Age >50 y, KPS ≥70 (*JCO* 2006;24:5711)

Staging
- Not applicable, typically dz is limited to CNS (Ann Arbor stage IE)
- Perform systemic evaluation to exclude systemic lymphoma & define EOD

Adequate performance status (>40%)
- **HD-MTX containing regimen:** Rec for all pts w/ goal of avoiding RT, especially for older pts. Combination regimens (MTX + cytarabine, MTX + temozolomide, MTX + procarbazine/vincristine) superior to single agent. Include rituximab unless CD20 (–) or T-cell lymphoma
- HD-MTX + Rituximab vs. HD-MTX: PFS of 26.7 mos vs. 4.5 mos (*Neurology* 2014;83:235)
- Phase II trial of HD-MTX, temozolomide, rituximab w/ consolidation cytarabine/etoposide: 66% CR w/ induction & median PFS of 2.4 y (*JCO* 2013;31:3061)
- **HD-MTX:** Optimal dose ≥ 3.5 mg/m^2
- Low dose WBRT after CR used w/ efficacy & less neurotox (*JCO* 2013;31:3971)
- **Ocular irradiation:** For intraocular lymphoma

Poor performance status (<40% despite steroid therapy)
- **HD-MTX unless contraindicated** (renal insufficiency, CrCl < 30 mL/min); small series shows tolerability even if elderly (>80 y) & poor PS (*J Neuro Oncol* 2012;14(10):1304)
- **WBRT:** Rarely curative alone, a/w significant neurotox in 25–35%, median survival 10–18 mos (*J Neuro Oncol* 1999;43:241)
- **CKD (CrCl < 30 mL/min):** No published series, consider non–MTX-containing 2nd-line regimens listed below as 1st-line tx

Investigational
- **Rituximab:** Has activity & has been combined w/ all upfront regimens
- **Intrathecal/intraventricular chemo:** Unclear benefit
- **HDT/ASCR:** Low level of evidence but appears very promising, consider thiotepa-based conditioning regimens (*JAMA Oncol* 2021;7(7):993)

HIV-positive PCNSL
- **HAART in conjunction HD-MTX vs. WBRT**

Relapsed/refractory disease
- No universal SOC in relapsed or refractory setting
- HD-MTX rechallenge (particularly if >1 y from initial HD-MTX therapy); small prospective & retrospective studies show high ORR, over half achieve 2nd CR (*J Neuro Oncol* 2014;117(1):161; *Clin Cancer Res* 2004;10(17):5643)
- Other less active chemo options include pemetrexed, topotecan, temozolomide +/– rituximab, HiDAC, dexamethasone/HiDAC/CIS
- Ibrutinib +/– rituximab/methotrexate: Ibrutinib monotherapy 560 mg daily w/ ORR 52%, though short median PFS at 4.8 mos (*Eur J Cancer* 2019;117:121) or 840 mg daily w/ ORR 77% & PFS of 4.6 mos (*Cancer Discov* 2017;7:1018). Combined ibrutinib/R/MTX w/ ORR 80% in small phase Ib study, longer median PFS (*Blood* 2019;133:436)
- Lenalidomide +/– rituximab: ORR 63%, median PFS 7.8 mos (*Blood* 2016;128:785)
- WBRT, if not used in 1st-line (though neurocognitive tox remains a concern)
- Consolidative HDC/ASCR can be considered

MGUS AND MULTIPLE MYELOMA (MM)

Definition

- **MGUS:** Asx premalignant clonal plasma cell (PC) disorder w/o evidence of other B-cell dz
  - **All criteria must be met:** <10% clonal bone marrow PCs (BMPCs), <3 g/dL M-protein, no "CRAB" features
- **Smoldering multiple myeloma (SMM):** Asx
  - **Criteria:** >3 g/dL serum M-protein or Bence-Jones protein ≥500 mg/24 h &/or clonal BMPC 10–59%; no "CRAB" features
- **MM:** Incurable, symptomatic malignant neoplasm of clonal PCs, arises from MGUS/SMM
  - **Criteria:** "CRAB" features or myeloma-defining events present (see below)
  - Other features: Monoclonal Ig (M-protein) in ~80% of MM, light chain/Bence-Jones myeloma 15–20%, nonsecretory myeloma 1–2%
- **Plasma cell leukemia:** Rare variant of MM (2–4% of MM) w/ aggressive course. Leukemic phase of MM → either 1° or 2° (antecedent MM), poor OS
- Related organ or tissue impairment: **"CRAB"**
  C = **C**alcium ↑ (Ca >11 mg/dL or >1 mg/dL above ULN)
  R = **R**enal insufficiency (CrCl <40 mL/min or serum Cr >2 mg/dL)
  A = **A**nemia (Hb <10 g/dL or >2 g/dL below lower limit of nl)
  B = **B**one lesions (≥1 osteolytic lesion on imaging)
- 2014 Int'l Myeloma Working Group (IMWG) **Myeloma-Defining Events (MDE): "SLiM"**
  S = **S**ixty percent: Clonal **BMPC ≥60%**
  Li = **Li**ght chains: Involved/uninvolved **serum free light chain ratio ≥100** & **involved serum-free light chain >10 mg/dL**
  M = **M**RI: **>1 focal lesion** on whole-body MRI (at least 5 mm in size)

2014 IMWG Criteria for Diagnosis of MM

	% Clonal BMPC (A)	M-Protein (B)	CRAB or MDE "SLiM-CRAB" ©
MGUS A & B & C	Clonal BMPC <10%	Serum M-protein <3 g/dL	No CRAB or MDE
SMM A &/or B & C	Clonal BMPC 10–59%	Serum M-protein ≥3 g/dL or urine M-protein >500 mg/24 h	No CRAB or MDE
MM A & B & C	Clonal BMPC ≥10% &/or bx-proven plasmacytoma[a]	± M-protein	≥1 CRAB &/or MDE
Solitary Plasmacytoma A & C	Solitary bx-proven plasmacytoma of soft tissue or bone & no clonal BMPC[a]	± M-protein	No CRAB
Plasma Cell Leukemia A & B & C	Peripheral blood PC ≥5%[b], clonal	± M-protein	± CRAB

[a]If solitary plasmacytoma & clonal BMPC <10%, diagnosis is solitary plasmacytoma with minimal marrow involvement.
[b]Original diagnostic criteria >2,000/uL and/or >20% subject to reexamination (*Leukemia* 2013;27:780); diagnose if ≥5% circulating peripheral blood PC in patient presenting with MM (*Blood Cancer J* 2021;11:192)

Epidemiology

- **MGUS:** ↑ incidence w/ age & in Western countries → ~3% of adults >50 y, ~7% in adults >85 y. IgG 55%, IgM 14%, IgA 9%. Male > female, ~0.5–1% /y progress to MM
  - Relatives of individuals w/ MGUS have increased risk of MGUS (RR 2.8–3.3)
  - Obesity a/w ↑ risk of MGUS (OR 1.8 [*Blood* 2010;116:1056]) & ↑ MGUS → MM progression (HR 1.9–2.6 [*Blood Adv* 2017;1:2186, *JNCI* 2016;109:djw264])
- **MM:** 1–2% of all cancers worldwide, 17% of hematologic malignancies (2nd most common). United States 2021: ~34,920 new cases, ~1.8% of new cancer cases, ~12,410 deaths
  - M:F ratio 1.4:1; median age at dx: 70 y. Risk of SMM → MM ~10–20% /y; ↑ incidence in African Americans & Afro-Caribbeans

- Risk of developing MM ~3.7× higher for persons w/ a 1st-degree relative w/ MM
- Exposure risks: Agent Orange, pesticides, World Trade Center 9/11 1st responders
- Obesity increases risk of death in MM (*NEJM* 2003;348:1625, *BJH* 2014;166:667)

Biology/Progression (*Lancet* 2021;397:410)

- **Pathogenesis:** Arises from postgerminal center PCs
  - Progression: MGUS → SMM → MM → PC leukemia
  - Multistep progression of **genetic & BM microenvironment changes**
    - Initiating event involves acquisition of hyperdiploidy or translocation involving IgH
    - Structural variations (chromothripsis, chromoplexy, templated insertions) play a role
    - Clonal events are present in early precursor dz MGUS/SMM
    - Genetic events increase (copy number abnormalities, 2° translocations, somatic muts) w/ progression to MM → converge to dysregulate cell cycle
    - BM microenvironment changes are a/w progression & include ↑ tumor-promoting immune cells & loss of cell-mediated immunity
    - APOBEC cytidine deaminases shape mutational landscape of precursor dz & are a/w progression & poor prog (*Nat Commun* 2021;12:1861)
- **MGUS:** Asx proliferation of monoclonal PCs from postgerminal center B cells
  - **Cytogenetics:** 50% **hyperdiploid** (gain of odd chrs)
  - Translocations at **IgH switch region (45–50%):** Chr 14(q32.33) → IgH gene enhancers/promoter juxtaposed in proximity to oncogene locus
  - Most common translocation partners: ***CCND1*** t(11;14); ***MMSET*** & ***FGFR3*** t(4;14); ***CCND3*** t(6;14), ***MAF*** (t14;16); ***MAFB*** (t14;20)
- **MM: Cytogenetics: Hyperdiploidy** & nonhyperdiploid (hypodiploid, near tetraploid, & pseudohypodiploid) & *IgH* **translocations** as in precursor dz
  - 2° events: *MYC* (8q24), del 1p, del 13, del 17p, gain 1q
  - **Adverse outcomes** a/w t(4;14), t(14;16), t(14;20), del 17p, gain 1q
  - Somatic muts affect **RAS/MAPK pathway** in ~50% of pts: *KRAS* (22%) ↑ risk of progression of SMM → MM (HR 3.5, *Nat Comm* 2021;12:293), *RAS* (17%), *BRAF* (8%)

Presentation

- **M-protein:** ~80%; **anemia:** 73% (BM infiltration, chronic dz, CKD); **bone pain:** 60%, pathologic fx/compression fx/osteoporosis 20–25%; **renal impairment:** 48% elevated Cr (light chains → tubular damage; dehydration; ↑ Ca; nephrotoxic meds)

Workup

- Initial H&P, BMP (esp. serum **Cr & Ca**), LFTs, CBC w/ diff, peripheral blood smear, SPEP/SIF, 24-h UPEP/UIF, SFLC, serum quantitative Ig, β_2-microglobulin, albumin, LDH, BM aspirate, & bx (w/ IHC, morphology, flow cytometry, & FISH: del 1p, del 13, del 17p, gain 1q, t(4;14), t(11;14), t(14;16), NGS if available, **whole-body PET/CT or MRI** preferred over skeletal survey due to ↑ sensitivity. In SMM, if skeletal survey neg, whole-body MR or PET/CT is indicated. Tissue bx if plasmacytoma
- **DDx:** MGUS, SMM, MM, PC leukemia, lymphoplasmacytic lymphoma (LPL)/WM, NHL, 1° amyloidosis, heavy-chain deposition dz, light-chain deposition dz, cryoglobulinemia, idiopathic cold agglutinin dz

Risk stratification

- **MGUS:** Factors a/w progression to MM or related malignancy: Abnl SFLC ratio (<0.26 or >1.65), M-protein ≥ 1.5 g/dL, non-IgG MGUS or reduction of 1 or 2 noninvolved Ig isotype levels (immunoparesis) (*Blood* 2005;106:812, *Blood* 2014;123:338)
- **SMM:** Mayo Clinic 2018 Model (20-2-20): BMPC > 20%, M-protein > 2 g/dL, FLC ratio >20; identifies high-risk SMM (*BCJ* 2018;8:59). PETHEMA Model (for MGUS & SMM): aberrant PC/BMPC >95%, DNA aneuploidy, immunoparesis; requires flow cytometry, not available universally (*Blood* 2007;110:2586). Significant discordance among models (*JAMA Oncol* 2021;7:132). Ongoing evaluation of genomic prognostic signatures

Staging MM

- **International staging system (ISS):** Uses **β_2-microglobulin (B2M) & albumin (Alb).** Prog determined from start of systemic tx
- **Revised ISS (R-ISS):** Adds **LDH & cytogenetic abnormalities (cyto abnl)** High-risk CA: del 17p &/or t(4;14) &/or t(14;16); standard-risk CA: No high-risk CA

ISS Criteria (*JCO* 2005;23:3412)		**R-ISS Criteria** (*JCO* 2015;33:2863)	
ISS Stage	**B2M & Alb**	**R-ISS Stage**	Includes **CA & LDH**
ISS-I	B2M <3.5 mg/L & Alb ≥3.5 mg/dL	R-ISS-I	ISS Stage I & standard-risk CA by FISH & LDH ≤ ULN
ISS-II	Not ISS stage I or III	R-ISS-II	Not R-ISS stage I or III
ISS-III	B2M ≥5.5 mg/L	R-ISS-III	ISS-III & high-risk CA or LDH > ULN

Initial treatment

- **MGUS:** No tx required. Monitor q3mos initially, then q6–12mos w/ clinician visit & labs
- **SMM:** No tx required. Monitor q3mos initially, then q6mos if low risk or q3mos if high risk. **Clinical trials** encouraged for high-risk SMM
- **Solitary osseous plasmacytoma:** IFRT 40–50 Gy in 1.8–2.0 Gy/fraction
- **Solitary extraosseous plasmacytoma:** IFRT 40–50 Gy in 1.8–2.0 Gy/fraction ± excision
- **Newly dx'd MM (NDMM):** Tx indicated. Eligibility vs. noneligibility for high-dose melphalan & auto SCT dictates tx choice. **MRD negativity** is major prognostic factor in MM & correlates w/ ↑ PFS & OS
- **Transplant-eligible induction tx:**
  - **Daratumumab (Dara)-VRd** (bortezomib/lenalidomide/dexamethasone), **KRd** (carfilzomib/lenalidomide/dexamethasone) or **VRd** are effective 1st-line tx
  - Response (see below for criteria): VRd ≥VGPR 28–77%, MRD negativity 6–50%; KRd ≥VGPR 74–90%, MRD negativity 54–73%; Dara-VRd ≥VGPR 72%, MRD negativity 21% (MRD by flow cytometry or NGS after 4–12 cycles) (*JAMA Oncol* 2015;1(6):746; *Lancet* 2017;389:519; *NEJM* 2017;376:1311; *Blood* 2018;132(suppl 1):121; *Lancet Oncology* 2020;21:1317; *Blood* 2020;136:936; *Blood* 2020;136:2513)
  - **CyBorD** (cyclophosphamide/bortezomib/dexamethasone, or VCd) is reasonable for rapid induction in pts w/ acute kidney injury; consider switching to VRd/KRd/Dara-VRd after 1–2 cycles
  - Arrange stem cell collection after completion of 4–6 cycles of induction tx
  - VRd + high-dose melphalan (HDM)-ASCT w/ significantly longer PFS vs. VRd alone, but no diff in OS (*NEJM* 2017;376:(14):1311)
  - Early vs. late HDM-ASCT equivalent OS at 5 y (*Leuk Lymphoma* 2013;54:1658)
  - Role of upfront transplant less clear in pts who achieve MRD negativity after induction (*Blood* 2018;132:2456)
- **Transplant-ineligible induction tx: Dara-Rd** (*NEJM* 2019;380:2104), **VRd** (*BCJ* 2020;10:53) or **KRd** if pt can tolerate triple tx. **IRd** (ixazomib/lenalidomide/dexamethasone) is oral alternative. **Rd** or **Vd** (bortezomib + low-dose dexamethasone) for doublet therapy
- **Maintenance tx:** Lenalidomide w/ longer PFS vs. placebo after ASCT (52.8 vs 23.5 mos) (*JCO* 2017;35:3279). Alternatives include bortezomib (*JCO* 2012;30:2946); daratumumab (*Lancet* 2020;395:132); ixazomib (*JCO* 2020;38:8527)

Approach to NDMM Treatment (*BMT* 2016;51:913)

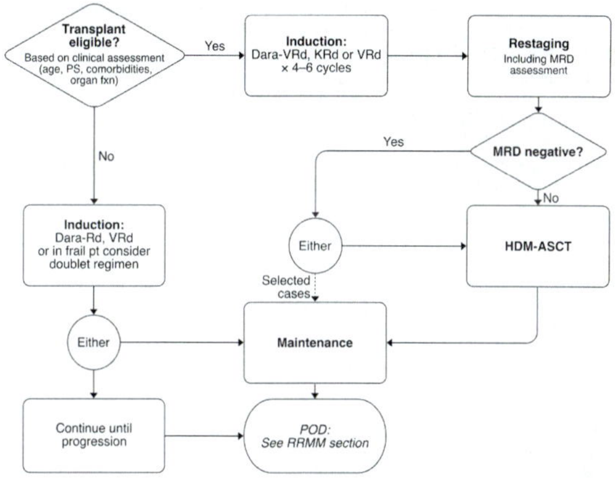

Supportive therapies

- **Anemia:** ESA if no response w/ tx or renal failure
- **Bone dz/fractures:** All pts on active MM tx should receive bisphosphonate (zoledronate, pamidronate); denosumab noninferior to zoledronate (*Lancet Oncol* 2018;19:370), useful as alternative esp. in pts w/ renal insufficiency (*JCO* 2017;35(suppl 15):8005)
- **Analgesia:** Steroids, bisphosphonates, IFRT, vertebro/kyphoplasty; avoid nephrotoxins

- **Infection ppx:** Vaccination, antimicrobials (consider viral, Pneumocystis, bacterial, fungal coverage), IVIg, G-CSF; use shingles ppx w/ proteasome inhibitors (PIs) & daratumumab
- **Thromboprophylaxis:** Most regimens including immunomodulator (IMiD; eg, lenalidomide) maintenance alone: ASA in nl-risk or DOAC in high-risk pts. DOAC (rivaroxaban or apixaban) w/ regimens including carfilzomib + IMiD (*NCCN* 2022)

Response and MRD criteria (*Lancet Oncol* 2016;17:e328)

- **IMWG uniform response criteria:**
  - **Stringent complete response (sCR):** CR + nl FLC ratio, absence of clonal PC in BMBx by IHC (κ/λ ratio ≤4:1 or ≥1:2 for κ & λ pts, respectively)
  - **CR:** Neg M-protein by SIF & UIF, disappearance of any soft tissue plasmacytomas & <5% PC in BM aspirate
  - **VGPR:** Detectable M-protein by SIF/UIF but not on SPEP/UPEP or ≥90% reduction in serum M-protein + urine M-protein <100 mg/24 h
  - **Partial response (PR):** ≥50% reduction of serum M-protein + reduction in 24-h urine M-protein by ≥90% or to <200 mg/24 h + ≥50% reduction in size of soft tissue plasmacytomas if present at baseline; if serum/urine M-protein unmeasurable, ≥50% reduction in involved & uninvolved FLC difference instead; if SFLC assay also unmeasurable, ≥50% reduction in BMPC% instead provided baseline BMPC >30%
  - **Minimal response (MR):** ≥25% but ≤49% reduction of serum M-protein + reduction in 24-h urine M-protein by 50–89% + ≥50% reduction in size of soft tissue plasmacytomas if present at baseline
  - **Stable dz (SD):** Not meeting criteria for CR, VGPR, PR, MR, or PD
  - **PD:**
    - 25% increase from lowest value of:
      - (a) Serum M-protein (absolute increase must be ≥0.5 g/dL, or increase ≥1 g/dL if lowest M component was ≥5 g/dL)
      - (b) Urine M-protein (absolute increase must be ≥200 mg/24 h)
      - (c) If serum/urine M-protein unmeasurable, involved & uninvolved FLC difference (absolute increase must be >10 mg/dL)
      - (d) If SFLC assay also unmeasurable, BMPC% (absolute increase must be ≥10%)
    - Appearance of a new lesion, ≥50% increase from nadir in size of >1 lesion, or ≥50% increase in longest diameter of previous lesion >1 cm in short axis
    - ≥50% increase in circulating PCs (minimum 200 cells/uL) if the only measure of dz
  - **Clinical relapse:** New CRAB criteria, hyperCA (>11 mg/dL), ↓ Hgb by ≥2 g/dL not related to tx or non-MM conditions, ↑ SCr by 2 mg/dL from start of tx that is related to MM, hyperviscosity due to serum paraprotein
- **IMWG MRD Criteria (requires sCR or CR):**
  - **Flow MRD-neg:** Absent phenotypically aberrant clonal PCs by flow cytometry on BM aspirate w/ minimum sensitivity 1 in 10^5 nucleated cells
  - **Sequencing MRD-neg:** Absent clonal PCs by NGS on BM aspirate w/ minimum sensitivity 1 in 10^5 nucleated cells
  - **Imaging + MRD-neg:** Flow &/or sequencing MRD-neg + neg PET/CT
  - **Sustained MRD-neg:** Imaging + MRD-neg confirmed ≥1 y apart

Treatment of relapsed/refractory MM (RRMM)

- Tx individualized, best sequence not yet defined
- If tolerated/available, 3-drug regimen more efficacious than 2-drug regimen
- Consider salvage ASCT if eligible, allo-SCT used rarely
- Changes in clonal tides allow for reuse of agents; recent tx is the most important factor when choosing next tx
- Other factors affecting tx choice include age, frailty, comorbidities, previous tox, cytogenetics, & aggressiveness of relapse
- Clinical trial enrollment highly rec
- Multiple agents approved:
  - **MAbs:** Anti-CD38 (daratumumab, isatuximab), anti-SLAMF7 (elotuzumab)
  - **IMiD:** Lenalidomide, pomalidomide, thalidomide
  - **PIs:** Bortezomib, carfilzomib, ixazomib
  - **Nuclear export inhibitor:** Selinexor
  - **Alkylators:** Bendamustine
  - **Ab-drug conjugate:** Anti-BMCA (belantamab mafodotin)
  - **CAR-T cells:** Anti-BMCA (idecabtagene vicleucel, idecabtagene vicleucel)

- Select investigational agents:
  - **CAR-T cells:** Multiple agents in trials, BMCA most common target; modifications include additional targets, cell source, transfer method, use of γ-secretase inhibitors; other CAR-T targets include GPRC5D, SLAMF7, CD38, CD138, TACI, CD56, Lewis Y, κ light chain
  - **Bispecific antibodies:** BCMA-CD3 most common, other combinations w/ CD3 include GPRC5D, CD38, FcRH5
  - **Venetoclax** if t(11;14) or BCL-2 overexpressing
  - Other agents include tumor vaccines, small-molecule inhibitors
- **Tox considerations** common to many tx: hematologic (may require dose reduction, consider G-CSF), immune compromise (consider ppx, routine vaccinations, IVIg), thrombosis (consider ppx)
- Select toxicities:
  - Bortezomib: Peripheral neuropathy (see also toxicities of PIs)
  - Carfilzomib: Hypertension, cardiac tox (see also toxicities of PIs)
  - Lenalidomide: Diarrhea, 2nd 1° malignancy (see also toxicities of IMiDs)
  - Belantamab mafodotin: Keratopathy
  - CAR-T cells: CRS, ICANS
  - IMiDs: Birth defects
  - Protease inhibitors: Thrombotic microangiopathy

Approach to RRMM Treatment (*Lancet Oncol* **2021;22:e105**)		
1st Relapse		
Not R-refractory	Preferred	DRd, KRd, DPd
	Alternatives	DKd, Isa-Kd, KPd, DVd, KCd, Kd, IRd, Elo-Rd, PVd
	if D/K/Isa unavailable	Rd, Pd, Vd, VCd, VTd, VMp
R-refractory	Preferred	DPd, DKd, Isa-Kd
	Alteratives	Isa-Pd, KPd, DVd, PVd, Kd, IPd
	If D/K/P/Isa unavailable	VCd, Vd, VMp
Later Relapse		
	Preferred	Any 1st-relapse regimen not yet used, DPd, DKd, Isa-Kd, Isa-Pd, KPd, Elo-Pd
	Alternatives	Anti-BMCA CAR-T (ide-cel, 4+ prior lines), Belamaf (4+), SVd, VdT-PACE, Benda
	If D/K/Elo unavailable	PCd, Pd
	Investigational	Bispecific Ab, other CAR-T, Ven (t(11;14))

Belamaf, belantamab mafodotin; Benda, bendamustine; C, cyclophosphamide; D, daratumumab; d, dexamethasone, Elo, elotuzumab; I, ixazomib; Isa, isatuximab; K, carfilzomib; M, melphalan; P, pomalidomide; p, prednisolone; PACE, cisplatin/doxorubicin/cyclophosphamide/etoposide; R, lenalidomide; S, selinexor; T, thalidomide; V, bortezomib; Ven, venetoclax.

WALDENSTRÖM MACROGLOBULINEMIA

Definition

- B-cell malignancy w/ BM infiltration by monoclonal **lymphoplasmacytic** cells **plus** an **IgM** monoclonal gammopathy. May have extramedullary involvement (LNs, liver, spleen, kidney, etc.)
- Considered an indolent lymphoma (LPL) per 2008 & 2016 WHO Classification of Lymphoid Neoplasms. The 2016 update incorporates MYD88 L265P mut (*Blood* 2016;127:2375)

Epidemiology

- **Overall incidence:** ~3/million persons/y
  - 1,500 new cases dx'd each y in the United States
- **Strong familial predisposition:** Most cases sporadic. By some reports ~20% WM pts have ≥1 1st-degree relative w/ B-cell neoplasm (*Ann Oncol* 2006;17:488; *Clin Cancer Res* 2007; 13:5063; *Blood* 2008;112:3052)

HCV: Implicated in some studies, esp w/ type II (mixed) cryoglobulinemia

IgM MGUS: Risk of progression to WM 2% per y in the first 10 y after dx & 1% per y thereafter (*NEJM* 2018;378:241)

Biology (*Best Pract Res Clin Haematol* 2016;29:135)

- **B-cell** arrested in germinal center, after somatic hypermutation, before terminal differentiation to PC. *VH* gene somatic mut. No isotype class switch
- **Del 6q:** Most common cytogenetic abnormality (~55%)
- ***BLIMP-1* (6q21)** regulates PC differentiation
- WM also a/w trisomy 4, trisomy 5, monosomy 8, & Del 20q
- **MYD88 exon 5 L265P** in ~ 90–95% of WM pts (*NEJM* 2012;367:826)
  - MYD88 adaptor protein → mediates **TLR-4** & **IL-1 receptor** signaling
  - >90% MYD88 locus (3p22) involved in WM: L265P or 3p22 gain (*Blood* 2013;121:4504) → ↑ IRAK-mediated **NF-κB** signaling & ↑ **JAK/STAT3** signaling
  - NF-κB chronic stimulation possibly earliest oncogenic event
- **CXCR4** *WHIM*–like mut in ~30–35% of WM/LPL pts. CXCR4 is a chemokine receptor, binds to ligand CXCL-12. CXCR4 mut inhibits internalization & prolongs activation → ↑ WM cell survival, migration, & adhesion (*Blood* 2014;123:1637)
- **BTK** is constitutively active in WM cells, likely through a MYD88–mediated mechanism
- **BCR** signaling hyperactive in WM cells compared to nl B cells (*Leukemia* 2016;30:1116)
- Activation of **PI3K/Akt/mTor** pathway w/o specific activating mut
- Likely strong role of external stimulation via BM microenvironment
  ↑ Cytokine & chemokine upregulation in WM (BLyS, IL-6, CD40 ligand, BAFF, APRIL, & SDF-1), ↑ BM angiogenesis factors
- NF-κB inhibition by PIs has preclinical & clinical efficacy

Pathology

- Defined as IgM LPL. Located mostly in BM. Small lymphocytes w/ evidence of plasmacytoid/PC differentiation. Clonally related PC population often seen
  Secretes IgM M-protein. Most LPL are WM (IgM). <5% are IgA or IgG
- Immunophenotype (IHC & flow cytometry): CD19+, CD20+, CD22+, CD79+, sIgM+ Up to 20% WM: CD5+, CD10+, or CD23+ (*Clin Lymphoma* 2005;5:246)

Disease manifestations

- Related to WM neoplastic cell **BM infiltration** &/or **physicochemical or immunologic** properties of IgM
- WM neoplastic cell burden mostly in **BM.** <15% p/w significant LAD or organomegaly. BM infiltration → **cytopenias**
  - IgM physiochemical/immunologic properties (*Blood* 2009;114:2375)
  - **Hyperviscosity:** IgM pentameric structure → HAs, CN palsies/neuro deficits, blurred vision, retinal hemorrhages, epistaxis, ICH, AMS, LE cramping
  - **Peripheral neuropathy:** IgM autoAb to (1) MAG, (2) GM1 or (3) nerve sheath sulfatide moieties → sensorimotor neuropathy, painful neuropathy, ataxic gait, foot drop
  - **Type I cryoglobulinemia** (up to 20%; 5% sx): IgM precipitation w/ cooling → Raynaud phenomenon, acrocyanosis, digital ulcers, purpura, & cold urticaria
  - **Type II cryoglobulinemia:** IgM against IgG F_c → purpura, arthralgias, renal failure, & sensorimotor neuropathies
  - **Cold agglutinins** (~10%): IgM against RBC Ag → AIHA, Raynaud phenomenon, acrocyanosis, & livedo reticularis
  - **Multiorgan dysfunction: IgM** amorphous aggregation & tissue deposition → Derm (bullae, papules, Schnitzler syn); GI (diarrhea, ↓ absorption, GIB); Renal (proteinuria, light chain deposition dz, renal failure)

- **Multiorgan dysfunction: Amyloid** deposition → fatigue, ↓ wt, edema, organomegaly, macroglossia, peripheral/autonomic neuropathy, CHF, cardiac dysrhythmias, proteinuria, renal failure, & liver dysfunction other ROS (*Blood* 2009;114:2375)
- Recurrent **sinopulmonary infxn** (↓ IgG & IgA)
- **Thrombosis** (APLA syn)
- **Bruising/bleeding diathesis** (↓ plats, acquired vWD)

Workup

- **Essential:** Hx & physical, CBC w/ diff, metabolic panel + LFTs, quantitative Igs (IgM level under 37°C bath if cryoglobulin +), SPEP, SIF, SFLC, β_2-microglobulin, serum viscosity, hepatitis B & C testing, unilateral BM aspirate & bx (aspirate heme-path review, flow cytometry, & cytogenetics—MYD88 L265P [10% of WM pts are wildtype]), & CT CAP
- **Nonessential:** Warranted/useful in certain circumstances → HIV, *CXCR4* muts (if plan for ibrutinib), serum viscosity, cryoglobulins, cold agglutinins, APLA syn Abs, anti-MAG & anti-GM1 Abs, electromyelogram, neurology consult, retinal exam (if ↑ viscosity s/s), fat pad bx w/ Congo-red stain or BMBx for amyloid, & MRI brain ± anti-Hu/anti-Hsp70 Abs (hearing loss), UPEP, UIF

Staging

- Revised ISSWM informs prog given CD20, BTK, & proteosome targeted tx
  Does not include cytogenetics or molecular parameters (*Leukemia* 2019;33:2654)

Revised ISSWM Criteria
Age ≤65 y (0 points)
Age 66–75 y (1 point)
Age >75 y (2 points)
β_2-Microglobulin >4 mg/L (1 point)
LDH >250 IU/L (1 point)
Serum albumin <3.5 g/dL (1 point)

Revised ISSWM Categories		
Score	**Risk**	**10-y OS**
0	Very low	84%
1	Low	59%
2	Intermediate	37%
3	High	19%
4–5	Very high	9%

Treatment

- WM is an indolent lymphoma → tx indicated only if sxs present:
  - Cytopenias, hyperviscosity, neuropathy, organomegaly, bulky LAD, cold agglutinin dz, cryoglobulinemia, amyloidosis, B sxs
- Not curable w/ conventional therapies (CT or HDT → ASCR)
- Like other indolent lymphomas, possibly curable w/ allo HSCT, but not rec in WM except for highly refractory dz; clinical trials encouraged
- ↑ Viscosity sxs, serum viscosity >3.5 cP, or IgM >5 g/dL → **urgent plasmapheresis before CT** (1–2 courses → ↓ IgM 30–60%).
- CT regimen choice first depends on if candidate for **ASCR**. If ASCR candidate → avoid nucleoside analogs (difficulty w/ stem-cell collection & ↑ risk of MDS/AML/dz transformation) & oral alkylators
- **BDR, DRC, R-bendamustine (BR), ibrutinib ± rituximab** preferred 1st-line options, can also be used as preferred options in relapsed/refractory setting. (R-CHOP → similar efficacy but ↑ tox compared to BR in indolent NHL including LPL) (*Blood* 2016;128(10):1321)
- **Ibrutinib** (BTK inhibitor): Major response in ~60% MYD88 & CXCR4 mutated tumors, SOC for relapsed/refractory WM (*NEJM* 2015;372:1430). Phase 3 INNOVATE trial supports ibrutinib + rituximab in both 1st & later lines (*Blood* 2018;132:149)
- **Anti-CD20 mAb** (rituximab) cornerstone of most regimens, but leads to ↑ IgM transiently (**IgM flare** ~40–50%) which may ↑ sxs, particularly hyperviscosity. Plasmapheresis before initiation of rituximab to prevent flare. Maintenance rituximab controversial, no PFS or OS benefit observed in prospective studies but found in retrospective studies (*Br J Haematol* 2011;154:357; *Br J Haematol* 2018;181:77)
- **Bortezomib** → rapid ↓ IgM, incommensurate to actual ↓ neoplastic cell burden due to ↓ protein synthesis. Highly effective in combination regimen. Be wary of worsening **neuropathy**. **Carfilzomib** neuropathy-sparing alternative to bortezomib. Be wary of cardiac tox
- HDT → ASCR: 45–65% DFS at 5 y. Not curative, oft used in chemosensitive, relapsed dz
- Complete response: No monoclonal protein by IFE, nl serum IgM, resolution of extramedullary dz, & no BM involvement (*Br J Haematol* 2013;160:171). Note anti-CD20 mAb ↑ IgM & bortezomib, ibrutinib, everolimus can ↓ IgM w/o correlation to tumor response; use BM studies to clarify if IgM levels discordant w/ clinical context
- Acalabrutinib & zanubrutinib recently added as tx option in relapsed/refractory setting (*Lancet Haematol* 2020;7(2):e112; *Blood* 2020;136:2027)

AMYLOIDOSIS

Definition

- Systemic amyloidosis is characterized by presence of proteins which have changed conformation to a **β-pleated sheet structure & form amyloid fibrils** that deposit in tissues & lead to organ failure
- At least 31 different protein precursors to amyloid fibrils have been identified. Most commonly dx'd subtype is **1° systemic light chain (AL) amyloidosis**

Classification of Amyloidosis		
Amyloid Type	**Amyloid Protein**	**Organ Systems**
AL ("1°")	Monoclonal κ or λ light chains	Renal, cardiac, GI, neuro, cutaneous, hepatic, pulm, MSK, heme
AA ("2°") a/w chronic illness	Serum amyloid A (SAA)	Renal, GI, hepatic, neuro, cutaneous
ALECT2	Leukocyte chemotactic factor 2 (LECT2)	Renal, less commonly hepatic, GI, etc.
ATTR variant (hereditary)[a]	Mut transthyretin (TTR)	Neuro, cardiac
ATTR wild-type[b]	Wild-type TTR, ANP	Cardiac, aorta, GI
Aβ_2M dialysis–assoc	Beta-2 microglobulin	MSK
Organ-specific	Various	Various: CNS, bladder, cutaneous, etc.

[a]Other forms of hereditary amyloidosis include AApoAI (mutant apolipoprotein AI) associated with liver and kidney involvement.
[b]Previously known as senile systemic amyloidosis.

Primary amyloidosis (AL)

- Rare, estimated at 1 case per 100,000 person/y in Western countries but the exact incidence is unknown
- Cellular basis is a **clonal B-cell disorder,** 98% due to plasma cell disorders w/ amyloid protein derived from Ig light-chain fragments (ratio of κ-to-λ clones is 1:4). Can occur in context of **MGUS** or **MM**
- 10–20% of pts w/ MM develop AL in the course of dz
- In 2% of cases, pathologic FLC is produced by LPL or other mature B-cell lymphomas

Clinical Manifestations of AL	
System	**Manifestations**
General	Fatigue, wt loss
Renal	Proteinuria (70% of pts), nephrotic syn, acute/chronic renal failure (much less common)
Cardiac	CMP—infiltrative & restrictive, CHF (most often diastolic dysfunction), conduction abnormalities, AF, orthostatic HoTN
GI	Bleeding (vascular fragility), gastroparesis, constipation, bacterial overgrowth, malabsorption, & intestinal pseudo-obstruction resulting from dysmotility Macroglossia → dysphagia
Neurologic	Mixed sensory & motor peripheral neuropathy (paresthesias, pain), carpal tunnel syn Autonomic dysfunction → bowel/bladder dysfunction, dysmotility, orthostasis, erectile dysfunction
Cutaneous	Waxy skin, nonpruritic papules; periorbital purpura ("raccoon eyes"), ecchymoses
Hepatic, Splenic	Hepatosplenomegaly
Musculoskeletal	Infiltration of skeletal muscles → macroglossia Arthralgias, arthritis due to amyloid deposition, "shoulder sign"
Hematologic	Factor X deficiency (2.5% of pts)

Diagnosis

- **Evaluate for monoclonal protein:** SPEP & IFE, UPEP & IFE, quantitative Ig, serum FLC
- **Fat pad bx** or **bx of involved organ:** Demonstrates presence of amyloid fibrils by Congo-red staining w/ classic apple-green birefringence under polarized light. Additional studies identify amyloid subtype. Identification of light chains in serum or urine w/o confirmation of tissue amyloid composition is inadequate for dx of AL amyloidosis as pt may have another form of amyloid & unrelated MGUS (*NEJM* 2002;346:1786); **tafamidis** now available as specific tx for ATTR cardiomyopathy (*NEJM* 2018;379:1007)
- **Cardiac:** NT-proBNP, troponin, EKG (low voltage, conduction abnormalities), echo (interventricular septal thickness >12 mm, BiV thickening, biatrial enlargement, diastolic dysfunction, intracardiac thrombus). Cardiovascular MRI sometimes indicated
- **Labs:** CBC, differential, comp metab panel, 24-h urine, Cr clearance, coagulation studies
- **Imaging:** Whole-body low-dose CT
- **BMBx & aspirate** (mildly ↑ clonal plasma cells, often 5–10%). Congo-red evaluation
- **Cytogenetic testing:** Chromosomal abnormalities: *IgH* translocations found in 75%: t(11;14) most common, also t(4;14), del(13q14), & gain 1q21
- If hereditary subtype suspected, **genetic testing** (eg, *TTR* gene)
- **Mass spectrometry:** Gold standard to identify amyloid subtype

Diagnostic criteria for AL amyloidosis (*Lancet Oncol* 2014;15:e538)

- Presence of an amyloid-related systemic syn
- Amyloid staining by **Congo red** in any tissue
- Evidence that amyloid is light chain related by direct exam of the amyloid (ie, IHC, immunogold EM, mass spectrometry)
- Evidence of a monoclonal plasma cell proliferative disorder

Cardiac amyloid staging and prognosis (*JCO* 2004;22:3751; *Blood* 2020;136:2620)

- Markers: NT-proBNP >332 ng/L, cardiac Tn-T >0.035 ng/mL (or cardiac Tn-I >0.01 ng/mL)

Stage	Definition	Median OS
I	No markers above cutoff	>10 y
II	One marker above cutoff	67 mos
IIIa	Both markers above cutoff & NT-proBNP <8,500 ng/L	15 mos
IIIb	Both markers above cutoff & NT-proBNP ≥8,500 ng/L	4 mos

- Poorer prog a/w t(11;14), *CCND1* (*Clin Lymph Myel Leuk* 2012;12(1):49); but t(11;14) a/w ↑ hematologic EFS to daratumumab (Dara)-containing salvage Rx (*Blood* 2020;135:1517)
- CV complications are most common cause of death

Treatment of AL amyloidosis

- **Goal:** Eliminate clonal plasma cells to ↓ production of Ig light chains
- **Initial therapy:** Dara SC, bortezomib, cyclophosphamide, dexamethasone (Dara-CyBorD) (*NEJM* 2021;385:46); CyBorD (less effective in pts w/ t(11;14)); bortezomib, melphalan, dexamethasone (BMDex) ↑ RR & OS compared to MDex (*JCO* 2020;38:3252); if contraindication to bortezomib & ASCT, options include lenalidomide-containing Rx
- Cardiac stage IIIb dz excluded from most trials, no standard Rx; monitor carefully, consider initially reduced doses or sequential introduction of agents; young pts w/ isolated severe cardiac involvement may be candidates for cardiac transplant before Rx
- **High-dose melphalan & ASCT:** In selected pts w/ limited organ dysfunction & good PS (*Blood* 1996;88:2801; *Ann Intern Med* 2001;134:746; *Ann Intern Med* 2004;140:85); risk-adapted melphalan & ASCT followed by bortezomib consolidation (*Leukemia* 2013;27:823); ~20% of pts eligible for ASCT at dx, reassess others after 2 cycles of systemic Rx
- **Tx response:** Hematologic response (hem resp) measured by ↓ in serum FLC (*JCO* 2012;30:4541); reversal of organ damage (*Leukemia* 2012;26:2317; *Blood* 2014;124:2325) often lags hem resp; composite hem resp & organ response (CHOR) (*Blood Cancer J* 2020;10:41)
- **Relapsed/refractory dz:** Δ Rx if absent very good PR (VGPR) after 2–3 cycles of initial Rx; Dara (*Blood* 2020;135:1531; *Blood* 2020;135:1541) or isatuximab if anti-CD38 Ab not used initially; if suboptimal response to Dara monotherapy, consider adding attenuated immunomodulator; consider retreating w/ bortezomib-based Rx in pts w/ good initial response; venetoclax for t(11;14) dz (*Blood Cancer J* 2021;11:10); other options include immunomodulator-containing regimens, ixazomib ± Dex (*JCO* 2020;38(15 suppl):8546); bendamustine & Dex phase 2 results promising (*JCO* 2020;38:1455)
- **Emerging therapies:** Antiamyloid fibril Ab CAEL-101 (*Blood* 2020;136(suppl 1):26), anti–plasma cell Rx w/ ADC under study
- **Supportive therapy** for cardiac failure, arrhythmias, nephrotic syn, & renal failure; caution w/ beta blockers & ACE inhibitors due to HoTN; mainstay is diuretics for CHF, amiodarone for AF; gabapentin or pregabalin for neuropathy

ESSENTIAL THROMBOCYTHEMIA

- Clonal hematopoietic disorder resulting in ↑ plts

Epidemiology

- **Incidence:** Median age at dx is 60 y. 1/5 of pts dx'd < age 40

Signs and symptoms

- Up to 50% of pts may be asx at dx
- **Sx:** Erythema, pain, burning, & occasional cyanosis in hands & feet (**erythromelalgia**), vasomotor sx (syncope, atypical CP light-headedness), & visual complaints (amaurosis fugax)
- 2° events: **Thrombosis,** both arterial & venous, may be initial presentation of dz **hemorrhage,** particularly in pts w/ plt count >1 million, may be initial manifestation

Exam and laboratory

- Common physical findings: None; organomegaly (eg, splenomegaly) uncommon
- **Lab findings:** Sustained plt count >450K

Diagnosis

- Other causes of thrombocytosis must be excluded to make dx
- Ddx: Reactive thrombocytosis (iron deficiency, inflammation, infxn, malignancy), MDS (*JAK2V617F* positive RARS-T can p/w thrombocytosis), MF (esp prefibrotic), PV, CML
- Prefibrotic MF is characterized by the absence of relevant reticulin fibrosis in BM, dual megakaryocyte & granulocyte proliferation, & megakaryocyte dysplasia. Diagnostic BM is integral to assess for fibrosis, spleen imaging may be helpful
- **WHO diagnostic criteria:** Dx requires either 1–3 & 4A or 1–3 & 4B. Presence of ↑ reticulin fibrosis excludes dx of ET
- FHx of thrombocytosis should be assessed for possibility of familial ET (rare AD disorder)

WHO Criteria for Diagnosis of Essential Thrombocythemia
1. Sustained plt count >450,000
2. BM showing ↑ numbers of enlarged mature megakaryocytes; no left-shift of granulopoiesis or erythropoiesis. Very rare minor increase (grade I) in reticulln fibers
3. Not meeting WHO criteria for PV, PMF, *BCR-ABL*+CML, MDS, or other myeloid neoplasm
4A. Acquired Mt of clonal marker (*JAK2, CALR,* or *MPL*)
4B. Presence of clonal marker or no reactive cause of thrombocytosis

Adapted from *Blood Cancer J* 2015;5:e337.

Genetics

- Mt in JAK-STAT pathway cause dz in majority of cases. ***JAK2V617F:*** Found in approx 50–60% of ET pts. However, not specific for dx of ET as occurs in other MPNs (*NEJM* 2013;369:2379); phenotypic shift possible in JAK2+ MPN (ET → PV)
- Mt in exon 10 of ***MPL*** (thrombopoietin receptor) found in up to 5–10% of remaining pts
- Mt in exon 9 of ***CALR*** (ER chaperone) activates MPL receptor; found in 67% of pts w/ nonmutated JAK2 or MPL, or 20–25% of overall pts (*NEJM* 2013;369:2379)
- Chromosomal alterations such as trisomy 8 or 9, or deletion of chr 20q or 13q may occur

Disease sequelae

- **Thrombotic events:** Clinical RFs for thrombosis not completely understood, but include age >60, h/o thrombosis, WBC $>11 \times 10^9$/L, CV RF (obesity, smoking). Presence of *JAK2V617F* also an RF
- **Hemorrhagic events:** RFs include plt count >1 million, or ASA >325 mg/daily. Pts w/ ↑ plt count at risk of **acquired vWD** (check vWF Ag, fxn, Ristocetin cofactor assay)
- **Dz evolution:** May evolve to post-ET, MF, or AML (5%). RF for POD incompletely understood. Single-center study indicates low Hb (female <12, male <13.5), age, plt count >1 million as factors for leukemic transformation (*Leukemia* 2007;21:270)

Disease Sequelae in Essential Thrombocythemia	
Thrombosis	Reported in roughly 10–20% of pts
Hemorrhage	Reported in roughly 5–35% of pts
Transformation to MF	↑ w/ dz duration: 3–10% in 1st decade after dx. 6–30% in 2nd decade after dx
Low risk	↑ w/ dz duration. 1–2.5% in 1st decade after dx. 5–8% in 2nd decade after dx

Risk Stratification for Thrombotic Events in Essential Thrombocythemia	
Risk Category	**Risk Factor(s)**
High risk	Age >60 &/or h/o thrombosis; +*JAK2* mut
Intermediate risk	Age >60; no h/o thrombosis; no *JAK2* mut
Low risk	Age <60; no h/o thrombosis; +*JAK2* mut
Very low risk	Age <60; no h/o thrombosis; no *JAK2* mut

Treatment

- **Cytoreductive Rx:** Used to reduce leukocyte count, plt count, spleen size, ameliorate dz-related sx, & to ↓ risk of thrombosis. Indicated for **high/intermediate-risk** pts & should be considered for **low-risk pts w/ *JAK2* mut**
  - **Hydroxyurea (HU)** proven to reduce thrombosis risk in ET w/ ARR ~20% for thrombosis w/ use of HU (*NEJM* 1995;332:1132). Titrate dose to clinical response or desired lab parameters. Contraindicated in pregnant pts. Main toxicities from HU include cytopenias oral/dermal (LE) ulcers, nail changes. No evidence to suggest HU causes increased risk of transformation to AML
  - **Anagrelide** can be used as 2nd-line Tx. Anagrelide plus ASA shown to be inferior to HU plus ASA in preventing thrombosis (*NEJM* 2005;353:33)
  - **Alpha-IFN** or **Pegylated IFN alpha-2a/2b** can be used for pts intolerant or refractory to HU (contraindicated in thyroid disorders or h/o depression, not contraindicated in pregnancy). Pegylation → ↑ half-life → less-frequent dosing & decreased s/e. ↑ Pegylation formulation (ro-peg IFN) under development. IFN under study for role in molecular response (↓ variant allele fraction *JAK2*, *CALR*, etc.)
  - **Pipobroman** alkylating agent, long-term exposure may be a/w ↑ risk of leukemic transformation, not available in the United States
- **Anti-plt Rx:** Retrospective data indicate ASA may reduce thrombotic risk in ET. Used w/ caution w/ plt count >1 million due to bleeding risk: R/o acquired vWD & use doses <100 mg/d. Hold ASA if ristocetin cofactor activity <30%. Dose 81–162 mg; higher doses may be used for +hx CAD/CV RFs
- **Symptomatic control:** Erythromelalgia may respond to ASA. Twice-daily ASA can be considered in pts w/ persistent vasomotor sx while on once-daily therapy
- **RF modification:** CV risk reduction/mitigation suggested; Tobacco cessation, wt loss, may ↓ thrombosis risk in pts w/ ET refractory cases

POLYCYTHEMIA VERA (PV)

Polycythemia vera (PV)
- Clonal hematopoietic disorder resulting in pathologically elevated red cell mass

Epidemiology
- Incidence: Median age at dx is 60 y. 1/3 of pts <age 50
- Survival largely depends on age, leukocyte count, & h/o thrombosis

Signs and symptoms
- **Sxs: Pruritus,** typically following shower or bath (aquagenic), erythema, pain, burning & occasional cyanosis in hands & feet **(erythromelalgia)**, GI sx (↑ prevalence of gastroduodenal lesions & *H. pylori* positivity), visual complaints (amaurosis fugax), abdominal discomfort, & decreased appetite 2/2 splenomegaly. Constitutional sxs (fever, wt loss, night sweats) may be seen but are more common in MF than PV
- 2° events: **Thrombosis,** both arterial & venous, may be initial presentation of dz. Can include mesenteric, portal, & splenic vein thrombosis. **Budd–Chiari** syn, **gouty arthritis** may be initial presenting sxs

Exam and laboratory
- **Physical findings:** Plethora (ruddy complexion), organomegaly (splenomegaly, hepatomegaly), evidence of previous thromboses, arthritis, gouty tophi
- **Lab findings:** Prominently elevated Hb/Hct & low EPO level. WBC & plt counts are variably increased

Diagnosis
- Causes of reactive (2°) polycythemia must be excluded including chronic hypoxia (smoking, altitude, arteriovenous malformation), EPO-producing tumors (RCC, HCC, hemangioblastoma), lung dz (COPD), sleep apnea, exogenous administration of EPO
- **WHO diagnostic criteria:** Dx requires **3 major criteria or 1st 2 major criteria plus the minor criterion**. BMBx is not required to make the dx if Hb >18.5 or Hct 55% in men, >Hb 16.5 or Hct 49.5% in women & other major/minor criteria are met, but may still be diagnostically & prognostically useful

WHO Criteria for the Diagnosis of Polycythemia Vera
Major Criteria
(1) Hgb >16.5 g/dL (men) or >16.0 (women) or Hct >49% (men) or >48% (women) or increased red cell mass >25% above mean nl predicted value
(2) BMBx demonstrating hypercellularity for age w/ prominent erythroid, granulocytic, & megakaryocytic proliferation w/ pleomorphic mature megakaryocytes
(3) Presence of *JAK2*V617F mut or *JAK2* exon 12 mut
Minor Criteria
Serum EPO levels below reference range

Swerdlow SH, Campo E, Harris NL, et al. *World Health Organization Classification of Tumours of Hematopoietic and Lymphoid Tissues*, revised 4th ed. IARC. Lyon 2017.

Genetics
- ***JAK2* V617F:** Found in >90% of pts (this finding is not specific for dx & is seen in other MPNs & in clonal hematopoiesis). *JAK2* exon 12 muts may also be seen. Muts in other genes causing PV are rare
- High *JAK2* V617F allele burden is an RF for thrombosis & progression, increase risk of progression or death

Natural history
- Median OS estimated at 24 y in pts <60 y old
- Thrombosis is 1° cause of early mortality & a major cause of morbidity
- Risk of progression to post-PV MF as well as to acute leukemia <10% at 20 y (*Am J Hematol* 2015;90:162)

Risk Stratification for Thrombotic Events in Polycythemia Vera	
High risk	Age ≥60 or h/o thrombosis
Low risk	Age <60 & no h/o thrombosis

Blood 2012;120:275.

Disease sequelae

- Thrombotic events: *Most common clinical consequence of PV*. RFs for thrombosis not completely understood but include age, h/o thrombosis, WBC >15 × 10^9/L, smoking (*Blood* 2007;109:5104)
- Dz evolution: May evolve to post-PV MF **("spent phase")**, MDS, or AML. WBC >15 × 10^9/L, *JAK2* V617F allele burden >50%, & presence of BM fibrosis increase the risk of progression

Disease Sequelae in Polycythemia Vera	
Thrombosis	3.4/100 pts per y[a]
Transformation to MF/acute leukemia	1.3/100 pts per y[b]

[a]*Ann Intern Med* 1995;123:656.
[b]*Blood* 2007;109:5104.

Treatment

- The 1° goals of tx are to prevent early mortality by preventing thrombosis & to relieve sxs of dz to improve QoL
- **Low (thrombotic) risk:** ASA (81–100 mg daily), phlebotomy (see below), optimally manage cardiovascular RFs
- **High risk:** All therapy for low risk as above + add cytoreductive therapy (see below)
- **Phlebotomy:** Keeping Hct below 45% reduces thrombosis risk (*NEJM* 2013;368:22). We recommend sex-specific goals of <45% for men & <42% for women
- **Medical therapy:** Lowers blood counts & relieves phlebotomy burden, decreases spleen size, ameliorates dz-related sx, decreases risk of thrombosis
  - **Hydroxyurea (HU)** common 1st-line cytoreductive agent. Titrate dose to clinical response or desired lab parameters. Unsafe in pregnancy. May increase risk of leukemic progression. Common s/e include mucositis, cytopenias
  - **Pegylated IFN alfa-2a** can also be used in 1st-line setting (contraindicated in thyroid disorders or h/o depression). Can induce BM remission (*Blood* 2013;122:893–901). Broad tox potential (CV, GI, derm, endocrine, psych), close monitoring required, potential for intolerance
  - **Ropeginterferon alfa-2b** induces more hematologic & molecular responses than HU w/ at least 2 y of therapy in early PV & is well tolerated (*Lancet Haematology* 2020;7;e196)
  - **Ruxolitinib** (JAK inhibitor) Consider **if resistant to HU** or intolerant. Decreases need for phlebotomy, decreases spleen size, improves B sxs (*NEJM* 2015;372:426)
- **Anti-plt therapy:** ASA (81–100 mg/d) reduces risk of thrombosis in pts w/ PV & should be initiated unless contraindicated (*NEJM* 2004;350:114)
- **Symptomatic control:** Sx such as erythromelalgia may respond to ASA. Pruritus may respond to photochemotherapy (psoralen & UVA light), IFN, or ruxolitinib. Anecdotal evidence of low-dose SSRI benefit in pruritus (*Blood* 2002;99:2627)
- **RF modification:** Guideline-directed cardiovascular risk reduction is rec for all pts w/ PV, including tobacco cessation

MYELOFIBROSIS

Epidemiology

- Prevalence of 16–18,500 people in the United States
- Median age of onset mid-60s
- Includes 1° MF as well as post-PV & post-ET MF

Signs and symptoms

- **Systemic sxs:** Fatigue, fevers, night sweats, wt loss, pruritus, early satiety
- **Organomegaly:** Hepatomegaly & **splenomegaly** (may be massive)

Physical and laboratory findings

- **CBC:** Anemia, thrombocytopenia common, thrombocytosis may also be seen early in dz. Leukopenia or leukocytosis may be seen. WBC differential may show left shift
- **Other labs:** Elevated LDH, alkaline phosphatase, & uric acid common
- **Blood smear: Leukoerythroblastosis** (nucleated RBCs, dacrocytes, myeloid left shift)
- **BMBx:** Prefibrotic MF vs. overt MF (2016 WHO classification)

Differential diagnosis

- **Other causes of BM fibrosis:** Other myeloid neoplasms, lymphoid neoplasms, metastatic malignancy, infxn, connective tissue disorder (lupus)
- **WHO criteria:** Requires meeting **all three major criteria & at least 1 minor criterion**

WHO 2016 Criteria for the Diagnosis of Prefibrotic Myelofibrosis

Major Criteria	Minor Criteria
Megakaryocyte proliferation & atypia w/ reticulin &/or collagen fibrosis, grade MF-1 or less. In absence of fibrosis, must have ↑ marrow cellularity, granulocyte proliferation, & ↓ erythropoiesis	Leukoerythroblastosis Leukocytosis ≥11,000
Does not meet WHO criteria for PV, CML, MDS, or other myeloid neoplasm	Elevated LDH
Presence of clonal marker such as *JAK2*, *CALR*, or *MPL* Mt or no evidence of reactive fibrosis in absence of clonal marker	Anemia Palpable splenomegaly

WHO 2016 Criteria for the Diagnosis of Overt Myelofibrosis

Major Criteria	Minor Criteria
Megakaryocyte proliferation & atypia w/ reticulin &/or collagen fibrosis, grade MF-2 or MF-3	Leukocytosis ≥11,000
Does not meet WHO criteria for PV, CML, MDS, or other myeloid neoplasm	Elevated LDH
Presence of clonal marker such as *JAK2*, *CALR*, or *MPL* Mt or no evidence of reactive fibrosis in absence of clonal marker	Anemia Palpable splenomegaly

Blood 2016;127:2391–2405.

Genetics

- **Driver muts:** Majority of pts have mut in one of *JAK2* (*JAK2* V617F in ~50%, *JAK2* exon 12 in ~15%), *CALR* (~25%), or *MPL* (~5%). Approx 10% of pts are "triple-negative" & have none of these muts. *CALR* muts are a/w improved survival relative to other muts
- Muts in *ASXL1*, *EZH2*, *IDH1/2*, *SRSF2*, Ras pathway are a/w worse prog (*Leukemia* 2013;27(9):1861; *Leukemia* 2020;34(3):799)

Disease sequelae

- **Transformation to acute leukemia:** Occurs in 20% of pts. Carries extremely poor prog w/ median survival of 2.7 mos. Factors a/w transformation include: Blasts ≥3%, plt <100, unfav karyotype (see DIPSS)
- **Extramedullary hematopoiesis:** May occur in areas such as near vertebral column, LNs, & can result in organomegaly, effusions, cord compression
- **Thrombotic events:** ↑ Risk of both arterial & venous thrombotic events
- **Bone & joint alterations:** May include osteosclerosis, gouty arthritis

Prognostication

- **IPSS:** Estimates survival from time of dx (*Blood* 2009;115:392)
- **DIPSS:** Can be used at any time **DIPSS-plus** additionally considers karyotype, transfusion, thrombocytopenia (*JCO* 2011;29(4):392)
- **Molecular IPSS (MIPSS)-70 & MIPSS70-plus** include molecular data ie, high-risk muts (*ASXL1*, *EZH2*, *IDH1/2*, *SRSF2*) (*JCO* 2018;36(4):310)

- **Lille system:** Based on Hb levels & presence of leukopenia or leukocytosis

International Prognostic Scoring System: Risk Factors & Scoring		Survival	
RF	**Points**	**Number of Points**	**Survival (mos)**
Constitutional sx	1	0 (low risk)	135
Age >65	1	1 (intermediate-1 risk)	95
Hb <10 g/dL	1	2 (intermediate-2 risk)	48
Leukocyte count >25,000	1	≥3 (High risk)	27
Circulating blasts ≥1%	1		

Blood 2011;117:3494.

Treatments and indications

- **AlloSCT:** Only **curative** intervention currently. Has been performed w/ both myeloablative & reduced-intensity conditioning regimens. Effect of splenectomy prior to transplant not clear but is sometimes performed. Hematologic recovery following transplant may be delayed due to fibrotic marrow environment
- **JAK inhibitors: Ruxolitinib** (JAK1/2 inhibitor) reduces spleen size & sx scores (*NEJM* 2012;366(9):787). S/e include anemia & thrombocytopenia. Withdrawal of drug can cause sx & inflammatory flare, therefore taper when discontinuing. **Fedratinib** has similar efficacy to ruxolitinib. Rare incidence of Wernicke encephalopathy: Replete thiamine prior to initiation. Can be used 1st line & retains 27–30% response rate 2nd line after ruxolitinib (*Lancet Hematol* 2017;4(7):E317, *Am J Hematol* 2020;95(6):594)
- **Other txs useful in specific circumstances**
  - **HU:** Can be used if reduction of high cell counts is needed
  - **Azacitidine:** May improve BM & spleen response when added to ruxolitinib therapy (*Blood* 2018;132(16):1664)
  - **Lenalidomide:** May improve hematologic parameters in pts w/ deletion of chr 5q as their 1° cytogenetic abnormality (*Leuk Res* 2008;32:1927–1930)
  - **Androgens:** Combination of danazol & prednisone or danazol monotherapy may improve anemia in some pts (*Ann Hematol* 2015;94:1791–1796)
  - **IFN alpha:** Induces hematologic responses in some pts (*Cancer* 2017;123:2680–2687)
  - **Radiation:** Focal radiation of spleen to treat splenomegaly or to sites of extramedullary hematopoiesis can be used to control dz sx
  - **Splenectomy:** Can be considered to reduce symptomatic splenomegaly, or relieve other assoc sequelae of splenomegaly such as thrombocytopenia & portal HTN

MASTOCYTOSIS

Classification

- **Cutaneous mastocytosis:** Limited to involvement of the skin. Includes *Urticaria Pigmentosa* (most common), telangiectasia macularis eruptiva perstans, diffuse cutaneous mastocytosis, solitary mastocytoma (*Am Soc Hematology Ed Prog* 2015;98)
- **Systemic mastocytosis:** Infiltration of extracutaneous organs (may have skin involvement as well). Consists of indolent systemic mastocysosis (ISM, most common), smoldering systemic mastocytosis (SSM), systemic mastocytosis w/ assoc hematologic non–mast cell (MC) lineage disorder (SM-AHND, can be myeloid or lymphoid), aggressive systemic mastocytosis (ASM) (organ dysfunction), mast cell leukemia (>20% abnl MCs on BM aspirate smear)
- **MC sarcoma:** Single destructive mast-cell–based mass, extremely rare

Signs and symptoms

- Sxs result from release of MC mediators
- Flushing, nausea, diarrhea, pruritus, syncope, **anaphylaxis, wheezing, bone/muscle pain**, neuropsychiatric sxs
- **Darier's Sign:** Erythema & urticaria upon rubbing skin infiltrated by MCs

Exam and laboratory

- **Physical findings:** Urticaria, rashes, splenomegaly, hepatomegaly
- **Lab findings:** Anemia, eosinophilia, thrombocytopenia, elevated serum tryptase, MCs w/ expression of CD25 in addition to nl markers

Diagnosis

- Must distinguish from other disorders w/ ↑ MCs, including chronic eosinophilic leukemia & myeloproliferative variant of hypereosinophilic syn
- Cutaneous mastocytosis dx'd by skin bx
- BMBx should be pursued in all adult pts & in those w/o cutaneous involvement but sx consistent w/ systemic mastocytosis & elevated tryptase
- Initial evaluation: *KIT D816V* mut (present in >90% of pts) should be performed
- Evaluation of serum tryptase (80% sensitive, 98% specific) & urinary histamine should be performed (elevated)
- Dx established by WHO criteria w/ either at least **1 major + 1 minor** or **3 minor** criteria fulfilled
  - **Major criteria:** Multifocal dense MC infiltrate (>15 MC/infiltrate)
  - **Minor criteria:** 25% spindle shaped MC in the infiltrate, 25% atypical MCs in the smear, presence of *KIT D816V*, expression of CD2/CD25 on MC, serum tryptase >20 ng/mL
- Evaluation for presence of "B" & "C" sxs

Mastocytosis-associated Symptoms	
"B" sx (Increased MC burden)	**"C" sx** (Impaired organ fxn)
>30% infiltration of BM by MCs (focal aggregates) & serum tryptase >200 ng/mL	Neutrophils <1,000 or Hgb <10 g/dL or Plt <100,000/μL
Dysmyelopoiesis or myeloproliferative changes that does not meet criteria for another hematologic malignancy	Palpable hepatomegaly w/ impaired liver fxn &/or portal hypertension
Hepatomegaly, splenomegaly, or LAN	Skeletal involvement: Osteolysis or osteoporosis
	Palpable splenomegaly & hypersplenism
	Malabsorption & wt loss due to GI MC infiltration

Leuk Res 2001;25:603.

Management

- Avoid triggers of MC activation: Avoid heat, humidity, stress, alcohol, medications
- Carry epinephrine in case of anaphylaxis
- H1- & H2-blockers for sxs of MC activation. Cromolyn sodium for GI sx (*Blood* 2013;121:3085)
- ASM: Prefer clinical trial or **midostaurin** (multikinase inhibition including *KIT*, 60% response rate) (*NEJM* 2016;374:2530). Other regimens: Cladribine, peginterferon alfa-2a +/– prednisone. **Imatinib** if *KIT D816V* mut testing is neg, or *Kit* status is unknown.

Avapritinib (a selective inhibitor of *KIT D816V*) FDA approved in 2021 for ASM w/ ORR 75% (PATHFINDER, *Nature Med* 2021;27:2192)
- Consider referral to specialized center w/ expertise in mastocytosis

Supportive Medications Utilized in Systemic Mastocytosis	
Rx	**Indication**
HR1 antagonist	Mediator-related sx
HR2 antagonist	GI tract sx
PPI	GI tract sx
Cromolyn sodium	GI tract sx
Bisphosphonates	Osteolysis, T score <–2
Glucocorticoids	Mediator-related sx not responsive to HR1/HR2 antagonists or mast-cell stabilizers
Allergen immunotherapy	Allergy
Epinephrine pen	Anaphylactic shock

Blood 2010;116:5812.

Systemic Mastocytosis	
Category	**Criteria**
ISM	Meets criteria for SM. No "B" or "C" sx
SSM	As above, but w/ two or more "B" sx
SM-AHNMD	Meets criteria for SM & other clonal non–MC hematologic disorders
ASM	Meets criteria for SM w/ one or more "C" sx
Mast cell leukemia	20% or greater immature MCs in BM aspirate

Blood 2016;127:2391.

Myeloproliferative Variant of Hypereosinophilic Syndrome

Diagnosis and classification
- **Blood eosinophilia ≥1,500/µL,** if absolute peripheral eosinophil count is >20,000/µL this is very specific for a 1° myeloproliferative hypereosinophila
- **Exclude 2° causes of eosinophilia:** Allergy/atopy, drug reaction, parasite (strongyloides), fungi (coccidiodomycosis, allergic bronchopulmonary aspergillosis), eosinophilic granulomatosis w/ polyangiits or other collagen vascular dz, eosinophilic pneumonia, adrenal insufficiency

Workup
- CBC, CMP, peripheral blood smear, serum tryptase, serum B12, LDH, quantitative Igs w/ IgE
- BMBx/aspirate for pathologic interpretation, flow cytometry, karyoptype, FISH or RT-PCR assessment of gene rearrangements, myeloid NGS panel. Consider sending genetic studies & flow cytometry from peripheral blood if not performing BMBx

Genetics
- Rearrangements involving *PDGFRA*, *PDGFRB*, *FGFR1*, *JAK2*, *ABL1*, or *FLT3* (including *FIP1L1-PDGFRA*, *FIP1L1-PDGFRB*, *PCM1-JAK2*) are hallmark features of myeloid/lymphoid neoplasms w/ eosinophilia & tyrosine kinase fusion genes. These rearrangements can also occur in the absence of eosinophilia (*Blood* 2016;127:2391)

Management
- **Monitor for end-organ damage:** Particularly cardiac & pulmonary
- Initial therapy: Steroids, HU, IFN-alpha. If *PCM1-JAK2*, may respond to JAK inhibitors
- ***PDGFR* rearrangements: Imatinib** is 1st-line therapy (*FIP1L1-PDGFRA* is particularly sensitive to low-dose Imatinib) (*Blood* 2007;109:4635)
- **AlloSCT** may be considered for refractory cases, high-risk genetic profile, &/or overlap syns w/ myelodysplasia

MYELODYSPLASTIC SYNDROMES

Epidemiology

- ~10,000 cases dx'd annually in the United States
- Incidence increases w/ age → Median age of onset ≥65 y/o; male predominance (~2:1)
- **RF:** Radiation or chemo → therapy-related MDS (t-MDS); latency period after alkylating agent or RT = 5–7 y & after topoisomerase II inhibitors = 1–3 y

Disease biology/pathogenesis *(NEJM 2020;383:1358)*

- MDS is a heterogeneous dz of acquired, **clonal** hematopoietic stem cell leading to ineffective hematopoiesis → **cytopenias & dysplastic changes in BM precursors & circulating blood cells**
- Several **cytogenetic abnormalities** are characteristic of MDS → +8, loss or partial deletions of chrs 5 or 7, del (20q)
- Mt in genes in **RNA splicing machinery** in ~50% of MDS (eg, *SF3B1* K700E a/w RS)
- **Leukemic transformation:** Evolution to AML varies greatly across subtypes → EB-2 (>50%), RS (<5%)

Clinical presentation

- Nonspecific sx such as fatigue, infxn, & bleeding d/t **anemia** (85%), **neutropenia** (50%), **thrombocytopenia** (25%), as well as **impaired granulocyte fxn**
- Occasionally a/w AI phenomenon (eg, vasculitis, ITP)

Diagnosis

- DDx: AML, MPN (overlap), aplastic anemia, PNH, viral infxn (HIV, hepatitis, parvovirus), nutritional deficiencies (B12, **copper/zinc**), EtOH, meds, lead or arsenic poisoning
- Most pts anemic, often w/ **macrocytosis (1/3 pts),** & have ≥1 other cytopenia
- Peripheral smear: **Oval macrocytes,** hyposegmented neutrophils (**pseudo-Pelger–Huët cells**), hypogranulated neutrophils
- BM: Typically, **hypercellular (paradoxical given low counts); ≥10% dysplasia in ≥1 lineage** (myeloid, erythroid, megakaryocytes)
- BM exam also used to quantify the **blast percentage,** to detect presence of RS (esp relevant if anemia only), & for immunophenotyping
- **Cytogenetic testing** (karyotype) mandatory; FISH performed for translocations of *MLL* (11q23) or *EVI1* (3q26)
- **Molecular testing:** RNA splicing factor muts in ~50% (*SF3B1, SRSF2, U2AF1, ZRSR2*), epigenetic regulators in ~45% (*TET2, ASXL-1, DNMT3A, EZH2, IDH1/2*), both epigenetic & RNA splicing factor in 25%, *TP53* in ~5%, other genes in ~15%

WHO classification (2016)

Classification	Incidence	Pathologic Features
MDS w/ SLD: Hb <10 g/dL, ANC <1.8 K/μL, or plt <100 K/μL	<5%	≥10% dysplasia in affected cell lineage <5% BM blasts; ≤1% PB blasts <15% RS (see below) No Auer rods; no monocytosis
MDS w/ RS (a sideroblast is iron ring around nucleus)	<5%	RS ≥15% of BM or ≥5% of erythroid elements (if SF3B1+)
MDS w/ multilineage dysplasia	**70%**	≥10% dysplasia in 2 or more cell lines & same exclusions as MDS w/ SLD
MDS w/ excess blasts-1 (EB-1)	25%	Blasts: 5–9% BM, 2–4% PB, & no Auer rods
MDS w/ excess blasts-2 (EB-2)		Blasts: 10–19% BM, 5–19% PB or any Auer rods
MDS w/ isolated del(5q) (5q-syn)	5%	<5% blasts; del(5q)
MDS, unclassifiable (MDS-U)	<5%	+cytogenetic abnormality but <10% dysplasia & <5% blasts

Recurrent structural cytogenetic abnormalities, such as t(15;17), t(8;21), inv(16)/t(16;16), *MLL* gene rearrangements, are considered diagnostic of AML regardless of BM blast count.

Unique subtypes of MDS

5q-syn

- Characterized by **progressive anemia,** preserved/elevated plt count, & **del(5q) as sole cytogenetic abnormality or w/ 1 other except del7q or -7**
- Female predominance; classically benign course w/ **low risk of transformation to AML**
- In addition to dyserythropoiesis, micromegakaryocytes present in most cases (80%)
- Excellent RR to **lenalidomide**, w/ most pts achieving red-cell transfusion-independence & some w/ complete cytogenetic response (*NEJM* 2006;355:1456)

Hypoplastic MDS

- Rare, can be difficult to distinguish from **aplastic anemia** (cytogenetics can be helpful)

MDS/MPN overlap syn (also see MPN section)

- Pts have coexisting features of marrow failure & proliferation; BM blast count <20%; requires absence of genetic abnormalities which would classify pts in another WHO category, such as such as *BCR–ABL, JAK-2, PDGFRα/β*
- **CMML:** Characterized by peripheral **monocytosis** (>1,000/µL for 3 mos), anemia & thrombocytopenia, dysplastic neutrophils, often **splenomegaly**
- **RARS-T** (RARS & thrombocytosis) → RARS + plt count >450 K/µL; frequently *JAK-2* V617Fpositive

Prognosis

- **IPSS score**—commonly used & best validated prognostic scoring system
- Correlates w/ OS & evolution to AML (*Blood* 1997;89:2079)

International Prognostic Scoring System (IPSS) Score					
	0	0.5	1	1.5	2
BM blasts (%)	<5	5–10	—	11–20	21–30[a]
Karyotype[b]	Good	Int	Poor	—	—
Cytopenias	0 or 1	2 or 3	—	—	—

[a]Now considered AML per 2008 WHO classification.
[b]Good, nl; -Y alone, del(5q) alone, del(20q) alone; Poor, complex karyotype (≥3 abnls) or chromosome 7 abnls; Intermediate, any other cytogenetic abnls.

Risk Group	Total Score	Median Survival	AML Risk (25%)
Low	0	5.7 y	9.4 y
Int-1	0.5–1	3.5 y	3.3 y
Int-2	1.5–2	1.2 y	1.1 y
High	≥2.5	0.4 y	0.2 y

- **Revised IPSS (IPSS-R) score:** Assigns greater prognostic significance to cytogenetics & utilizes 5 rather than 3 prognostic subgroups; uses modified cytopenia thresholds—neutropenia as <800/uL vs. <1,800/uL (*Blood* 2012;120:2454)
- Complex karyotype & t-MDS have poor prog, as do Mts in *TP53, EZH2, ETV6, RUNX1* & *ASXL1* (*NEJM* 2011:364:2496); poor outcomes observed w/ *TP53* Mts are specific to biallelic *TP53* loss but not monoallelic *TP53* Mts (*Nature Med* 2020;26:1549)

Treatment

- Must consider age, PS, & IPSS score/risk status, & transplant candidacy
- IPSS Low/Int-1 risk: Supportive care incl **ESAs** (epoetin alfa or darbepoetin; esp if EPO level <500); consider ESA + G-CSF for RARS; **lenalidomide**—esp for 5q-syn (*Blood* 2011;118(14):3765–3776) but also others (*JCO* 2016;34:2988)
  - If progression → hypomethylating agents (azacytidine or decitabine); **Luspatercept** for transfusion dependent MDS w/ either RS or SF3B1 Mts (*NEJM* 2020;382:140)
- IPSS Int-2/High risk: **Hypomethylating agents** → survival benefit compared to BSC & some pts achieve CR (9–17%) (*Lancet Oncol* 2009;10:223; *Cancer* 2006;106:1794); possible increased efficacy in *TET2* to azacytidine (*Blood* 2014;124:2705) & *TP53* to decitabine (*NEJM* 2016;375:2023); decitabine/cedazuridine recently approved as alternative all oral formulation (*Blood* 2000;136:674)
- **Allo transplant** is only curative strategy & leads to improved OS compared to drug therapy alone in higher-risk MDS (BMTCTN 1102 trial; *Blood* 2021;138(suppl_1):75)
- Hypoplastic MDS → can be treated like aplastic anemia w/ **ATG & cyclosporine** (*JCO* 2008;26:2505)
- **Supportive care** (regardless of risk & Rx strategy): RBC & plt transfusions, Antimicrobial therapy as needed. Iron chelation Rx if needed (esp if transplant candidate)
- **Promising novel agents:** NEDD8 activating enzyme inhibitor pevonedistat, bcl-2 mimetic venetoclax, anti-CD47 Ab magrolimab, anti-TIM3 Ab sabatolimab (all in phase III trial testing in combination w/ azacytidine); telomerase inhibitor imetelstat

ACUTE MYELOID LEUKEMIA (AML)

Epidemiology

- Incidence: Estimated 20,240 new cases in the United States in 2021 (11,400 deaths)
- Most common leukemia in adults; median age at dx: **68 y**
- **RF:** Cytotoxic chemo, benzene, smoking, DS (trisomy 21), rare congenital syns (eg, severe congenital neutropenia, Shwachman–Diamond, dyskeratosis congenita, Fanconi anemia; Li–Fraumeni, Klinefelter, Noonan syn)

Disease biology/natural history

- Heterogeneous clonal disorder of hematopoietic stem or progenitor cells (**blasts**)
- Many genotypic variants (many w/ prognostic relevance)
- **W/ tx:** ↑ blasts in BM & circulation & ↓ ANC/Hb/plt; typically, fatal in wk to mos d/t BM failure (**infxn**, bleeding) or organ infiltration

Clinical presentation/emergencies

- Presenting s/s reflect ↓ hematopoiesis: Most commonly fatigue &/or infxn
- Most pts pancytopenic w/ circulating blasts at dx → ~50% ↓ or nl WBC; ~20% WBC >100K/μL
- **Coagulopathy:** Very common in **APL** & frequent cause of early death (cerebral hemorrhage) → early admin of ATRA critical at 1st suspicion of APL (ie, in the ER)
- **TLS** (more common w/ ALL but can occur in AML): Ppx w/ IVF & allopurinol, Rx includes IVF, forced diuresis, rasburicase, HD if severe
- **Leukostasis** poss if WBC >50K/μL → vascular occlusion/hemorrhage (microcirculation) → visual Δ/retinopathy, **dyspnea**/pulm infiltrates, myocardial ischemia, **TIA/CVA** → Rx w/ IVF, TLS ppx/tx, **cytoreduction:** Chemo, hydrea, or leukapheresis if chemo delayed
- CNS involvement in 2–3% of cases (RF: ↑ WBC, relapsed APL); work-up incl eye exam, CT/MRI, usu defer LP until CR1 unless symptomatic (theoretical risk of CNS seeding)

Diagnosis

- BM **aspirate** & bx w/ flow cytometry, cytogenetics/FISH & molecular studies (*KIT, FLT3, NPM1, CEBPA, IDH1, IDH2, TP53* are standard)
- AML confirmed if **≥20%** myeloblasts in BM or blood; blast percentage can be <20% for AML if the following translocations are present: t(15;17), t(8;21), or t(16;16)
- R/o ALL → morphology (**Auer rods** are pathognomonic for AML; N:C ratio often higher in ALL); immunophenotyping by IHC/flow; cytogenetics/molecular genetic studies
- Common myeloid Ag: **CD13, CD33, CD34, CD117, MPO**

WHO Classification of AML (*Blood* 2016;127:2391)	
W/ recurrent genetic abnormalities	**Core-binding factor (CBF)** leukemias → t(8;21), inv(16)/t(16;16); APL w/ *PML-RARA; KMT2A (MLL)*/11q23 abnls; t(6;9); inv(3)/t(3;3)[a]; t(1;22)[b]; *NPM1*; biallelic *CEBPA* Mts; Provisional: AML w/ *BCR-ABL1* & AML w/ mutated *RUNX1*
W/ myelodysplasia-related changes	H/o MDS; or present MDS-related cytogenetic abnormality except del(9q); or morphologic multilineage dysplasia (≥50% dysplastic cells in ≥2 cell lines) w/o *NPM1* or biallelic *CEBPA* Mts
Tx-related myeloid neoplasms (~10–15% of AML)	RT/alkylating agents → monosomies or deletions of chr 5 or 7; onset ~5–10 y after exposure; more common type Topoisomerase II inhib (eg, etoposide, anthracyclines) → 11q23 abnls, t(15;17), t(8;21); typically 1–5 y after exposure
NOS	W/o maturation, w/ min differentiation, w/ maturation, w/ myelomonocytic, monoblastic, or monocytic differentiation **less common** → pure erythroid, megakaryoblastic, or basophilic leukemia; acute panmyelosis w/ MF (rare)
Myeloid sarcoma[c] (chloromas)	Extramedullary involvement may antedate BM dz (more common w/ monocytic differentiation)

[a]3q21q26 syndrome/*EVI1* gene rearrangements → a/w thrombocytosis & very poor prognosis.
[b]Very rare, megakaryoblastic phenotype, infant leukemia.
[c]Treat as systemic AML (*Blood* 2011;118:3785).

Prognosis

Determined primarily by **age & cytogenetic/molecular risk**

- Age >60 y is an independent poor-risk feature
- Poor-risk factors: Poor PS, high-presenting WBC, antecedent hematologic disorder, tx-related AML
- Good risk: **APL** (10–15% of all AML), (+)**CBF** (~12%)
- Most pts have an intermediate or unfavorable risk at presentation
- **MRD** by flow cytometry even w/ morphologic CR predicts poor outcomes w/ allo-HCT d/t high rates of relapse (*JCO* 2016;34;329); molecular MRD (*NPM1* RT-PCR) also emerging as powerful prognostic factor (*NEJM* 2016;374:422)

AML genetics and risk (*Blood* 2010;116:354; *NEJM* 2016;374:2209)

2017 ELN risk classification by genetics (*Blood* 2017;129:424)

Risk Status	Cytogenetics	Molecular Abnormalities
Favorable risk	CBF: inv(16) or t(16;16) or t(8;21) APL: t(15;17)	*NPM1* & *FLT3*–; *NPM1* & *FLT3–ITD*$^{low a}$; *CEBPA* (biallelic)
Intermediate risk	Nl **(~45% pts);** +8; t(9;11)	*NPM1* & *FLT3–ITD*$^{high a}$
Poor risk	Complex cytogenetics (≥3 clonal abnls); monosomal; –5/5q–; –7/7q–; 11q23; inv(3)/t(3;3); t(6;9); t(9;22)	Wild type *NPM1* & *FLT3–ITD*$^{high a}$; *RUNX1*; *TP53*; *ASXL-1*

[a]low, low allelic ratio (<0.5); high, high allelic ratio (≥0.5).

- Favorable karyotypic abnls are considered favorable regardless of other cytogenetic abnls
- *c-KIT* Mt unfavorable in t(8;21) (*c-KIT* Mt prog less established in inv(16)/t(16;16))
- *IDH1/2* prog controversial—some data suggest *NPM1* & *IDH* co-Mt in nl cytogenetics w/o *FLT3-ITD* → very favorable (*NEJM* 2012;366:1079); Other data suggest *NPM1* & *IDH* co-Mt in nl cytogenetics w/o FLT3-ITD confer adverse prog (*JCO* 2010;28:3762)
- **Monosomal karyotype** (≥2 monosomies or 1 w/ other structural abnl) carries an extremely poor prog (*JCO* 2008;26:4791)

Treatment

- **Assess if candidate for intensive induction chemo** based on age & comorbidities (Ferrara criteria: *Leukemia* 2013;27:997)

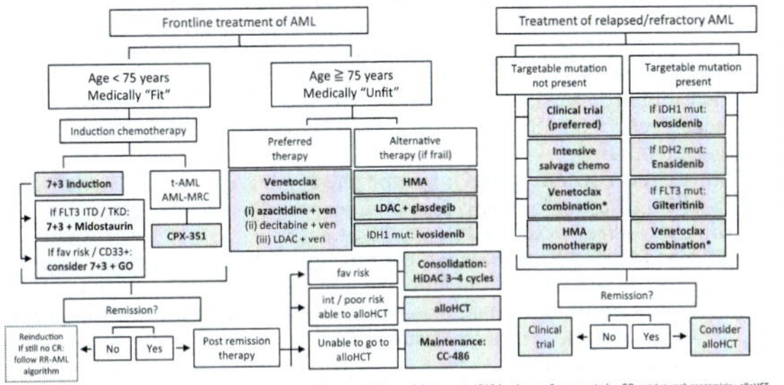

t-AML, treatment related AML; s-AML, AML-MRC, AML with myelodysplasia related changes; HMA, hypomethylating agents; LDAC, low dose ara-C; ven, venetoclax; GO, gemtuzumab ozogamicin; alloHCT, allogeneic hematopoietic stem cell transplant; HiDAC, high dose ara-C; fav, favorable; int, intermediate; RR, relapsed/refractory.
*Currently FDA approved in frontline AML but not FDA approved in R/R AML.

- **Frontline tx of AML (age <75 & medically "fit" for intensive chemo)**
  - **Induction chemo** (7 + 3): 7 d of infusional **cytarabine** & 3 d of **dauno or idarubicin;** RCTs confirmed **high-dose dauno** (90 mg/m^2) superior (**OS benefit**) to standard dose (45 mg/m^2) (*NEJM* 2009;361:1249); dauno 90 mg/m^2 superior to 45 mg/m^2 across cytogenetic/molecular subgroups incl complex cytogenetics & *FLT3-ITD* (*Blood* 2016;127:1551); for >60 y dauno 90 mg/m^2 has OS benefit only in 60–65 y or CBF (*NEJM* 2009;361:1235); can use dauno 60 mg/m^2 in older pts w/ good PS & cardiac fx
  - **(7+3) + Midostaurin** (multikinase inhibitor incl FLT3): Midostaurin + chemo OS benefit over chemo alone (*NEJM* 2017;377:454); SOC in *FLT3* mut AML
  - **(7+3) + GO ozogamicin** (ab–drug conjugate to CD33 linked to calicheamicin): reapproved based on ALFA-0701 trial & large meta-analysis showing OS benefit over chemo alone in favorable risk CD33+ AML (*Lancet* 2012;379:1508; *Lancet Oncol* 2014;15:986)

- **CPX-351** (liposomal formulation of cytarabine & dauno in 5:1 molar ratio): OS benefit over 7+3 (dauno 60 mg/m^2) in pts w/ therapy-related AML (t-AML) & AML w/ myelodysplasia-related changes (AML-MRC) (*JCO* 2018;36:2684)
- **Assessment of response:** D 14 BMBx remains SOC to document hypoplasia following induction; BMBx upon peripheral count recovery to confirm CR **(<5% blasts);** persistent cytopenias >28 d after chemo → likely residual leukemia; can repeat 1 course of induction or alternative regimen if no CR
- **Postremission tx dictated by AML risk status, age, comorbidities, PS, candidacy for allo-HCT, donor status:** Favorable-risk AML CR1 → consolidation Rx; intermediate or poor-risk AML → consider allo-HCT in CR1 if appropriate candidate vs. consolidation Rx; if not eligible for allo-HCT → consider maintenance therapy w/ CC-486
- **Consolidation Rx: HiDAC** → optimal dose under debate → younger pts current standard 3 g/m^2 × 6 (q12h d 1,3,5) for 3–4 cycles in favorable risk; **cerebellar tox** rare but potential SE; **modify dose in older pts;** use steroid eye drops QID until 24-h postcompletion of HiDAC to reduce risk of keratoconjunctivitis; No proven benefit to multiple courses of HiDAC, esp. in older pts & non-CBF leukemias
- **Allo-HCT:** In appropriate pts (unfavorable or intermediate-risk prog) w/ suitable donor (RIC for pts >60 y)—best results for allo-HCT in CR1; MUD & matched related-donor HCT now similar outcomes; UCB has expanded donor pool (*Blood* 2010;116:4693); Haploidentical + posttransplant cytoxan promising (*Blood* 2015;126:1033); auto-HCT **rarely** used, though may benefit pts w/ favorable or intermediate risk who received high-dose dauno (*Blood* 2011;117:5306)
- **Maintenance Rx:** Oral azacytidine (CC-486, Onureg) maintenance therapy showed OS advantage over placebo in pts who achieved remission after induction therapy but could not complete intensive consolidation chemo or were not candidates for allo-HCT (*NEJM* 2020;383:2526)
- **Supportive care:** IVF, abx for F+N, antimold antifungal ppx if prolonged neutropenia, TLS ppx w/ allopurinol (rasburicase if ↑ UA & risk for tumor lysis), RBC & plt transfusions, hydrea if ↑ WBCs (leukapheresis rarely needed)

- **Frontline tx of AML (age ≥75 y or medically "unfit" for intensive chemo)**
  - **Bcl-2 mimetic venetoclax** in combination w/ **azacitidine** (*NEJM* 2020;383:617) or **decitabine** (*Blood* 2019;133:7) or **low-dose ara-C** (*JCO* 2019;37:1277); OS advantage for venetoclax + azacitidine over azacitidine alone (*NEJM* 2020;383:617)
  - **Hypomethylating agents** (HMA) alone (azacitidine, decitabine) → benefit in older pts not candidates for intensive chemo (*JCO* 2010;28:562) or venetoclax. Decitabine w/ very high ORR in pts w/ *TP53* Mts (100%, n = 21), though responses transient (*NEJM* 2016;375:2023)
  - **IDH1 inhibitor ivosidenib** in frail AML pts w/ an *IDH1* mut (*Blood* 2020;135:463), if not frail prefer venetoclax combination given high-response rate in *IDH* mut AML (*Blood* 2020;135:791)
  - **Shh receptor-smoothened inhibitor glasdegib** in combination w/ low-dose Ara-C; OS advantage over low-dose ara-C alone (*Leukemia* 2019;33:379)
- **Tx of relapsed/refractory AML** (*Blood* 2020;136:1023)
  - If fit & no targetable mut: **Salvage chemo** (eg, MEC → mitoxantrone, etoposide, cytarabine; or fludarabine, high-dose cytarabine, G-CSF, idarubicin → FLAG-IDA) vs. **venetoclax combination** (*Blood Advances* 2021;5:1552) vs. **hypomethylating agents** (*Blood Advances* 2018;2:923) vs. **clinical trial** (preferred) → goal to achieve CR2 & consider consolidation w/ allo-HCT
  - If targetable mut: Prefer targeted therapy or venetoclax combination as alternative; *FLT3-ITD* or *TKD* mut → gilteritinib (*NEJM* 2019;381:1728); *IDH1* mut → ivosidenib (*NEJM* 2018;378:2386); *IDH2* mut → enasidenib (*Blood* 217;130:722)

Outcomes (*Blood* 2005;106:1154; *JCO* 2009;27:61; *Blood* 2020;136:1023)

- ~70–80% of younger pts (<60 y) & ~40–50% of older pts (>60 y) will achieve CR w/ induction chemo (+CR correlates w/ survival)
- Long-term OS ~35–40% in younger adults; better prog in APL & CBF leukemias
- Older pts have poor prog (OS ~10–15%), d/t medical comorbidities & underlying dz biology/genetics (eg, ↑ risk of antecedent MDS, monosomal karyotype)

Promising selected investigational agents

- Venetoclax combinations: Multiple trials combining venetoclax w/ intensive chemo, targeted therapy (IDH & FLT3 inhibitors) & IO
- Novel targeted therapy: Menin inhibitor, TP53 activator (APR-246), RARα agonist, others
- IO: DART (flotetuzumab), immune checkpoint inhibitors (anti-CD47 ab magrolimab, anti-TIM3 ab sabatolimab), CAR T cells

Acute promyelocytic leukemia (APL)

- Unique subtype of AML w/ **excellent prog & distinct biology**
- Characterized by **atypical promyelocytes** (considered "blast equivalents" in APL)
- Driven/defined by translocation of RAR gene (t(15;17)) → aberrant fusion protein ***PML-RARα*** → blocks nl myeloid differentiation at promyelocyte stage
- **Early death** often from characteristic **coagulopathy** → start ATRA early, aggressively, correct w/ FFP, cryoprecipitate (fibrinogen >150 mg/dL), & PLT (plt >50K/µL)
- Most pts now cured w/ differentiating tx **ATRA** & **ATO** → almost all achieve CR, OS ~90%
  - Greatest barrier to cure remains early death largely from coagulopathy
- APL risk groups: **WBC ≤ 10K/µL low risk; WBC > 10K/µL high risk**
- Low-risk APL tx: **ATRA+ATO** for both induction/consolidation—ATRA+ATO 2-y DFS 97% for low risk; no chemo or maintenance needed (*NEJM* 2013;369:111)
- High-risk APL tx: **Chemo needed**—several combination ATRA + chemo ± ATO regimens:
  - **Standard Rx:** Induction w/ **ATRA+idarubicin+ATO** → consolidation w/ ATRA+ATO → maintenance w/ ATRA, 6-MP, oral MTX (*Lancet Haematol* 2015;2:e357); **auto-HCT** if relapse; chemo free protocols for high-risk APL (incorporating a single dose of GO ozogamicin) are an alternative (*Lancet Oncol* 2017;16:1295; *Blood* 2017;129:1275)
- **Differentiation syn:** Fever, edema, serositis, ARDS, HoTN → Rx w/ high-dose steroids, & temporary cessation of ATRA/ATO (potentially life-threatening); consider ppx w/ steroids in high-risk APL
- **Risk of CNS relapse:** Consider IT chemo ppx during consolidation in high-risk APL

ACUTE LYMPHOBLASTIC LEUKEMIA/LYMPHOMA

Lymphoblastic neoplasms

- Can present as leukemia or lymphoma, but are treated the same
  - ALL: ≥20% BM blasts
  - LBL: <20% BM blasts + mass lesion
- ALL/LBL can be further classified by lineage → precursor **B** or **T** cell ALL
- >6,500 cases annually in the United States (2% of all lymphoid neoplasms); more common in children & adolescents; higher incidence in Hispanics; T-ALL/LBL w/ male predominance

Clinical presentation

- Aggressive malignancy p/w pancytopenia & circulating blasts; common s/s → B-sxs, fatigue, pallor, infxn, bleeding, bony pain, adenopathy, splenomegaly
- **Anterior mediastinal mass** → suggests **T**-ALL; ***NOTCH*** gene Mt: Important role T-ALL
- **CNS involvement**: Usu cranial neuropathies/leukemic meningitis, but can be mass lesion (headache); more common T-ALL (requires IT chemo ± cranial radiation)
- TLS more common in ALL > AML (see TLS section); DIC & leukostasis rare but can occur

Diagnosis and disease biology

- BM morphology: Hypercellular marrow usu replaced w/ lymphoblasts (unless LBL) → **absence** of granules/Auer rods; must obtain flow cytometry & cytogenetics

WHO Classification of ALL

Subtype	Frequency (Adults)	Immunophenotype
Precursor B cell	75%	(+) TdT; (+) CD19; (+) CD22; (–) CD3; variable CD10, CD20, CD79a
Precursor T cell	20%	(+) TdT; (+) cCD3; (+) CD7; (–) CD10; variable CD1a, CD2, sCD3, CD4, CD5, CD8

- B-ALL: **T(9;22)/Ph chr** by FISH or molecular testing affects tx/prog
- **"Ph-like"** (BCR-ABL1-like) B-ALL (~25%): Lack t(9;22) but have similar **gene expression profile** to Ph+ B-ALL; ↓ response to standard CT & ↓ OS (*NEJM* 2014;371(11):1005)
- Early T-precursor (ETP) ALL: Resembles immature thymic immigrants from BM w/ similar muts/gene exp as myeloid/stem cells; CD1a$^-$, CD8$^-$, CD5$^{dim/-}$ & ≥1 stem cell/myeloid marker; ↓ OS w/ standard CT in some series (*Lancet Oncol* 2009;10(2):147)
- Assess for sanctuary sites: **LP in all pts;** image 1st in pts w/ neurologic s/s; **IT chemo** is part of standard tx; usu given w/ diagnostic LP (as CNS involvement common & to prevent seeding from circulating blasts/traumatic tap); testis exam at dx
- CT chest to r/o mediastinal mass (if T-cell lineage); TTE before anthracyclines

Prognosis

- **Better in children;** most children w/ ALL are cured w/ chemo alone (see **Pediatrics** section)
- >85% of adult pts will achieve morphologic CR
- The cure rate in **adult** ALL remains ~35–40% but varies depending on prognostic features, ranging from 10–30% w/ unfavorable-risk features to 50–70% w/ favorable-risk features
- **MRD** (see below), strongly predicts DFS/OS in pts achieving morphologic CR
- Favorable prognostic features: **Children/adolescents/younger adults;** WBC <30 K/µL for pre–B-cell ALL; <100 K/µL for T-ALL; **rapid achievement of MRD-CR;** hyperdiploidy (>50 chrs); t(12;21) → more common in childhood ALL
- Poor prognostic features: Infants (<1 y) & **older adults; t(9;22)/Ph chr** (TKI therapy has transformed therapy & prog is evolving); **t(4;11);** hypodiploidy (<45 chrs); Ph-like; *MLL*-rearrangement

MRD assessment

- **MRD:** Absence of morphologic ALL w/ only dz detected by highly sensitive techniques; ideally assessed from **1st pull** of BM aspirate
- **Techniques: RT-PCR** for *BCR-ABL1* (sensitivity < 0.001%); quantitative PCR for T-cell receptor or Ig gene rearrangement (sensitivity < 0.001%); multiparameter flow cytometry w/ abnl blast population (sensitivity < 0.01%)

Principles of treatment of Ph– B or T ALL

- **Induction:** Many published combination regimens; NCCN suggest 1st-line clinical trial
  - **HyperCVAD** regimen commonly used in adults; alternates between parts A & B
    - Part A: Hyperfractionated cyclophosphamide, doxorubicin, vincristine, dexamethasone
    - Part B: HD-MTX & high-dose cytarabine

- Pediatric-inspired regimens based on BFM model:
  - Regimens include anthracyclines, cyclophosphamide, cytarabine, vincristine, steroids, **asparaginase;** 2-phase induction & planned "re-induction"
  - **Asparaginase related tox:** Hepatic tox, hypersensitivity, pancreatitis, hypertriglyceridiemia, thrombosis
- After induction, repetitive courses of **postremission** chemo (consolidation/intensification) over 6–8 mos, followed by **maintenance** chemo (2–3 y)
- **Relapsed/Refractory** (R/R) Ph-ALL: Salvage therapy followed by allo-HCT if appropriate. Outside of salvage chemo, other options for R/R ALL include:
  - **Blinatumomab:** CD3/CD19-targeted BiTE effective in R/R (*NEJM* 2017;376:836) or MRD+ B-ALL (*Blood* 2018;131:1522); watch for CRS/neurotox
  - **Inotuzumab ozogamicin:** CD22-targeted ab–drug conjugate effective in R/R B-ALL; risks include hepatic tox/SOS (*NEJM* 2016;375:740)
  - CD19-targeted **CAR T cells** (see **CAR T Therapy** chapter) effective in R/R B-ALL; tisagenlecleucel approved for pts age <26 y; others under investigation
  - **Nelarabine** (standard), venetoclax, daratumumab, everolimus (invest) for R/R T-ALL

Principles of treatment of Ph+ ALL (~25% of adult ALL)

- Defined by **t(9;22) → BCR-ABL1 fusion gene;** usu **p190 subtype** (p210 = usu CML)
- More common in older adults (>40% pts age ≥60) & historically a/w poorer prog
- As w/ Ph–B-ALL, can use **MRD** status (incl qPCR for BCR-ABL1) to assess response
- R/R Ph+ ALL: Adv generation TKIs & use of other salvage therapies

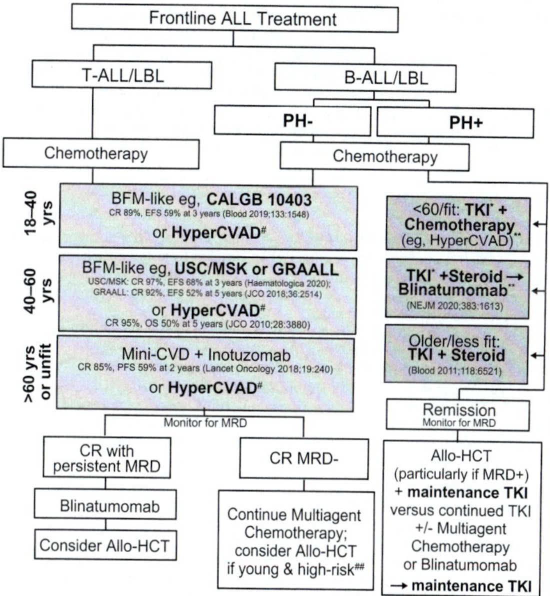

*2nd or 3rd generation TKI + CT may be more potent than imatinib + CT in frontline setting (*Haematologica 2015;100:653; Lancet Oncol 2015;16:1547*)
**TKI + lower-intensity chemo may be reasonable (*Blood 2015;125:3711*).
#Rituximab may improve DFS in CD20+ B-ALL (*NEJM 2016;375:1044*).
##High-risk features such as Ph-like, MLL-rearrangement, ETP, hypodiploid.

CHRONIC MYELOGENOUS LEUKEMIA (CML)

Epidemiology
- Classified as an MPN
- A dysregulated production & uncontrolled proliferation of **mature/maturing granulocytes**
- **15–20% of adult leukemias,** approx 5,000 new cases/y in the United States, 1–2 cases per 100,000 adults, median age ~64 (United States), younger median age in Asia/Africa

Pathology
- **CBC:** WBC elevated, median ~80 K/μL; anemia (40–60%), plts nl or elevated (600–700k)
  Differential & smear: Full spectrum of myeloid forms ('left shift'-eg, blasts, myelocytes, metamylocytes, neutrophils, etc.); basophilia ± eosinophilia also common (>90%)
- **BMBx:** Hypercellular, granulocytic hyperplasia, small megakaryocytes w/ hypolobated nuclei, blasts variable (% defines dz phase)

Clinical features
- 30–50% of cases asx—found incidentally on routine CBC (eg, leukocytosis)
- Other: Fatigue, sweats, wt loss, easy bleeding/bruising, splenomegaly (w/early satiety, abd fullness)
- Three general dz phases exist; progression can be either biphasic or triphasic

Phase	Features (WHO)
CP/Chronic (3–5 y duration pre-TKI)	**85% of pts** present in CP, often w/o sx, no criteria for accelerated or blast crisis
AP/Accelerated Phase (12–18 mos duration pre-TKI)	≥1 of the following is present: **10–19% blasts** in peripheral blood or BM, PB basophils ≥20%, plt <100,000/μL (unrelated to tx), plt <100,000 *or* >1 million/μL (unresponsive to tx), progressive splenomegaly or ↑ WBC (unresponsive to tx), cytogenetic clonal evolution (eg, additional chromosomal abnormalities beyond Ph+)
BC/Blast Crisis (3–9 mos duration pre-TKI)	Resembles acute leukemia: Myeloid or lymphoid blasts, **≥20% peripheral blood or BM blasts,** clusters of blasts on BMBx, or extramedullary blastic infiltrates (eg, myeloid/granulocytic sarcoma)

*Revised WHO Criteria for myeloid neoplasms & acute leukemias (*Blood* 2016;127(20):2391).

Biology
- **Philadelphia (Ph) chr: *BCR–ABL1*** gene fusion, reciprocal translocation between chrs 9 (*ABL1*) & 22 (*BCR*) –> t(9;22)(q34;q11), identified by karyotype/FISH (noncryptic) in 95% of cases → encodes constitutively activated tyrosine kinase central to CML pathogenesis → progression to AP/BC based on clonal evolution, likely additional molecular changes, *ABL* kinase muts
- Three types of **fusion proteins** based on location of breakpoint in BCR gene:
  - **p210:** Classic breakpoint (>95% of pts); (also seen in 30% Ph+ ALL)
  - **p230:** Alternative breakpoint; found in only rare cases (<1%)
  - **p190:** Also rare (<1%); (common breakpoint in Ph+ ALL, 70%)
- NOTE: A minority of pts (<5%) may harbor a **variant** translocation (eg, t(9;14;22)) → testing at dx by both cytogenetics (karyotype, FISH) & molecular (PCR) important; need to confirm fusion type (eg, p210) & splice type (e13 vs. e14a2) → impact on response

Molecular diagnostics
- **BMBx:** Advised at dx for CP, if questions of AP/BC (anytime) & loss/failure of cytogenetic response
- **Cytogenetics:** Testing for *BCR-ABL1* (& to identify any additional chromosomal abnormalities), repeat if significant ↑ qPCR or minimal ↓ (eg, loss of CCyR, CHR)
- **FISH:** For *BCR–ABL1* fusion gene; historically poorer prog w/ 9q deletion
- **Quantitative RT-PCR (qPCR):** Fusion mRNA product, most sensitive technique to detect MRD; used extensively to monitor therapy response (early into deep remission)
- Kinase domain mutational analysis: Not obtained at dx (unless BC), only if failure of TKI

Prognosis
- Stage of dz at dx is strongest predictor of outcome (CP vs. AP/BC)
- OS approximates age-matched nl life expectancy (if dx'd in CP) in TKI era
- Various scoring systems devised to predict outcomes at dx:
  - **Sokal score:** Categories: Low vs. intermediate vs. high; calculated from % peripheral blasts, plt count, spleen size, age (*Blood* 1984;63:789)
  - **ELTS (EUTOS long term survival score):** Categories: Low vs. intermediate vs. high; same elements as Sokal; different weighting, imatinib-based (*Leukemia* 2020;34(8):2138)

Front-line therapy

- Significant majority of CP CML pts achieve excellent response to up-front TKIs
  - **Imatinib:** 400 mg daily (may ↑ dose to 800 mg daily w/ suboptimal response but caution w/ s/e); longest safety data, OS similar to 2 g TKI (*NEJM* 2017;376:917)
  - **Nilotinib** (*NEJM* 2010;362:2251), **dasatinib** (*NEJM* 2010;362:2260) or **bosutinib** (*JCO* 2018;36(3):231) may be used **front-line** (preferred if **int/high-risk Sokal**) or if goal is to achieve tx-free remission (TFR); 2nd-gen TKI results in faster/deeper cytogenetic response but no effect on 5-yr PFS/OS (*JCO* 2016;34(20):2333–2340)
    - Consider baseline cardiovascular (CV) w/u prior to tx as well as QTc monitoring
    - Avoid nilotinib in pts w/ severe DM, uncontrolled CVD
    - Avoid dasatinib in pts w/ limited pulm reserve or PAH
    - Bosutinib is a/w LFT ↑/diarrhea, latter minimized w/ titration
- **Presentation in AP:** 2nd /3rd gen TKI (dasatinib, bosutinib, nilotinib, or ponatinib) & consideration of alloSCT rec

Resistance/progressive disease on TKI

- Evaluate adherence, drug–drug interactions, reconsider comorbidities (esp. CV) if switch
- TKI resistance frequently a/w **point mts in *BCR–ABL1*** kinase domain (eg, T315I, Y253H, etc.) → check for *BCR–ABL1* resistance mts, & repeat BMBx w/ cytogenetics if w/o CyR
- Consider switching to a different TKI (can ↑ dose of imatinib to 800 mg but caution w/ s/e). Resistance mut & s/e profile can guide choice of alt TKI. **Ponatinib**—only effective TKI against T315I resistance mt; assoc w/ HTN, pancreatitis, arterial/venous thrombosis. Dose ↓ to 15 mg w/ response, to mitigate these effects. CV monitoring impt
- **AlloSCT:** Now used mainly if adv stage dz at dx, progression to AP/BC w/ 2nd CP restored or CP TKI-refractory dz, especially w/ T315I mut

Response evaluation

- Response types: **Hematologic** (CBC/clinical-spleen ↓), **cytogenetic** (*BCR-ABL1* by karyotype & FISH), & **molecular** (*BCR–ABL1* qPCR in PB)

Response	Description
Complete Hematologic Response (CHR)	WBC <10K/µL w/ no immature granulocytes & <5% basophils; plt <450K/µL; no s/s (↓ spleen)
Cytogenetic Response	**% of Ph+ cells by metaphase karyotyping/FISH:**
Major **(MCyR):**	0–35%
- Complete **(CCyR):**	0
- Partial **(PCyR):**	%1–35%
Minor **(mCyR):**	>35%
Molecular Response	**Assessed by qPCR:**
Early **(EMR):**	*BCR–ABL1* ≤10% on the intl scale (IS) by **3 mos on tx**
Major **(MMR):**	≥3-log ↓ in *BCR–ABL1* transcript levels (eg, **≤0.1%** IS)
Deep (DMR/MR4)	*BCR–ABL1* transcript levels **≤0.01%** IS)
Complete **(CMR/MR4.5)**	*BCR–ABL1* transcript *undetectable* using assays w/ sensitivity of ≥4.5-log reduction from the IS standardized baseline (eg, **≤0.0032%** IS)

Per National Comprehensive Cancer Network (NCCN) 2021 guidelines version 1

- **qPCR:** Obtain at dx, then q3mos until MMR, then q3–6mos thereafter (q3mos preferred to document deep MR for TFR)
- *BCR-ABL1* qPCR ≤10% at 3 mos on TKI, as well as rate of decline (halving time) predictive of improved long-term PFS & OS & lower rates of transformation
- TKI discontinuation can be trialed after prolonged remission in select CML pts (*Lancet Oncol* 2010;11:1029, *JAMA Oncol* 2021;7:42, *Lancet Haematol* 2015;2:e528, NCCN Guidelines version 1. 2021). Consider for pts on TKI for ≥3 y & sustained DMR/MR4 ≥2 y. Adequate monitoring (monthly until 6mos → q2mos until 12 mos, q3mos thereafter) is essential

Recommendations for follow-up therapy

Follow-up	Response (by qPCR)	Treatment Recs
3 mos	• *BCR–ABL1* ≤10% (IS) • *BCR–ABL1* >10% (IS)	• Continue same TKI • Consider switch to alternate TKI
12 mos	• *BCR–ABL1* ≤1% (IS) • *BCR–ABL1* >1–10% (IS) • *BCR–ABL1* >10% (IS)	• Continue same TKI • Consider switch to alternate TKI • Switch TKI & consider alloSCT
18 mos	• *BCR–ABL1* ≤0.1% (IS) • *BCR–ABL1* >0.1–1% (IS) • *BCR–ABL1* >1% (IS)	• Continue same TKI • Consider switch to alternate TKI • Switch TKI & consider alloSCT

Changes in single qPCR results should not prompt changes in Rx; repeat in 1–3 mos.

CHRONIC LYMPHOCYTIC LEUKEMIA (CLL)

Definitions (*Blood* 2018;131(25):2745; *NEJM* 2020;383(5):460)

- Chronic lymphoproliferation & accumulation of monoclonal, functionally incompetent mature CD5+ B-lymphocytes in BM, blood, LNs & spleen
- **Monoclonal B cell lymphocytosis (MBL):** <5,000 x 10^9/L clonal B lymphocytes w/o organomegaly or nodal involvement or cytopenia; progresses to CLL requiring tx ~1–2% per y; manage w/ observation
- **Chronic lymphocytic leukemia (CLL):** >5,000 x 10^9/L clonal B lymphocytes in PB for at least 3 mos, clonality of B cells must be confirmed by flow cytometry
- **Small lymphocytic leukemia (SLL):** <5,000 x 10^9/L lymphocytes in PB w/ CLL-phenotype by flow cytometry + LAN; no cytopenia caused by marrow infiltrate; if requires tx, is managed like CLL
- **B prolymphocytic leukemia (B-PLL):** ≥55% prolymphocytes in PB

Epidemiology

- Most common adult leukemia in Western countries; average age at CLL dx = 72 y; more common in males than females (*NEJM* 2020;383(5):460)

Clinical presentation (*NEJM* 2020;383(5):460)

- Heterogeneous presentation & dz course; ~30% of pts never require tx
- Some pts are asx at presentation w/ dx discovered on CBC obtained for other reasons; other pts p/w B-sxs from CLL (fevers, drenching NS, unintentional wt loss, fatigue), recurrent infxns
- May have AI complications (eg, ITP or AIHA) w/o CLL progression; if ITP or AIHA in isolation, may manage w/ steroids & not CLL-directed therapy

Diagnostic evaluation (*Blood* 2018;131(25):2745; *NEJM* 2020;383(5):460)

- **PB flow cytometry:** B cells are CD5+ & coexpress CD19, CD20 (usu dim), CD23; clone either kappa or lambda Ig light chain-restricted; other markers incl CD200 may help w/ dx
- **FISH for t(11;14):** Rec at dx to r/o MCL; can be performed on PB (if circulating clone detectable), LN or BM
- **Bx:** LN or BMBx required only if no circulating clone in blood or to establish dx if LAN potentially suspicious for other dz process (lymphoma or solid tumor); BM indicated if unexplained cytopenias or atypical flow cytometry profile not diagnostic of CLL or other leukemia/lymphoma; LN bx always indicated if clinical &/or radiographic suspicion of transformation
- **Hx:** Assess for B-sxs, fatigue, infxns, rapidly progressive sxs (may signify transformation)
- **PE:** Attention to LNs & examination for hepatosplenomegaly
- **Imaging:** Not always indicated. CT CAP may be helpful as baseline for SLL pts to assess LAN not palpable on PE; PET CT useful if suspicion for transformation
- **Other laboratory evaluation:** CBC w/ differential, CMP, Hep B & C serologies, HIV in anticipation of IST; Coombs test, LDH, haptoglobin if suspicion for hemolytic anemia; beta-2-microglobulin & LDH, serum Ig levels
- **Further prognostic testing:** Not required at dx, but SOC to perform prior to tx initiation & w/ each subsequent line of therapy
  - **Cytogenetics:** FISH (or SNP array): Performed for common chromosomal abnormalities incl del17p, del13q, trisomy 12, del11q; karyotype if available
  - **Molecular testing:** *IGHV* mutational status & *TP53* mutational status imperative

CLL Staging			
Rai	**Description**	**Binet**	**Description**
0	Lymphocytosis	A	<3 involved sites w/o cytopenias
I	+ LAN	B	≥3 involved sites w/o cytopenias
II	+ Splenomegaly		
III	+ Anemia[a] (Hgb <11)	C	Anemia[a] (Hgb <10) or Thrombocytopenia[a] (Plt <100K)
IV	+ Thrombocytopenia[a] (plt <100K)		

[a]Due to progressive CLL & not autoimmune or other causes (*Blood* 1975;46(2):219; *Cancer* 1981;48(1):198).

Indications for treatment: iwCLL criteria (*Blood* 2018;131(25):2745)

iwCLL criteria for initiation of therapy: 1 or more of the following:

- Progressive marrow failure d/t CLL manifesting as worsening anemia of thrombocytopenia; in general, Hgb < 10 & plt <100,000 are used as guides but not strict cut-offs. Alternative causes of cytopenias should be ruled out
- Progressive, symptomatic, or massive (≥6 cm below costal margin) splenomegaly
- Progressive, symptomatic, or massive (≥10-cm diameter) LNs
- Progressive lymphocytosis w/ >50% increase over 2 mos or doubling over 6 mos; no cutoff ALC & should not be used as single reason for tx initiation; leukostasis is rare
- AI complications of CLL (eg, ITP, AIHA) not responsive to steroids
- Extranodal involvement causing sxs (eg, kidney, lung, spine, cutaneous)
- Dz-related sxs: Unintentional wt loss, fatigue, fevers, NS (alternative causes should be ruled out)

Clinical pearls: Principles of management

- Observation: Rec for pts not meeting iwCLL criteria for tx; CBC, history, & physical exam q3–6 mos depending on dz burden & tempo
- Novel agents provide durable & deep responses for many pts; incurable dz aside from alloSCT

Front-line treatment

- **No single standard approach.** Molecular/cytogenetic features guide options, but therapy selection ultimately depends on pt-specific comorbidities & tox profiles
- **CIT:** Fludarabine, cyclophosphamide, & rituximab (FCR) appropriate in young, fit pts w/ mutated *IGHV* status, although novel agent-based approaches are also appropriate
  - Pts w/ the following should **not receive CIT:**
    - Del17p &/or *TP53* mut, given historically poor responses (*Blood* 2014;123:3247)
    - Unmutated *IGHV*; comparative trials show improved survival w/ novel agents over CIT for these pts (*NEJM* 2019;380:2225, *Leukemia* 2020;34:787, *Lancet* 2020;395:1278)
- **BTKi +/– antiCD20 ab therapy:** Oral medications given continuously until progression or unacceptable tox; approved for initial therapy for all CLL pts, regardless of cytogenetic &/or molecular profile (*NEJM* 2015;373:2475, *Leukemia* 2020:34:787, *NEJM* 2018;379:2517, *NEJM* 2016;374:323, *Lancet* 2020;395:1278)
  - Ibrutinib typically NOT administered w/ anti-CD20 ab therapy given no benefit (*NEJM* 2018;379:2517)
  - Acalabrutinib may be administered w/ obinutuzumab (*Lancet* 2020;395:1278)
- **Venetoclax (BCL-2 inhibitor):** Approved for all pts in front-line setting in combination w/ obinutuzumab as a fixed-duration therapy (12 mos); deep responses possible (undetectable "minimal residual dz") (*NEJM* 2019;380:2225)

Treatment of relapsed and/or refractory CLL

- **Sequencing of subsequent therapies depends on initial therapy & reason for discontinuation**
- **Prior BTKi:** 1. Discontinued d/t intolerance: May try alternative BTKi (eg, ibrutinib → acalabrutinib (*Haematologica* 2021;106(9):2364) 2. Discontinued d/t progressive CLL: venetoclax +/– rituximab (*NEJM* 2018;378:1107); PI3Ki (idelalisib, duvelisib) also approved (*NEJM* 2014;370:997, *Blood* 2018;132:2446)
- **Prior Venetoclax:** Ibrutinib or acalabrutinib (*Clin Cancer Res* 2020;26:3589); PI3Ki option
- **Prior BTKi & Venetoclax: PI3Ki** option, responses generally not durable (*Clin Cancer Res* 2020;26:3589); consider clinical trials if available
- **AlloSCT:** Only curative tx for CLL; if pt young, fit, & responding to therapy, should be considered in the relapsed &/or refractory setting
- **CIT:** No data for relapse after tx w/ novel agents, but could be considered in pts w/ *IGHV* mut & *TP53* intact

Supportive care & other disease complications (*Blood* 2018;131(25):2745; *NEJM* 2020;383(5):460)

- **Immunodeficiency:** Infxns related to underlying immunodeficiency from dz major complication, txs may also increase risk of infxns; IVIG may be used as prophylaxis in pts w/ recurrent sinopulmonary infxns & IgG level <500
- **Vaccinations:** Recommend annual influenza, PCV13, & PPSV23, recombinant zoster, COVID-19 vaccinations; pts may have suboptimal vaccine responses (*Blood* 2021;137(2):185; *Blood* 2021;137(23):3165); live vaccines are contraindicated
- **2° CAs:** Increased risk of **cutaneous malignancies & 2° CAs**. Recommend annual total body skin examination w/ dermatologist & routine age-appropriate CA screening

Richter transformation (RT) (*Blood* 2018;131(25):2761)

- Transformation of CLL to more aggressive lymphoma; occurs in about ~5% of pts; most commonly DLBCL; less commonly, HL; overall poor prog
- Suspect w/ rapid dz progression, B-sxs; PET CT imaging helpful to guide bx; dx must be confirmed by bx; may be clonally related or unrelated
- **All pts require tx;** no single SOC; often will treat DLBCL type w/ R-CHOP or R-EPOCH-based therapy; clinical trials ongoing investigating novel agents; in fit pts, for clonally related RT, goal is consolidation w/ alloSCT

Key toxicities associated with treatment

- **BTK inhibitors:** Atrial fibrillation, bleeding, arthralgias, headache (acalabrutinib), opportunistic infxns, rash (*Leukemia* 2020:34:787, *Lancet* 2020;395:1278)
- **Venetoclax:** TLS, requires 5-wk dose-escalation w/ hydration & close lab monitoring, pts are risk-stratified to determine whether dose escalation occurs inpt or outpt, cytopenias (*NEJM* 2019;380:2225)
- **PI3K inhibitors:** Diarrhea, colitis, pneumonitis, liver enzyme elevations, opportunistic infxns (*NEJM* 2014;370: 997, *Blood* 2018;132:2446)
- **Obinutuzumab:** Infusion-related reactions, cytopenias (*Blood* 2016;127:79)
- **FCR:** Therapy-related MDS/AML (late), infxn (*Blood* 2016;127:303)

Hairy cell leukemia (HCL)

- ~2% of all leukemias; 600–800 cases/y in the United States (*Blood* 2006;107:265)
- Median age of onset 52 y; strong male predominance (~4:1) & Caucasians

Pathogenesis/disease biology

- HCL is an **indolent B-cell LPD**
- Expresses common **mature B-cell Ag** (CD19, **CD20, CD22, CD25,** monotypic surface Ig) & does not express CD21 (an immature B-cell marker)
- Characterized by aberrant expression of non–B-cell markers **(CD11c, CD103, CD123)**
- Cytogenetic anomalies seen in ~2/3 of pts (commonly chr 5, 7, or 13)
- ***BRAF* V600E** seen in virtually all classical HCL (*NEJM* 2011;364:2305); the mut originates in hematopoietic stem cells (*Sci Tr Med* 2014;6:238). Mt is typically hetero- or hemizygous. Rare exon 11 *BRAF* Mts can also occur in HCLc (*BRJH* 2014;165(4):529)

Clinical presentation

- Constitutional sx, abdominal fullness/discomfort from **massive splenomegaly,** symptomatic or asx **cytopenias** (bleeding/easy bruising; recurrent infxn)
- Almost all pts (≥80%) have palpable splenomegaly; LAN & B-sxs usu not present

Diagnosis

- PB smear: Small–medium-sized mononuclear cells w/ eccentric nuclei, absent nucleoli, & finger-like **cytoplasmic projections**/indistinct borders (**hairy cells**)
- BMBx: Usu hypercellular w/ infiltrating hairy cells; abundant cytoplasm surrounding nuclei may give **"fried egg"** appearance; often abundant mast cells; ↑ reticulin fibrosis common & may make marrow **inaspirable/"dry-tap"**
- Immunophenotyping (flow cytometry): CD19, CD20, CD22, aberrant CD11c, CD25 (IL2RA), CD103, CD123. Also, the majority of cases are Annexin A1+ by IHC
- *BRAF* V600E considered one of the diagnostic criteria (though not required) in WHO 2016
- DDx: CLL, SMZL, PLL, or **HCL variant** = Distinct biologic entity though morphologic features of both HCL & PLL (eg, cytoplasmic projections & prominent nucleoli); ↑ WBC; lacks CD25/CD123 expression; CD27(+); annexin A1 neg; *BRAF* wild-type; ~50% *MAP2K1* (MEK1) mut (*Nat Genet* 2014;46:8)

Figure 26-1 Peripheral blood smear showing classical hairy cells.

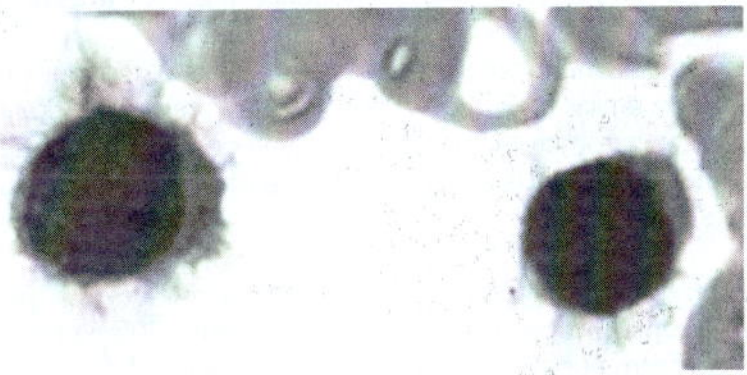

Treatment

- **Indications for tx:** Significant cytopenias (Hb <11 g/dL, ANC <1,000/μL, plt <100,000/μL); sx splenomegaly; constitutional sx (wt loss, etc.)
- 1st line: **Purine analogs,** eg, cladribine & pentostatin, have revolutionized tx of HCL
  - **Cladribine:** 1 cycle → excellent OS (≥95% at 5+ y); 95% CR rate; median 1st response is 98 mos; 37% will ultimately relapse at a median time of 42 mos. Re-tx is effective for relapse (*JCO* 2003;21:891). Cladribine is a/w ↑ rate of 2° hematologic malignancy; given as continuous infusion (0.1 mg/kg/d) over 7 d; alternative is daily bolus (0.14 mg/kg/d over 2 h) for 5 d
  - **Pentostatin** is given q2wk until max response
  - Most common s/e is **fever** (60–70%), a/w F/N & prolonged immunosuppression
  - Rituximab + cladribine can lead to deeper MRD(–) responses (*JCO* 2020;38:1527)
- **Relapsed dz:**
  - **Cladribine** re-tx w/ 1 cycle is often effective (~70%) w/ duration of CR1 = CR2; subsequent remission durations shorten
  - **Vemurafenib** w/ 98% ORR & ~40% CR rate in R/R setting (*NEJM* 2015;373:1733); potential further benefit when combined w/ rituximab (*NEJM* 2021;384(19):1810). Tox = rash, arthralgia, LFT abnormalities, w/c be modulated by dose ↓
  - **Moxetumomab pasudotox:** Anti-CD22 antibody approved if >2 prior lines, incl purine analog. 34% MRD(–) CR rate (*Leukemia* 2018;32:1768)
- Clinical trials of BRAF/MEKi & BRAF/anti-CD20 combinations are ongoing

B-cell prolymphocytic leukemia (B-PLL)

- Clonal disorder of medium-sized, high IgM+ B cells (as opposed to CLL—small, IgM dim); *MYC* & *p53* alterations are seen at >50% each, most cases are complex-karyotype
- Very rare, <1% of B-cell leukemias, usu affects older adults (median age 69 y/o)
- Pts typically p/w **leukocytosis** (commonly >100,000/µL), anemia ± thrombocytopenia, **++splenomegaly,** B sxs (wt loss, fever, NS), infrequently LAD

Dx

- **B-prolymphocytes** must comprise **≥55% of total lymphocytes** in the PB
- PB smear: Numerous "prolymphocytes" → medium-sized cells w/ moderately abundant, slightly basophilic cytoplasm, moderately condensed chromatin, & a single **prominent nucleolus**
- DDx includes more common B-cell malignancies such as CLL & leukemic phase of MCL
- Distinguish from variant HCL & T-PLL (w/c can have similar morphologic appearance & clinical presentation) by immunophenotyping & clonal rearrangement of Ig genes
- Immunophenotype: Bright expression of **surface Ig** w/ **light-chain restriction**, **bright CD20** (in contrast to CLL). (+) CD19, CD22, CD79a, & FMC7; weak or absent CD5, CD23; absent CD103, CD11c
- Cytogenetics/FISH (r/o MCL) → t(11;14) or cyclin D1+ by IHC

Prog/Treatment (*Mayo Clin Proc* 2005;80:1660)

- Clinical course can be indolent in a rare subgroup, but often progressive & resistant to chemo w/ **median OS ~3–5 y**
- **del(17p)/*p53*** alterations a/w **poor response/survival,** similar to CLL
- If *p53* WT, usu treat w/a CLL-like regimen such as **FCR** (fludarabine, cyclophosphamide, rituximab) or BR (bendamustine, rituximab); if *p53* altered, likely chemoresistant, & therefore initial tx is usu w/ ibrutinib. Alemtuzumab is alternative option via compassionate use
- Consider **splenectomy**/splenic irradiation for refractory, sx splenomegaly
- In younger pts w/ good PS, strongly consider **allo-HCT** since dz will relapse
- **Relapsed/refractory:** Alemtuzumab, ibrutinib, idelalisib, venetoclax, anti-CD20. No SOC

T-cell prolymphocytic leukemia (T-PLL)

- Clonal disorder of postthymic, mature T cells (prolymphocytes)
- Genetics: Rearrangements of ***TCL1* family genes** (*TCL1A, TCL1B, MTCP1*) in >90% of cases I, inv(14)(q11q32). 50% haploinsufficient for ***CDKN1B***. 80% have deletions/missense w/in the *ATM* locus (11q23). ↑ incidence in pts w/ **ataxia telangiectasia** d/t *ATM* alteration, age of onset 20–30 y
- Rare, ~2% of mature lymphocytic leukemias, usu affects older adults (male 2:1 ratio)
- Clinical presentation similar to B-PLL w/ leukocytosis (often >100,000/µL), cytopenias, & splenomegaly, but hepatomegaly & LAD more common in T-PLL, can also see extranodal involvement of **skin & serositis** (periorbital & conjunctival edema characteristic when seen) is common (25%)
- **Dx**
  - **Morphology:** Monomorphic, medium-sized "prolymphocytes," **prominent nucleolus**, cytoplasmic protrusions; small-cell variant (20%); rare Sézary cell–like variant (cerebriform nuclei) w/ irregular nuclear outline (5%)
  - Immunophenotyping: Bright expression of CD52**,** pan–T-cell markers (CD2, CD3, CD7). Can either individually express CD4, CD8, or express both (25%)
  - IHC will show increased expression of Tcl1. TdT is neg, unlike T-ALL
  - Clonal *TCR* gene rearrangement (TRB &/or TRG)
  - Distinguish from MF/SS, T-cell LGL leukemia, & ATLL by morphology, immunophenotype, genetics, & labs (ATLL is HTLV-1 virus positive)

Prog/Tx (*Blood* 2019;134:1132)

- **Worse prog** than B-PLL, but subset (~15%) still can have an indolent phase potentially lasting y, rapidly progressive thereafter w/ median OS <1 y
- **Alemtuzumab** (anti-CD52 Ab, Campath) is tx of choice: Good RR (~60% CR; >90% ORR). Relapse almost always occurs (median dur of response for responders < 2 y). Pentostatin can be added for pts w/ suboptimal response to alemtuzumab alone
- Alemtuzumab depletes T-cell niche & very **immunosuppressive** (high risk of PJP, CMV reactivation, etc.)
- Must consolidate w/ **allo HSCT** in appropriate candidates for chance of cure
- **Relapsed/refractory:** Can consider repeat alemtuzumab (must reassess CD52 expression), pentostatin, bendamustine, nelarabine. BCL2i, HDACi, JAK3i under study

CLONAL HEMATOPOIESIS (CH)

Clonal hematopoiesis of indeterminate potential (CHIP)

- Presence of a somatic mutation a/w hematologic neoplasia at a variant allele frequency (VAF) of at least 2%
- Absence of definitive morphologic evidence of a hematologic neoplasm
- Normal peripheral blood counts

Epidemiology

- Incidence increases w/ age. Rare in subjects <40, common (>10%) in those >70, & found in >20% of those over 90
- *DNMT3A* is the most commonly mutated gene in CHIP, followed by *TET2* & *ASXL1*
- Nearly all adults have detectable clonal cell populations when ultrasensitive detection methods are used (*Nat Comm* 2016:12484)
- Risk factors: Age, cytotoxic chemotherapy, radiation therapy, smoking
- Subjects w/ CHIP have shorter overall survival due in part to 2-fold increased risk of cardiovascular mortality (*NEJM* 2017;377:111–121)

Clinical presentation

- CHIP is often an incidental finding in pts undergoing workup for other conditions
- Pts w/ clonal cytopenias of uncertain significance (CCUS) will have cytopenia-related symptoms (fatigue, bleeding/bruising, infections)

Diagnosis

- Diagnosis is most commonly made by a targeted oligo capture & high-throughput sequencing assay performed on peripheral blood or bone marrow
- Evaluation of DNA from nonhematopoietic tissue (nails, dermal fibroblasts) is useful to exclude germline mutations particular for high VAF (40–60%) &/or rare mutations
- Bone marrow examination is not required to diagnose CHIP, but can be useful in excluding a myeloid neoplasm

Classification

	Idiopathic Cytopenias of Uncertain Significance (ICUS)	Clonal Hematopoiesis of Indeterminate Potential (CHIP)	Clonal Cytopenias of Uncertain Significance (CCUS)	Myelodysplastic Syndrome (MDS)
Clonality	No	Yes	Yes	Yes
Dysplasia	No	No	No	Yes
Cytopenias	Yes	No	Yes	Yes
Risk	Very low	Generally low	High (to MDS)	Variable (to AML)

Blood 2015;126:9–16.

Risk of progression

- Clonal hematopoiesis alone increases risk of a hematologic malignancy ~10–15-fold although absolute risk remains low in most individuals w/ single small clones
- Features associated w/ increased risk of progression (*Nat Comm* 2021:338): (1) high-risk mutations in *TP53*, splicing factors (*SF3B1*, *SRSF2*, *U2AF1*, *ZRSR2*), or *IDH1/2*; (2) mutation VAF >10%; (3) multiple mutations; (4) co-occurrence of mosaic chromosomal alteration; (5) abnormal red blood cell indices
- CCUS confers high risk of progression to myelodysplastic syndrome (MDS)

CH in the context of oncologic treatment

- **CH & chemotherapy:** Pt w/ highest-risk CHIP categories who receive chemotherapy may have up to 15% risk of hematologic malignancy over 10 y (*Nat Genetics* 2020;52:1219)
- **CH & allogeneic hematopoietic stem cell transplant (HSCT):** Pretransplant CHIP increases risk of therapy-related myeloid neoplasm w/ autologous HSCT (*JCO* 2017;35:1598). Some transplant centers screen for & avoid donors w/ CH though data to justify this approach is lacking

Management

- No safe & effective tx exists to eliminate clonality
- Optimize guideline-directed cardiovascular risk management
- Monitor complete blood count at least annually; obtain bone marrow biopsy for cytopenias
- Consider referral to specialized CH clinic

Description

- High-dose therapy & autologous stem cell transplant (ASCT) rely on cytotoxic effects of HDC/radiation to treat hematologic malignancies followed by infusion of **auto** stem cells to "rescue" from profound pancytopenia (generally no significant graft-vs.-malignancy effect)
- Tx intent (curative vs. palliative) depends on dz

Most Common Indications	
Disease	**Indication**
Multiple myeloma (MM)	Most common indication for ASCT. Generally palliative intent Up-front consolidation following response to induction chemo or for relapsed/refractory dz (IFM 2009 trial, *Blood* 2020;136:39; EMN02/HO95 MM trial, *Lancet Haematol* 2020;7:e456)
Hodgkin lymphoma (HL)	Chemo-sensitive relapsed dz. Curative intent (*Cochrane Database Syst Rev* 2013;CD009411)
DLBCL	Chemo-sensitive relapsed dz. Curative intent (Parma Trial, *NEJM* 1995;333:1540; CORAL study, *JCO* 2010;28:4184)
CNS Lymphoma (DLBCL)	Chemo-sensitive relapsed dz or for up-front consolidation. Curative intent (*Blood* 2015;125:1403)
Follicular lymphoma (FL)	Chemo-sensitive early relapsed dz or dz that has progressed to clinically aggressive histology (eg, DLBCL) (*JCO* 2013;31:1164; LymphoCare Study, *BBMT* 2018;24:1163)
Peripheral T-cell lymphoma	Consolidation in first CR or for chemo-sensitive relapsed dz. Curative intent (*Blood* 2012;30:3093; *JCO* 2013;31:3100)
Mantle cell lymphoma	Consolidation in first CR or for chemo-sensitive relapsed dz (*BJH* 2012;158:355; *Blood* 2005;105:2677)
Ig light chain (AL) amyloidosis	Consolidation following initial response to chemo or for relapsed dz. Palliative intent (*Blood* 2015;126:2345)

ASBMT Guidelines: Indications for Auto- & Allo-HCT (*BBMT* 2020;26:1247).

Pretransplant evaluation

To establish extent of dz & assess pt comorbidities:

- **Hx:** KPS, prior therapy, drug allergies, prior infxn, & social support
- **Physical exam:** Comprehensive—oral cavity/skin for nidus for infxn, CNS exam, assessment of LAN
- **Labs:** CBC, chemistries w/ liver & renal fxn, 24-h urine for accurate Cr clearance
- **Imaging:** CXR or CT chest
- **Cardiac fxn:** EKG & ECHO (or MUGA)
- **PFT** including DLCO
- Dz-specific **restaging studies:** BMA/bx, CT or PET/CT in pts w/ certain lymphomas, & SPEP/UPEP w/ IFE, serum FLCs & skeletal assessment in pts w/ MM
- Transplant-related mortality for SCT can be estimated using the **HCT-CI** (*BBMT* 2015;21:1479)
- **Comprehensive geriatric assessment** in older pts

Stem cell source

- Stem cells should be **collected prior to exposure to an alkylator** (eg, melphalan), nitrogen mustard or purine analog as these agents are stem cell toxic
- Collection is done by **PBSC apheresis** following G-CSF ± plerixafor or chemomobilization (BM harvesting only very rarely used for ASCT)
- Collected CD34+ stem cells are cryopreserved until time of transplant

Conditioning regimens

- All conditioning regimens are myeloablative & combine HDC ± **radiation** given prior to stem cell infusion to eradicate dz
- **Melphalan-based regimens** are commonly used for the tx of plasma cell dyscrasias & lymphoma (commonly treated w/ BEAM: BCNU, Etoposide, Ara-C, Melphalan)

Engraftment

- Expansion of HSC in the BM resulting in normalization of blood counts/immune recovery
- **Time to engraftment** varies based on conditioning regimen & stem cell graft source
  PBSC grafts engraft more quickly than BM grafts (which generally have lower cell dose)

Transplant complications and outcomes

- Major complications include, but are not limited to:

Complication	Description
Infxns	Less likely c/w allogeneic transplant d/t ↓ time to engraftment & no post-ASCT immunosuppression However, pts are still at risk prior to engraftment
Oral/GI mucositis	Injury to alimentary tract mucosa commonly a/w conditioning regimen tox. **Tx:** Pain medications & IVF/TPN
Organ toxicities	A result of direct regimen-related toxicities from conditioning **Acute/Sub-acute:** SOS/VOD, pulmonary (IPS, DAH), cardiac, & renal injury **Late (chronic):** Infertility, cataracts, 2° malignancies (below)
Engraftment syn	Characterized by rash, fever, capillary leak/pulm edema, renal failure, etc. (*BBMT* 2015;21:2061) **Tx:** Systemic glucocorticoids
"Auto-GVHD"	Rare occurrence post ASCT, similar to acute GVHD after allo-HCT. Usu mild & self-limiting (*BBMT* 2015;21:2061)
2° malignancies	↑ Incidence of **nonmelanoma skin CA, other solid tumors, hematologic malignancies** Risk is higher w/ TBI-based conditioning regimens Post-HSCT **oropharyngeal CA** may have more aggressive behavior w/ poorer prog when compared to those in non-HCT pts

- **Relapse:** In addition to close clinical & lab follow-up, BMA/bx &/or PET/CT (depending on dz) is generally done at routine intervals posttransplant to r/o relapsed dz
- **Main Causes of Death after ASCT:** 1° dz (relapse) is most common cause of death, followed by infxn, organ failure, & "other" causes (Phelan, R., CIBMTR Summary Slides, 2020)

Post-transplant maintenance therapy

- Post-ASCT maintenance therapy may be given for selected dzs, eg:
  - Lenalidomide maintenance improves PFS & OS for MM (*JCO* 2016 [suppl; abstr 8001]; *NEJM* 2014;371:895)
  - Rituximab maintenance showed no benefit for DLBCL based on randomized phase III data (CORAL study, *JCO* 2010;28:4184), but showed PFS benefit in FL (EBMT LYM1 study, *JCO* 2013;31:1624) & PFS & OS benefit in MCL (particularly in younger pts) (*NEJM* 2017;377:1250)
  - BV maintenance in 1° refractory or unfav relapsed HL pts not previously exposed to BV showed PFS benefit in a randomized phase III study (AETHERA, *Lancet* 2015;385:1853)

Prognosis

- Prog varies & is dependent upon many factors which include:
  Dz type & initial stage
  Pre-ASCT dz status (eg, chemosensitivity in lymphoma)
  Conditioning regimen
  HCT-CI (*BBMT* 2015;21:1479)
  Pre-ASCT functional status

Healthy living ("Survivorship") posttransplant

- Systematic long-term follow-up of HCT pts who are at risk for multiple possible late complications is essential
- See: "Recommended Screening & Preventive Practices for Long-term Survivors after Hematopoietic Cell Transplantation" (*BMT* 2012;47:337)

Description

- Consists of **conditioning regimen** (chemo &/or RT to eradicate dz & achieve immunosuppression to prevent graft rejection) → followed by infusion of **donor HSC allograft** to replenish hematopoietic system & further eradicate dz via **graft-vs.-tumor effect**
- Indications: In general, dzs that would not benefit from additional standard tx or are resistant to chemo (*BBMT* 2015;21:1863), eg, **selected malignancies** (high-risk or rel/ref acute & chronic leukemias, HL & NHL, plasma cell dyscrasias, MDS, MPN); aplastic anemia & other marrow failure states, PNH, thalassemia, sickle cell dz, SCID

Pretransplant evaluation

- **Hx:** PS, comorbidities, prior Rx, drug allergies, prior infxn, social support system, FHx/sibling info
- **PE:** Assess oral cavity/skin for nidus for infxn, CNS exam, assessment of LAN & HSM
- **Labs:** CBC, chemistries w/ liver & renal fxn, ABO, viral serologies (esp CMV)
- **Other diagnostics:** CXR or CT chest, ECG & study of **cardiac fxn** (echo or MUGA), **PFTs** including DLCO; dz-specific **restaging studies** (BMA/Bx, imaging as indicated)

HLA matching and graft sources

- Tissue-type matching between the donor & recipient at 3+ loci. Mismatch ↑ risk of rejection & GVHD
- HLA genes fall in two categories: Type I = HLA-A, -B, -C; type II = -DRB1, -DQB1, -DPB1
- 6/6 = matched at A, B, DR; 8/8 = also C; 10/10 = also DQ; 12/12 = also DP
- Donors may be related or unrelated; in general, gold standard = 8/8 related donor; direct prospective comparisons re: optimal "alternative" donor are lacking (see below)
- **Graft sources:**
  - **PBSC:** Apheresis from donor after mobilization w/ G-CSF; higher CD34 cell dose, more rapid engraftment vs. BM
  - **BM:** Must be harvested from donor under general anesthesia; a/w lower cGVHD, higher long-term QoL vs. PBSC (*NEJM* 2012;367:1487; *JAMA Oncol* 2016;2:1583)
  - **Cord blood**

Graft Sources in Absence of Matched Related Donor		
Unrelated Donor	**Cord Blood (CB)**	**Haploidentical**
BM or PBSC from URDs identified through NMDP **Advantages** • W/ improved HLA typing, outcomes w/ 8/8-matched URD have become closer to those w/ MRD (eg, *Leukemia* 2010;24:1276) **Disadvantages** • Higher GVHD vs. related, especially if mismatch • Longer process of procuring graft • Likelihood of matched URD highly dependent on race (*NEJM* 2014;371:339)	Banked; suitable units identified through NMDP **Advantages** • Immunologically naïve → can tolerate higher degrees of mismatch • Graft can be procured quickly if HCT is urgent • More likely to identify CB units for non-Caucasian pts **Disadvantages** • Low cell dose (can be overcome w/ double-unit CBT, procurement of backup graft in case of rejection) • Slower engraftment	BM or PBSC from half-matched related donor **Advantages** • Most pts will have at least 1 potential donor • Advent of post-HCT Cy to deplete alloreactive T cells has reduced risk of GVHD & rejection • Lower cost of procurement than URD or CB • ↓ rates of cGVHD compared to even MRD; ↓ rates of aGVHD compared to MUD & MMUD (*JAMA Oncol* 2019;5:1739) **Disadvantages** • Less long-term data

Conditioning regimens (*BBMT* 2009;15:1628)

- **MAC:** Expected to destroy hematopoietic cells in the BM → results in pancytopenia that is long-lasting, usu irreversible, & in most instances fatal unless hematopoiesis restored by infusion of HSCs
  - Eg, TBI ≥5 Gy single dose or ≥8 Gy fractionated; Bu ≥8 mg/kg PO or IV equivalent

- **Nonmyeloablative (NMA):** Cause minimal cytopenia but significant lymphopenia; following administration of allo-HSCs → engrafting donor T cells will eventually eliminate host hematopoietic cells allowing establishment of donor hematopoiesis (*JCO* 2005;23:1993)
  - Eg, Flu + Cy w/ or w/o ATG, TBI ≤2 Gy w/ or w/o purine analog
- **Reduced intensity conditioning (RIC):** Intermediate in intensity, result in cytopenias that may be prolonged & result in significant morbidity/mortality, eg, Bu ≤9 mg/kg PO, melphalan ≤140 mg/m^2

Engraftment

- Expansion of HSC in recipient BM results in (1) normalization of blood counts, (2) recovery of the immune system that is donor-derived
- **Definition:** 3 consecutive days of ANC ≥0.5 × 10^9/L
- Time to engraftment depends on conditioning regimen (ablative vs. NMA), HSC graft source & characteristics (longer time to engraftment w/ cord blood grafts, BM)
- Graft failure: Can be 1° (failure to attain ANC >0.5) or 2° (ANC <0.5 for 7 d after initial engraftment, w/o response to growth factor & in absence of relapse)

Complications of Allogeneic Transplantation

Complication	Features
Organ tox	Usu related to conditioning regimen. Selected specific toxicities: **TBI:** GI, pulm, hepatic; long-term: Endocrinopathies, cataracts **Bu:** Seizure (requires ppx), pulm, hepatic/SOS **Cy:** Cardiac, hemorrhagic cystitis
Infxn	Neutropenia w/ conditioning, prolonged use of immunosuppression for GVHD ppx or tx ↑ risk of infxn; **prophylactic antibacterials, antivirals, & antifungals** necessary prior to engraftment; **revaccination** necessary d/t loss of acquired immunity
GVHD	See below
SOS/ VOD	Hepatocyte injury & obstruction in hepatic vein sinuses → jaundice, painful hepatomegaly, & fluid retention are hallmarks; anticoagulants/ ursodiol used for prevention; **defibrotide** = 1st approved tx for severe SOS (*Blood* 2016;127:1656)
Mucositis	Injury to oral/esophageal mucosa commonly a/w conditioning regimen tox, treat w/ pain medications & IVF/TPN
Oral & skin carcinoma	Post-HCT oral CA may have more aggressive behavior & poorer prog c/w oral CA in non-HCT pts
PTLD	Uncontrolled proliferation of B cells (typically of donor origin) post-infxn w/ **EBV** → calcineurin inhibitors can prevent T-cell–mediated control of B-cell proliferation; depletion of T cells by **anti–T-cell Ab** (ATG, ALG, OKT3) in the prev or tx of transplant rejection further ↑ the risk of developing PTLD; may spontaneously regress on reduction/cessation of immunosuppressant & can be treated w/ **rituximab,** DL, or EBV-targeted CTLs

Graft-versus-host disease (GvHD)

Graft T-lymphocytes react to Ag presented on the MHC of the host

- **Acute GvHD** typically occurs in the first 3 mos post-HCT, attacking skin, GI, or hepatic cells; first-line tx = corticosteroids. Grading depends on stage of each organ's involvement (see tables)
- **Chronic GvHD** occurs later & can affect numerous organ systems, autoimmune-like features (*BBMT* 2015;21:389)
- Approaches to prevent GVHD: CNIs (CSA, tacrolimus), **antimetabolites** (MTX), **antiproliferatives** (mycophenolic acid), **mTOR inhibitors** (sirolimus), **T-cell depletion** (ATG, alemtuzumab, PTCy, ex vivo graft manipulation)
- Toxicities of GVHD ppx: Nephrotox, TMA, HTN/PRES w/ CNIs; mucositis, hepatotox w/ MTX

Staging and Overall Grading of Acute GvHD				
Stage	**Skin**	**<Liver**	**Lower GI**	**Upper GI**
1	Maculopapular rash <25% of BSA	TB 2.1–3.0	Diarrhea 501–1,000 mL/d	Persistent n/v or anorexia
2	25–50% of BSA	TB 3.1–6.0	1,001–1,500 mL/d	
3	>50% of BSA	TB 6.1–15.0	>1,500 mL/d	
4	Generalized erythroderma w/ bullae &/or desquamation	TB >15.0	Severe abd pain &/ or ileus	

	Skin	Liver	Lower GI	Upper GI
I	1			
II	2	1–2	1–2	1
III	3	3	3	
IV	4	4	4	

BJH 1997;97:855.

Prognosis

- **Relapse:** In addition to frequent clinical/lab follow-up, BMA/Bx &/or surveillance imaging is rec at 1, 3, 6, 12, 18 & 24 mos post-HCT to determine chimerism & r/o relapsed dz
- Most common causes of death post-HCT: (1) relapse, (2) GvHD, (3) infxn
- Prog varies dependent on dz type, stage, stem cell source, HLA-matched status, conditioning regimen, pt age/comorbidities
- Prognostic tools (*Bone Marrow Transplantation* 2016;51:1283):
  - **HCT-Comorbidity Index** (*Blood* 2005;106:2912) estimates nonrelapse mortality
  - Transplant-specific **Dz Risk Index** (*Blood* 2014;123:3664) stratifies pts by dz features

Sites of hematopoiesis

- BM is the principal site of hematopoiesis in adults, predominantly in pelvis, vertebrae, ribs, sternum, & skull
- During fetal development sites include yolk sac → liver → spleen → BM

Stem cell niche

- In the BM, HSCs develop in a complex microenvironment of stromal cells (fibroblasts, smooth muscle cells, endothelial cells, adipocytes, osteoblasts, osteoclast, & macrophages) & extracellular matrix
- Unique sites w/in the marrow, termed niches, favor HSC self-renewal vs. differentiation

The hematopoietic hierarchy

- **HSCs:** Cardinal features: (1) Pluripotency (can give rise to all mature blood cell types) & (2) self-renewal capacity
- HSCs give rise to 2 kinds of multipotent cells, the CLPs & CMPs

Figure 28-1 Hierarchal map of hematopoietic development.

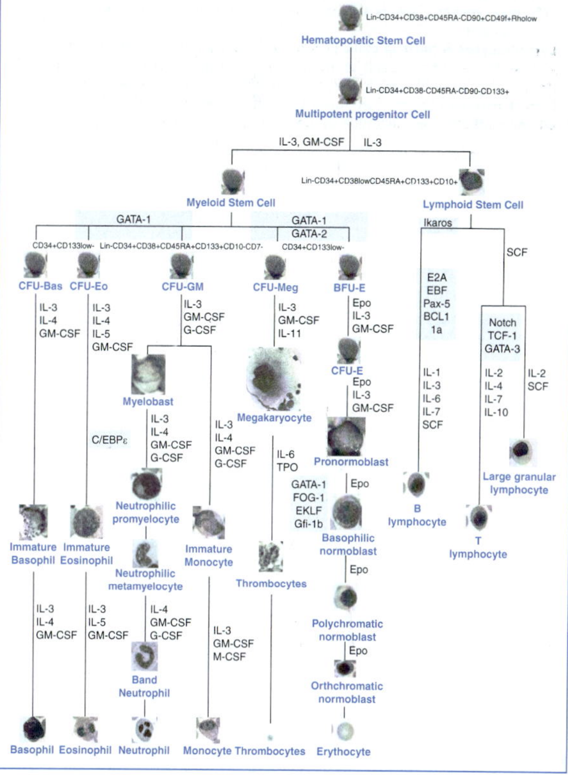

Bone marrow examination (see section BM Aspirates/Biopsies)

Interpretation of bone marrow aspirate and biopsy

Morphology: BM is comprised of hematopoietic tissue islands & adipose cells surrounded by vascular sinuses. The ratio of fat cells to hematopoietic elements is 1:1 in adults but increases w/ age. Thin-walled sinusoids are lined by endothelial cells & differentiated blood cells enter the circulation by transcellular migration through endothelial cells.

- **Cellularity:** 100—Pt Age = Nl % cellularity
- **Myeloid: Erythroid Ratio:** Nl range 1.2:1 to 5:1. Assess on bx or aspirate. >5:1 ratio—physiologic stress (infxn), <1.2:1 ratio—erythroid response to anemia (hemolysis)
- **Megakaryocytes:** Assess number & appearance. Nl cells are large, multilobulated, irregularly lobed nuclei
- **Myeloid & erythroid maturation.** Excess blasts (>5%) or differentiation arrest suggestive of myeloid neoplasm
- **Dysplasia:** Nuclear & cytoplasmic blebs, dysmorphic nuclei
  - **Erythroid dysplasia:** Multinucleated-erythroid precursors, nuclear-cytoplasmic dyssynchrony, ringed sideroblasts
  - **Myeloid dysplasia:** Hypersegmented neutrophils, hyposegmented neutrophils (Pseudo-Pelger–Huet), hypogranular neutrophils, Auer rods, dysmorphic granules (basophilic & eosinophilic granules in eos)
  - **Megakaryocyte dysplasia:** Hyper/hypolobulated megakaryocytes, micromegakaryocytes
- **Lymphocytes & plasma cells:** Benign lymphoid population, more T cells than B cells. Abnl, such as a monotonous B-cell lymphocyte population, is suggestive of lymphoma. Plasma cells <2% of BM cells in nl adult, increased % in plasma cell dyscrasia
- **Iron stores:** Can be increased (hemochromatosis) or decreased (IDA)
- **Other cells:** marrow infiltration by tumor or fibrosis ("myelophthisis")

Definition (*ASH-SAP* 2010;1:109)

↓ RBC mass Hb <13 g/dL (men), <12 g/dL (nonpregnant women), <11 g/dL (pregnant women) caused by decreased RBC production (commonly w/ low reticulocyte index <2)
Morphologic classification of anemia as Microcytic (MCV <80 fL), Normocytic (MCV 80–100 fL), or Macrocytic (MCV >100 fL) constrains differential dx

Mechanism	Egs
Nutritional deficiency	↓ Fe, ↓ Folate, ↓ Cu, ↓ Vit B_{12}, ↓ A, ↓ B_6, ↓ E; ↑ Zn (a/w↓ Cu)
Functional nutritional deficiency	Anemia of chronic inflammation; drugs; increased RBC turnover (bleeding, hemolysis)
Sideroblastic anemia	Congenital; acquired (MDS, Pb tox, drugs, ↓ Cu)
Hemoglobinopathy	α Thalassemia & β thalassemia (see "Hemoglobinopathy" chapter)
Endocrinopathy	↓ Thyroid, ↓ androgens, ↓ cortisol; ↑ PTH
EPO deficiency/resistance	CKD, ESRD, EPO autoAbs, EPO/ESA resistance & ↓↓↓ protein
Infxn	Parvovirus, HIV, CMV, EBV, HHV-6, HBV, HCV, sepsis
Drugs → ± pure red cell aplasia/ aplastic anemia	Chloramphenicol, phenytoin/antiepileptics, gold salts, isoniazid, rifampin, EPO (autoAb), lindane, SMX-TMP, cytotoxic chemo, sulfasalazine
IgG autoAb against erythroblasts → pure red cell aplasia	Transient erythroblastopenia
BM infiltration/fibrosis myelophthisic anemia	Met solid tumor, myeloid/lymphoid neoplasm, MF, osteopetrosis, Gaucher dz, granulomatous dzs
Immune-mediated pure red cell aplasia/aplastic anemia	Idiopathic, thymoma, LPD, rheumatologic/AI dz, ABO-mismatched allo-HSCT
1° BM failure/d/o	PNH, DBA, DKC, Fanconi anemia, SBDS, Amegakaryocytic thrombocytopenia
Toxins	EtOH; benzene
Enzymopathy	Hereditary orotic aciduria; Lesch–Nyhan syn

Fe deficiency anemia (*NEJM* 2015; 372 (19):1832)

Most common anemia worldwide, affects >2 billion people. Prevalence is ~30% in menstruating females & 38% in pregnant females
Developed world: Premenopausal women: Menstrual blood loss. Adult men: GIB
Infancy: Dietary deficiency (def): (High milk intake w/o Fe supplementation)
Children: Diet def. Developing World: GIB (parasitic infxn)
Rapid infancy growth. Pregnancy/lactation (↑ Fe demand)

- **Malabsorption:** Celiac dz, gastric bypass, *H. pylori,* achlorhydria (↑ w/ age), gastric/duodenal infiltration or resection. Abnl transferrin fxn
- **S/S:** Fatigue, dizziness, orthostasis. Pica (uncommon), stomatitis, glossitis, koilonychia, esophageal webs: Plummer–Vinson Syn (rare)
- **PB smear:** Microcytosis hypochromia, anisopoikilocytosis, ↑ RDW. Cigar/pencil RBC ± reactive thrombocytosis (EPO cross-reacts w/ TPO receptor)
- **Lab eval:** ↓↓ Ferritin (<15 μg/L diagnostic; >100 μg/L unlikely). High nl to ↑ TIBC. ↓↓ transferrin sat (<20%), serum Fe <40 μg/L ↑ RDW. Other: ↓ Hepcidin. ↑ Soluble transferrin receptor. Retic-He (>32 essentially r/o Fe Def) (*Am J Clin Path* 2014;142:506)
- **Tx: Uncomplicated/mild Fe deficiency:** PO Fe. Ferrous salts ↑ solubility & absorption but ↑ GI tox. Ascorbic acid → ↑ absorption. ↓ Absorption w/ antacids, full meals, whole grains, tannins, & Ca supplements. Fe sulfate = 66 mg elemental Fe per 325 mg tab
  Complicated Fe deficiency: Parenteral Fe when ↓ absorption, gastric, or duodenal resection, ↑ Fe deficit &/or PO Fe intolerance
  Fe sucrose & Fe gluconate: ↓↓↓ Rate anaphylaxis → no test dose. Generally, requires repeated dosing for full repletion
  Fe dextran: Can replete Fe in one infusion (not rec). ↑ Risk anaphylaxis (11.3/1,000,000) → small test dose required
  Fe carboxymaltose: ↓↓↓ Rate anaphylaxis. No test dose. 2 doses only. Can cause hypophosphatemia

Fe derisomaltose/isomaltoside (Monoferric): Single infusion. Test dose not required. Can result in a more rapid & more pronounced hematologic response compared with Fe sucrose (*Am J Hematol* 2019;94(9):1007)

Response: ↑ Retics after 4–7 d, Hb increase expected to being 1–2 wk post-tx. Anemia responds over wk. Ferritin ~ Fe store

Anemia of chronic inflammation (AOCI) (*NEJM* 2005;352:1011)

- Hypoproliferative anemia (functional Fe def) a/w chronic inflammation: Connective tissue dz, autoimmunity, chronic infxn, malignancy, trauma/surgery, critical illness
- Mild/mod (Hb rarely <7 g/dL) anemia. Sometimes ↑ ESR/CRP
- **Pathogenesis:** ↑ Cytokines (TNFα, IL-1, IL-6, IFNs) → ↓ response to EPO in RBC precursor
  Altered Fe metabolism ↑ IL-6 → ↑ hepcidin → ↓ intestinal Fe absorption/↓ Fe release from enterocytes → ↓ plasma Fe/Fe def
- **Dx:** Nl chromic. Nl/↓ MCV. Nl to ↑ RDW. ↓ to nl Fe. ↓ to low nl TIBC. ↓ Fe sat Nl to ↑↑ ferritin. Experimental: Nl sol transferrin receptor/↑ Hepcidin (*Blood* 2016;127:2809)
- **Tx:** Treat 1° condition. Correct nutritional deficiencies if present. Consider EPO administration if severe particularly in palliative setting

Megaloblastic anemia (*NEJM* 2013;368:149)

Impaired DNA synthesis → RBC lineage usu affected before other cells

Blood smear: ↑ MCV earliest sign. Hypersegmented PMNs (≥5% w/ 5 lobes & some w/ ≥6 lobes). Macroovalocytes. Cabot rings. Promegaloblasts. ↑↑ MCV but may be nl if concurrent microcytic process

BM: Nuclear: Cytoplasm dyssynchrony, giant bands. Other labs: ↑ LDH, ↑ indirect bilirubin → intramedullary hemolysis

- **Folate deficiency:** Duodenum/proximal jejunum absorption. No neuro sxs
  Etiologies: ↓ Intake, ↓ absorption, ↑ use (chronic hemolysis), drug interaction
  ↑ Risk in alcoholics, elderly, TPN w/o supplemental folate, duodenal or jejunal resection/infiltration, celiac dz, chronic hemolysis
  Dx: ↓ Serum folate ± RBC folate (may better reflect folate def but also ↓ in B_{12} def), ↑ homocysteine, nl methylmalonic acid
  Tx: R/o ↓ B_{12} before replete folate. ↓ Folate: ↑ doses PO folate (1–5 mg/d). Ppx prenatal/pregnancy
- **B_{12} deficiency:** Multiple steps for dietary B_{12} absorption in terminal ileum
  ↓ Intake (no animal products/vegans). Hypochlorydia (age, PPIs, atrophic gastritis). ↓ pancreatic proteases. ↓ Binding B_{12} & intrinsic factor (bacterial overgrowth, *Diphyllobothrium*, pernicious anemia, gastric resection). ↓ Absorption w/ meds (cholestyramine, colchicine, metformin). Ileal resection/dysfunction (Celiac, NHL, Crohn, etc.)
  A/w neuropsych sxs: ↓ Vibriosensation, spastic paralysis, psychosis/dementia
  Full B_{12} stores generally take >1 y to deplete (slower than folate depletion)
  Dx: Subclinical B_{12} Def (↑ in elderly): Low nl B_{12}, ↑ homocysteine, ↑ MMA
  Clinical B_{12} Def: ↓ B_{12}, ↑↑ homocysteine, ↑↑ MMA
  Tx: Oral B_{12} or intramuscular B_{12} 1 mg/d × 14 d → 1 mg/wk until anemia resolves → 1 mg/mo. Monitor for hypokalemia w/ repletion
  Some respond to PO B_{12}. Quick Δ to parenteral B_{12} if PO not working
- **Other megaloblastic anemias:** Pyrimidine Analog (5-FU), purine analog (AZA), DNA synthesis Inhibitor (cytarabine), antifolate (MTX), RNA reductase inhibitor (hydrea), PPI, NO, antiepileptic, zidovudine
- **Macrocytic anemias w/ similar morphologic Δ's:** Myelodysplasia, erythroleukemia, Lesch–Nyhan syn, hereditary orotic aciduria

Other nutritional deficiencies (see table)

↑ **Starvation/anorexia nervosa:** Normochromic/normocytic anemia → BM necrosis

↓ **Cu:** Malnourished infants/adults ± TPN. Postbariatric surgery/gastrectomy. ↑ Zn intake → ↓ Cu absorbed → reversible myelodysplasia/sideroblastic anemia

HEMOLYTIC ANEMIAS

General overview and clinical pearls (*ASH-SAP* 2010;1:133; Go and Kuo, *ASH-SAP* 2019)

- **Definition:** RBC destruction & ↓ RBC lifespan (nl ~120 d)
  Compensated hemolysis: BM response is adequate (↑ erythropoiesis) → no ↓ Hgb; **Decompensated hemolysis:** ↓ Hgb
  Classification:
  - **Acute vs. chronic**
  - **Intrinsic vs. extrinsic** factors w/ respect to the RBC itself
  - **Intravascular vs. extravascular** (commonly both intravascular & extravascular hemolysis)
  - **Inherited vs. acquired causes**
- **Approach to pt w/ suspected hemolysis:** Preliminary diagnostic workup: CBC, CMP incl. indirect bilirubin, LDH, haptoglobin, reticulocyte count, PB smear
- **Laboratory findings:** ↓ Hgb (if decompensated), ↑ indirect bilirubin, ↑ LDH, ↓ haptoglobin, ↑ reticulocyte count (will vary based on BM response)
- **If hemolysis, further diagnostic workup warranted:** Coombs/DAT testing, G6PD testing, FHx, medications, infectious workup, PNH clone
- **Sxs:** Fatigue, dyspnea, chest pain, dark urine; **Physical exam:** Conjunctival pallor, jaundice (+/– splenomegaly)
- **Extravascular:** RBC destruction in liver & spleen, can have splenomegaly
- **Intravascular S/S:** RBC destruction in vessels, may have hemoglobinuria
- **Coombs test positive:** Suggestive of AIHA (see section below)
- **Schistocytes:** Consider cardiac valve/device hemolysis, MAHA or TMA incl. DIC, TTP, HUS, HELLP, CA

Selected causes of hemolytic anemias

Hemolytic Anemia	Site	Etiology	Development
Thalassemias (α, β)	Intrinsic	Quantitative hemoglobinopathy	Inherited
Sickle cell dz (Hgb SS, SB°, SB+, SC)	Intrinsic	Qualitative hemoglobinopathy (Hb S) ± quantitative hbopathy (β Thal)	Inherited
Hgb E, C, D	Intrinsic	Qualitative hemoglobinopathy	Inherited
Hgb H	Intrinsic	Quantitative hemoglobinopathy	Inherited/acquired
Unstable Hgb	Intrinsic	Qualitative hemoglobinopathy	Inherited
Methemoglobinemia	Intrinsic	Qualitative hemoglobinopathy	Inherited/acquired
HS, HE, HPP, Rh deficiency (Null)	Intrinsic	Membrane abnormality	Inherited
Acanthocytosis, stomatocytosis	Intrinsic	Membrane abnormality	Inherited/acquired
↓ PK/other glycolytic enzyme	Intrinsic	Glycolytic enzymopathy	Inherited/acquired
↓ G6PD/other HMP shunt enzyme	Intrinsic	HMP shunt enzymopathy	Inherited
AIHA, drug-induced	Extrinsic	Immune-mediated	Acquired
Paroxysmal nocturnal hemoglobinuria	Intrinsic	Membrane Abnormality	Acquired
Microangiopathic hemolytic anemia	Extrinsic	Trauma-microvascular	Inherited/acquired
Macrovascular/prosthesis	Extrinsic	Trauma-macrovascular	Acquired
Toxins: Pb, Cu, Drugs, spider/snake venom	Extrinsic	Direct toxic effect	Acquired
Malaria, babesia	Extrinsic	Intracellular infxn	Acquired
Clostridium, gram neg rods, gram positive cocci	Extrinsic	Direct toxic effect	Acquired
Mycoplasma, EBV, CMV, HSV	Extrinsic	Immune-mediated; cold AIHA	Acquired
Hypersplenism	Extrinsic	Entrapment/RE system	Acquired

Autoimmune hemolytic anemia (AIHA) (*ASH-SAP* 2010;1:133; Go and Kuo, *ASH-SAP* 2019)

- **Suspect w/ positive DAT test;** may have warm autoAb (most common, ~80–90% of cases, Ab bind RBC at 37°C), cold autoAb (Ab bind at cold temperatures), or mixed (both warm & cold autoAb present)
  1° (no underlying cause) vs. 2° (underlying condition) AIHA

Warm autoimmune hemolytic anemia (Go and Kuo, *ASH-SAP* 2019; *Blood* 2021;137(10):1283; *NEJM* 2019;381(7):647)

- Ab-mediated RBC destruction by IgG autoAb +/− complement activation; IgG-coated RBCs → removed by splenic mϕ w/ F_c receptors; RBC destruction by ADCC
- Treg cells, cytokines, & BM response impact clinical presentation & response
- Microspherocytes
- Occasional neg DAT w/ AIHA; false-positive DAT may occur (IVIG, daratumumab)
- Assoc conditions: LPDs/NHL, particularly CLL, SLE, ulcerative colitis, drug-induced
- BMBx: Not always required, but rec in 1st relapse & may be helpful in underlying lymphoproliferative disorder (LPD), other condition

Tx:

- **1st-line tx w/ steroids:** Majority of pts respond (80–90%); dose depends on acuity & severity
- **2nd-line txs:** Rituximab, IVIG (acute setting), splenectomy, PLEX if no response (acute setting, severe cases); **Later line:** Immunosuppression: Typically used following rituximab: Cyclosporine, azathioprine, sirolimus, Cy, mycophenolate, danazol; other drugs have been reported in the literature/ongoing trials

Cold autoimmune hemolytic anemia (Go and Kuo, *ASH-SAP* 2019; *Blood* 2021;137(10):1295)

- **Cold autoAb:** Mostly **IgM** autoAb, a/w agglutination
  RBC destruction from complement fixation → removal by splenic mϕ/hepatic Kupffer cells
- 1°: **Cold agglutinin Dz (CAD): DAT** positive for C3d, neg or weakly positive IgG; Cold agglutinins made by clonal B cells; usu IgM kappa population; not all pts require tx; if tx required (sxs, labs): 1st line: Bendamustine & rituximab (fit pt) or rituximab monotherapy; 2nd line: Sutimlimab in clinical trials; bortezmib; steroids are generally not effective in CAD
- **2° cold agglutinins:** Postinfectious (EBV, mycoplasma); B-cell LPD
- **Cold hemolysins:** Paroxysmal cold hemoglobinuria, 2° paroxysmal cold hemoglobinuria (peds viral infxns, syphilis)

Drug-induced hemolytic anemia (Go and Kuo, *ASH-SAP* 2019)

- Hx-taking is key; multiple drugs may cause RBC immune destruction through multiple mechanisms (hapten or drug adsorption, ternary-immune complex, autoAb, nonimmunologic prot adsorption, other mechanisms)
- Numerous drugs may cause eg, penicillin derivatives, cephalosporins, NSAIDs
- Discontinue offending drug

Fragmentation anemias (Go and Kuo, *ASH-SAP* 2019)

Hemolysis w/in the vessels: Mechanical RBC destruction; PB smear w/ schistocytes
Types: MAHA (damage to microvasculature/endothelial injury); TMA; destruction by shear force, RBC trauma

Microangiopathic hemolytic anemia (MAHA) (Go and Kuo, *ASH-SAP* 2019)

- Includes: CA-assoc MAHA, atypical HUS, TTP, DIC, Kasabach–Meritt syn, foot strike hemolysis, HELLP
- **CA assoc MAHA:** Supportive mgmt & treat underlying malignancy, may be a /w progression of dz (*Blood* 2021;137(1):3104)
- **DIC:** Causes include sepsis, CA, esp APML but solid tumors as well, obstetric complications; Labs: Elevated PT, PTT, INR, thrombin time, decreased fibrinogen, increased D-dimer; a/w increased risk of bleeding & thrombosis; mgmt: Supportive care incl. blood products as needed. Definitive mgmt requires tx of underlying cause
- **TTP:** MAHA, low platelets, often w/ renal failure, fever, & CNS involvement, but also may impact other organs incl. GI tract & heart. Severe ADAMTS13 deficiency → ultralarge VWF multimers; life-threatening & cannot miss dx. Test for ADAMTS13 activity, hemolysis labs, renal fxn, troponin, EKG. PLEX should be started if high-clinical suspicion w/o waiting for ADAMTS13 result; PLASMIC score may be used to help guide PLEX initiation decision (*Lancet Haematol* 2017;4(4):e157; *Blood* 2017;129(2):2836). Use of caplacizumab may be considered w/ PLEX (*NEJM* 2019;380(4):346)
- **HUS:** Hemolysis, thrombocytopenia, renal failure; typical HUS a/w Shiga toxin *E. Coli* & Shigella infxn

- **Complement-mediated hemolytic uremic syn (atypical HUS):** Alternative complement-pathway defect; tx: Eculizumab (*NEJM* 2013;368:2169)
- **HELLP:** Majority 3rd trimester of pregnancy, proteinuria, HTN, hemolysis, liver fxn abnormalities, thrombocytopenia; tx: Obstetrics consultation; magnesium sulfate administration; HTN mgmt, & delivery of fetus per obstetrician (*Blood* 2013;121(1):38; *American Journal of Obstetrics and Gynecology* 2011;205(3):191)

Other fragmentation anemias (Go and Kuo, ASH-SAP 2019)

Macrovascular: Cardiac valve/vascular prosthesis, aneurysms, intraaortic balloon pump, malignant HTN, scleroderma renal crisis

Infectious causes of hemolytic anemia (Go and Kuo, *ASH-SAP* 2019)

- EBV, mycoplasma (AIHA, see above)
- *C. perfringens, C. septicum*: Alpha toxin leads to RBC hemolysis; gram positive & gram-neg bacterial infxns: May lead to hemolytic anemia
- Viral infxns (HIV, influenza A, HSV, CMV, HCV, etc): Also may lead to AIHA
- Parasitic infxns (malaria—plasmodium species, intraerythrocyte infxn w/ *P. falciparum* most severe hemolysis), Babesiosis (warm AIHA)

Defects of the RBC membrane (Go and Kuo, *ASH-SAP* 2019)

- **Hereditary spherocytosis:** RBCs w/ increased osmotic fragility; many muts may lead to HS; mild forms—pigmented gallstones, more severe-aplastic crisis; hyperhemolytic crisis; increased MCHC; prot deficiencies (spectrin, ankyrin, band 3, prot 4.2) & dysfunction (beta-spectrin abnormalities); spherocytes on blood smear & may confirm w/ eosin-5–maleimide binding assay; definitive tx is splenectomy
- **Hereditary elliptocytosis (HE) & hereditary pyropoikilocytosis (HPP):** Many genetic defects; 3 main subtypes: Common HE (biconcave elliptocytes), spherocytic HE (HE/HS hybrid), Southeast-Asian ovalocytosis (spoon-shaped erythrocyte morphology); typically elliptocytes are present, dominant inheritance pattern; tx not always necessary, can treat hemolytic anemia w/ splenectomy if needed
- **Stomatocytosis:** Inherited & acquired disorders may lead to stomatocytes (wide slit in center of RBC)
- **Rh deficiency (null syn):** Absent or reduced Rh antigen; hemolytic anemia; increased osmotic fragility

G6PD deficiency (*ASH-SAP* 2010;1:133, *Lancet* 2008;371:64; Go and Kuo, *ASH-SAP* 2019)

- G6PD is an X-linked gene; leads to ↓ G6PD in males; lyonization pattern determines female phenotypic variance
- Coombs neg hemolytic anemia
- HMP shunt 1st enzyme: ↓ G6PD → ↓ NADPH → ↓ renewal reduced glutathione → ↑ RBC/Hgb oxidant stress susceptibility → extravascular + ↑↑ intravascular hemolysis w/ ↑↑ oxidant + ↓↓ G6PD.
- PB smear: Eccentrocytes, bite cells, Heinz bodies

Other defects of RBC enzymes (*ASH-SAP* 2010;1:133)

- **Other HMP shunt: Rare**-phosphogluconate dehydrogenase; glutathione reductase
- **Glycolysis:** ↓ **PK** >80% hemolytic anemias a/w glycolysis. ↑ Northern & Eastern Europeans. Nl osmotic fragility/MCV. Diagnosed w/ quantitative RBC enzyme analysis
- Tx depends on severity. Consider folate supplementation & splenectomy
- **Wilson dz:** ↑ Copper inhibits hexokinase → acquired hexokinase deficiency
- **Nucleotide metabolism abnormality:** ↓ Pyrimidine-5′–NT (Pb tox) & ↓ adenosine deaminase

Germline hemoglobinopathies: see "Hemoglobinopathies" chapter

PNH: See "Anemias of Underproduction" chapter

- Consider in DDx for Coombs neg (DAT neg) hemolytic anemia

HEMOGLOBINOPATHIES

Physiology

- Hb = 2 pairs of 2 globin chains. Adults normally have majority HbA = $\alpha2\beta2$; also HbA2 = $\alpha2\delta2$; HbF = $\alpha2\gamma2$
- Globin gene muts change quantity &/or structure of α & β globin leading to insufficient Hb, abnl Hb, &/or tox from imbalanced globin expression; protect from malaria (*Nature* 1986;321:744)
- Nomenclature: $\alpha°$ or $\beta°$ = no expression; α+ or β+ = partial expression, milder phenotype
- Dx: PB smear, Hb electrophoresis, genetic testing

Alpha thalassemia

- **Genetics:** 2 loci on each Chr 16; $\alpha\alpha/\alpha\alpha$ = Nl. Mt: α–/α– = trans, $\alpha\alpha$/– – = cis
- **Epidemiology:** Increased incidence in populations from South/Southeast Asia (cis deletion), Sub-Saharan Africa (trans deletion), Mediterranean, Middle East
- **Alpha thal (0),** Homozygous = –/– = Hb Bart's ($\gamma4$ tetramers) → *hydrops fetalis*, incompatible w/ extrauterine life. Incidence ↑ in Asian descent d/t ↑ cis deletion
- **Alpha thal major** = α–/– → HbH dz ($\beta4$ tetramers) = neonatal jaundice secondary to lack of HbF; HSM, hemolytic anemia, chronic leg ulcers
- **Alpha thal trait** = α–/α– or $\alpha\alpha$/– → mild microcytic anemia, ↓ mean corpuscular Hb (MCH)
- **Alpha hal minima** = $\alpha\alpha/\alpha$– → Silent carrier, no hematologic manifestations
- **Hemoglobin constant spring** = α–/– CS → Nondeletional form of alpha-thalassemia

Beta thalassemia

- **Genetics:** 1 locus on Chr 11; β/β = Nl. AR inheritance
- **Epidemiology:** Highest in Mediterranean, N. Africa, Middle East, W. Asia
- **Beta thal major,** eg, $\beta°/\beta°$ = Cooley Anemia. Jaundice >6 mos after ↓ HbF, ineffective/extramedullary hematopoiesis → skeletal abnormalities, characteristic facies; poor growth; extravascular hemolysis → HSM, biliary stones. Transfusion dependence → allo-Abs & iron overload. Susceptibility to *Yersinia* infxn; Parvo B19 → aplastic crisis. Chronic hypoxia → pulm HTN, cardiac tox
- **Beta thal minor/trait,** eg, β/β+ or $\beta/\beta°$—mild anemia w/ microcytosis. MCV/RBC ratio <13 (Mentzer index). RDW nl. Typically free of severe sxs
- **Beta thal intermedia,** eg, $\beta°/\beta$+—varying degrees of anemia & transfusion dependence, hepatospenlomegaly
- **Tx:** Splenectomy, chronic transfusion, iron chelation, folate supplementation. Only curative option is allo-SCT (*NEJM* 2005;353:1135). Gene therapy clinical trials ongoing

Hemoglobin C disease

- **Genetics:** β-globin gene Glutamate 6 → Lysine mut. AR
- **Epidemiology:** ↑ freq in Black pts (2% carrier, 1:6,000 homozygous)
- **Dx:** Mild hemolytic anemia; PB smear: Microcytes, target cells, RBCs w/ HbC crystal inclusions; hemoglobin electrophoresis

Hemoglobin E disease

- **Genetics:** β-globin gene: Glutamate 26 → Lysine. AR
- **Epidemiology:** Highest in Southeast Asia; ↑ freq in US from immigration
- **Dx:** Mild hemolytic anemia, microcytosis, RBC targeting, splenomegaly (rare)

*Compound heterozygosity of HbC or HbE w/ other α- or β-globin Mt leads to phenotype w/ variable clinical severity (*ASH Education Book* 2007;1:79)

Electrophoresis Patterns in Hemoglobinopathies

	Hb A (α2a2) (%)	HbA2 (α2c2) (%)	HbF (α2f2) (%)	HbH (a4) (%)	Hb Barts (f4) (%)
Nl	>95	2–3	<1	0	0
Alpha Thal (0)	0	0	0	<10	>90
Alpha Thal Major	60–90	2–3	0	5–30	2–5
Alpha Thal Trait	95	3–4	<1	0	0
Beta Thal Major	0–5	0–5	>90	0	0
Beta Thal Intermedia	5–90	0–5	10–90[a]	0	0
Beta Thal Minor	90–95	3–10	2–3	0	0

[a]Variable depending on severity of Mt

Sickle cell disease

- **Genetics:** Beta globin—6th aa: Glutamine → Valine = HbS. AR. Hereditary persistence of fetal hemoglobin (HPFH) is protective. Compound heterozygosity w/ other β-chain muts causes a spectrum of dz severity (HbS/β^0 is often severe, $HbS/\beta+$, HbSC generally milder)

- **Epidemiology:** Most common monogenic d/o. Black pts 1:400–600 S/S dz. 8% Carrier rate A/S high prevalence Sub-Saharan Africa, Mediterranean basin, Middle East, & India 2/2 protection that the sickle cell trait provides against severe malaria (*NEJM* 2017;376:1561–1573). Couples at risk should be offered hemoglobinopathy testing early in pregnancy & newborn screening
- **Pathophysiology:** Polymerization→ damages the RBC → hemolytic anemia, blocked small blood vessels → VOC

Sickle cell VOC

- **Pain**—treat w/ O_2, fluids, analgesia
- **Acute chest syn:** Major source of **mortality**. Dx'd by new infiltrate, often w/ pain, tachypnea, hypoxia, confusion, fever
  Triggers: Prior VOC, infxn, fat embolism, cold weather, air pollution, high altitude
  Tx: Exchange or simple transfusion (HbS <30%), O_2, maintain euvolemia. Broad spectrum ABX
- **Exchange transfusion:** Adding donor HbA removes HbS (goal <30%); often requires apheresis catheter, ICU-level care. Indicated for CVA, sev. acute chest, refractory priapism, end-organ dysfunction

Acute anemia in sickle cell disease

- **Exacerbation of hemoglobinopathy:** Hemolytic anemia → ↑ LDH, ↑ unconjugated bili., ↓ hapto, ↑ retic. Neg *DAT*. Often occurs w/ VOC as above
- DHTR: 5–15 d after transfusion, d/t **alloimmunization;** up to 50% have Ab against minor blood Ag (*Blood* 2012;120:528). Dx w/ positive **DAT in elution**. Prev: Minimize transfusions, perform extended-Ag matching (Rh, Kell, Duffy, Kidd, MNS groups)
- **Hyperhemolytic crisis**—↑↑ hemolysis d/t DHTR against pt's own RBCs. Elevated retics. Consider immunosuppressive therapy w/ steroids +/– IVIG
- **Splenic sequestration:** Esp in younger pts; sev. HSM, life-threatening rapid drop in Hb may → shock
- **Aplastic crisis:** Retic <1% despite brisk hemolysis; often **Parvo B19** triggered

Multiorgan sequelae of sickle cell disease

- **Cardiopulmonary:** Cardiomegaly, pulm HTN (major cause of *mortality*) (*Blood* 2016;127:820)
- **Endocrine:** Delayed puberty, growth delay, short stature
- **GU:** Priapism → impotence; tx intracavernous aspiration, phenylephrine
- **Hepatobiliary:** Pigment gallstones; frequently require cholecytectomy, sickle hepatopathy
- **ID:** Functional asplenia → ↑↑ risk encapsulated bacterial infxn (*S. pneumo, H. flu, Neisseria; Salmonella*, & *S. aureus* osteo)
- **Musculoskeletal:** Dactylitis in infancy**,** avascular necrosis of femur/humerus, osteomyelitis
- **Neuro:** *High risk of CVA*; screen w/ transcranial Doppler in children (*NEJM* 1992;326:605); if abnl → simple transfusion to ↓ HbS <30% (*NEJM* 1998;339:5) ↓ risk by >90%. Acute tx: Exchange transfusion. Chronic tx: Simple transfusion & chelation superior to hydroxyurea (*Blood* 2012;119:3925)
- **Ophtho:** Proliferative retinopathy → detachment, ↑↑ risk *w/ HbSC* dz
- **Renal:** Hematuria, papillary necrosis, CKD, RTA, nephrogenic DI, isosthenuria
- **Skin:** Chronic leg ulcers, poor wound healing

Chronic management of sickle cell disease

- **Vaccinations**—CDC rec: Pneumococcal 13-valent × 1, pneumococcal polysaccharide q5y × 2 (>8 wk s/p 13-valent), meningococcal, influenza; consider HAV, HBV; *H. flu*
- **Medical therapy:**
  Hydrea ↑ HbF, ↓ VOC risk, strokes, & prolongs survival (*NEJM* 1995;332:1317)
  L-glutamine decreases pain crises (*NEJM* 2018;379:226–235)
  Folate supplementation in all pts given ↑ RBC turnover
  Iron chelation (deferoxamine, deferasirox) for chronic iron overload
  Penicillin ppx indicated in children to prevent pneumococcal sepsis
  Crizanlizumab anti-P-selectin Ab, decreases VOC frequency (*NEJM* 2017;376:429–439)
  Voxelotor inhibitor of Hb polymerization, decreases hemolysis (*NEJM* 2019;381:509–519)
- **Simple transfusion:** Adding HbA → dilutes HbS. Minimize use; avoid goal hemoglobin or use liberalized goal hemoglobin (5 or 6 g/dL rather than 7 or 8) except in setting of CVA, acute chest, or severe organ dysfunction. Extended-Ag matching to decrease alloimmunization. Consider prophylactic preoperative transfusion prior to surgery
- **Curative tx:** NMA-matched related (*NEJM* 2009;361:2309) or alternative donor allo-SCT (*Blood* 2014;123:3089). Gene therapy in sickle cell dz is an active area of clinical investigation (*NEJM* 2021;384:205–215; *NEJM* 2021;384:252–256)

HYPERCOAGULABLE STATES

Hypercoagulable states

- **Inherited:** FVL, PTG G20210A, prot C/S, AT deficiency, other genetic determinants
- **Acquired:** Surgery, malignancy, APS, hormonal (pregnancy, OCPs), drugs (IMIDs), etc.

Factor V Leiden (FVL)

- **Epidemiology: Most common inherited thrombophilia in white pts** (~5%)
- **Genetics:** Single point mut → factor V R506Q; AD, 99% heterozygous
- **Pathophys:** Factor V is procoagulant, inactivated by activated prot C (APC), mutated site of inactivation → APC resistance → ↑ coag, ↓ AC
- **Thrombosis risk: VTE** for heterozygote = 7–10× wt (*Lancet* 1993;342:1503), homozygote >80× wt (*Blood* 1995;85:1504), unclear if ↑ risk of recurrent VTE (*NEJM* 1999;341:801), only 5–20% of pts w/ FVL develop clinically apparent VTE in lifetime
- **Dx:** APC resistance assay = suggestive; PCR for FVL mut = definitive & preferred

Prothrombin G20210A

- **Epidemiology:** 2–7% white pts, uncommon in Asians, Africans, Hispanics
- **Genetics:** Guanine → adenine point mut in 3′ untranslated region; AD
- **Pathophys:** Mut → ↑ mRNA half-life → 30% increased prothrombin levels
- **Thrombosis risk: VTE** ~3× wt (*Blood* 1996;88:3698), no ↑ risk of arterial thrombosis
- **Dx:** PCR G20210A variant

Protein C deficiency

- **Epidemiology:** 0.2 to 0.5%, no known ethnic or geographic disparity
- **Genetics:** AD, >160 mts in *PROC* gene → quantitative or qualitative defects
- **Pathophys:** APC inactivates coag factors; Type I: ↓ Prot C Ag level; Type II: Nl prot C Ag level, ↓ activity → ↓ APC cleavage of FVa, FVIIIa → ↑ thrombosis
- **Thrombosis risk: VTE** risk ~10× wt, no ↑ risk of arterial thrombosis, ↑ risk of **warfarin skin necrosis** (**mgmt:** Stop Vit K antagonists → start UFH + IV Vit K + FFP), homozygotes → neonatal purpura fulminans or stillbirth
- **Dx:** Plasma prot C level, fxn assay preferred (detects ↓ Ag & ↓ fxn), **warfarin ↓s level**

Protein S deficiency

- **Epidemiology:** Rare, 1:1,000–1:3,000, no known ethnic or geographic disparity
- **Genetics:** Mts in *PROS 1* gene; AD, rarely homozygous
- **Pathophys:** Cofactor of prot C; Type I: ↓ Total Ag, free Ag, fxn; Type II: Nl total & free Ag, ↓ fxn; Type III: Nl total Ag, ↓ free Ag, ↓ fxn; all → ↓ APC cleavage of FVa, FVIIIa
- **Thrombosis risk: VTE** risk ~30× wt, no ↑ risk of arterial thrombosis. **Warfarin skin necrosis** & neonatal purpura fulminans or stillbirth similar to prot C deficiency
- **Dx:** Plasma prot S Ag (total, free) & fxn levels, no defined cutoffs (depends on assay), **warfarin ↓s level, acute thrombosis can ↓ levels**

Antithrombin (AT, formerly AT III) deficiency

- **Epidemiology:** Rare, 1:2,000–1:5,000, no known ethnic or geographic disparity
- **Genetics:** AD w/ variable penetrance, >100 mts
- **Pathophys:** AT is an AC (inhibits thrombin, etc.), mts or acquired (liver failure, DIC, VOD) → ↓ inhibition of coag enzymes; heparin resistance (heparin binds AT → ↑ AT activity); Type 1: ↓ AT Ag level + fxn; Type 2: Nl AT Ag level, ↓ fxn
- **Thrombosis risk: VTE** risk ~15–20×, **heparin resistance** (can give AT concentrate)
- **Dx:** Decreased plasma AT fxn (preferred) & Ag levels, **heparin & thrombosis ↓ levels**

Methylene tetrahydrofolate reductase (MTHFR) polymorphisms

- **Epidemiology:** Up to 10% of population have polymorphism in MTHFR gene
- **Genetics:** 2 most common polymorphisms are C677T & A1298C
- **Pathophys:** Polymorphism → ↓ activity; if homozygous & ↓ folate → ↑ serum homocysteine
- **Thrombosis risk:** Controversial, may have ↑ risk if very ↑ homocysteine

Antiphospholipid antibody syndrome (APS)

- **Definition:** Syn of **(+) AP Ab & thrombosis or other clinical sequelae** (see table); "primary" if no predisposing condition, "secondary" APS if coexisting condition
- **Epidemiology:** 1–5% have (+) Ab but far fewer have syn
- **Pathophys:** AI, Abs against prots & phospholipids → ↑ risk of thrombi; paradoxical prolonged PTT in vitro; exact mechanisms unclear
- **Clinical manifestations & dx:** See table, be aware of false positives: Syphilis, Lyme, viral, others; **"catastrophic APS"** = TMA w/ 3+ organ dysfxn <1 wk & (+) Ab; ~20% mortality
- **Tx: Warfarin w/ goal INR 2.5** (*J Thromb Haemost* 2005;3:848), **do not use DOACs** (*Ann Intern Med* 2019;171:685), indefinite AC if prior clot, add ASA in select pts, pregnant women should see high-risk OB, catastrophic: AC, steroids, PLEX, IVIG

Revised Classification (Sydney Criteria) for APS (*J Thromb Haemost* 2006;4:295)		
Clinical criteria (at least 1)	**Thrombosis:** ≥1 venous, arterial, or small vessel clot	If pathologic dx, no underlying vessel wall inflammation
	Fetal loss: ≥3 <10 wks or ≥1 loss ≥10 wks	Excluding chromosomal abnl, fetal malformations, or other underlying etiologies
	Placental insufficiency: ≥1 preterm labor <34 wks due to pre/eclampsia or placental insufficiency	
Lab criteria (at least 1)	**β2 Glycoprotein I** IgG, IgM **Anticardiolipin Ab** IgG, IgM **Lupus anticoagulant (LA) activity**	Medium or high titer on 2 occasions, >12 wk apart

Heparin-induced thrombocytopenia and thrombosis (HITT)

- **Definition: Life-threatening** syn of thrombosis, ↓ plt & (+) HIT Ab
- **Epidemiology:** Highest w/ surgical pts, UFH > LMWH (but can be **any** product, dose, schedule), up to 5% of pts w/ 4+ days of heparin exposure
- **Pathophysiology:** Ab against PF4: Heparin complex → activates plt → thrombosis
- **Clinical manifestations:** Type I: Mild transient ↓ plts, direct effect of heparin, clinically insignificant; **type II: Thrombocytopenia** (85–90% of pts, usu >30–50% drop plt in 5–15 days) &/or **venous** > **arterial thrombi** (limb ischemia, MI, adrenal necrosis), if heparin exposure w/in prior 100 d, onset may be sooner (w/in 24 h) + faster decline
- **Dx:** Clinical suspicion → **use 4T score to guide workup** (*J Thromb Haemost* 2006;4:759)
  → Score 0–3: Low probability (<1%) → evaluate for other causes
  → Score 4–5: Intermediate probability (~10%) & Score 6–8: High probability (~50%) → Send HIT Ab ELISA, functional assay (SRA, HIPA), use institutional policy
- **Tx: Stop heparin** immediately & **start nonheparin AC except warfarin** until plt normalize, **screen for DVT,** continue AC at least 4 wks, 3 mos if clot; list allergy

Malignancy-associated thrombosis

- **Epidemiology:** ~1% per person-year (*PLoS Med* 2012;9:e1001275); highest in pancreas, brain, lung; ↑ risk if chemo, RT, surgery, mets (*J Thromb Thrombolysis* 2016;41:81)
- **Pathophys:** ↑ Cytokines, tissue factor, & others, ↑ neutrophil extracellular traps, ↓ mobility
- **Tx: DOACs** (avoid if GI/GU lesion, liver dz, drug interaction); **LMWH** > **UFH** (*Cochrane* 2018;1:CD006649; *NEJM* 2003;349:146); avoid VKA

DOAC for VTE Treatment in Malignancy			
Agent	**Control**	**Outcomes (vs. control)**	**Notes**
apixaban	dalteparin	**Recurrence:** 5.6% vs. 7.9% (HR 0.63, 95% CI 0.37–1.07) **Major bleed:** 3.8% vs. 4.0% (HR 0.82, 95% CI 0.40–1.69)	NI trial, met NI endpt (*NEJM* 2020;382:1599)
rivaroxaban	dalteparin	**Recurrence:** 4% vs. 11% (HR 0.43, 95% CI 0.19–0.99) **Major bleed:** 6% vs. 4% (HR 1.83, 95% CI 0.68–4.96)	Excess clinically relevant nonmajor UGI bleeds (*JCO* 2018;36:2017)
edoxaban	dalteparin	**Recurrence:** 7.9% vs. 11.3% (HR –, 95% CI – 7.0–0.2) **Major bleed:** 6.9% vs. 4% (HR –, 95% CI 0.1–5.6)	Edoxaban given after 5 days of LMWH, met NI endpt (*NEJM* 2018;378:615)

- **Duration:** At least 6 mos, potentially indefinite if active malignancy
- **Prevention:** Guidelines differ, **select pts w/ Khorana score ≥2;** use Khorana score to assess risk (variables: Site of tumor, pre-tx plt, HGB, pre-tx WBC, BMI); **AVERT** (*NEJM* 2019;380:711): Apixaban vs. placebo for Khorana ≥2 ↓ VTE but ↑ major bleed; **CASSINI** (*NEJM* 2019;380:720): Rivaroxaban vs. placebo for Khorana ≥2 ↓ VTE but ↑ major bleed, ↓ risk of VTE not sig, pts screened w/ ultrasound upon enrollment (different than AVERT)

Treatment of venous thromboembolism (VTE) in patients without cancer

- Generally by standard approach, in presence or absence of hypercoagulable state
- Rx: DOACs preferred (rivaroxaban, apixaban, edoxaban, dabigatran) due to convenience, other: UFH, LMWH, fondaparinux, & VKA based on comorbidities & drug interactions
- **Duration:** Individualize, weigh risks/benefits of recurrent VTE vs. bleeding; generally, 1st provoked = at least 3 mos, 1st unprovoked = consider indefinite (*Blood Adv* 2020;4:4693), can also switch to long-term low-dose tx w/ rivaroxaban or apixaban (lower risk of bleeding)

PORPHYRIAS

Definition

- Metabolic disorders caused by altered activity of enzymes w/in the heme biosynthetic pathway leading to the accumulation of porphyrins or porphyrin precursors

Genetics

- Often due to genetic muts in the heme biosynthetic pathway, but can also be caused by acquired functional deficiencies of these enzymes
- Dz-causing muts are often private or shared / only a few other families

Epidemiology

- Rare dzs, affect fewer than 20,000 people in the United States
- *Most common* porphyria is porphyria cutanea tarda (PCT), prevalence of 1 in 10,000

Classification of the porphyrias

- **Hepatic or erythropoietic** depending on whether the site of initial production & accumulation of pathway intermediates is in the liver or BM
- **Acute or cutaneous** based upon the 1° clinical manifestation, although overlaps exist
  - Acute:
    - Acute intermittent porphyria (AIP) delta-ALA deficiency porphyria (ADP), hereditary corprophyria (HCP), & variegate porphyria (VP)
    - Cause attacks w/ visceral complaints &/or neurologic complications, can be life-threatening (*J Clin Neurosci* 2011;18:1147) a/welevations in the porphyrin precursors delta-ALA & PBG
- Cutaneous:
  - Photosensitivity due to activation of porphyrins in the skin upon exposure to UV-A
  - Chronic blistering skin lesions

Diagnosis

- Consider porphyria in the DDx of otherwise unexplained abdominal complaints &/or neurologic sxs, particularly if recurrent
- **Labs:** Porphyrin precursors ALA & PBG (AIP, HCP, VP only), as well as porphyrins in urine, plasma, erythrocytes, & feces

Porphyria subtypes

- **AIP:** AD inheritance, deficient enzyme is PBG deaminase, many people w/ genetic mut never develop sx, often manifests after puberty (*J Clin Pathol* 2012;65:976)
- **Delta-ALA deficiency porphyria (ADP):** AR inheritance, extremely rare
- **HCP:** AD form of hepatic porphyria, similar to AIP except that some pts develop photosensitivity
- **VP:** AD, common among white South Africans, hepatic porphyria; may have photosensitivity
- **PCT:** Hepatic porphyria, deficiency of UROD enzyme, 75% acquired, 25% familial dz, mainly p/w skin manifestations
  - Sporadic PCT is a/w hepatitis C, HIV, & EtOH (*Liver Int* 2012;32:880)
- **Erythropoietic protoporphyria (EPP) or protoporphyria:** Mut in ferrochelatase gene (FECH), presents in early childhood, characterized by photosensitivity
- **X-linked dominant protoporphyria (XLDPP or XLP):** Similar to EPP, due to gain of fxn mut in delta-ALA synthase-2 gene (ALAS2) on chr X
- **Congenital erythropoietic porphyria (CEP):** AR, rare, a/w photosensitivity
- **Hepatoerythropoeitic porphyria (HEP):** AR deficiency of UROD, rare, skin blistering that usu begins in infancy

Treatment

- Acute porphyrias should be treated urgently w/ hemin or glucose in order to avoid a prolonged or fatal attack (*Ann Intern Med* 2005;142:439–450)
- PCT: Iron reduction & hydroxychloroquine (*Clin Gastroenterol Hepatol* 2012;10(12):1402–1409)
- AIP: Givosiran (RNAi directed against ALAS1) decreases delta-ALA & reduces acute attacks (*NEJM* 2020;382:2289–2301)
- Avoidance of sunlight is rec
  - In those pts who have photosensitivity, such pts w/ CEP & EPP
  - Skin blistering, as in pts w/ VP & HCP

BLEEDING DIATHESES

Clinical manifestations

- **1° Hemostasis (plt/vascular/VWF dysfunction):** Typically, immediate mucocutaneous bleeding (epistaxis, gingival bleeding). Petechiae, small superficial ecchymoses, menorrhagia
- **2° Hemostasis (factor deficiency):** Often deep tissue bleeding; sxs can be delayed. Larger ecchymoses w/ organ, intracranial, muscle, or joint bleeds

Diagnostic approach

- Obtain pt's bleeding hx, FHx, medication use, & perform PE
- Initial tests: CBC, PT & aPTT
- Peripheral smear, fibrinogen, plt screening aggregation, specific factor levels, mixing studies for inhibitor, or other special tests (see below) will also aid in identifying etiology

Disorders of blood vessels

- Bleeding or bruising may result from blood vessels that are not formed properly or do not fxn properly
- Genetic
  - Hemorrhagic telangiectasia (**Osler–Weber–Rendu syn**): AD inheritance. Fragile vascular telangiectasias result in recurrent bleeding episodes, particularly GI & oral–pharyngeal
  - **Ehlers–Danlos syn:** Defect in collagen synthesis resulting in weak, elastic collagen w/in blood vessels that causes them to be more prone to injury. May be AD or AR inheritance depending on type of Ehler–Danlos syn
- Acquired: Allergic, infectious, renal insufficiency, chronic glucocorticoids, vitamin C def

Disorders of platelets (see section on Platelet disorders)

Disorders of coagulation factors: Hereditary single factor defects

- **Von Willebrand's disease (VWD):** Most common inherited bleeding d/o (~1% prevalence) (*NEJM* 2016;375:2067)
  - VWF involved in plt adhesion & carries factor VIII in plasma
  - Dx: 1st-level tests are VWF antigen (VWF:Ag), plt-binding activity of VWF (VWF:RCo), & factor VIII activity (FVIII:C); if all abnl, confirms VWD
    2nd-levels tests determine subtype: Ristocetin-induced plt aggregation (RIPA), VWF-FVIII binding activity (VWF:FVIIIB), VWF propeptide (VWFpp), & multimer analysis

vWD Variants

Variant	Description	Diagnostic Pattern
Type 1 (70% of cases)	Partial quantitative deficiency of VWF; uniform ↓ in all VWF multimers. Can be due to ↓ production or ↑ clearance	VWF:RCo <30 IU/dl Ratio of VWF:RCo to VWF:Ag >0.6 Ratio of VIII:C to VWF:Ag >0.6 Nl RIPA & multimers VWF:Ag <5 IU/dl abd VWFpp >5 IU/dl (severe type 1)
Type 2—qualitative deficiency of VWF		
Type 2A (15% of cases)	↓ large multimers due to defective cleavage (ADAMTS13) or defective assembly & transport	VWF:RCo <30 IU/dl Ratio of VWF:RCo to VWF:Ag ≤0.6 Loss of high molecular weight multimers RIPA nl or reduced
Type 2B (Plt type, 5% of cases)	↑ GPIb binding of large multimers → ↓ circulating large multimers	VWF:RCo <30 IU/dl Ratio of VWF:RCo to VWF:Ag ≤0.6 Loss of HMW multimers RIPA enhanced
Type 2M (rare)	↓ GPIb binding to VWF → uniform ↓ in all VWF multimers	VWF:RCo <30 IU/dl Ratio of VWF:RCo to VWF:Ag ≤0.6 Nl Multimers
Type 2N (rare)	Defective factor VIII binding, nl VWF multimers & activity	Ratio of VIII:C to VWF:Ag ≤0.6 VWF:FVIIIB reduced
Type 3 (rare)	↓↓↓ or undetectable VWF → severe bleeding	VWF:Ag <5 IU/dl VWFpp <5 IU/dl Multimer & RIPA absent

Treatment

1. DDAVP (300 μg i.n. or 0.3 μg/kg i.v. or s.c.) for minor bleeds/surgery (contraindicated in type 2B dz) → release of endogenous stores of VW
2. Antifibrinolytic agents (tranexamic & aminocaproic acid) as required for mucosal-based surgery or bleeding
3. VWF concentrates or recombinant VWF for major bleeds/surgery. Less effective in subtype 2, ineffective in type 3 (needs plasma-derived concentrates that contain VWF & FVIII). Concern for thrombosis in type 2b (plt type)

- **Hemophilia A** (↓ FVIII) & **B** (↓ FIX): X-linked recessive. Delayed bleeding, deep muscle bleeds. Hemarthrosis most common event. Also ICH & oral mucosal bleeding
  - Severity depends on factor level: <1% severe (spontaneous bleeding), 1–5% moderate (bleeding w/ mild injury), 5–25% mild (bleeding w/ surgery or trauma); hemostatic level at >30% & nl is 50–150%
  - Affected males: All daughters are carriers & no sons are affected
  - Female carriers: 50% risk of carrier daughter; 50% risk of affected son
  - 30% of cases result from new spontaneous mut
  - Complications of bleeding: Flexion contractures, joint arthritis/arthropathy, chronic pain, muscle atrophy, compartment syn, neurological impairment
  - Dx: Factor level <40%
  - Tx: Factor replacement (*NEJM* 2020;382:29–40)
    - Factor VIII: 1 unit/kg → 2% ↑ in level, BID dosing
    - Factor IX: 1 unit/kg → 1% ↑ in level, QD dosing
    - Fc fusion prot versions can reduce FVIII dosing to QD & FIX to weekly
    - On demand: Goal of 40–50% for minor & 80–100% for major bleeding
    - Prophylactic: FVIII 20–50+ u/kg /dose; FIX 20–100+ u/kg /dose
    - In North America, 1° ppx is SOC; downsides of ppx are frequent venipunctures, lifelong therapy, infxn, & formation of inhibitors (20–30% of sev. hemophilia A & 1–4% of sev. hemophilia B pts)
    - Can use plasma-derived concentrates containing VWF or recombinant factor VIII; rVIII is more likely to develop inhibitory Abs (*NEJM* 2016;374:2054)
    - After development of inhibitor, can treat w/ rFVIIa (90–120 μg/kg bolus Q2h), PCC, or emicizumab (*NEJM* 2017;377:809–818)
  - Gene therapy ↑ circulating factor IX to 1–6% of nl & in high-dose group, conferred a 9% reduction in bleeding episodes & use of prophylactic factor IX concentrate (*NEJM* 2014;371:1994). SPK-9001 (AAV8 vector-derived Padua-variant FIX:C) ↑ circulating factor IX to >30% in 7 pts w/o immunosuppression or neutralizing Abs (*NEJM* 2017;377:2215–2227)
  - Adjunctive therapy: Fibrinolysis inhibitors or DDAVP (for mild dz)
  - **Hemophilia C** (↓ FVI): AR, 1/500 AJ
    - Tx: Recombinant XI & plasma-derived XI are not available in the United States. Use FFP
  - **Factor XIII deficiency:** AR, 1/500 AJ
    - Tx: Plasma-derived or recombinant factor XIII
  - **Fibrinogen:** Congenital fibrinogen deficiency
    - Tx: RiaSTAP human fibrinogen concentrate
  - **PAI-1 deficiency:** AR, dx by measuring PAI activity
    - Tx: Fibrinolysis inhibitors
  - **Alpha-2 antiplasmin:** AR, dx by measuring α2 antiplasmin level
    - Tx: FFP & fibrinolysis inhibitors

Disorders of coagulation factors: Acquired single factor defects

- **Factor VIII:** Inhibitors 2/2 malignancy (eg, lung, prostate, H&N), also postpartum
  - Tx: Prednisone, cyclophosphamide, or RTX
- **VWF:** Inhibitors 2/2 MGUS, MPN, Wilms tumor, Heyde syn. Adsorbed by plt in ET
  - Tx: DDAVP (0.3 μg/kg) – > FVIII/VWF conc (40 FVIII U/kg) –> IVIG (1 g/kg)
- **Factor V:** Inhibitors 2/2 beta lactams, bovine thrombin (prev used in surgeries)
  - Tx: Plt transfusion (factor V bound to plt are not affected by inhibitor)
- **Factor X:** Adsorbed by fibril in amyloidosis. Tx: FFP, PCC

Disorders of coagulation factors: Multifactor defects

- Liver dz (*NEJM* 2011;365:147), DIC 2/2 sepsis or malignancy (eg, APL & prostate CA), vitamin K deficiency, snake venom, & anticoagulants

Disorder	F V	F VII	F VIII	F X
Liver Dysfunction	↓	↓	Nl or ↑	↓
Vitamin K Deficiency	Nl	↓	Nl	↓
DIC	↓	↓	↓	↓

- Tx: Treat underlying cause
- Cryoprecipitate if fibrinogen <100 in DIC
- Warfarin overdose can be treated w/ vitamin K (IV 10 mg) depending on INR (low dose oral optional if INR 4.5–10). If acute major bleeding → PCC; FFP if PCC not available
- DOAC reversal: For dabigatran reversal, use Idarucizumab; Andexanet for reversal of Xa inhibitors (apixaban, endoxaban, rivaroxaban) based on dose & timing of the factor Xa inhibitor or 4-factor PCC
- Do not correct coagulopathy from snake bite until antivenom administered

For all coagulopathies, antifibrinolytic agents **can serve as an adjunctive tx**

PLATELET DISORDERS

Normal platelet function—hemostasis

- **Production:** Regulated by hormone TPO secreted from liver & acting on megakaryocytes in BM; 1×10^{11} produced daily, circulate for 7–10 d
- **Adhesion:** Endothelial injury → plt activation & binding via GPIb–IX to VWF or via GPVI, integrin $\alpha 2\beta 1$ to the subendothelial matrix (eg, collagen)
- **Aggregation:** Activated GPIIb–IIIa binds VWF & fibrinogen to form clumps → ADP & serotonin released from granules → additional plt recruited
- **Pseudothrombocytopenia:** Falsely ↓ plt count due to plt clumping, seen on peripheral smear; mgmt: Collect blood in non-EDTA, citrate- or heparin-containing tube

Thrombocytopenia (plt <150,000/μL)

- **Clinical S/S:** Mucocutaneous bleeding, petechia, ecchymosis, epistaxis; when severe, can lead to life-threatening hemorrhage, but usu not until <10K

Underproduction	Peripheral Destruction	Other
1°: **BM disorders:** Aplastic anemia, drugs, EtOH, radiation, postinfectious (eg, HCV, EBV, parvovirus, VZV, mumps, rubella), MDS/leukemia, metastatic CA, MF, granulomatous dzs, ↓ vitamin B12, ↓ folate **Inherited syns:** (*Blood* 2004;103(2);390) Fanconi anemia, DKC, MYH9-related dzs, Mediterranean variant	**Immune mediated:** *1°*: ITP 2°: Drugs (quinine, vancomycin, GPIIb–IIIa inhibitors), vaccines (COVID-19), infxn (HIV, HCV, EBV, *H. pylori*), SLE, APS, lymphoproliferative disorders, posttransfusion purpura, IgA deficiency, common variable immune deficiency, ALPS, neonatal alloimmune thrombocytopenia **Nonimmune:** MAHA (DIC, HUS, TTP), vasculitis, preeclampsia, HELLP syn, HD, cardiac bypass, IABP, hemangiomas	Sequestration: Hypersplenism Infectious: Ehrlichiosis, babesiosis, RMSF, etc. Misc: Liver dz (↓ TPO) hypothermia, vWD type 2B

Heparin-induced thrombocytopenia (HIT) (see also Hypercoagulability chapter)

- **Nonimmune** (type I): Transient thrombocytopenia; plt nadir >100,000/μL ~1–4 d after starting heparin; may continue heparin & observe, caution to not confuse w/ early onset HIT w/ earlier fall due to prior exposure to heparin in last 3 mos
- **Immune** (type II): Median plt nadir 50–60K, 5–10 d after starting heparin, earlier fall if prior exposure to heparin in last 3 mos, bovine > porcine UFH > LMWH; pathogenesis: Ab to PF4-heparin Ab complex → thrombocytopenia & prothrombotic state w/ life- & limb-threatening arterial & venous clots; plt activation NOT destruction
- **Labs:** Ab testing indicated if 4Ts Score (*J Thromb Haemost* 2006;4:759) is **intermediate or high;** +HIT Ab (PF4/heparin ELISA, highly sensitive, ~90% specific); confirm by **functional** plt activation (serotonin release) assay (>90% specific) if ELISA optical density >0.4
- **Additional evaluation:** Doppler U/S of the lower extremities to r/o subclinical DVT; U/S of upper extremity if indwelling CVC
- **Tx of immune HIT** (*NEJM* 2015;373:252): **Discontinue all heparin products;** start alternative anticoag (argatroban, bivalirudin, fondaparinux, rivaroxaban) until plt nl
  - Once plt >150K & stable, can begin VKA: MUST overlap w/ argatroban for 5 d to avoid venous limb gangrene; warfarin is contraindicated as initial rx of HIT; if pt already on warfarin, must reverse w/ vitamin K when starting HIT tx; can use DOAC instead of VKA
  - Tx duration = DVT tx duration; if no thrombus, treat for 3 mos
  - Refractory: Consider PLEX (esp. if heparin needed for surgery, *J Clin Apher* 2011;26:219), IVIg (*Expert Rev Hematol* 2019;12:685)
  - If heparinoid product **needed** in future, recheck Ab: If neg **&** >3 mos since HIT dx, can BRIEFLY use intraop heparin

4Ts Clinical Scoring System of Suspected Immune HIT				
Points	**Thrombocytopenia**	**Timing of ↓ plt**	**Thrombosis**	**Other Causes**
2	↓ >50% & nadir ≥20K	5–10 d after heparin (1 d if prior heparin w/in 30 d)	New clot, skin necrosis, or rxn after IVB	None
1	↓ 30–50% or nadir 10–19K	Unclear w/in 5–10 d or after 10 d or w/in 1 d (if prior heparin)	Recurrent, progressive, or suspected; nonnecrotic skin lesions	Possible
0	↓ <30% or nadir <10K	<4 d w/o recent heparin	None	Definite
Score: Low (0–3); intermediate (4–5); high (6–8)				

Immune thrombocytopenia (ITP)

- *1°* immune plt destruction; dx of exclusion
- **Presentation:** Variable bleeding sx, may be asx
- **Dx:** Isolated ↓ plt, large plt on peripheral smear; R/o 2° etiologies, esp. HIV, HCV; BMBx no longer rec, except for atypical presentations, presplenectomy or refractory dz
- **Tx:** Should be centered on pt values & preferences. Consider **observation** if asx & plt count >20–30 × 10^9/L; hospitalize initial presentation w/ plt count of <20 × 10^9/L, active bleeding or other variables (anticoag)
- **Emergency tx of bleeding:** Plt transfusion + IVIg 1g/kg/d × 2–3 d + methylprednisolone 1 g/d × 3 d; ± adjunctive aminocaproic acid (inhibits plasmin activation & stabilizes thrombus); if refractory, consider emergency splenectomy

Treatment of ITP in Adults		
Setting	**Treatment**	**Notes**
Initial	**Steroids:** Dex 40 mg PO × 4 d (max 3–4 cycles) better ORR vs. prednisone 1 mg/kg. If giving pred. & responding, goal taper off by 6 wks of tx (*Blood Adv* 2019;3:3780–3817)	50–75% respond, but long-term s/e <20% have sustained remission ↓ FcR on Mϕ ↓ anti-plt Ab production
	IVIg 1 g/kg/d × 1–2 d or 0.4 g/kg/d × 5 d	If **bleeding** or steroid-**refractory** ↓ fcR on Mϕ ↓ anti-plt Ab production
	Anti-Rh(D) Ig	Ab-coated RBCs overwhelm Mϕ FcR
Subsequent/ persistent	**Rituximab** (anti-CD20 MAb)	↓ Plt clearance **Finite tx**
	Romiplostim, eltrombopag, avatrombopag	TPO-RA; 80–95% response rate (*Lancet* 2008;371:395), insuff. evidence to rec. upfront
	Splenectomy	↓ plt clearance ~65% long-term remission
	Fostamatinib	SYK inhibitor; rate of stable plt >50K = 18% in heavily pre-tx pts (*Am J Hematol* 2018 Jul;93[7]:921–930)
	Danazol, vincristine	↓ Plt clearance
	AZA, cyclophosphamide, 6MP, MMF, dapsone, CSA	Immunosuppressants ↓ anti-plt Ab production

Thrombotic microangiopathies

- Characterized by occlusive microvascular dz, often w/ intraluminal thrombus formation. Clinically, TMA p/w triad of MAHA, decr plt, & organ ischemia/damage
- MAHA ≡ DAT(–) hemolytic anemia, ↑ LDH, ↑ indirect bili, ↓ hapto, reticulocytosis, schistocytes
- **HUS:** A/w enterohemorrhagic *E. coli* & bloody diarrhea usu in children; **HUS Triad:** Thrombocytopenia + MAHA + renal failure; Shiga toxin binds/activates renal endothelium & plt → intrarenal microthrombi; D0 = severe abd pain, nonbloody diarrhea → D3 = bloody diarrhea → by D7 = 90% recover, 10% develop HUS

- **Complement-mediated TMA (cmTMA, previously "atypical HUS")**; disrupted regulation of the complement system d/t (1) muts in complement genes or (2) autoantibodies against complement regulatory prots
- **TTP:** Deficient ADAMTS13 → uncleaved large VWF multimers bind plt & form thrombi; etiologies: Idiopathic/immune, drugs (quinine, ticlopidine, clopidogrel, CSA, tacro, gem), pregnancy, HSCT, HIV, AI dz, familial (Upshaw–Shulman syn)
- **TTP pentad:** Thrombocytopenia + MAHA ± renal failure ± fever ± ΔMS; **pentad present in ≤25% of cases;** presence of MAHA & thrombocytopenia w/o other apparent course sufficient to diagnose TTP; can also use PLASMIC risk prediction score to determine likelihood of TTP (https://www.mdcalc.com/plasmic-score-ttp)
- **Dx:** ↓ Plt (<20K) + MAHA; neg Coombs, nl PT/PTT, & fibrinogen; ADAMTS-13 deficiency (typically <10%); ADAMTS-13 gene sequencing for congenital TTP
- **DDx:** DIC, vasculitis/connective tissue disorders, scleroderma renal crisis, APS, malignant HTN, preeclampsia/HELLP syn, disseminated malignancy
- **Tx of TTP: Emergent (w/i 4–8 h of presentation) plasma exchange** (1–1.5 plasma volumes daily) + steroids until plt >150K, LDH nl, & sx resolve (*NEJM* 1991;325:393); if delay in initiating PLEX, **transfuse** FFP; once dx confirmed, rx rituximab + caplacizumab (unless congenital); plt transfusion contraindicated unless life-threatening bleed
- **Tx of HUS:** Supportive if *E. coli*-assoc, avoid abx; use of eculizumab reported in severe 2011 HUS outbreak in Europe (*NEJM* 2011;364:2561)
- **Tx of cmTMA:** Consider PLEX (temporizing measure); once dx confirmed (evidence of increased activation of alternative complement pathway or +complement mut), tx w/ complement inhibitors (eculizumab, ravilizumab) generally indefinitely

Thrombocytopenia in the critically Ill

- Commonly multifactorial etiology; occurs in up to 50% of ICU pts; severe (<50K) in 5–20%
- DDx: Critical illness itself, medications, sepsis, hemodilution/massive transfusion, extracorporeal circuit, TMA, blood loss/massive trauma
- Plt transfusion a/w ↑ thrombosis risk (*J Crit Care* 2005;20:348)
- Avoid plt transfusion unless bleeding, procedure, or <20K

Qualitative platelet disorders

Acquired Platelet Function Disorders	
Adhesion defects	Uremia, acquired vWD (often due to underlying LPD)
Aggregation defects	Medications: Ticlopidine, clopidogrel, GP IIb/IIIA antagonists, high dose β-lactam abx, SSRI, herbal supplements Dysproteinemias: Myeloma, amyloidosis
Granule defects	MPN, acute leukemias, liver dz, cardiopulmonary bypass Medications: ASA, NSAIDs, SSRI

Inherited Platelet Function Disorders		
Defect	**Inheritance**	**Description**
Adhesion defects		
Bernard–Soulier	AR	Defective GPIb-IX-V complex
DiGeorge syn	22q11.2 deletion	↓ & large plt; multiple abnormalities
Aggregation defects		
Glanzmann	AR	↓ or qualitative defect in GPIIb/IIIA
Granule defects		
Chediak–Higashi	AR	↓ δ-granules, immunodeficiency
Hermansky–Pudlak	AR	↓ δ-granules, oculocutaneous albinism

Testing platelet function (practical-haemostasis.com/Platelets/platelet_function_testing_introduction.html)

- **When to suspect a platelet d/o?** Consider ISTH-BAT = validated scoring system for predicting the presence of an inherited bleeding d/o (*J Thromb Haemost* 2020;18:73)
- **Morphology** on smear: Giant plt in Bernard–Soulier, small plt in Wiskott–Aldrich syn
- **PFA-100:** Broad screen for plt dysfunction
- **Plt aggregation assays:** Diagnose plt disorders (incl. meds) according to response to ADP & other agonists (collagen, thrombin, epinephrine, ristocetin & arachidonic acid)
- **VerifyNow:** Plt aggregation test to monitor anti-GPIIB/IIIa rx (*Thromb Haemost* 2009;102:404)
- **Electron microscopy:** Visualize plt granules & diagnose defects therein
- **Flow cytometry:** Abnormalities in platelet cell surface markers seen in Bernard Soulier (CD42) & Glanzmann thrombasthenia (CD41, CD61)

Transfusion Products		
Product	**Indication**	
RBC	1 unit RBC ↑ Hgb ~1 g/dL 1 unit = ~350 cc	• RBC transfusion threshold of Hb < 7 g/dL is rec for hospitalized adult pts who are hemodynamically stable • RBC transfusion threshold of < Hb 8 g/dL is rec for pts undergoing orthopedic surgery, cardiac surgery, & those w/ preexisting cardiovascular dz (*JAMA* 2016;316[1]:2025–2035)
Plts	Suspended in an appropriate volume of the original plasma Either apheresis-derived (majority) or whole blood derived Apheresis plts offer advantage of fewer donor exposures. One unit of Apheresis Plts usu contains ≥3.0×10^{11} plts & is the therapeutic equivalent of 4–6 whole blood-derived units	Bleeding due to thrombocytopenia or plt functional abnormalities Prophylactic plt transfusion for hospitalized adult pts w/ plt count ≤10×10^9 cells/L Prophylactic plt transfusion for low-risk procedures w/ plt count ≤20×10^9 cells/L Prophylactic plt transfusion for LP w/ a plt count ≤50×10^9 cells/L Prophylactic plt transfusion for major elective non-neuraxial surgery w/ plt count ≤50×10^9 cells/L Pts who are plt refractory due to HLA-alloimmunization may be supported by transfusion of plts from donors lacking the targeted epitopes by phenotyping donors & providing HLA-matched plts (*Ann of Intern Med* 2015;162:205–213)
FFP, PF24 & Thawed Plasma	FFP contains plasma prots including all coagulation factors at levels close to those of nl plasma; it is frozen w/in 8 h of collection 1 unit = ~200 cc PF24 is plasma frozen w/in 24 h of collection Thawed plasma is derived from FFP/PF24, thawed & maintained at 1–6°C for up to 5 d. Provides readily available source of plasma	Mgmt of preoperative or bleeding pts who require replacement of multiple plasma coagulation factors (eg, liver dz, DIC) Pts undergoing massive transfusion who have clinically significant coagulation deficiencies Pts taking warfarin who are bleeding or need to undergo an invasive procedure before Vit K could reverse the warfarin effect or who need only transient reversal of warfarin effect Transfusion or plasma exchange in TTP pts Pts w/ selected coagulation factor deficiencies, congenital or acquired, for which no specific coagulation concentrates are available Only FFP should be used to replace FV or FVIII, as other types of plasma have decreased levels of these factors Pts w/ rare specific plasma prot deficiencies, such as C1 inhibitor, when recombinant products are unavailable. (Circular of information (COI) for the use of human blood & blood components, AABB 2017)

Cryoprecipitated Cryopercipitated Antihemophilic Factor (AHF)	Cold-insoluble portion of FFP that precipitates when FFP is thawed at 1–6°C Contains fibrinogen, VWF, Factor VIII, XIII, & fibronectin 1 unit = 5–20 cc	Used in the control of bleeding a/w fibrinogen deficiency & to treat FXIII deficiency when volume considerations preclude the use of frozen plasma & recombinant prots are not available 2nd-line therapy for vWD z & hemophilia A May be considered for control of uremic bleeding after other modalities have failed Indications for use as a source of fibronectin are not clear. (COI for the use of human blood & blood components, AABB 2017)
Granulocytes	Contain numerous leukocytes (usu $>1.0 \times 10^{10}$), plts, & 20–50 cc of RBCs Need to be administered w/in 24 h of collection Final product 200–300 cc	Neutropenia w/ infxn, unresponsive to appropriate antibiotics Pt who received an average dose per transfusion of $\geq 0.6 \times 10^9$ granulocytes per kg tended to have better outcomes Overall, benefit remains controversial (*Blood* 2015;26:2153)

Preparations of Transfusion Products

Technique	Indication
Leukocyte reduced (LR)	Contains $<5 \times 10^6$ leukocytes; leukocytes are a/w HLA alloimmunization, febrile nonhemolytic transfusion rxns, & carry risk of CMV infxn Considered CMV-reduced risk & an alternative to CMV-neg components Indicated for HSCT candidates or those chronically transfused
IRR	Prevents donor T-cell proliferation & transfusion-assoc GVHD Primarily indicated for pt w/ significant immune deficiencies (eg, hematologic malignancies, congenital immunodeficiencies, HSCT)
PAS	Conventional plts are coadministered w/ donor plasma. In PAS plt, ~65% of the donor plasma is replaced w/ PAS, thereby reducing anti-A & anti-B titers & lowering the risks of donor plasma-related adverse rxns such as, allergic transfusion rxn
Pathogen reduction (PR)	The process of treating the blood component soon after collection in order to inactivate any remaining infectious agents May be expected to (1) materially reduce the risk of transfusion-transmitted infections, (2) eliminate the need for serologic testing for CMV by production of CMV-reduced risk components, (3) eliminate the need for irradiation to prevent GVHD
CMV-neg	Cellular blood products from CMV-neg donors Indicated in CMV-neg pts considered at risk for severe CMV infxn, including HSCT, severe immunodeficiency, & neonates
Washed products	Washing is done to mitigate complications a/w residual plasma in the unit. Washed components are indicated for (1) pts who have had severe allergic or anaphylactic rxns to blood transfusion, washed RBCs should be used for intrauterine transfusions

COI for the use of human blood & blood components, AABB 2017, *AABB Tech. Manual* 20th ed. 2020.

SCREENING TESTS IN HEMOSTASIS

Clinical scenarios suggestive of bleeding disorders

- **1° hemostasis (plt-type bleed):** Mucocutaneous bleeding (mucosal membranes, menorrhagia, petechiae, & ecchymoses) suggests thrombocytopenia, plt dysfunction, vWD, or vascular causes
- **2° hemostasis (coagulation-type bleed):** Deep tissue, hematomas, &/or delayed bleeding suggests factor deficiency/dysfunction

Prothrombin time (PT)

- Measures **extrinsic** (FVII) & **common** pathways (FII, V, X, & fibrinogen)
- **INR** is a normalized result that allows for inter-laboratory comparison: INR should be used for pts on warfarin. **Note:** Reagent contains neutralizing agent for therapeutic doses of heparin

Causes of isolated prolonged PT

- **Vit K deficiency**—Vit K is needed for synthesis of FII, VII, IX, X, protein C & protein S; **causes:** Inadequate intake, malabsorption, & prolonged antibiotic use; deficiency affects FVII first (shortest $t_{1/2}$)
- **Liver dz**—factors synthesized in liver
- **Anticoagulants:**
  Warfarin—causes Vit K deficiency → prevents γ-carboxylation of coag factors
  Other anticoagulants—rivaroxaban, apixaban, & edoxaban directly inhibit FXa & dabigatran directly inhibits thrombin

Activated partial thromboplastin time (aPTT)

- Measures the **intrinsic** (FVIII, IX, XI, XII, prekallikrein, high-molecular–wt kininogen) & **common** (FII, V, X, & fibrinogen) pathways

Causes of isolated prolonged aPTT

- **Factor deficiencies of clinical relevance**—VIII, IX, & X
- **Specific factor inhibitors**—acquired hemophilia (anti-VIII & anti-IX)
- **Nonspecific inhibitors**—lupus anticoagulant (LAC, antiphospholipid Ab), indirect inhibitors (MM, lymphoproliferative neoplasms), heparins

Combined prolongation of PT and aPTT

- Deficiency or inhibition of factor(s) in the common pathway or of multiple factors, DIC/consumption, severe liver dz, dysfibrinogenemia, hypofibrinogenemia, excessive warfarin AC or severe/prolonged Vit K deficiency (*Mayo Clin Proc* 2007;82:864)

Fibrinogen

- **Low**—Causes: DIC, thrombolytic therapy, liver dz (↓ synthesis), tx w/ L-asparaginase (*Note: Direct thrombin inhibitors (dabigatran) & UFH may falsely ↓ fibrinogen assay results*)
- **High**—acute phase, pregnancy, oral contraceptives, malignancy

D-dimer

- Product of plasmin-mediated lysis of cross-linked fibrin
- Current gen. of D-dimer assays are VERY specific biomarker indicating the presence of fibrin formation (ie, *in vivo* clot); sensitive, but not specific for presence of activation of the coag system *in vivo*
- Neg D-dimer result is useful to r/o VTE in low-risk setting. Positive result is nonspecific & may occur in the setting of multiple conditions

Common antithrombotic medications

Mechanism	Drug	PT	PTT	½ Life	Metabolism	Reversal
Potentiates activity of ATIII	UFH	—	↑	1.5 h	Hepatic	Protamine
Indirect Xa inhibitors	Enoxaparin	—	↑ or none	4.5 h	Renal	Protamine (NB limited reversal)
	Fondaparinux	—	↑ or none	17–21 h	Renal	No established agent
Vit K antagonist	Warfarin	↑	No	40 h	Hepatic	See below; vit K, 4-PCC
Direct thrombin inhibitor	Dabigatran	↑	↑	12–17 h	Renal 80%, Potent P-gp inducers/ inhibitors	Idarucizumab
Direct Xa inhibitors	Rivaroxaban	↑	↑	5–9 h	66% renal, CYP3A4, P-gp inducers/ inhibitors	Andexanet alfa
	Apixaban	↑	↑	12 h	25% renal, CYP3A4, P-gp inducers/ inhibitors	
	Edoxaban	↑	↑	10–14 h	50% renal	
Irreversible COX-1 inhibitor	Aspirin	—	—	2–5 h	Hepatic, 0 order kinetics	No established agent Possible benefit from plt administration 8–20 h after last dose
Irreversible $P2Y_{12}$ inhibitors	Clopidogrel	—	—	7–8 h	Hepatic	No established agent Possible benefit from plt tfn 4 half-lives after last dose
	Prasugrel	—	—	2–15 h	Hepatic	
Reversible $P2Y_{12}$ inhibitor	Ticagrelor	—	—	7–8.5 h	Hepatic	No established agent Plt activity recovery after 4 half-lives

Derived from package inserts for each agent.

Warfarin reversal

Figure 28-2 Warfarin reversal.

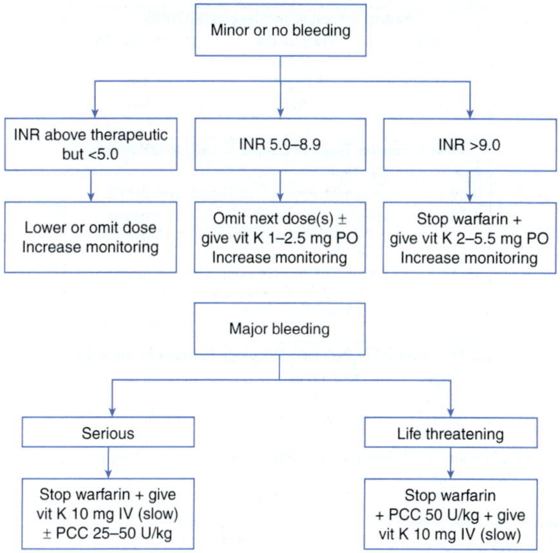

- **Administration of vit K:**
  In pts w/ mild to moderately elevated INR w/o major bleeding, give vit K orally rather than intravenously (Grade 1A) (*Chest Journal* 2008;133:160S)

Additional tests

- **Mixing study** (mixes pt plasma w/ nl plasma): Correction = factor deficiency, no correction = inhibitor
- **Types of inhibitors:** (1) immediate-acting inhibitors (often **LAC,** contamination w/ anticoagulants), (2) inhibitors requiring 37°C incubation for 1–2 h (suspect specific-factor inhibitor), (3) & specific-factor inhibitor. Follow up by ordering LAC or specific factor assay(s) if applicable (*Clin Lab Med* 2009;29:229). Note: Weak inhibitors may be diluted by nl plasma leading to correction & inaccurate interpretation

Bleeding disorders with normal PT/aPTT

- **VWD:** May have mild FVIII deficiency, not low enough to detect w/ elevated aPTT
- **Rare bleeding disorders may have nl. PT/aPTT:**
  FXIII deficiency = insufficient fibrin cross-linking, recurrent spontaneous abortion, delayed wound healing
  Deficiency of α2-antiplasmin or plasminogen activator inhibitor (PAI-1) (excessive fibrinolysis)

GENERAL PEDIATRIC CONSIDERATIONS

Epidemiology (*CA Cancer J Clin* 2020;70:7; *NCHS Data Brief* 2016;257:1)

Pediatric Cancer Incidence USA 2020		
Age	**Dx'd w/ CA**	**Deaths d/t CA**
0–19 y	16,850	1,730
0–14 y	11,050	1,190
15–19 y	5,800	540

Most Common Types of Cancer in the United States	
Age	**CA Type**
0–19 y	Leukemias, Brain & CNS Tumors, Lymphomas
0–14 y	Leukemias, Brain & CNS Tumors, Lymphomas, Neuroblastoma, Kidney Tumors, Malignant Bone Tumors
15–19 y	Brain & CNS Tumors, Lymphomas, Leukemias, Thyroid CA, Gonadal Germ Cell Tumors, Malignant Bone Tumors

5-Year Survival in Pediatric Oncology Patients in the USA		
Age	**Mid 1970s**	**2010–2016**
0–14 y	58%	84.1%
15–19 y	68%	85.3%

Causes of cancer in children and young adults (*NEJM* 2015;373:2336)
- Up to 8.5% d/t germline mts
- Not commonly caused by environmental exposures

Cancer chemotherapy for children and young adults
- Physiologic differences in children affect drug distribution
  - ↓ Renal blood flow, GFR, tubular function → ↓ renal excretion
  - ↓ Hepatic drug-metabolizing enzymes, biliary excretion → ↓ metabolic clearance, biliary clearance
  - ↓ Gastric acid secretion, motility → variable drug absorption
  - ↑ Blood volume, extracellular fluid volume, total body water, fat composition → ↑ distribution volume

Radiation therapy principles in pediatric oncology (*Radiology* 1975;114:155)
- Craniospinal irradiation in children <3–5 y a/w decr IQ performance
- Irradiation of the pituitary gland & hypothalamus a/w ↓ growth hormone production & short stature, precocious puberty, & ovarian failure
- Doses of irradiation >20 Gy to the epiphyseal plate impedes bone growth & integrity
- Risk of 2° malignant neoplasms

Transfusion of blood products in pediatric oncology (Pizzo, P. (2011). *Principles and Practice of Pediatric Oncology* (6th Ed.). Lippincott; *J clin Oncol* 2018;36:283)
- RBC transfusion parameters for hemodynamically stable pts: Hb <7 g/dL
- Plt transfusion parameters $<10 \times 10^9$/L

For surgical or invasive procedures: $<40–50 \times 10^9$/L

For bone marrow aspirations/biopsies & removal of CVCs: $<20 \times 10^9$/L
- Irradiation of RBCs & plts for all immunocompromised pts prevents TA-GVHD
- CMV negative, leukoreduced RBCs & plts rec for pts w/ immune deficiencies, premature infants, & CMV seronegative stem cell transplant recipients

Blood Product Dosing Guidelines for Pediatric Pts		
RBCs	10–15 mL/kg	Hb ↑ 2–3 g/dL
Plts	5–10 mL/kg	Plt ↑ 50,000–100,000/µL
FFP	10–15 mL/kg	Factor activity ↑ 15–20%
Cryoprecipitate	1–2 units/10 kg	Fibrinogen ↑ 60–100 mg/dL

Special consideration for AYA (see also AYA chapter)
- Ages 15–39 y
- <10% rate of clinical trial enrollment
- Improvement in survival outcomes lags behind that of younger children
- Assent to tx &/or clinical trial enrollment begins at age 7 y

Special consideration for infants
- Chemo dose reduction for infants <6 kg: Dose calculated on mg/kg basis (dose in mg/m^2 divided by 30)
- Transient myeloproliferative disorder (TMD) a/w trisomy 21: Myeloproliferative disorder manifesting in early infancy w/ hepatosplenomegaly, leukocytosis, & circulating myeloblasts. Self-resolving. Chemo indicated for respiratory failure. Leukemic infiltrate results in hepatic fibrosis. 20–30% of infants w/ TMD will develop AMKL by 3 y of age

Survivorship
Referral to survivorship specialist is rec for all pts treated for pediatric malignancies (see Survivorship chapter).

PEDIATRIC ONCOLOGIC EMERGENCIES

Fever and neutropenia (*J Clin Oncol* 2017;35:2082–2094)

- Fever: Single oral temperature ≥38.3°C, an oral temperature ≥38.0°C for longer than 1 h, or an oral temperature ≥38.0°C × 2 during a 12-h period
- ANC = total WBC × (% PMNs + % bands)/100

Degree of Neutropenia	ANC (cell/µL)
Mild neutropenia	1,000–1,500
Moderate neutropenia	500–1,000
Severe neutropenia	<500

- Tx: Antibiotics w/in **1** h of fever (a/w decr ICU stay)
- Initial therapy w/ antipseudomonal beta-lactam/4th generation cephalosporin monotherapy
- Combination therapy w/ vancomycin for hemodynamic instability, concern or gram-positive bacterial infxn
- Consideration of anaerobic coverage for rectal/abd pain
- G-CSF in pediatrics can lead to decr duration of febrile neutropenia & length of hospital stay (*Pediatr Blood Cancer* 2005;45:274–280)

Tumor lysis syndrome (*NEJM* 2011;364:1844–1854)

- Defined as metabolic abnormalities (hyperkalemia, hyperphosphatemia, hypocalcemia, hyperuricemia) d/t rapid cellular turnover, a/w incr. creatinine, seizures, cardiac dysrhythmia, or death (see Tumor Lysis Syndrome chapter)

Clinical Presentation	
Hyperkalemia	Weakness, dysrhythmias
Hyperphosphatemia	Hypocalcemia, renal failure
Hypocalcemia	Seizures, mental status changes, tetany
Hyperuricemia	UA nephropathy, oliguria, renal failure
Treatment Principles	
Prevention of AKI	Hydration &/or diuretics
Prevention of UA formation	Allopurinol
Incr. UA excretion	Recombinant urate oxidase (Rasburicase)
Prevention of cardiac dysrhythmias d/t electrolyte abnormalities	Sodium polystyrene sulfonate, glucose w/ insulin/beta agonists, calcium gluconate
Mgmt of severe AKI	Continuous renal-replacement therapies
Close monitoring during time period of risk for tumor lysis syn	Electrolyte, creatinine, UA, urine output q4–6h for high-risk pts

Hyperleukocytosis (*Blood Rev* 2012;26(3):117–122)

- WBC >100,000/µL inducing leukostasis, tumor lysis syn, DIC
- Incidence: 5–20% of children w/ new dx of ALL or AML
- Leukostasis (vascular obstruction d/t high leukocyte count) presents in CNS (confusion, dizziness, headache, delirium) & pulmonary system (dyspnea, tachypnea, hypoxea)

Treatment Principles	
Supportive care	Aggressive hydration, allopurinol, respiratory support as needed for tumor lysis syn, treat underlying coagulopathy
Cytoreduction	Leukapheresis, induction chemo, hydroxyurea. Consider cranial irradiation for leukostasis & neurologic sxs

Mediastinal masses (*Anes Clin* 2001;19:559–579)

- Pts w/ a mediastinal mass are at risk for acute cardiopulmonary arrest w/ supine positioning & sedation
- Appropriate airway mgmt & close monitoring w/ anesthesia specialists should be arranged for definitive imaging & bx

Spinal cord compression (*NEJM* 2017;376:1358–1369)

- Oncologic emergency that may lead to permanent paralysis, can present w/ localized pain &/or various neurologic signs (hyperreflexia, Babinski sign, limb paralysis, urinary retention/incontinence, loss of sensation)
- Most frequently seen in pts w/ sarcoma, neuroblastoma, lymphoma
- Evaluation w/ MRI w/ gadolinium, emergent consultation w/ Neurosurgery, Neurology, & Radiation Oncology
- Tx: Surgical decompression, glucocorticoids, radiotherapy, control of local tumor growth

SVC syndrome (*NEJM* 2007;356:1862–1869)

- Compression or obstruction of SVC d/t space occupying lesion or thrombus
- Commonly seen in lymphoma, germ-cell CA, thymoma
- Presents w/ facial edema, cough, dyspnea, dysphagia, wheezing, hoarseness, facial edema, rarely w/ chest pain or pleural/pericardial effusions
- Dx: Combination of clinical hx & contrast enhanced CT chest to distinguish b/w extrinsic compression versus thrombosis. Tissue sample to identify malignant process
- Tx principles: Relieve obstruction, treat underlying malignancy
- Supportive care (elevate head of bed, consider diuretics or glucocorticoids), radiotherapy, systemic chemo

PEDIATRIC HEMATOLOGIC MALIGNANCIES

Acute lymphoblastic leukemia (ALL): (For presentation, disease biology, & diagnosis, see adult ALL chapter)

Epidemiology

- Accounts for ¼ of all childhood malignancies → most common pediatric CA
- ~3,000 children dx'd annually in the United States
- Incidence: 2–5 cases per 100,000 children; ↑ in ages 2–5; M > F

Prognosis

- 5-y EFS & 5-y OS for childhood ALL ~90%, w/ variation based on prognostic features
- Unfavorable prognostic factors: Age ≥10 y or <1 y, presenting WBC count ≥50,000/mm³, CNS dz at dx, cytogenetic/molecular features incl. hypodiploidy, *BCR-ABL1*, *KMT2A* rearrangements, *iAMP21*, *IKZF1* deletions, Philadelphia-like ALL, & high EOI MRD (>0.01%)

Treatment

Regimen/Study	Subtype	Intervention	EFS/DFS (%)	OS (%)
COG AALL0932 (*J Clin Oncol* 2021;39:1437)	SR B-cell ALL	Lower exposure to VCR/DEX in Maintenance: VCR/DEX pulses q12wks	95.1	98.6
COG AALL0232 (*J Clin Oncol* 2016;34:2380)	HR B-cell ALL	HD MTX for pts w/ HR B ALL; DEX during induction for younger pts	79.6	88.9
COG AALL0434 (*J Clin Oncol* 2020;38:3282)	T-cell ALL	Addition of nelarabine	88.2	90.3
DFCI 05-001 (*Lancet Oncol* 2015;16:1677)	B-cell ALL	Pegaspargase consolidation	85	91
St. Jude Total 16 (*J Clin Oncol* 2019;37:3377)	B & T ALL	↑ IT chemo in induction	88.2	94.1
BFM ALL 2000 (*Blood* 2016;17:2101)	B &T ALL	Dexamethasone in induction improves survival	83.9	90.3
UK2003 (*Lancet Oncol* 2013;14:199)	LR B & T ALL	Reduced tx based on low MRD at EOI	94.4	97.9

Acute myeloid leukemia (AML): (For presentation, disease biology, & diagnosis, see adult AML chapter)

Epidemiology

- Accounts for ~25% of pediatric leukemias
- 500–600 new cases annually in the United States; 10,000 new cases each year worldwide
- Incidence: 5–7 cases/million people annually; ↑ in children <2 y & adolescents 15–20 y/o

Risk factors

- **Environmental exposures:** See section on adult AML
- **Inherited disorders:** Trisomy 21, Trisomy 8, Fanconi anemia, Bloom syn, Li–Fraumeni syn, Dyskeratosis congenita, severe congenital neutropenia, NF 1, CEBPA-mediated AML, Shwachman–Diamond syn, DBA, Familial plt d/o, congenital amegakaryocytic thrombocytopenia, TAR syn
- **Acquired disorders:** Severe aplastic anemia, acquired amegakaryocytic thrombocytopenia, PNH

Prognosis

Risk Status	Host Factors	Clinical Factors	Cytogenetic/Molecular Abnormalities
Favorable	Trisomy 21; Age <4 y	CR; No MRD at EOI	Inv(16)(p13.1q22)/t(16;16)(p13.1;q22); *CBFB-MYH11* t(8;21)(q22;q22.1); *RUNX1-RUNX1T1* *NPM1* mt Biallelic *CEBPα* mt
Unfavorable		WBC >100 k/μL; Persistent dz; +MRD at EOI	Monosomy 5 Monosomy 7 Deletion 5q *FLT3*-ITD w/ high allelic ratio

- **MRD** is a strong predictor of relapse; multidimensional flow cytometry (MDF) & PCR are used to detect MRD → improved detection compared to morphologic assessments

Treatment

- **Induction:** 1–2 cycles of anthracycline (daunorubicin or idarubicin) or mitoxantrone + low-dose or high-dose cytarabine; ± fludarabine or etoposide → goal to induce CR
- **Consolidation:** 2–3 cycles of high-dose cytarabine ± 2nd agent (mitoxantrone, amsacrine, or etoposide)
- **IT chemo:** Prophylaxis or tx
- **AlloHCT:** For pts w/ high-risk features, usually after 2–3 cycles of chemo & once in CR

Regimen/Study	Intervention/Outcome	EFS (%)	OS (%)
COG AAML0531 (*J Clin Oncol* 2014;32:3021)	GO + chemo improves EFS by reducing RR in pediatric AML	53.1	69.4
MRC AML12 (*Br J Hematol* 2011;3:366)	4 courses of chemo are adequate; equal CR rates w/ daunorubicin or mitoxantrone in Induction	54	63
AML-BFM 2004 (*Blood* 2013;122:37)	Liposomal daunorubicin has antileukemic activity similar to idarubicin & causes less tx-related mortality	59	76

Myelodysplastic syndrome (MDS): <5% of childhood malignancies

- Occur in context of inherited BM failure syn or germ line syn (*GATA2, ETV6, SRP72, SAMD9, SAMD9-L*)
- Cytogenetic aberrations: Monosomy 7 (30% of patients), trisomies 8 & 21, & del20q
- **AlloHCT** is the only curative option, IPSS-R score not validated in pediatrics
- **Transient abnormal myelopoiesis (TAM)** occurs in 1/3 of neonates w/ DS & is a/w an acquired mt in *GATA 1*; most undergo spontaneous remission, ~20% evolve to ML-DS by acquiring additional oncogenic mts in *GATA 1* mutant cells

Juvenile myelomonocytic leukemia (JMML)

- **2–3% of childhood hematologic malignancies**

Epidemiology

- Incidence: 1.2 million children affected annually; median age at presentation is 2 y; M > F

Diagnostic criteria

Clinical/hematologic features (all 4 of below)	**Genetic studies** (≥1 of below)	**For pts w/out a genetic feature** (≥2 of below)
PB monocyte count >1 × 10^9/L; blast in PB & BM < 20%; splenomegaly; absence of *BCR-ABL* fusion	Somatic mt in *PTPN11, K-RAS*, or *N-RAS*; dx of *NF1*/germline *NF1* mt; or germline *CBL* mt & loss of heterozygosity of *CBL*	Monosomy 7 or any other chromosomal abnormality; HbF ↑ for age; myeloid precursors on PB smear; GM-CSF hypersensitivity in colony assay; hyperphosphorylation of STAT5

Treatment

- **AlloHCT** cures >50% of pts, rec for pts w/ NF1, somatic *PTPN11, K-RAS*, & most *N-RAS* mts; pts w/ germline *CBL* mts → spontaneous regression

Hodgkin lymphoma (HL): (For presentation, disease biology, & diagnosis, see adult HL chapter)

Epidemiology

- In industrialized countries, peaks in middle-to-late 20s
- EBV detected in variable frequencies, from 3–100% depending on histologic subtypes & HIV status; more common in children <10 y/o living in low-income countries

Treatment

Risk Group	Stage	Therapy
Low	IA-IB-IIA	ABVD × 3 +/– RT AVPC × 3 +/– RT COPP-ABV × 4 +/– RT VAMP × 4 +/– RT OPPA/OEPA × 2 +/– RT
Intermediate	IA/IIA w/ bulk IB w/ or w/out bulk IIB w/out bulk IIIA	ABVE-PC × 4 +/– RT
High	IIIB, IVA/B IIB w/ bulk	ABVE-PC × 5 +/– RT ABVD × 6 +/– RT

A: doxorubicin; B: bleomycin; V: vinblastine or vincristine; D: dacarbazine; P: prednisone; C: cyclophosphamide; O: vincristine; P: procarbazine; M: methotrexate; E: etoposide

- No uniform system of prognostic stratification exists in pediatric HL; different consortia have established different risk categories, & different studies have identified clinical prognostic factors; these have not been validated across various tx regimens
- Current studies assessing **immunotherapy** as upfront therapy in combination w/ standard chemo for both low-risk & high-risk dz incl. brentuximab vedotin (antibody-drug conjugate targeting CD30) as well as pembrolizumab & nivolumab (immune checkpoint inhibitors targeting PD-1)

Non-Hodgkin lymphoma (NHL): (For presentation, disease biology, & diagnosis, see adult NHL chapter)

Epidemiology

- Accounts for 7% of all childhood malignancies in children <20 y/o
- Incidence: 750–800 new cases in the United States each year; M > F

Characteristics and treatment of common NHL subtypes

Subtype	Cytogenetic/ Molecular Aberrations	Regimen & Reference	Intervention	EFS (%)	OS (%)
Mature B- cell NHL (Burkitt, Burkitt-like, & DLBCL)	*c-myc* translocations; 11q mts; *BCL-6* & *BCL-2* translocations; *IRF4* rearrangements	BFM LMB-96 (*Blood* 2007; 109:2773)	↓ Therapy for pts w/ unresected Stage I/II B-NHL (↓ cyclophosphamide & doxorubicin)	98.4	
		COG ANHL1131 (*NEJM* 2020; 382:2207)	Standard LMB chemo + rituximab for pts w/ Stage III/IV dz	94	95
Anaplastic large cell	*NPM-ALK* fusion; *TPM3-ALK* fusion	COG ANHL0131 (*PBC* 2014; 61:2236)		74	84
		ALCL99 (*JCO* 2010;28:3987)		71	94
Precursor/ lymphoblastic	*NOTCH1*, *FBXW7*, *CDKN2A*, *PTEN*, & *KMT2D* mts; LOH 6q	See treatment of pediatric ALL			

Langerhans cell histiocytosis (LCH)

Epidemiology

- Incidence: 4.6 cases per 1 million children; ↑ in children of Hispanic ethnicity; highest incidence <1 y/o

Pathogenesis

- Clonal neoplastic proliferation w/ expression of CD1a, CD207 (Langerin), & S100
- *BRAF* V600 mt found in ~57% of LCH lesions→ ↑ rapidly accelerated fibrosarcoma kinase activity → activation of RAS-RAF-MEK-ERK-MAP kinase pathway

Clinical Group	Description	Tx
Single-system	1 system involved	
Single bone lesion		Curettage + steroid injection
Skin	Seborrheic scalp rash; candida-type rash in the scalp, groin, abdomen, back, or chest	Observation alone; topical therapy, systemic therapy w/ 6MP & MTX if extensive
CNS-risk lesion	Lesions in 1 craniofacial bone ± intracranial soft tissue extension	Vinblastine + prednisone × 12 mos
Isolated CNS-LCH	Space-occupying lesions of CNS	Vinblastine & prednisone, Cladribine, cytarabine, clofarabine
Multifocal bone dz or bone +1 other site	2+ lesions in 2+ different bones or bone + other site (nonrisk)	Vinblastine + prednisone × 12 mos
Multisystem	2+ systems involved	Induction therapy w/ vinblastine + prednisone × 6 wks Continuation therapy w/ vinblastine + prednisone for total 12 mos + 6MP if risk organ involvement
W/ risk organ involvement	Liver, spleen, &/or BM	
W/out risk organ involvement	W/out liver, spleen &/or BM	

BONE MARROW FAILURE SYNDROMES

Bone marrow failure (BMF)

- **Definition:** Decr or defective production of ≥1 hematopoietic cell lineage (erythroid, granulocyte/monocyte, &/or megakaryocytic)
  Pts can present w/ either single- or multilineage cytopenia

Classification	
Acquired Aplastic Anemia	**Inherited Bone Marrow Failure Syndromes (IBMFS)**
Idiopathic aplastic anemia	Fanconi anemia
2° aplastic anemia (B12 or folate deficiency, infxns, medications, toxins, radiation) Autoimmune disorders	Dyskeratosis congenita Shwachman–Diamond Syn Diamond–Blackfan anemia Severe congenital neutropenia Congenital amegakaryocytic thrombocytopenia

Aplastic anemia (AA)

Definition: Presence of at least 2-lineage cytopenia w/ a hypocellular marrow w/out infiltration or fibrosis (*NEJM* 2018:379(17):1643-1656)

Classification: Acquired or inherited

- **Acquired:** 2° aplastic anemia, autoimmune dzs, eosinophilic fasciitis, hyperimmunoglobulinemia, thymoma, thymic carcinoma, paroxysmal nocturnal hemoglobinuria (PNH), pregnancy, idiopathic
- **Inherited:** Fanconi anemia, dyskeratosis congenita, Schwachman–Diamond syn, reticular dysgenesis, congenital amegakaryocytic thrombocytopenia, preleukemia (eg, monosomy 7)

Epidemiology: Approximately 600 new cases/y in the United States (*Blood* 1987;70(6):1718–1721)

- Biphasic distribution of aplastic anemia w/ 1st peak b/w 15–25 y, & a 2nd peak in pts older than 65 y of age

Signs & sxs: Pallor, petechiae, ecchymoses, rarely fever

- Physical examination: Often benign; can have signs of bleeding diathesis, fatigue.
  Laboratory work-up: Persistent pancytopenia

Dx: (*NEJM* 1982:306(11):645–652; *NEJM* 1982:306(12):712–718; AIEOP, *Blood Cells Mol Dis* 2015;55(1):40–47)

1. *Peripheral blood*: CBC w/ differential, blood smear & reticulocyte count, Comprehensive metabolic Profile (CMP), LDH, Folic Acid, Vitamin B12, Serology/virus PCR: Parvovirus, CMV, EBV, HHV6, Hepatitis A, B & C, Antinuclear Antibody (ANA) & Anti-ds-DNA.
2. *BMA & trephine bx*: Karyotype/cytogenetics/FISH (chromosome 5, 7, 8), flow cytometry for CD34, T & B cells
3. *Genetic testing* for IBMFS incl. DEB testing & telomere lengths (see IBMFS sections below)
4. *Other*: PNH screen by peripheral blood flow cytometry for GPI linked CD55/59 or FLAER

Grading of severity:

- Nonsevere AA: Hypocellular marrow w/ peripheral cytopenias not meeting criteria for severe or very severe AA
- Severe & very severe AA: BM cellularity <25% (or <30% of nl cellularity for age determined by marrow bx, or 25–50% w/ hematopoietic cells <30%) & at least 2 of the following:

Grading of Severity			
	ANC (×10⁹/L)	**Plts (×10⁹/L)**	**ARC (×10⁹/L)**
Severe	<500	<20	<60
Very Severe	<200	<20	<60

Counts must be persistent and other causes for cytopenias must be ruled out. ANC: Absolute Neutrophil Count, ARC: Absolute Reticulocyte Count

Tx: (*NEJM* 1982;306(11):645–652; *NEJM* 1982;306(12):712–718; AIEOP, *Blood Cells Mol Dis* 55(1):40–47)

- **Supportive care:** Leukoreduced & irradiated transfused blood products to reduce risks of febrile reactions, CMV infxn, & transfusion-assoc GVHD
- **Hematopoietic stem cell transplant (HCT):** Only definitive cure for AA
  Pts w/ an HLA-matched related donor – HCT at dx to avoid transfusion or HLA sensitization, iron overload, & infxns
  Pts w/out a suitable related donor – 1st-line immunosuppresive therapy (IST)

- **IST w/ equine antithymocyte globulin (hATG) & CsA:** 70–80% of children have a hematologic response, & 30% of those who respond will relapse & go on to receive another course of IST. 20–30% of pts will show evidence of clonal expansion w/ subsequent MDS. If relapse or no response: Consider HCT instead of 2nd IST
- **Eltrombopag:** Response rates of 40–50% in pts refractory to IST
- **Eltrombopag + hATG + CsA:** Higher overall & complete hematologic response (complete response in the longest tx cohort of 94%)

Outcomes: Fatal in 90% at 1 y for untreated pts w/ severe aplastic anemia
HCT from matched sibling donor (MSD) & MUD: 90% long term survival & cure
IST: Overall survival ~81–93% but risk for relapse, progression to MDS or Acute Myeloid Leukemia (AML)

Inherited bone marrow failure syndromes (IBMFS)

(Bone Marrow Failure. Hematology/Oncology Clinics. Editor: Colin A. Sieff. August 2018. Hematology Basic Principles and Practice. Edition 6. Chapter 28. Elsevier 2013. The EBMT Handbook. Hematopoietic Stem Cell Transplantation and Cellular Therapies. Springer. 2019)

Fanconi anemia

- **Genetics:** 22 known FA gene mts: *FANCA, FANCB, FANCC, FANCD1 (BRCA2), FANCE, FANCF, FANCG, FANCI, FANCJ, FANCL, FANCM, FANCN, FANCP, FANCS, RAD51CXPF* Defective DNA repair, DNA fragility, chromosomal breakage d/o
- **Inheritance pattern:** Autosomal recessive (>98%), rarely autosomal dominant (1–2%), (*RAD51*), X-linked recessive (*FANCB*)
- **Hematology/oncology:** Thrombocytopenia in 1st decade, anemia, neutropenia, pancytopenia, MDS, AML, solid tumors (head & neck, esophagus, female genital tract)
- **Dx:** Clinical. Chromosomal breakage analysis or cell-cycle arrest by mitomycin C or diepoxybutane. Molecular sequencing
- **Clinical features:** Mean age at dx – 7 y. Skeletal anomalies: (Aplastic or hypoplastic radii & absent or extra thumbs.) Congenital malformations of the kidneys, gonads, CNS, heart, gastrointestinal tract, skin pigmentation, endocrinopathy, reduced fertility, cytopenias/marrow failure, extreme sensitivity to radiation & chemo

Shwachman–Diamond syndrome (SBDS)

- **Genetics:** Biallelic *SBDS* mts (chromosome 7q11), defect in ribosomal maturation
- **Inheritance pattern:** Autosomal recessive heterozygous/compound heterozygous *SBDS* mts
- **Hematology/oncology:** Neutropenia, anemia, thrombocytopenia, MDS, AML
- **Dx:** Clinical: Low serum trypsinogen (age <3 y) or low serum pancreatic isoamylase (age >3 y). Molecular sequencing
- **Clinical features:** Presents in infancy, skeletal anomalies, exocrine–pancreatic insufficiency/failure to thrive, predisposition to infxn, hepatomegaly/elevated AST & ALT, dental anomalies, cytopenias/marrow failure

Dyskeratosis congenita (DKC)/telomere disorders *(GeneReviews® [Internet]. Seattle (WA): University of Washington, Seattle; 1993–2021)*

- **Genetics:** AR – *ACD, CTC1, NHP2, NOP10, PARN, RTEL1, STN1, TERT, WRAP5*
  AD – *ACD, RTEL1, TERC, TERT < TINF2, NAF1.*
  Defects in proteins involved in telomere stability
- **Inheritance pattern:** X-linked–*DKC1* (20–25%), AR (4–18%), AD (20–45%)
- **Hematology/oncology:** Thrombocytopenia, macrocytic anemia, pancytopenia. MDS, Leukemia (AML > ALL), HNSCC, solid tumors of gastrointestinal tract, skin cancer
- **Dx:** Clinical: Telomere lengths (<1st percentile for age in 4/6 subsets), Molecular sequencing *(Hematol Oncol Clin North Am* 2018;32(4):657–668; *Clin Cancer Res* 2017;23(11):e23–e31)
- **Clinical features:** Median presentation ~age 15
  BM failure & *classic triad (abnl skin pigmentation, nail dystrophy oral leukoplakia)*, hepatic cirrhosis, vascular anomalies, pulmonary fibrosis

Congenital amegakaryocytic thrombocytopenia

- **Genetics:** *MPL* gene (1p34), Mts TPO receptor (c-MPL)
- **Inheritance pattern:** AR
- **Hematology/oncology:** Thrombocytopenia, pancytopenia, AML
- **Dx:** Clinical. Molecular sequencing
  - **Clinical features:** Presents at birth or during 1st mo of life, perinatal intracranial hemorrhage, mucocutaneous bleeding. No congenital malformations, BMF

Diamond–Blackfan anemia (congenital pure red cell aplasia)

- **Genetics:** *RPS19* (chromosome19q13.2), *RPL5, RPL11, RPL35A, RPS10, RPS17, RPS24, RPS26.* Defects in proteins involved in ribosomal synthesis
- **Inheritance pattern:** AD (10–25% familial; rest sporadic)

- **Hematology/oncology:** Macrocytic anemia, reticulocytopenia, erythroid hypoplasia in marrow, MDS, AML, osteosarcoma (0.9%)
- **Dx:** Clinical: High erythrocyte adenosine deaminase activity, persistent fetal hemoglobin, erythroid paucity in marrow evaluation. Molecular sequencing
- **Clinical features:** Presents in early infancy (<1 y), growth retardation, congenital malformations (30–50%)

Kostmann syndrome/severe congenital neutropenia

- **Genetics:** Kostmann syn: *HAX1* mt (chromosome 1q21.3)
  Severe congenital neutropenia: *ELANE* (*ELA2*) (chromosome 19p13.3)
  Mts in the gene encoding a mitochondrial protein
- **Inheritance pattern:** AR
- **Hematology/oncology:** Neutropenia, MDS, AML
- **Dx:** Severe neutropenia (ANC <500/mm^3 on 3 CBCs in a mo)
  Promyelocytic–myelocytic arrest in marrow evaluation. Molecular sequencing
- **Clinical features:** Presents in infancy, mean dx age 3 y, recurrent fever +/– mucocutaneous infxns, +/– dysmorphic features

Thrombocytopenia absent radii syndrome

- **Genetics:** *RBM8A gene RBM8A gene RBM8A RBM8A* gene (chromosome 1q21.1 micro deletion)
- **Inheritance pattern:** AR, compound heterozygous
- **Hematology/oncology:** Thrombocytopenia
- **Dx:** Clinical. Severe thrombocytopenia
- **Clinical features:** Presents in early infancy, bilateral absence of radii w/ thumbs present, skeletal anomalies, cardiac anomalies, cow milk intolerance.

Molecular sequencing: sequential gene testing, next generation sequencing, whole exome sequencing.

Tx

	1st Line	Other	HCT	HCT Outcomes	Post-HCT Issues	Gene Therapy Targets
Fanconi Anemia	Supportive Care	Androgens Eltrombopag	Yes	OS at 5-y post HCT for MSD: 78% MUD: 65%	SCC	*FANCA (experimental)*
Dyskeratosis Congenita	Supportive Care	Androgens	Yes	5-y survival: 57% 10-y survival: 23%	Lung, Liver, GI late effects SCC	Telomere Lengthening *(experimental)*
Shwachman–Diamond Syn	Supportive Care, G-CSF		Yes		Liver Pancreas Issues	
Diamond–Blackfan anemia	Steroids	Eltrombopag	Yes	MUD: OS: 70–85%	Osteosarcoma	
Severe Congenital Neutropenia	G-CSF		Only MDS	OS: 82%		
Amegakarocytic Thrombocytopenia	Supportive Care Transfusions	Androgens Eltrombopag	Yes	5-y OS: 77%		
Thrombocytopenia Absent Radii Syn	Supportive Platelet transfusions		Yes			

SCC: Squamous cell carcinoma, GI: Gastrointestinal, MDS: Myelodysplastic Syndrome, AA: Aplastic Anemia, HCT: Hematopoietic Stem Cell Transplantation, G-CSF: Granulocyte colony stimulating factor, OS: Overall Survival, MUD: Matched Unrelated Donor, MSD: Matched Sibling Donor.

Pediatric indications for transplant

- **Autologous:** Rescue BM from severe pancytopenia after high-dose tx of malignancy
- **Standard of care:** NB (all high-risk), lymphoma (HL or NHL, chemosensitive relapsed dz in CR/VGPR), medulloblastoma (as per Head Start protocols to avoid RT, or for relapse), retinoblastoma (PR/CR2), germ cell tumors (PR/CR2)
- **Case-specific/on protocol:** Wilms tumor, Ewing sarcoma
- **Allogeneic:** Conditioning to eradicate dz or correct hematopoietic or immunologic defect → donor HSC infusion to replace/GVL effect

Category	Examples
Hematologic Malignancies	ALL, AML, CML, MDS, R/R lymphomas
Inborn Errors of Metabolism[a,b] (*Front Pediatr* 2019;7:433)	Hurler syn, MLD, GLD, ALD, Osteopetrosis
Hemoglobinopathies	Sickle cell dz, Thalassemia
1° Immunodeficiency Disorders	SCID, CID, Wiskott–Aldrich dz, LAD, CGD, Chediak–Higashi
1° Immune Regulatory Disorders	HLH, IPEX, ALPS, IBD, Rheumatologic d/o
BM Failure (see Bone Marrow Failure chapter)	Diamond Blackfan anemia[c], Fanconi anemia[c], Dyskeratosis congenita[c], Shwachman Diamond syn[c], Congenital neutropenia[c], Congenital amegakaryocytic thrombocytopenia[c], PNH[d], Aplastic anemia[d]

[a]*Highest success in pre-symptomatic phase.*
[b]*Other indications not listed here may be investigational.*
[c]*Inherited conditions.*
[d]*Acquired conditions.*

Pediatric pretransplant evaluation

- **H&P:** Comorbidities, allergies, FHx of genetic conditions
- **Labs:** CBC, renal & liver fxn, infectious dz markers
- **Other diagnostics:** Dz evaluate (eg, BMA/BMBx, LP, PET scan, MRI), cardiac evaluate (EKG, ECHO), pulmonary evaluate (SpO2, PFTs if able), occult infectious evaluate (CT CAP/sinus), dental clearance (evaluate for any nidus of infxn)

Pediatric graft sources

- BM is preferred over PBSC as the graft source for conventional HCT in pediatrics (*NEJM* 2012;367(16):1487–96; *J Clin Oncol* 2004;22(24):4872–80; *BMT* 2017;52(7):1071–1073)
- **PB:** ↑ CD34 count, most active CD3, ↓ rejection risk, early count recovery, ↑ GVHD
- **BM:** Mod CD34 count, active CD3, ↓ rejection risk, mod count recovery, moderate GVHD risk
- **UCB:** ↓ CD34 count, naïve CD3, mod rejection risk, late count recovery, ↓ GVHD

Pediatric transplant donors

- Refer to the Stem Cell Transplant section in adults for additional information on HLA typing, donors, etc.
- **HLA-matched related (eg, sibling):** Gold standard; lowest risk of GVHD & graft rejection; careful evaluation if pt may have heritable indication for transplant
- **HLA-matched unrelated:** MUD (8/8 or 10/10) not inferior to MRD re: EFS for pts w/ hematologic malignancies (*BBMT* 2012;18(8):1204–10); younger > older donor
- **HLA-mismatched related (eg, parent):** Haploidentical donor; most frequently combined w/ PTCy GVHD ppx; evaluate donor NK alloreactivity (for leukemia control) & recipient anti-HLA antibodies (for rejection risk)
- **HLA-mismatched unrelated donor:** Highest risk of GVHD & graft rejection
- **UCB:** Rapid availability, relatively naïve immune system → ↑ tolerability for HLA mismatch in the recipient, limited cell dose → delayed hematopoietic recovery

Pediatric GVHD prophylaxis

- **CNI+MTX:** Most common combo used for pts receiving MAC/BM graft
- **CNI+MMF:** Most commonly used for pts receiving UCB or RIC; reduced mucositis & facilitates engraftment compared to CNI+MTX (*BBMT* 2010;16(7):937-47)
- **PTCy:** Most commonly used for pts receiving haplo HCT (*BBMT* 2016;22(1):112–8); also consider in MUD for CNI-free GVHD ppx (BMT CTN 1301 Progress II Trial, *JCO* epub 2021)
- **T-cell depletion:** CD34+ selection or TCR-αβ depletion (usually w/ CD19 depletion); ↓ GVHD w/o add'l drugs, delayed immune reconstitution, ↑ infxn

Pediatric conditioning regimens

- Generally, MAC for pediatric pts, especially for malignancy; RIC for some PIDs or heavily pretreated pts; minimal use of NMA in pediatrics
- **Forms:** Chemo, TBI, serotherapy
- **Purposes:** Myeloablation (TBI, Bu, Mel, Thio), immunosuppression (TBI, Cy, Flu, Thio), antileukemic activity (TBI, Clo, Flu Bu-AML, Cy, Thio)
- Refer to the HCT section in adults for additional information on conditioning intensity

Considerations unique to pediatrics

- Vascular access, extracorporeal circuit volume, & blood flow rates are **limiting factors for PBSC collection** in small children donors
- Smaller pt size makes **UCB a more valuable source** than in adults. Favor single over double CBU in pediatrics unless limited by cell dose based on randomized trial w/ incr. GVHD & similar relapse (BMT CTN 0501, *NEJM* 2014 30;371(18):1685–94)
- **TBI** is generally not used for conditioning in pts ≤36 mos of age (ideally not ≤60 mos) d/t neurodevelopmental & growth concerns, & recipients of prior RT
- **Nonmalignant transplants:** More common in pediatrics than adults; consider when stable mixed donor–host chimerism might be sufficient & consider RIC
- **Ethical considerations:** Minor donors (independent donor advocate), creation of "savior children" w/ PGD selection for HLA-matched & unaffected siblings
- **Validated pediatric disease risk index (DRI):** Stratifies acute leukemia pts by age, dz status at transplant, & cytogenetic risk (*Blood* 2021;137(7):983–993)

Pediatric transplant complications

Infxns: 0–30 d: All bacterial, candida, RSV, HSV; 1–3 mos: Aspergillus, CMV, AdV, HHV6, VZV, EBV, toxo, PJP; 3–6 mos: CMV, AdV, HHV6, VZV, EBV, toxo, PJP

Engraftment syn:

- **RFs:** Rapid engraftment, cord blood, HLA mismatch
- **Sx: Fever, rash, capillary leak** w/ noncardiogenic pulmonary edema, fluid retention, liver dysfxn, renal insufficiency, transient encephalopathy
- **Tx:** High-dose corticosteroids followed by rapid taper

GVHD: Donor T lymphocytes activate & respond to HLA differences on recipient's tissue

- **RF:** Unrelated donor, HLA mismatch, female donors, older donors, PBSC graft
- **Ppx:** CNI+MTX or CNI+MMF; T-cell depletion (CD34+ or TCR-αβ depletion); either may also include ATG/alemtuzumab; PTCy (+CNI)

	Signs/Sxs	Txs
Acute GVHD <100 d *BJH* 1997;97:855 *Refer to the GVHD section in adults for additional information*	Skin: Rash, erythroderma, bullae, desquamation Liver: Jaundice, ↑ bilirubin Upper GI: N/V, anorexia Lower GI: Diarrhea, cramping, ileus, hematochezia	1st line: Steroids (topical &/or systemic) 2nd line: Ruxolitinib (≥12 y: REACH2, *NEJM*. 2020;382(19): 1800–1810), MSCs (*BBMT* 2020;(5): 845–854), ECP, infliximab (GI), alpha-1 antitrypsin
Chronic GVHD >100 d *Blood* 2017;129(1):30–37 *GVHD after 100 d includes classic chronic, acute-chronic overlap, & late acute*	Consider involvement of: Skin, joints/fascia, mouth, liver, upper/lower GI, esophagus, lungs, & eyes Score each organ system to determine **global severity score** Mild: 1–2 organs/sites, score ≤1, not involving lungs Moderate: ≥3 organs w/ score 1, or 1 organ w/ score 2, or lung score 1 Severe: ≥1 organ w/ score 3, or lung score 2: Usually extensive involvement, limiting ADLs	1st line: Steroids – Skin: Topical steroids, topical CNI, NB-UVB, acitretin - Pulm: FAM (fluticasone, azithromycin, montelukast) - GI: PO budesonide - MSK: PT/OT - Eyes: Tears, CSA/steroid gtts 2nd line: Ruxolitinib 3rd line: ECP, infliximab, ibrutinib (≥18 y) (*Blood* 2017;130(21):2243–2250; *BBMT* 2019;25(10):2002–2007)

- Skin GVHD: Use age-appropriate "rule of nines" for BSA in children
- Lower GI GVHD: Grade 1 = 280–555 mL/m^2/d; grade 2 = 556–833 mL/m^2/d; grade 3 = >833 mL/m^2/d diarrhea for children

Transplant-assoc thrombotic microangiopathy (*Blood Adv* 2021;5(1):1–11; *Blood* 2020;135(13):1049–1057)

- **RF:** RT, GVHD, unrelated donor, HLA mismatch, CNI, infxns

- **Sx: Microangiopathic hemolytic anemia, thrombocytopenia,** terminal complement activation (↑ sC5b-9), **proteinuria, hypertension,** renal dysfxn, other organ failures (CNS, GI, pulmonary), polyserositis
- **Tx:** Replace CNI/sirolimus w/ alternative GVHD ppx (eg, abatacept, steroids), eculizumab, plasma exchange

SOS/VOD:

- **RF:** Prior ozogamicin containing mAbs (inotuzimab/gemtuzumab), NB, infants, prior abd RT, prior HSCT, busulfan + 2nd alkylator, hepatic fibrosis, or iron overload
- **Sx:** Classically, Baltimore/Seattle criteria: RUQ pain, hepatomegaly, ↑ bilirubin, wt gain w/ ascites, coagulopathy, ultimately multiorgan failure; **pediatric-specific dx & severity criteria** are defined & include refractory thrombocytopenia, ascites, renal dysfxn; ↑ bilirubin late finding (*BMT* 2018;53:138–145)
- **Ppx:** Ursodiol, defibrotide used in some settings (*Lancet* 2012;379(9823):1301–1309)
- **Tx:** Defibrotide, consider pulse HD steroids. Supportive care for severe dz may include paracentesis or abd drain, renal replacement therapy, O_2/ventilatory support, blood product support

Post-transplant lymphoproliferative d/o: Usually donor-derived, monomorphic, & DLBCL morphology; monitor for EBV viremia & treat preemptively; evaluate w/ PET

- **RF:** EBV seropositive, UCB, haplo-identical, T-cell depleted, GVHD
- **Tx:** Rituximab, ↓ immunosuppression, EBV CTLs, DLI, RT; resect limited dz (tonsils)

Late complications: 2° malignancies (solid tumors from TBI, 2° leukemias, SCC from cGVHD), endocrine dysfxn (growth & hypothalamic-pituitary, thyroid, gonadal/reproductive, skeletal)

Cellular therapies in pediatrics

- **DLI:** Infusion of donor lymphocytes to mount graft-versus-tumor response in recipient (eg, tx of CML relapse after HCT)
- **CAR T cells:** Only FDA-approved product in pediatrics is tisagenlecleucel for CD19+ R/R B-cell ALL; toxicities include CRS, ICANS, infxn, TLS (*BBMT* 2019;25(4):625–638)
- **CTLs:** Infusion of allo or auto CTLs for elimination of viral or tumor targets (ie, viral targets: Phase III trials: EBV, CMV, AdV, BK, HHV6; tumor targets: Phase II trials: PRAME, WT1, survivin)

Post-transplant maintenance therapy

- Indicated for certain dzs: TKI for Ph+ ALL, CML if evidence of BCR-ABL, sorafenib/other TKI for *FLT3*-ITD AML (*BMT* 2019;54:1518–1520), brentuximab post-auto maintenance for HL (extrapolated from adults-AETHERA trial)
- Post-transplant azacytidine has been evaluated in pediatric AML pts but difficult to complete in practice d/t tolerance (*Pediatr Transplant* 2019;23(4):e13423)

Management of post-transplant relapse

- Universally poor outcomes for relapses <6 mos post-transplant
- >6 mo consider 2nd transplant if in CR, no ongoing GVHD, resolution of other toxicities

LOW GRADE ASTROCYTOMA AND OPTIC PATHWAY GLIOMA (OPG)

Epidemiology/risk factors
- Most common pediatric brain tumor (<15 y/o) w/ 14 new cases/1,000,000/y in United States
- RFs: NF1 (20% of OPG), Tuberous sclerosis (subependymal giant cell astrocytoma [SEGA])

Disease biology/pathology
- Insidious growth pattern (WHO Grade I/II), locally invasive. Cerebellar location > supratentorial & deep midline structures > optic pathway. ~90% of OPG are low grade gliomas (LGGs) & classified based on location as anterior or posterior visual pathway & NF1 germline or sporadic
- **Prognostic considerations:** ↓ PFS a/w: Age <1 y at dx, subtotal resection (brainstem/ deep thalamus), or high-risk **molecular alteration type** (see below)
- **Molecular considerations:** RAS/MAPK pathway is activated near universally in pLGG w/ 2 types of alterations (*J Clin Oncol* 2017;35:2934–2941)—(1) Rearrangement-driven pLGG (***BRAF-KIAA1549* fusion** is the most common alteration across pLGG, RTK fusion) & is considered low risk (*Nat Genet* 2013;45:927–932 & (2) single nucleotide variant (SNV)-driven pLGG (*BRAF* V600E, *FGFR1*) is considered intermediate/high-risk group, esp. in the presence of co-deletions (*CDKN2A*) (*J Clin Oncol* 2017;35:2934–2941)

Clinical presentation and diagnosis/workup
- Morning headache/emesis, CN palsies, seizures, focal motor deficits, visual field deficits, & precocious puberty (OPGs), Diencephalic syn (hypothalamic)
- OPG: Dx based on neuroimaging (bx if atypical) & ophthalmologic assessment
- Nonoptic pathway LGG: Bx, MR brain, MR spine (only if clinical sxs)

Treatment and outcomes/prognosis
- **Surgery:** Maximal safe resection, or bx if not feasible; typically not required in OPG.
- **Adjuvant tx:** Consider if recurrent, symptomatic or visual decline (OPG)
- **Chemo:** Carboplatin/vincristine or carboplatin monotherapy (low hypersensitivity)
- **Biologic therapy:** Emerging as preferred 2nd-line therapy w/ good response rates. MEK Inhibitor for *BRAF-KIAA1549* or *NF1* pLGG, BRAF Inhibitor for *BRAF* V600E mt. (*J Clin Oncol* 2017;35:2934–2941; *Nat Genet* 2013;45:927–932)
- **Radiation:** Effective but toxicity discourages upfront use. Avoided in NF1 given risk of stroke, moyamoya. Usually reserved for older pts w/ multiple recurrent dz
- LGG w/ GTR: Favorable 5-y PFS >90% & OS 99%; better prognosis in NF1-OPG

HIGH GRADE ASTROCYTOMA

Epidemiology/risk factors
- 10% of all pediatric CNS neoplasms. RFs: RT, CMMRD, Li–Fraumeni (*TP53*), NF1 (*Nature* 2012;482:226–231)

Disease biology/pathology
- Arise in the cerebral hemispheres, midline, & posterior fossa. Clinically aggressive, regionally invasive tumors. WHO grade III (anaplastic astrocytoma) & IV (glioblastoma)
- **Clinical prognostic considerations**: GTR a/w improved survival
- **Molecular/genetic considerations:** *MGMT* promoter methylation status—Clinical utility unclear in pediatrics, not independently prognostic (*N Engl J Med* 2005;352:997–100. *Neuro Oncol* 2011;13:317–323). Unknown if predictive d/t lack of RCTs). *H3K27* mutant diffuse midline glioma (DMG)—highly aggressive subset & generally considered WHO grade IV regardless of histology, w/ deep midline locations (incl. DIPG) (*Acta Neuropathol* 2015;129:669–678)

Clinical presentation and diagnosis/workup for staging
- Seizures, focal motor deficits, DIPG classic triad of long tract signs
- Workup: Brain MRI (w/in 72 h postop), MR spine (2 wks postop)

Treatment and outcomes/prognosis
- **Surgery:** Goal is maximal safe resection, or bx
- **Radiation:** Focal irradiation standard for all pHGG (except infant)
- **Chemo:** RT w/ alkylator-based chemo considered standard of care (temozolomide used most often) (*N Engl J Med* 2005;352:987–996; *Lancet* 2017;1645–1653)
  - DIPG: Consider bx for atypical presentation or for molecular profiling. No medical therapy has demonstrated benefit

- HGG, *BRAF* V600E mutated: BRAF & MEK inhibitor combination (investigational) (*Acta Neuropathol* 2015;129:669–678)
- HGG, hypermutant/CMMRD: TMZ refractory, Immune checkpoint inhibitor (investigational) (*J Clin Oncol* 2016;34:2206–2211)
- HGG, infant: RT avoided, carboplatin/etoposide or "BABY POG" regimen, targeted therapies if *NTRK/ALK/ROS* fusion detected (*NEJM* 1993;328:1725–1731)

- HGG 2 y OS <20%, DIPG: OS <1 y (<10% of pts survive >2 y)

MEDULLOBLASTOMA (MB)

Epidemiology

- 20% childhood brain tumors w/ 6 cases per 1,000,000/y (*J Clin Oncol* 2012;30:2648). Mean age: 6 y

Disease biology/natural history

- Highly malignant embryonal CNS (Small, round blue cell) tumor arising in cerebellum/posterior fossa. Mode of spread: Local invasion & CSF seeding
- 4 Histological groups: Classic, desmoplastic/nodular, & MB w/ extensive nodularity (generally SHH subgroup), large cell/anaplastic MB(LCA) (WHO 2016)
- Heterogeneous biology categorized into 4 major molecular subgroups seen in table (*Acta Neuropathol* 2016;131:821–831; *Nat Rev Dis Primers* 2019;5:1–20; *Brain Tumors in Children, Medulloblastoma chapter*, 2018)

Molecular Subgroups of Medulloblastoma

Molecular Subgroup	**WNT (10%)**	**SHH (30%)**	**Group3 (25%)**	**Group4 (35%)**
Age	Child/AYA	Infancy/AYA	Early Childhood	Childhood
Metastasis at dx	5%	15%	40%	35%
5-y OS	95%	75%	50%	75%
Genetic driver	*CTNNB1* *DDX3X*	*PTCH1, SUFU* *TP53*	*MYC/MYCN* *PVT*	*KDM6A* *SNCAIP*
Syndrome	FAP	Gorlin, GPR16 ELP1, Li–Fraumeni	*BRCA1/2* *PALB2*	*BRCA1/2* *PALB2*

Clinical presentation and diagnostic workup/staging

- Increasing ICP 2° to obstructive hydrocephalus, ataxia, dysmetria
- Diagnostic bx/resection, MRI brain (w/in 72 h postop). MRI spine w/ contrast (preop or 2 wks postop); LP w/ CSF cytology (2 wks postop) for staging. See M staging in table below (*Nat Rev Dis Primers* 2019;5:1–20)
- Clinical staging into risk groups for tx stratification, described in Table (*Acta Neuropathol* 2016;131:821–831)

M Staging in Medulloblastoma

Stage M0	No evidence metastasis
Stage M1	Microscopic tumor cells present in CSF
Stage M2	Gross nodular seeding in cerebral subarachnoid space/ventricles
Stage M3	Gross nodular seeding in spinal subarachnoid space
Stage M4	Extraneural metastasis (extremely rare, especially at initial presentation)

Clinical Staging by Age, Residual Tumor Size, Metastases, Histology

≥3 y, <1.5 cm^3 residual tumor, M0, no anaplasia
≥3 y, ≥1.5 cm^3 residual tumor, M1–M4, anaplasia (focal/diffuse)
<3 y, any M stage, +/– residual tumor, any histology

Treatment and outcomes/prognosis

- **Multimodal approach w/ surgery** (maximal safe surgical resection), CSI, chemo (*Nat Rev Dis Primers* 2019;5:1)
- **CSI:** SR: 2,340 cGy CSI w/ boost to tumor bed to dose of 5,400–5,580 cGy; HR: 3,600 cGy CSI w/ boost to tumor bed to dose of 5,400–5,580 cGy (*J Clin Oncol* 2006;24:4203; *Nat Rev Dis Primers* 2019;5:11)
- **Chemo:** Multiagent post RT (platinum containing regimen)
- **Infant risk group:** SHH or group 3. Irradiation sparing strategies. SHH subgroup have favorable survival w/ inclusion of intraventricular chemo (HIT-SKK'92) or Head start (high-dose chemo w/ stem cell rescue) but group 3 have poor survival (*Brain Tumors in Children, Medulloblastoma chapter*, 2018)

- **WNT subgroup:** De-escalation w/ reduced CSI & chemo under investigation.
- **PFS/cerebellar mutism:** 25% pts s/p resection (impaired language/emotional liability) (*Brain Tumors in Children, Medulloblastoma chapter*, 2018)
- 5-y EFS & OS for SR: 75–90%. 5-y OS for HR: 40–60%; Infants: 50–70%

EPENDYMOMA

Epidemiology and disease biology

- Glial tumors arising from ependymal lining of ventricular system. 2/3rd in posterior fossa. (*Neuro Oncol* 2018;20:450)
- WHO grading: Myxopapillary (Grade II); classic (Grade II); anaplastic (Grade III) (*J Neuro Oncol* 2017;135:202; *Neuro Oncol* 2021;23:1231–1251)
- 9 molecular subgroups across 3 anatomic areas: Spinal ependymoma (SP) includes MYCN-amplified; supratentorial (ST) includes *ZFTA* & *YAP1* fusion groups. Posterior fossa (PF) includes A & B groups (*Cancer Cell* 2015;27:728–743; *Neuro Oncol* 2021;23:1231–1251)

Diagnosis/workup

- MR brain & spine, LP for CSF cytology (*Neuro Oncol* 2018;20:446)

Treatment and outcomes/prognosis

- **Surgery:** Maximal safe surgical resection & **Focal irradiation** ~54–59.4 Gy following surgery if >1 yo; **Chemo:** No clear role, cytoreduction to facilitate GTR (*Neuro Oncol* 2018;20:447)
- 10-y OS 54–68% (*J Neuro Oncol* 2017;135:207). Outcomes vary by molecular subgroup (PF-B > PF-A, YAP > ZFTA) (*Cancer Cell* 2015;27:728–743)
- Poor prognostic factors: STR; 1q25 gain; 6q loss (PF-EPN-A); *CDKN2A/B* deletion (*EPN-ZFTA*) (*Clin Cancer Res* 2012;18:201)

MALIGNANT BONE TUMORS

Factor	Osteosarcoma	Ewing Sarcoma (ES)
Epidemiology (NIH Pub. 99-4649)	~400 cases per year	~200 cases per year
	More common in African Americans	More common in Caucasians
	Usually in long bones (~50% distal femur or proximal tibia)	Can be in bone or soft tissue (most commonly in the pelvis)
RFs	Previous radiation	Caucasian race
	Mt in *RB1* or *TP53*	Association w/ congenital hernia
X-Ray findings	Mixed sclerotic & lucent metaphyseal lesion w/ periosteal reaction	Periosteal reaction or calcification in soft tissue
	"Sunburst" appearance	"Onion-skinning"
Pathology	Osteoid production – various subtypes	Small round blue cell
		Positive staining for CD99
		EWSR1-FLI1 fusion t(11;22)(q24;q12) is most common mt

Clinical manifestations

- Most common sx is pain, sometimes related to trauma, not relieved by NSAIDs
- Palpable mass w/ swelling & loss of function of nearby joint
- Fever, wt loss, or constitutional sxs in advanced ES (*J Clin Oncol* 2000;18:4)

Diagnosis/staging

- Initially x-ray followed by MRI for better characterization
- Bx required to confirm dx
- Staged based on presence or absence of mets
- Noncontrast spiral CT of the chest to evaluate for pulmonary mets
- Bone scintigraphy to evaluate for bone mets or PET/CT to evaluate for bone or other mets
- BM evaluation can be considered in ES, but its role is controversial
- Most common sites of mets: Lungs or bone in both tumor types; BM in ES

Tx	
Osteosarcoma	Initial chemo consists of high-dose methotrexate, cisplatin & doxorubicin; ifosfamide & etoposide can be used in relapse
	Surgical resection of all detectable areas of dz incl. mets
	Insensitive to radiation
Ewing sarcoma	Initial chemo consists of cycles of vincristine, doxorubicin, & cyclophosphamide w/ ifosfamide & etoposide; irinotecan w/ temozolomide or cyclophosphamide w/ topotecan for relapse
	Incr. dose intensity by interval compression or incr. chemo dosage leads to improved outcomes
	Surgical resection, radiation, or both to primary tumor & mets
	Whole lung radiation for radiographically detectable pulmonary mets

Prognosis	
Osteosarcoma	EFS about 70% for localized dz (extremity tumors better than axial) (*J Clin Oncol* 2005;23:2004)
	EFS less than 20% for primary metastatic dz, better if only pulmonary mets (*Cancer* 2005;104:1100)
	90% or more tumor necrosis in response to neoadjuvant chemo a/w improved outcome
Ewing sarcoma	EFS approaching 75% for localized dz (*J Clin Oncol* 2012;33:4150)
	EFS about 20% for metastatic dz, better if only pulmonary mets (*J Clin Oncol* 2004;22:2873)

SOFT TISSUE SARCOMAS

Rhabdomyosarcoma

- **Epidemiology/RFs**
- 40% of all pediatric soft tissue sarcomas; uncommon in adults (*Cancer* 2009;115:4218)
- 3.5% of all tumors in children ages 0–14 (*Cancer* 2009;115:4218)
- **Histology & subtypes** (*Am J Pathol* 2009;174:550)
- Malignant tumor of mesenchymal origin
- Embryonal rhabdomyosarcoma—60–70% of cases
- Alveolar rhabdomyosarcoma—30% of cases; characterized by translocation b/w *FOXO1* & *PAX3* or *PAX7* genes (*Pediatr Blood Cancer* 2016;63:634)
- Other: Spindle cell/sclerosing (commonly paratesticular), pleomorphic (uncommon in children)

Initial workup:

- **Location:** – 1° sites can be disparate incl. GU tract (31%), head/neck region (25%), or extremities (13%) (*J Clin Oncol* 2001;19:3091)

Imaging

- CT chest to assess for pulmonary metastasis, MRI, or CT of the 1° site w/ evaluation of regional LNs, & whole-body PET scan to evaluate extent of dz
- Bilateral BM bxs for selected pts

Staging (*J Clin Oncol* 2003;21:78)

- Involves assignment of stage, clinical group, & risk group
- Stage determined by tumor site (favorable/unfavorable), size, presence of regional LN involvement, met
- Group determined by initial surgical procedure (resection/bx), margin, & LN involvement
- Risk group determined by histologic subtype, stage, & group

Tx

- Systemic chemo w/ local control (RT, surgical resection) (*J Pediatr Hematol Oncol* 2001;23:215)
- Intensity & duration of chemo dependent on risk group (*J Clin Oncol* 2014;32:3547)

Nonrhabdomyosarcomatous soft tissue sarcomas

Epidemiology/RFs

- Includes dozens of subtypes incl. fibrosarcomas, leiomyosarcomas, synovial sarcomas, desmoplastic small round cell tumors, alveolar soft part sarcomas, liposarcomas, nerve sheath tumors, Kaposi sarcoma (*Oncologist* 2008;13:668)
- Dependent on tumor type, arises from connective tissue, peripheral nervous system, smooth muscle, or vascular tissue

Initial workup

- Evaluate location/sxs
- Can develop in any part of the body, although most commonly in trunk/extremities (*J Pediatr Surg* 1992;27:241)
- Typically asx solid mass; systemic sxs rare

Imaging

- CT or MRI of 1° site, CT chest (to assess for pulmonary met), whole-body PET to evaluate extent of dz
- Core-needle bx or open incisional bx depending on location of mass

Staging

- Multiple staging systems, although 3 general risk groups accepted: (*Lancet Oncol* 2020;21:145)
- Low risk: Nonmetastatic R0, R1 low-grade tumor, or <5 cm high-grade tumor
- Intermediate risk: Nonmetastatic R0 or R1 >5 cm high-grade tumor, or unresected tumor (any grade/size)
- High risk: Metastatic tumor

Tx

- Dependent on risk group & resectability of tumor (*Lancet Oncol* 2020;21:145)
- Low risk: Surgical resection or radiotherapy alone
- Intermediate risk: Chemoradiotherapy (w/ consideration of neoadjuvant chemoradiotherapy if unresected)
- High risk: Surgery, chemoradiotherapy

NEUROBLASTOMA (NB)

Epidemiology

- Most common extracranial solid tumor of childhood: 650 cases per year in the United States, median age at diagnosis 18 mos, 90% dx'd before age 10 (*Paediatr Perinat Epidemiol* 2009;23(2):125–143)
- **RF:** Familial neuroblastoma d/t germline mts only accounts for 1–2 % of cases (mts in *ALK*, *PHOX2B*). NB cases are also detected in CA predisposition syn: Costello syn, Noonan syn, Turner syn, Beckwith–Weidemann syn, Simpson–Golabi–Behemel syn, Neurofibromatosis Type 1, Li–Fraumeni, Fanconi anemia & some chromosomal breakage syn (*Curr Opin Genet Dev* 2017;42:81)

Disease biology/natural history

- Tumor of the sympathetic nervous system arising anywhere along the sympathetic chain. Most 1° tumors occur in the adrenal gland, other common sites of origin include chest, neck, & pelvis
- 1 of the small round blue cell tumors of childhood (*Lancet* 2007;369:2106)

Clinical presentation/emergencies

- Clinical presentation: Abd mass, hypertension, Horner syn, subcutaneous skin nodules, proptosis/periorbital ecchymosis, bone pain, pancytopenia, fever. Opsoclonus-myoclonus-ataxia syn: Rare paraneoplastic presentation w/ cerebellar ataxia, or opsoclonus-myoclonus
- Emergency presentations: Cord compression w/ paralysis, SVC syn (see Cancer Complications, Radiation Oncology Emergencies, Pediatric Oncology Emergencies chapters)

Diagnosis/extent of disease evaluation (*J Clin Oncol* 2009;27:289)

- Tumor imaging: Cross-sectional imaging w/ CT/MRI of 1° & metastatic sites
  Radiolabeled ^{123}I-MIBG: ~90% of NB cases are MIBG avid (PET if MIBG-nonavid)
- Labs: CBC, CMP, LDH, Urine catecholamines: VMA, HVA
- Tumor tissue sampling: Bx to confirm dx, determine MYCN copy number, DNA index, presence of chromosomal aberrations; bone marrow aspirates/biopsies

International NB Risk Group Staging System (INRG) Staging for Risk Stratification	
L1	Localized dz, no image-defined RFs
L2	Locoregional tumor, ≥1 image-defined RF
M	Distant met (except MS, see below)
MS	Met confined to skin, liver, &/or BM (<10% involvement) in children < 18 mos of age

Recurrent genetic abnormalities (*Nat Genet* 2013;5:279)

- 50–60% have whole chromosomal gains causing hyperdiploid DNA content (a/w favorable prognosis in <12 mos), or segmental chromosomal aberrations w/ diploid content (inferior prognosis in 12–24 mos)
- Recurrent alterations include: *MYCN* amplification, loss of 1p, 11q deletion, gain of 17q, *ATRX* mt, *TERT* overexpression, *NRAS/KRAS* mts
- *MYCN* gene amplification: Detected in ~20% of all NB, enriched among pts w/ high-risk dz (~40%). Strong predictor of poorer prognosis across all dz stages (*J Clin Oncol* 2009;27:365)

Risk stratification (*J Clin Oncol* 2019;37:10012)

Low Risk	INRG L1, MS Any age (for MS <18 mos) No *MYCN* amplification
Intermediate Risk	INRG L2 or INRG M w/ favorable tumor biology & <18 mos No *MYCN* amplification
High Risk	Any INRG w/ *MYCN* amplification INRG M ≥18 mos

Spontaneous regression (*J Clin Oncol* 2000;18:477)

- Can be seen in infants, particularly those w/ MS pattern of metastatic spread
- Infants w/ asx, small, low-stage adrenal neuroblastoma can be observed

Treatment (*J Clin Oncol* 2019;37:3243)

Low Risk **>95% survival**	Surgery + Observation
	Chemo (life or organ threatening sxs, recurrent/progressive dz) +/− surgery
	Observation w/out bx (perinatal small adrenal tumor)
	Radiation (emergency therapy)
Intermediate-Risk **70–90% survival**	Chemo +/− surgery
	Surgery + observation
	Radiation
High-Risk **50% survival**	Chemo, surgery, tandem transplant,, radiation, immunotherapy w/ anti-gd2 antibody +/− isotretinoin (*JAMA* 2019;322:746)

Prognosis

Prognostic features include age at dx, tumor histology (INPC/Shimada: Favorable or unfavorable histology), *MYCN* status, DNA index (ploidy), stage of dz, response to tx, lactate dehydrogenase, & ferritin levels (*J Clin Oncol* 2011;29:3286)

Recurrent/refractory disease

High risk: Tx options include chemoimmunotherapy (most commonly irinotecan, temozolomide, anti-gd2 immunotherapy), ^{131}I-MIBG therapy, ALK inhibitors in pts w/ ALK mts, intermediate- or high-dose chemo. +/− surgery & radiation (*Oncoimmunology* 2015;4:e1016704)

HEPATIC AND RENAL TUMORS

Most common pediatric hepatic/renal tumors

	Hepatoblastoma	Wilms Tumor
Epidemiology	- 100 cases/y in the United States - Rapidly increasing in prevalence by 5%/y - Median age of 18 mos - Low birth wt & prematurity are important RF as well as CA predisposition (BWS, FAP) (*Oncologist* 2008;13(7):812–820)	- 500 cases/y in the United States - Median age of 3 y for unilateral cases & 2 y for bilateral cases - 5–10% of cases are bilateral & 10% of cases w/ CA predisposition (WAGR, Denys–Drash, BWS)
Histology	- Arise from hepatocyte precursors - Majority are of mixed epithelial subtype; 2 prognostically relevant rare subtypes are pure fetal (excellent outcome) & small cell undifferentiated (poor outcome; hepatic rhabdoid tumor) (*Mod Pathol* 2014;27(3):472–491)	- Arise from nephrogenic precursors which may include blastemal, epithelial, & stromal elements - Distinguished by absence (favorable; 90%) or presence (unfavorable; 10%) of anaplastic cells which can be focal or diffuse (*Pediatr Dev Pathol* 2005;8(3):320–338)
Genetics	- Nearly all cases have activation of WNT/β-catenin signaling pathway, most often via point mt or deletion in *CTNNB1* (*Hepatology* 2017;65(1):104–121)	- 1/3 of favorable cases have a mt in *WT1, CTNNB1, or WTX* genes - LOH 1p, LOH 16q, & 1q gain are unfavorable cytogenetic findings - 1/2 of unfavorable cases have *TP53* loss of fxn (*J Med Genet* 2006;43(9):705–715; *Nat Genet* 2017;49(10):1487–1494)
Presentation	Asx abd mass, wt loss, >90% w/ elevated AFP	Asx abd mass +/– hypertension, hematuria
Diagnosis	Imaging (U/S, CT/MRI), tumor markers (AFP, b-hCG), bx	Imaging (U/S, CT/MRI), nonspecific labs (consider vWF given risk of a VWD)
Staging	- Surgical (1: Complete resection w/ clear margin, 2: Gross resection w/ microscopic margins, 3: Gross resection w/ nodal involvement or spillage, 4: Metastatic dz) - Radiographic (PRETEXT: I: 3 contiguous sectors not involved, II: 2 contiguous sectors not involved, III: 1 contiguous sector not involved, IV: All 4 sectors involved). Annotation factors: VPEFR (vena cava, portal bifurcation, extrahepatic contiguous extension, focal liver tumor, rupture) (*Lancet Oncol* 2017;18:122)	I: Completely resected; tumor confined w/ in capsule II: Completely resected; penetration of capsule or invasion of renal vasculature III: Incomplete resection or regional LN involvement IV: Distant mets (lung most common site) V: Bilateral kidney involvement (*J Clin Oncol* 2006;24(15):2352–2358)

Treatment	- Very low risk (pure fetal, resectable up-front) is treated w/ resection alone (no chemo) - All other pts receive cisplatin-based chemo regimens - 20–30% have resectable dz at dx - Consider liver transplant in pts w/ unresectable tumors w/out distant mets	- Very low risk (<2 y, <550 gm tumor, stage I) receive resection alone (no chemo) - All other pts receive (usually) upfront surgery, chemo +/− radiotherapy depending on stage/histology &, for favorable histology: The presence of high-risk cytogenetics
Prognosis	- Dependent on histologic subtype, PRETEXT (lower is better), AFP (<100 ng/mL is poor), Age (younger is better) - Generally, OS >90% (*Curr Opin Pediatr* 2014;26(1):19–28)	- Dependent on histologic subtype, staging, molecular features, age (<2 y better) - FH: 5 y OS >90%; UH: OS 30–80% (*J Clin Oncol* 2006;24(15):2352–2358)

Less common hepatic tumors (*Clinical Liver Disease* 2018,753–772)

- **Hepatocellular carcinoma:** 2nd most common pediatric hepatic malignancy, more common in AYA; AFP elevated in 70% cases, managed analogously to adult HCC **(see HCC chapter)** w/ chemo, TKIs, immunotherapy; Adolescents commonly have distinct fibrolamellar subtype characterized by a *DNAJB1-PRKACA* fusion
- **Undifferentiated embryonal sarcoma:** 3rd most common pediatric hepatic malignancy, peak incidence b/w 6–10 y/o, AFP not incr., managed analogously to other sarcomas

Less common renal tumors

- **Clear cell sarcoma:** 2nd most common pediatric renal tumor, age overlaps w/ WT; t(10;17)(q22;p13) or *BCOR* internal tandem duplication; can metastasize to brain & bones, treat w/ more intensive chemo than FHWT
- **Congenital mesoblastic nephroma:** Usually dx'd in neonatal period, low malignant potential, complete nephrectomy for tx w/ OS >95%; for unresectable cases consider TRK inhibition since many of these have *NTRK3* fusions (*Pediatr Blood Can* 2017;64(7))
- **Malignant rhabdoid tumor:** Most pts <2 y, loss of *SMARCB1* results in INI1 protein loss, poor prognosis w/ OS <25%, usually aggressive/metastatic at dx, treat w/ more intensive chemo than FHWT; 1/3 of pts will be genetically predisposed (*J Clin Oncol* 2005;23(30):7641–7645)
- **Renal cell carcinoma:** Rare in childhood, 50% of cases involve unique translocation at Xp11.2; can be a/w VHL, tuberous sclerosis, prior oncologic tx; In adolescent boys > girls w/ sickle trait & a renal mass, concern for renal medullary carcinoma, which has very poor outcomes (*J Urol* 2015;193(4):1336–1341)

RETINOBLASTOMA (RB)

Epidemiology and disease biology

- Incidence: Estimated 4 cases per 1 million children younger than 15 y
- Unilateral dz: Median age of dx is 24 mos
- Bilateral dz: Median age of dx is 10 mos

Genetics (*Clin Cancer Res* 2017;23(13):e98–e106)

- Heritable (40%): *RB1* gene germline mt, unilateral or bilateral. Early age of dx
- Nonheritable (60%): Somatic allele mt, unilateral

Clinical presentation/emergencies

- Bilateral dz typically present in 1st 12 mos
- Presentation w/ leukocoria or strabismus (intraocular) or proptosis (extraocular)
- Late presentation includes bupthalmosis, hypopyon, orbital cellulitis
- Pathognomonic mt: Loss of fxn in RB1 gene on chromosome 13q

Diagnosis

- Dilated eye examination, especially number, location, size of tumor, vitreal seeding
- Ocular U/S & MRI Orbit/Brain to differentiate RB from other cause of leukocoria
- Bone scan, BM, LP if suspected extraocular dz or high-risk path in enucleated eye (massive choroidal invasion, optic nerve involvement beyond lamina cribrosa)

International Retinoblatoma Staging System (*Ped Blood Cancer* 2006;47[6]:801–805)

Stage	Description
Stage 0	Pts treated conservatively
Stage I	Eye enucleated, completely resected histologically
Stage II	Eye enucleated, microscopic residual tumor
Stage III	Regional extension a. Overt orbital dz b. Preauricular or cervical LN extension
Stage IV Metastatic dz	a. Hematogenous met (w/out CNS involvement) 1. Single Lesion 2. Multiple lesions b. CNS extension (w/ or w/out any other site of regional or metastatic dz) 1. Prechiasmatic lesion 2. CNS mass 3. Leptomeningeal & CSF dz

Treatment of intraocular retinoblastoma

- Enucleation of large tumors, +/– adjuvant chemo based on path risk
- When eye & vision can be saved, eye salvage w/ chemoreduction w/ systemic or ophthalmic artery infusion chemo +/– intravitreal chemo
- Local txs: Cryotherapy, thermotherapy, plaque RT

Treatment of extraocular retinoblastoma

- Platinum based chemo, enucleation, RT (45–50 Gy) +/– auto HSCT

Outcome, mortality, and late effects

- 5-y survival rate of 96%. Survival decreases w/ extraocular dz
- Pts w/ germline *RB1* mts are at risk for subsequent neoplasms, especially osteosarcoma, soft tissue sarcoma, melanoma
  - Dose dependent a/w radiation
- Late effects: Visual field defects, strabismus, potential for hearing loss after systemic carboplatin, therapy-related AML. Facial deformity & subsequent neoplasms after RT

Screening

- Positive family h/o RB, early fundus exam under general anesthesia & genetic evaluation
- Known or presumed germline *RB1* mt monthly exams for 1st y of life

Trilateral retinoblastoma (*Lancet Oncol* 2014;15(10):1157–1167)

- Bilateral RB + intracranial midline tumor (ie, pineoblastoma), 5–15% of children w/ heritable RB, dismal prognosis

GERM CELL TUMORS

Epidemiology

- Incidence: Rare in children <15 yo, representing 3% of new dxs (primarily 0–4 y); 14% of CA in adolescents b/w 15–19 y, reflecting a bimodal age distribution
- **RF:** Klinefelter (47XXY), Swyer (46XY), Turner (46X or XO) syn; cryptorchidism

Disease biology/natural history

- Embryologically, the primordial germ cell is a pluripotent cell which migrates & proliferates along the genital ridge destined to form gonadal & extragondal tissues
- GCTs are derived from the aberrant differentiation of the primordial germ cell & can be classified broadly as a teratoma (mature or immature) or a malignant GCT
  - Can be further classified by involvement of extragonadal sites (E), ovary (O) or testes (T)

Teratoma:

- Mature teratoma (EOT): Differentiated tissue derived from all 3 germ layers; benign
- Immature teratoma (EOT): All 3 germ cell layers but containing immature neuroepithelial tissue graded in degree from 0–3; uncertain malignant potential, +/– AFP ↑

Malignant GCT (often mixed histology w/ 1+ subtype):

- Yolk sac (endodermal sinus) tumor (EOT): Most common MGCT in young children; AFP ↑
- Choriocarcinoma (EOT): Arising from placental chorion cells; β HcG ↑
- Embryonal carcinoma (ET): No elevation in tumor markers
- Germinoma: Seminoma (T), dysgerminoma (O), gonadoblastoma (OT), germinoma (E)

Clinical presentation/diagnosis

- Dependent on 1° location & presence of mets; Mediastinal: Chest pain, shortness of breath, pleural effusion; Testicular: Painful/painless irregular mass, hydrocele; Ovarian: Pain, mass; CNS: Headache, diabetes insipidus
- Serum markers (AFP, β HCG, LDH); imaging dictated by site, CT scan/MRI/US
- Cytogenetics: Loss of 1p, 4, 6q; gain 1q (0–14 yo); Isochrosome 12; loss 1p, 11,13, 18; gain: 7, 8, 21 (15–39 y)

Staging

- Multiple systems: COG uses postsurgical classification for young children (EOT) vs. IGCCC (T)/ FIGO (O) for AYA/Adult. MaGIC-common risk stratification for staging in pediatrics (*J Oncol Pract* 2019;15:433)

COG Staging

Stage	T	O	E
I	Complete resection, negative nodes	Limited to ovary (peritoneal negative)	Complete resection w/ negative margins
II	Transscrotal Bx, microscopic dz in scrotum/cord, failure of markers to normalize	Microscopic residual, peritoneal evaluate negative, failure of serum markers to normalize	Microscopic residual dz, LN negative
III	RP LN involved, no extra-abd	LN involvement, contiguous visceral involvement (omentum, intestine, bladder), peritoneal +	LN involvement, gross residual dz
IV	Distant mets, incl. liver	Distant mets, incl. liver	Distant mets, incl. liver

MaGIC risk stratification

Risk Group	Site	Stage	Age (Years)
Low	Testis, Ovary, Extragonadal	I	Any
Standard 1	Testis, Ovary, Extragonadal	II–IV	<11
Standard 2	Testis (IGCCC good risk)	II–IV	>11
	Ovary	II–IV	>11
	Extragonadal	II	>11
Poor	Testis (IGCCC intermediate/ poor risk)	II–IV	>11
	Ovary	IV	>11
	Extragonadal	III–IV	>11

Treatment

- Conventionally involves use of platinum-based chemo
- COG AGCT1531-ongoing phase III trial: Surveillance (low risk) vs. combination bleomycin, etoposide & cisplatin/ carboplatin in treating pediatric pts w/ extracranial GCT

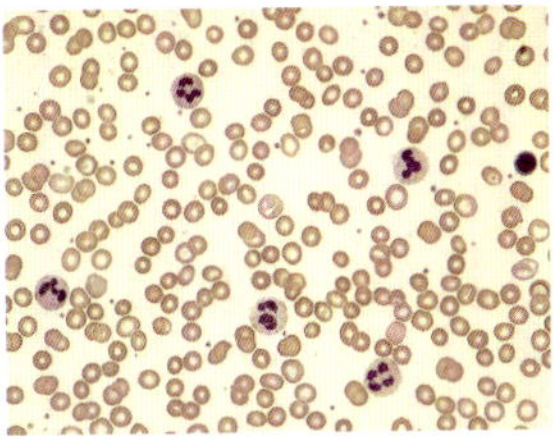

1. Normal peripheral blood: Smear contains granulocytes, a relatively uniform red cell population, and platelets.

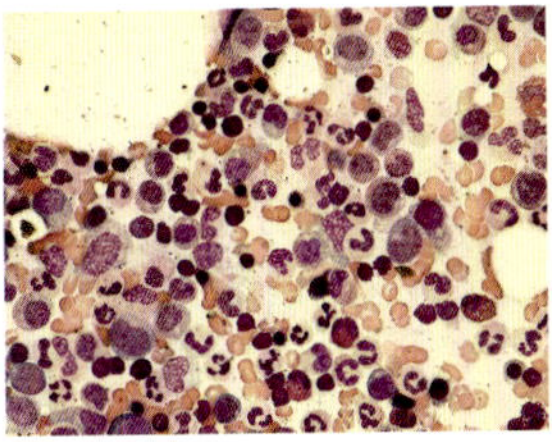

2. Normal bone marrow aspirate: Heterogeneous population with maturing elements in multiple lineages.

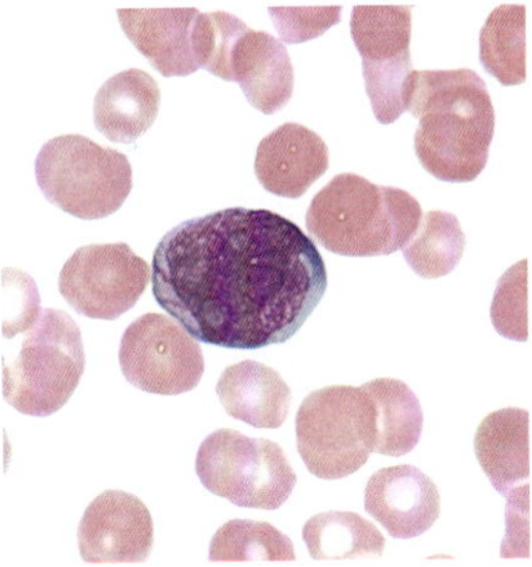

3. Myeloid blast with Auer rods: Immature cell with high nuclear cytoplasmic ratio and distinctive cytoplasmic inclusions.

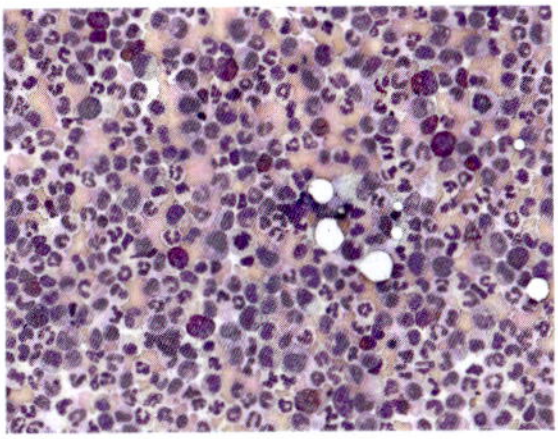

4. Chronic myelogenous leukemia—bone marrow aspirate: Hypercellular aspirate with increased M:E ratio and eosinophilia.

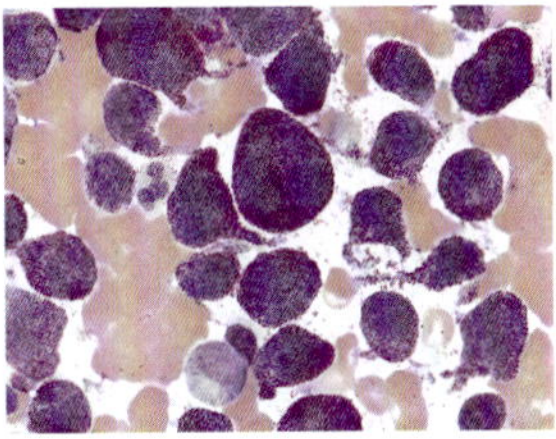

5. Mast cell leukemia—bone marrow aspirate: Irregular, immature cells with metachromatic staining granules.

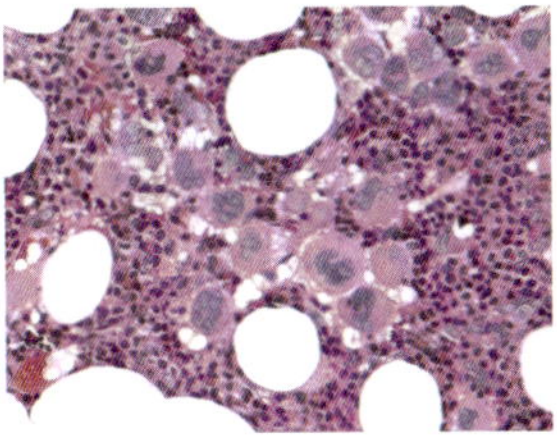

6. Essential thrombocythemia—bone marrow biopsy: Megakaryocytes are increased and appear in clusters.

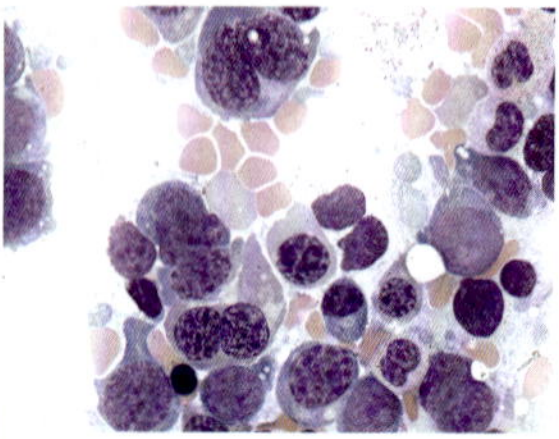

7. Myelodysplastic syndrome—bone marrow aspirate: Dysplastic erythroid elements are increased and display nuclear cytoplasmic asynchrony.

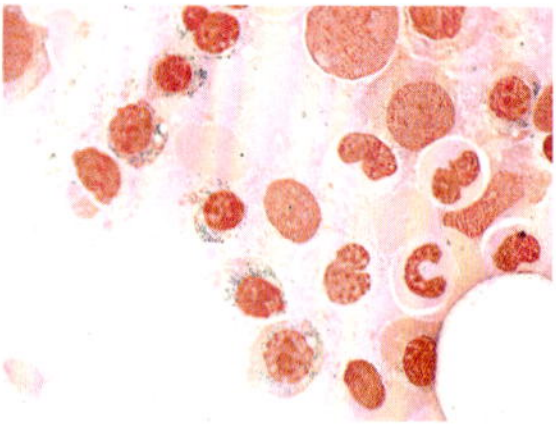

8. Ring sideroblasts (MDS)—bone marrow aspirate with iron stain: Iron stain demonstrates abnormal localization in the perinuclear mitochondria.

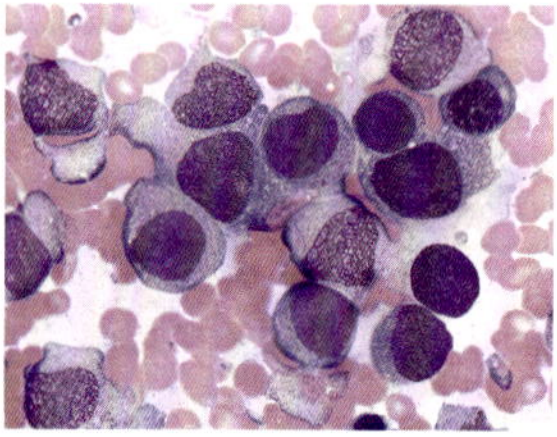

9. Acute monocytic leukemia—bone marrow aspirate: Blasts appear regular with ample cytoplasm.

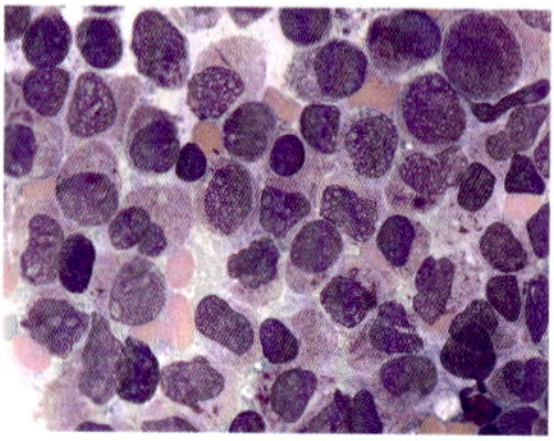

10. Acute promyelocytic leukemia—bone marrow aspirate: Heavy granulation obscures the nuclear cytoplasmic border.

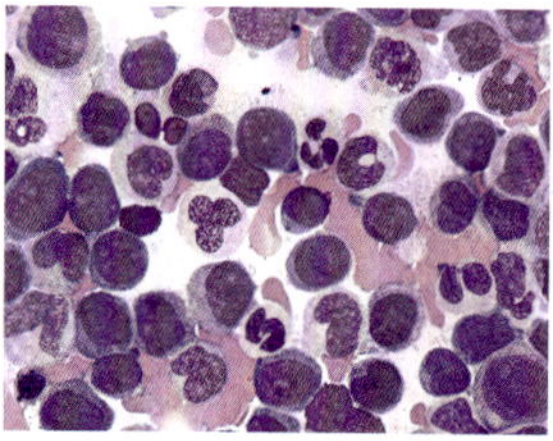

11. Acute myeloid leukemia with myelodysplasia-related changes—bone marrow aspirate: Blasts are increased with dysplastic changes in other lineages.

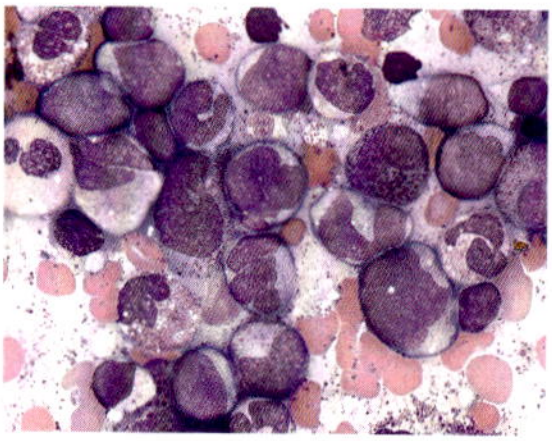

12. Acute myelomonocytic leukemia—bone marrow aspirate: Marrow contains both immature monocytic and myeloid elements with characteristic basoeosinophils.

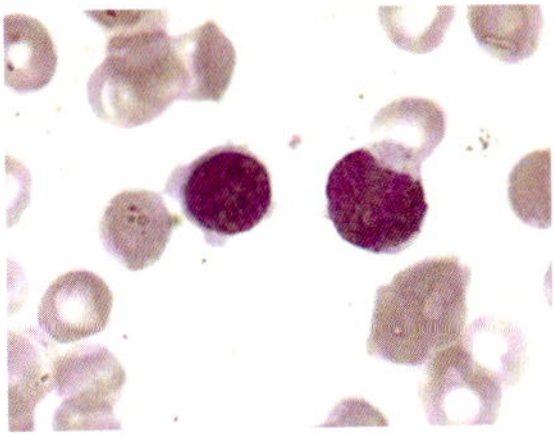

13. Acute megakaryocytic leukemia—bone marrow aspirate: Blasts are undifferentiated with cytoplasmic blebs.

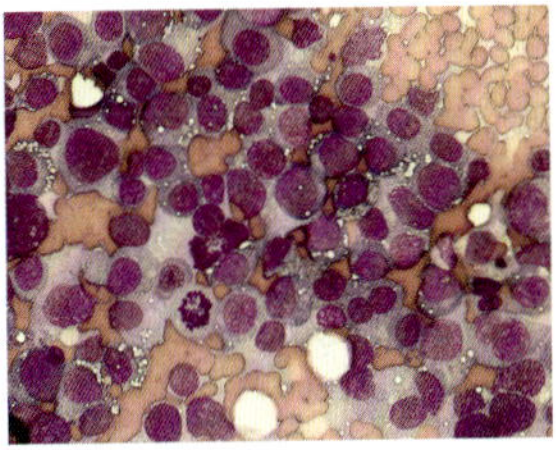

14. Pure erythroid leukemia—bone marrow aspirate: Proerythroblasts predominate the marrow.

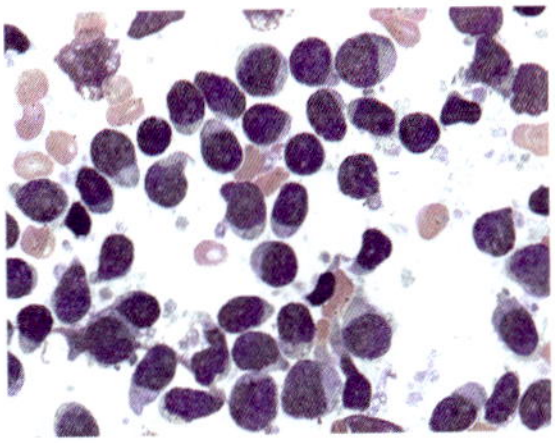

15. Blastic plasmacytoid dendritic cell neoplasm—bone marrow aspirate: Rare disorder is classified with the myeloid leukemias.

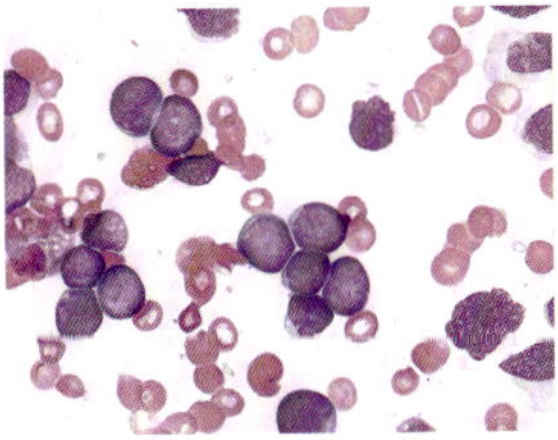

16. Acute lymphoblastic leukemia—bone marrow aspirate: Blasts with scant cytoplasm and smooth nuclear chromatin.

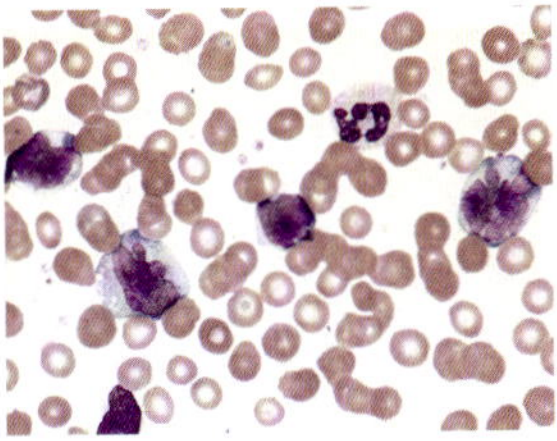

17. Adult T-cell leukemia/lymphoma—peripheral blood: Characteristic "flower cells" circulate in the blood.

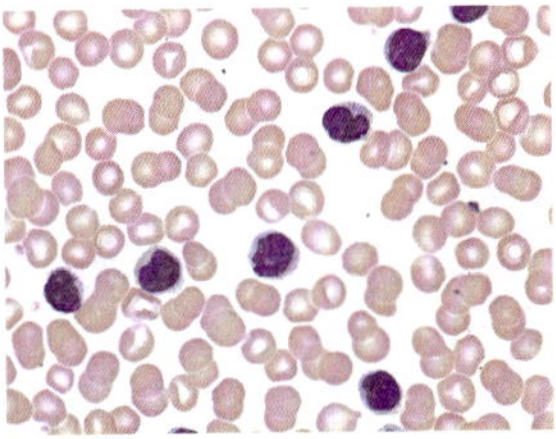

18. T-cell prolymphocytic leukemia—peripheral blood: Malignant cells often have indistinct nucleoli and irregular nuclear contours.

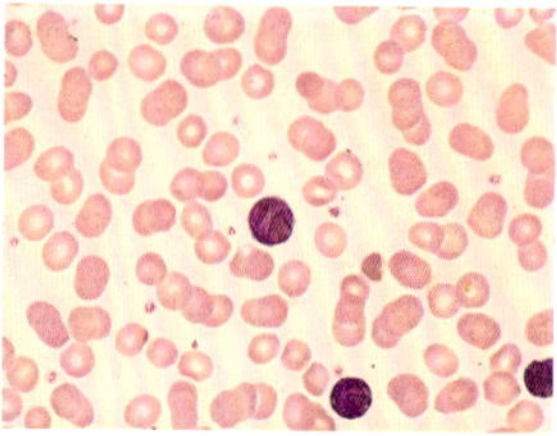

19. Sézary syndrome—peripheral blood: Cells have folded, irregular nuclei.

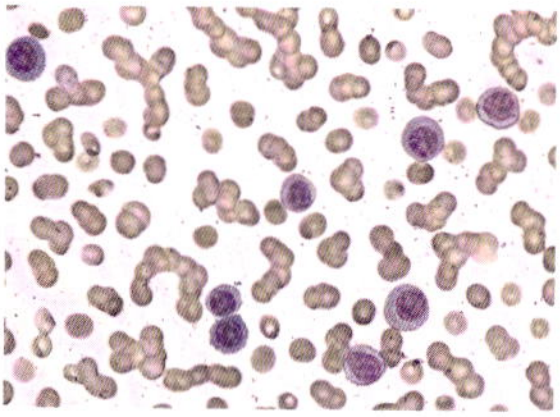

20. Plasma cell leukemia—peripheral blood; circulating plasma cells are often accompanied by rouleaux formation in the red blood cells.

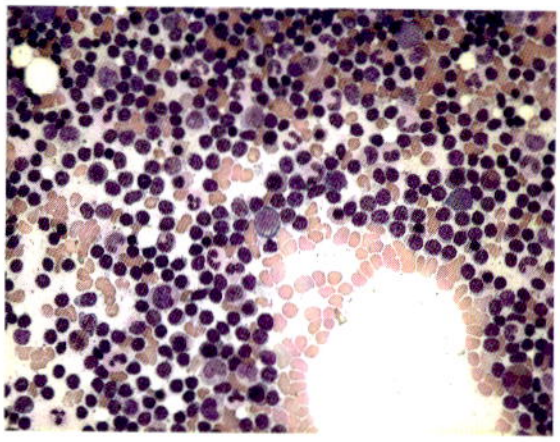

21. Chronic lymphocytic leukemia—bone marrow aspirate: Marrow replaced by well-differentiated lymphocytes.

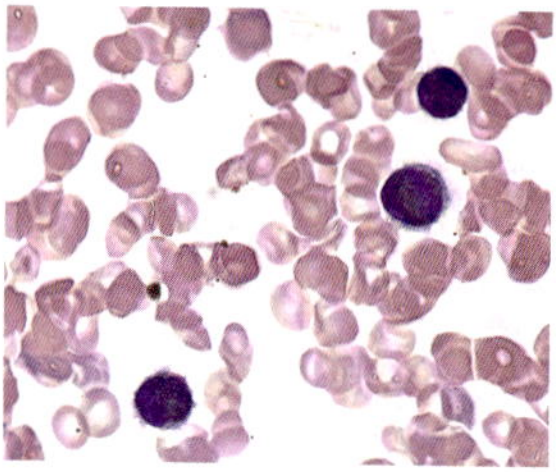

22. Hairy cell leukemia—bone marrow aspirate: Cells have characteristic cytoplasmic projections.

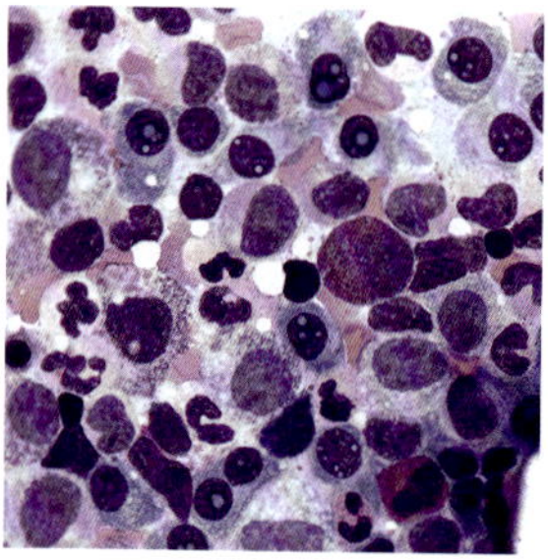

23. Multiple myeloma with Dutcher bodies—bone marrow aspirate: Sheets of plasma cells with distinctive nuclear inclusions.

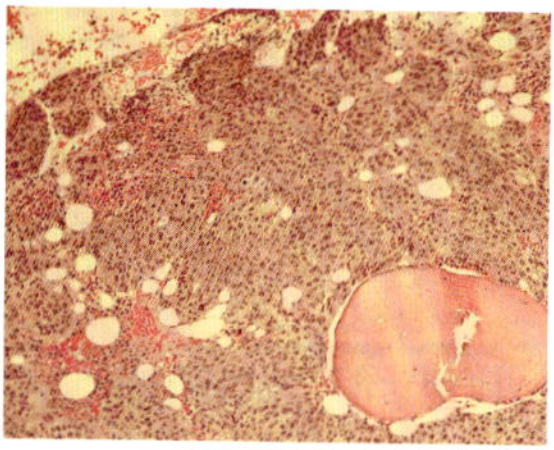

24. Metastatic breast cancer—bone marrow biopsy: Tumor cells disrupt the normal marrow architecture.

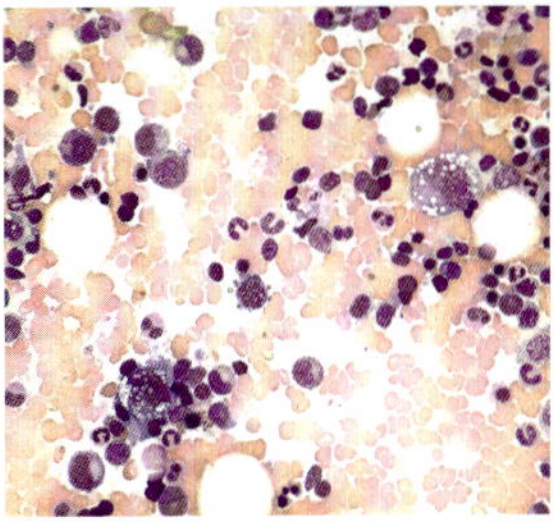

25. Anaplastic large cell lymphoma: Bone marrow aspirate contains large pleomorphic lymphoma cells scattered among normal hematopoietic elements.

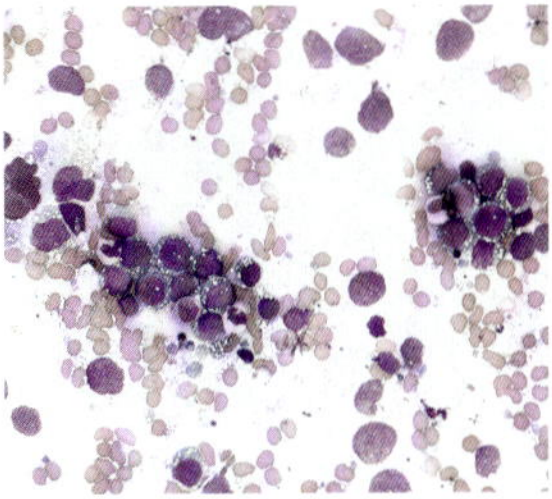

26. Burkitt lymphoma: Lymphoma cells are deeply basophilic with characteristic vacuolization.

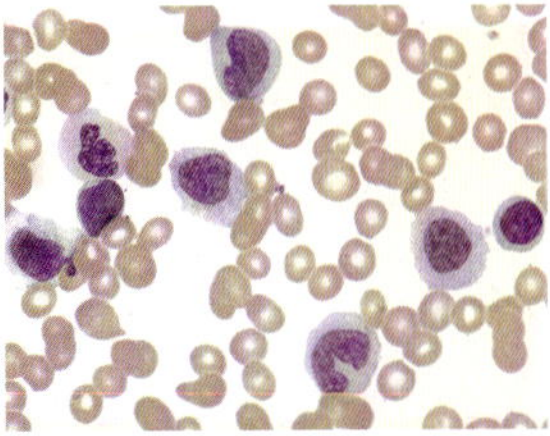

27. Chronic myelomonocytic leukemia: Monocytes are increased in the peripheral blood. Some appear immature while others are dysplastic.

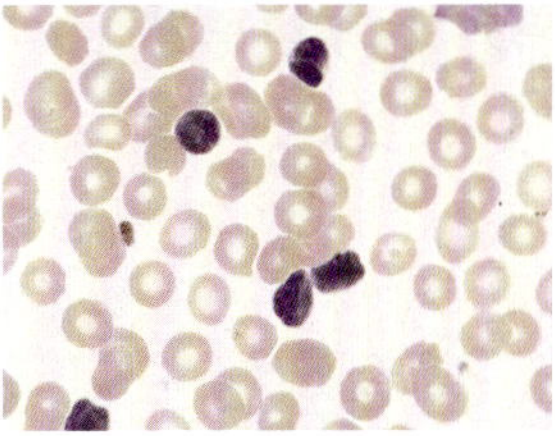

28. Follicular lymphoma: Involvement can be difficult to ascertain in the bone marrow aspirate. Here there are few small lymphocytes with cleaved/clefted nuclei.

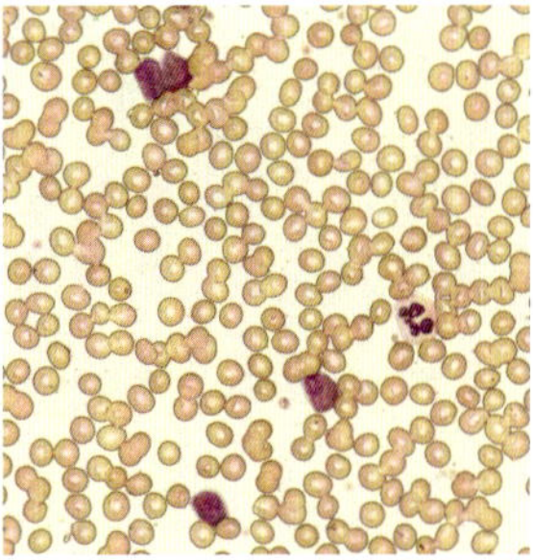

29. Mantle cell lymphoma: Lymphoma cells circulating in the peripheral blood are larger than normal lymphocytes and have a smooth appearance to the nuclear chromatin.

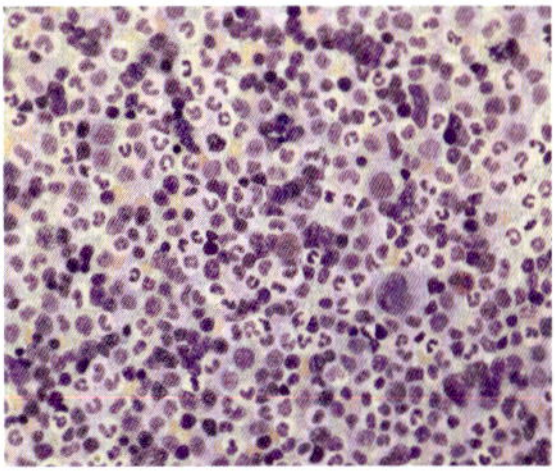

30. Myeloproliferative neoplasm: Bone marrow aspirate has a marked increase in the M:E ratio. Dysplastic myeloid forms with abnormal lobulation of the nuclei or hypogranulation of the cytoplasm are also noted.

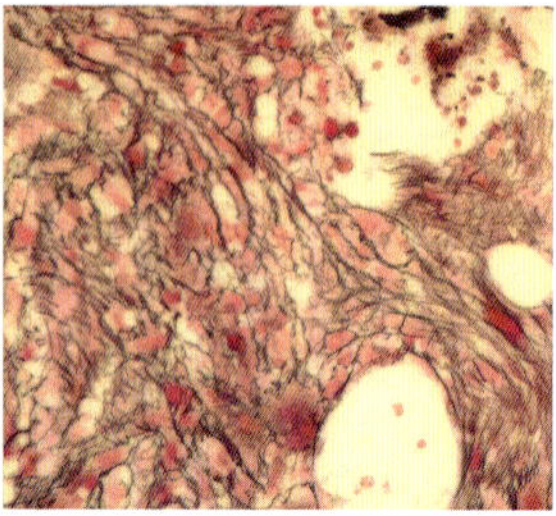

31. Primary myelofibrosis: Silver stain of the biopsy reveals marked reticulin fibrosis.

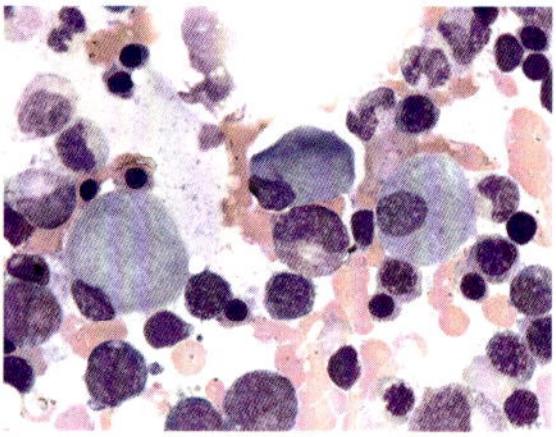

32. Pseudo-Gaucher cells: These are histiocytes with abundant pale blue fibrillar cytoplasm. They can be found in marrow of patients with CML or other myeloproliferative/myelodysplastic disorders.

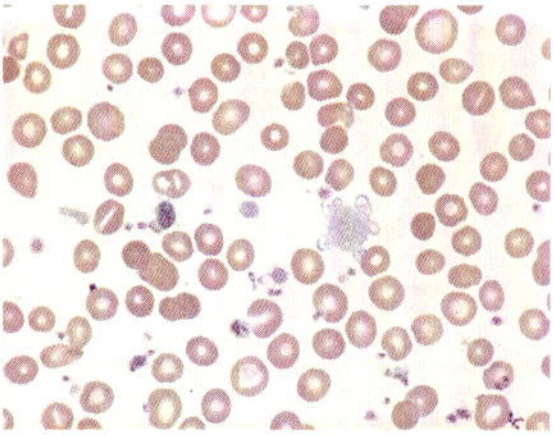

33. Abnormal platelets: A variety of giant platelet forms are noted in this peripheral smear from a patient with a myeloproliferative neoplasm.

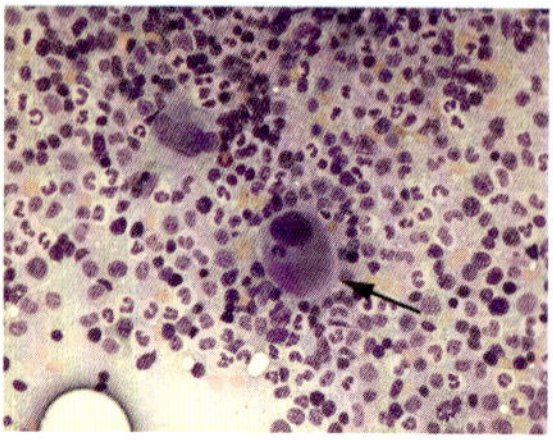

34. Megakaryocytic emperipolesis: *Arrow* marks megakaryocyte where a neutrophil can be seen transiting through the cytoplasm. This is not a distinct pathologic finding although it may be increased in certain disease like myelofibrosis.

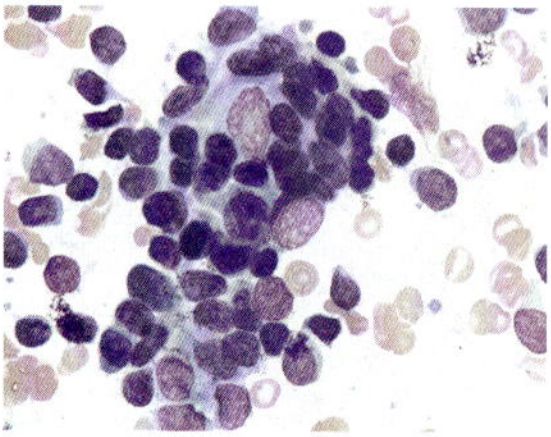

35. Hemophagocytic lymphohistiocytosis: In this pediatric case, histiocytes in the bone marrow are engulfing large numbers of lymphocytes.

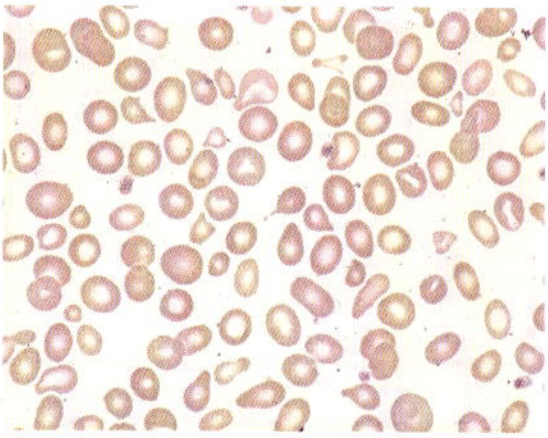

36. Anisocytosis/Poikilocytosis: Peripheral smear with wide variation in red cell size and shape. Such findings can be seen in hemoglobinopathies of myelodysplastic syndromes.

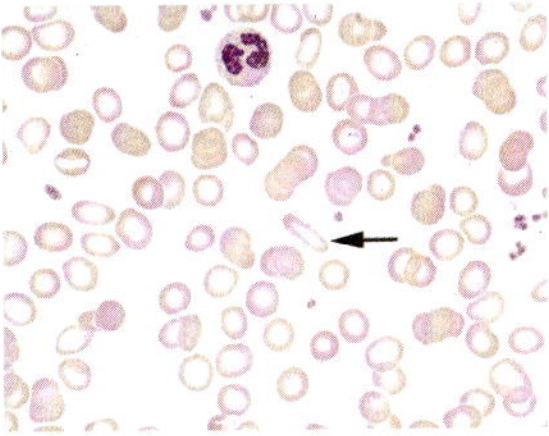

37. Iron deficiency anemia: Peripheral smear with hypochromic red cells and microcytes. *Arrow* marks a "pencil" cell.

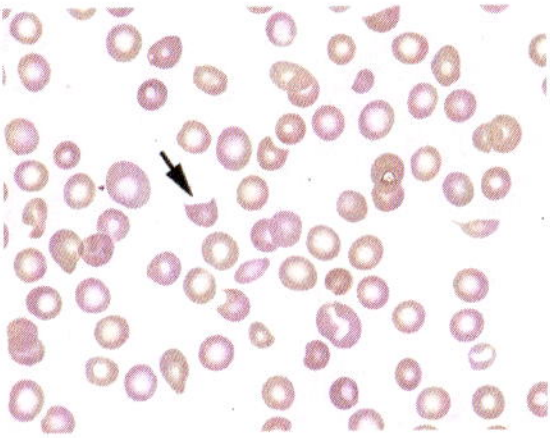

38. Schistocytes: *Arrow* marks classic schistocyte or "helmet cell" in this patient with a microangiopathic hemolytic anemia. Horn cells and other fragmented forms are also seen.

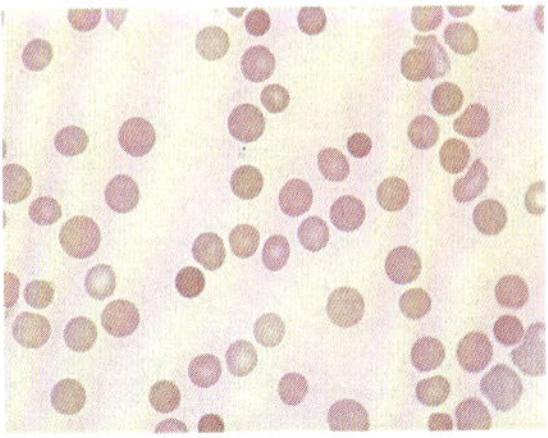

39. Spherocytes: These red cells lack the classic central pallor of normal erythrocytes. These forms are the result of membrane loss which causes a decrease in cytoplasm to cell surface ratio.

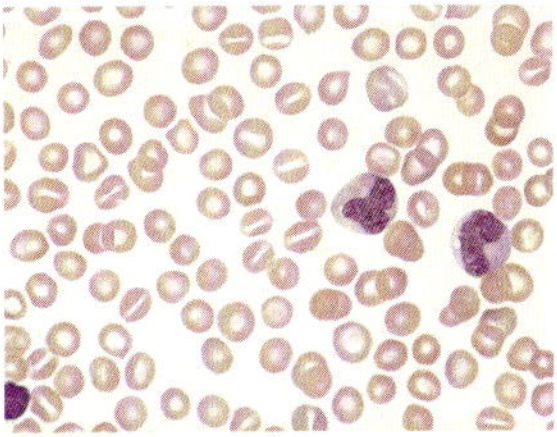

40. Stomatocytes: These red cells have a slit like central area of pallor as opposed to the round shape seen in normal erythrocytes. They can been seen in a form of inherited hemolytic anemia or in reaction to some drugs.

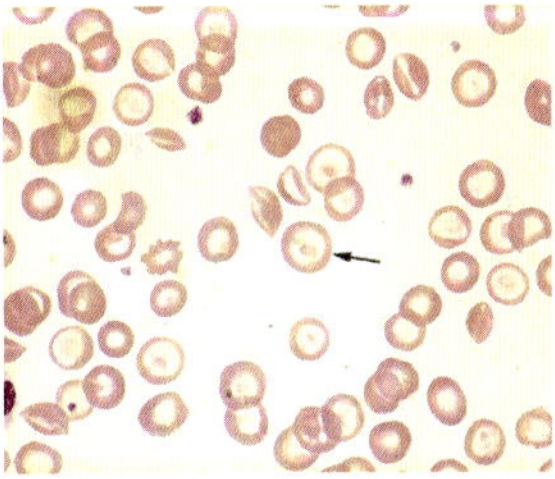

41. Target cells: In these cells, the central area of pallor has a cluster of hemoglobin located in the middle given the characteristic shape when the cell is seen in two dimensions.

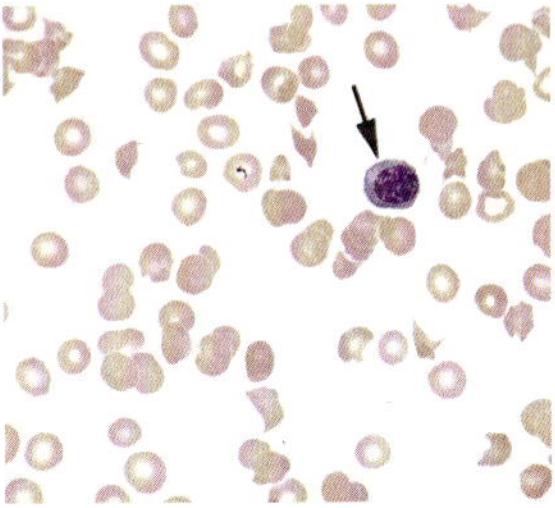

42. Nucleated red blood cell: *Arrow* marks nucleated red blood cell precursor circulating in the peripheral blood. These forms can be seen in conditions with increased red cell turnover when the marrow is stressed.

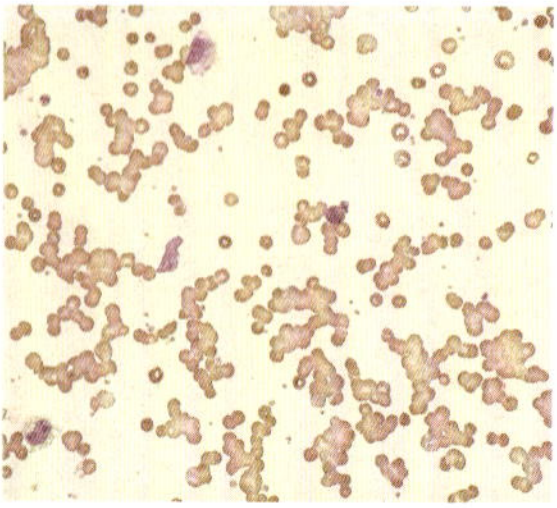

43. Cold agglutinin disease: Red cells are clumped together in response to cold temperature which eventually results in hemolysis. This disorder can occur in primary and secondary forms.

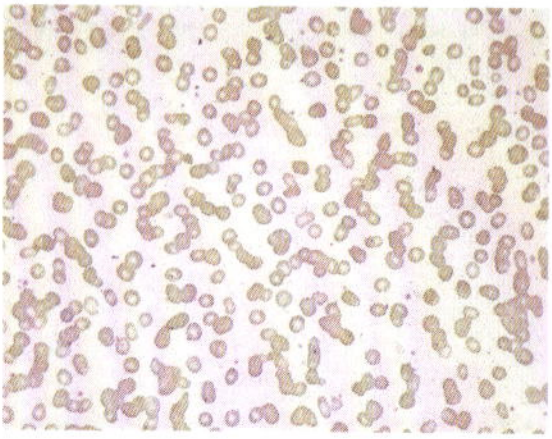

44. Rouleaux: Red cells stick together like "stacks of coins." These findings can been seen in disorders like multiple myeloma or Waldenstrom macroglobulinemia where increase in paraproteins cause the result cells to adhere to one another.

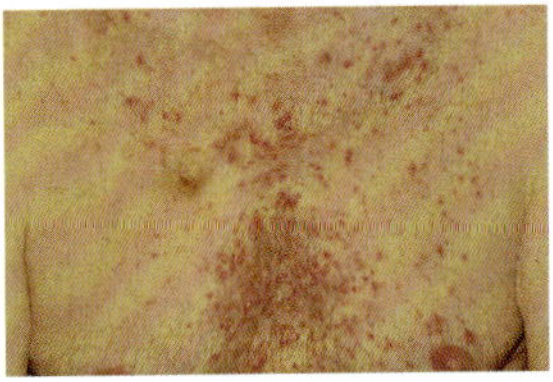

1. Papulopustular (acneiform) rash grade 2, related to EGFR inhibitor (erlotinib, afatinib, dacomitinib, cetuximab, panitumumab) therapy. Treatment consists of low/medium-potency topical corticosteroids (alclometasone, triamcinolone), oral antibiotics (minocycline 100 mg a day/ doxycycline 100 mg bid); and systemic corticosteroids (prednisone 0.5 mg/kg/day for 7 days) for grade 3 acneiform rash. Bacterial cultures are recommended when secondary infections are suspected, to guide antibiotic therapy.

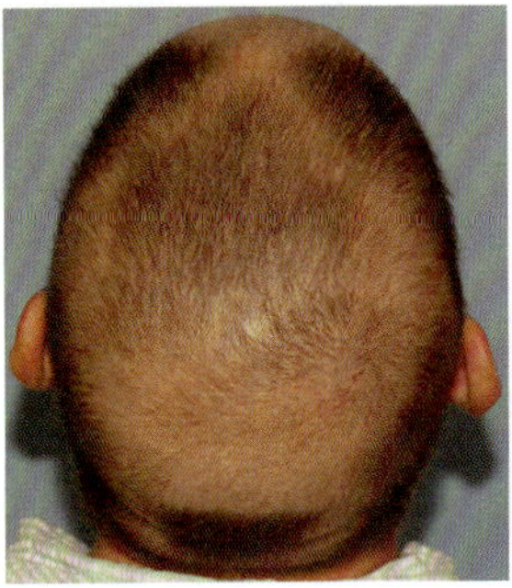

2. Persistent radiotherapy induced alopecia grade 2. Treatment for grade 1 consists of topical minoxidil foam 5% twice daily or oral minoxidil 1.25 mg daily. Treatment for grade 2 consists of scalp reconstruction (eg, simple excision or flaps, tissue expansion) or hair transplant (if not severe skin damage).

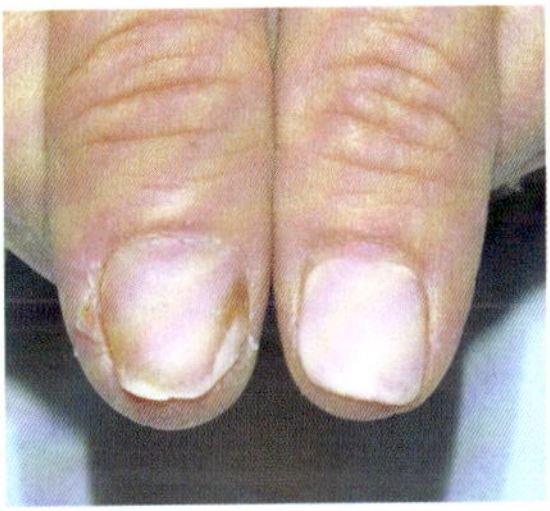

3. Paronychia grade 2, related to EGFR inhibitor (afatinib, lapatinib, erlotinib, cetuximab, osimertinib, panitumumab) therapy. Treatment consists of topical antibiotic (mupirocin, polysporin)/antiseptic (povidone/iodine) ointments, chemical cauterization with silver nitrate, and oral antibiotics when secondary infections are suspected or confirmed with microbial cultures.

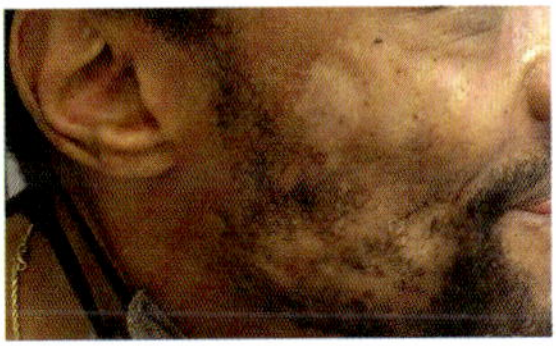

4. Vitiligo-like skin hypopigmentation/ depigmentation grade 1, after treatment with nivolumab. Treatment consists of photoprotection.

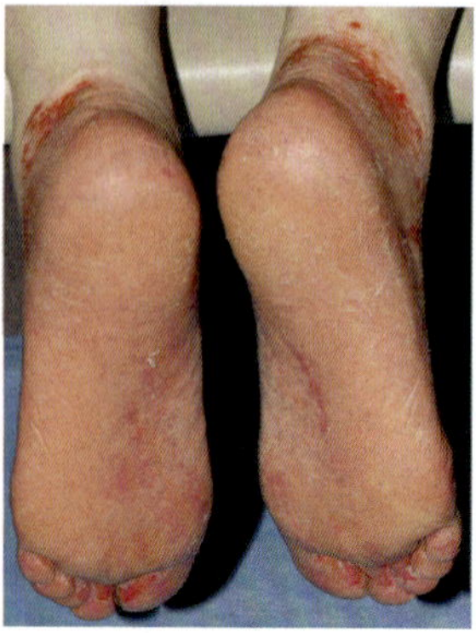

5. Palmar–plantar erythrodysesthesia (PPE) syndrome (also known as hand–foot skin reaction) grade 2, with blisters and hyperkeratosis related to multikinase inhibitor therapy (sorafenib, cabozantinib, lenvatinib, sunitinib, regorafenib, axitinib, pazopanib). Treatment consists of topical moisturizing keratolytic emollients (6% salicylic acid or 40% urea) as prophylaxis, high-potency topical corticosteroids (clobetasol), and anesthetics (lidocaine, prilocaine).

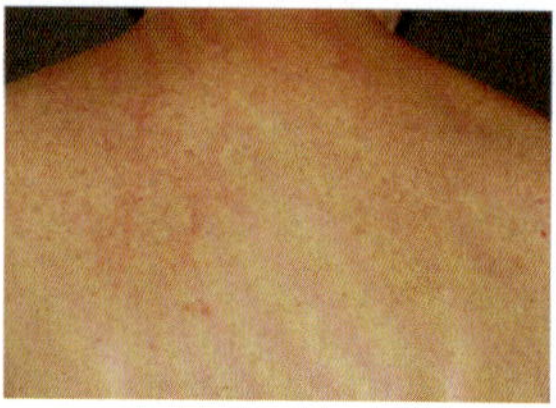

6. Pruritus and urticaria from immune checkpoint inhibitors. Treatment consists of high-potency topical corticosteroids twice daily, GABA analogs, oral antihistamines, and omalizumab or dupilumab.

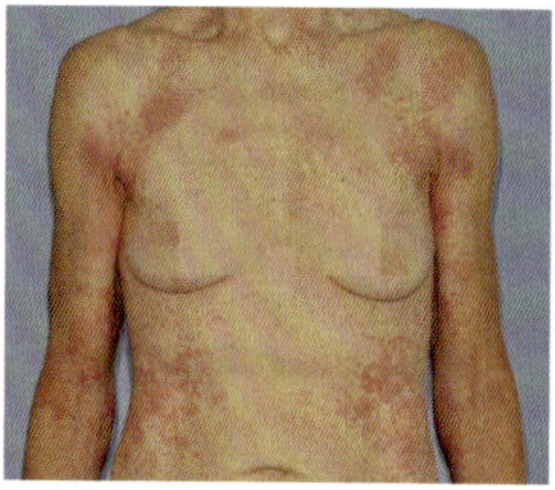

7. Maculopapular rash grade 3, related to BRAF inhibitor (vemurafenib) therapy, may occur with various TKIs (alpelisib). Treatment consists of topical/oral corticosteroids and for associated pruritus, oral antihistamines (loratadine, cetirizine, fexofenadine during the day and hydroxyzine, diphenhydramine at night).

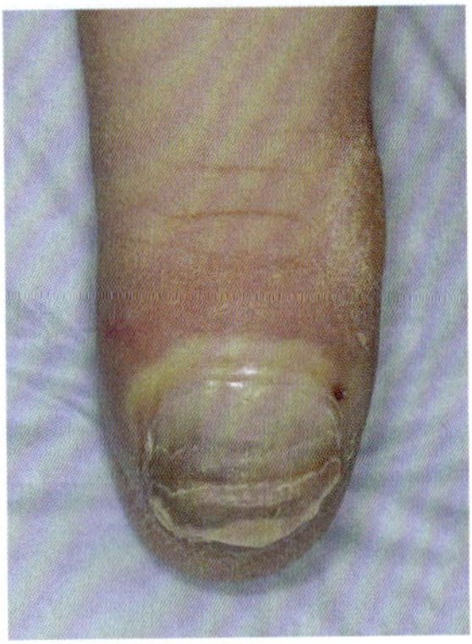

8. Nail loss (onycholysis) grade 2, related to taxane (paclitaxel, docetaxel) therapy. Treatment consists of antiseptic soaks (white vinegar in cool tap water 1:1 for 15 minutes daily), culture-driven oral antibiotics, and incision and drainage of the proximal nail fold abscess; prevention with frozen glove and sock therapy during chemotherapy administration.

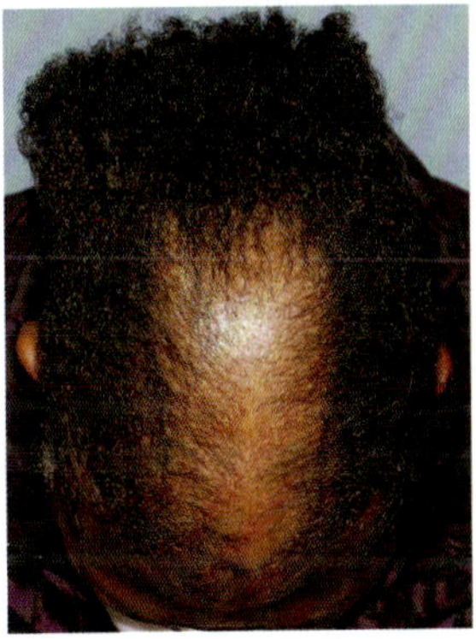

9. Alopecia grade 1, persistent after completion of taxane (paclitaxel, docetaxel) therapy. Treatment consists of topical minoxidil 2–5% twice daily and biotin 2.5 mg a day. Evaluation for other abnormalities that may contribute to alopecia are also recommended (serum TSH, vitamin D, ferritin, zinc levels).

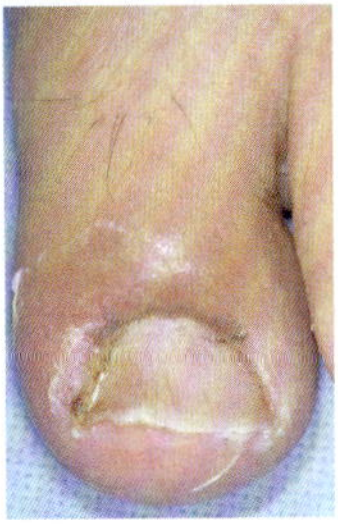

10. Paronychia grade 2, related to mTOR inhibitor (temsirolimus, everolimus) therapy. Treatment consists of topical antibiotics (mupirocin, polysporin)/antiseptic (povidone/iodine) ointments and partial or complete nail avulsion. For thin or brittle nails from mTOR inhibitors, daily use of polyurea urethane gel (Nuvail) or (hydrosoluble nail lacquer (Genadur) and PO biotin 2.5 mg a day.

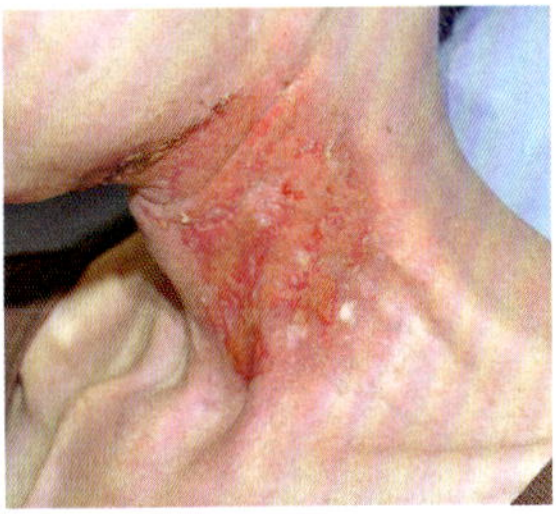

11. Radiation dermatitis (RD) grade 2, related to radiation therapy. More frequent and severe during treatment of head and neck, breast, and genitourinary cancers and with concurrent chemotherapy or targeted therapy. Prevention consists of topical corticosteroids (mometasone, betamethasone) or antibiotics (silver sulfadiazine for breast, silver leaf nylon dressing for anal cancers). Once developed, secondary infections are common, so bacterial cultures are recommended to guide choice of oral antibiotic therapy.

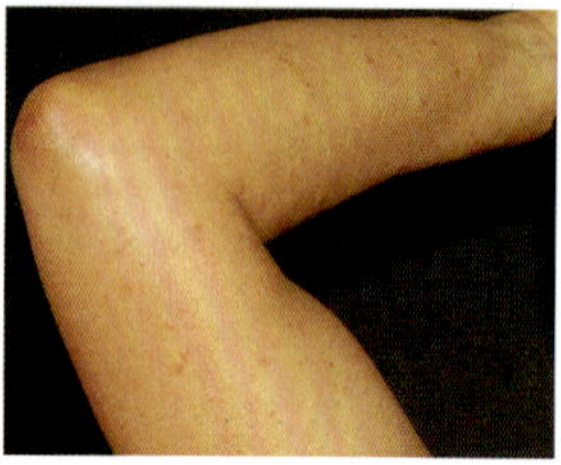

12. Maculopapular rash grade 3, related to immune checkpoint inhibitor therapy (ipilimumab, pembrolizumab, nivolumab, atezolizumab). Treatment consists of medium/high-potency topical corticosteroids for grades 1/2. Add oral corticosteroids and antihistamines for grade 3.

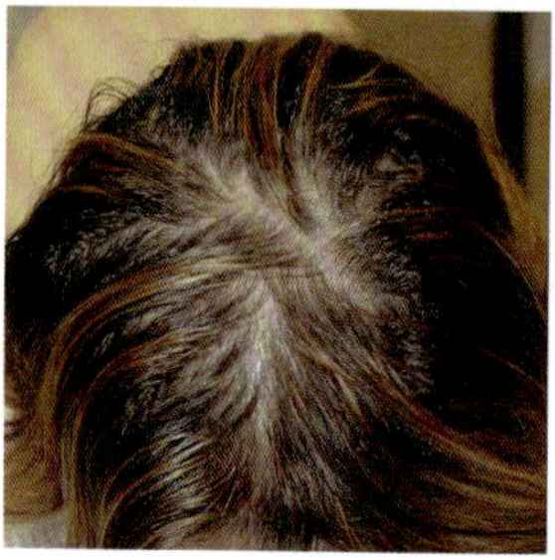

13. Alopecia grade 1, related to hormonal (tamoxifen, aromatase inhibitors) therapy. Treatment consists of oral minoxidil 1.25 mg a day and ketoconazole 2% shampoo twice weekly. Evaluation for other abnormalities that may contribute to alopecia are also recommended (serum TSH, vitamin D, ferritin, zinc levels).

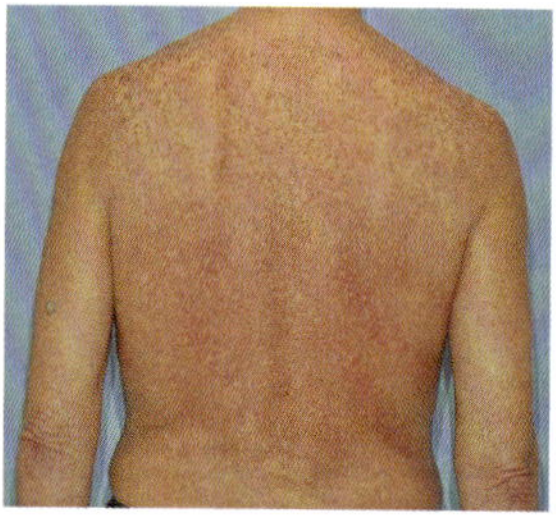

14. Maculopapular rash grade 2, post stem cell transplantation. Treatment consists of topical/oral corticosteroids and antihistamines.

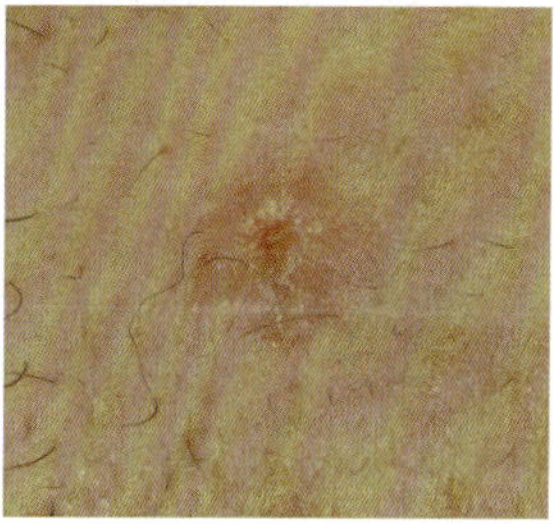

15. Basal cell carcinoma (BCC) on the upper lip. Most common type of nonmelanoma skin cancer, with over 2 million cases diagnosed per year. Frequently occurring on the face, head, neck and upper trunk, photo-exposed areas, or in areas of prior radiation therapy. Treatment is usually topical (ie, imiquimod, tazarotene) or local therapy (eg, laser therapy) for superficial BCCs; whereas surgical excision is the most common therapy for other BCCs. BCCs are the most common second primary malignancy in childhood cancer survivors, especially in areas that received radiation therapy.

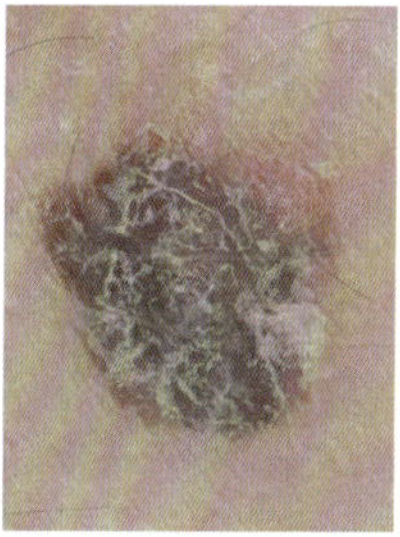

16. Melanoma representing only 8% of all skin cancers but nearly 80% of skin cancer–related deaths. Dermoscopy significantly aids in diagnosis and the initial treatment modality is surgical excision. Tumor thickness, mitotic rates, and ulceration are the most important prognostic factors.

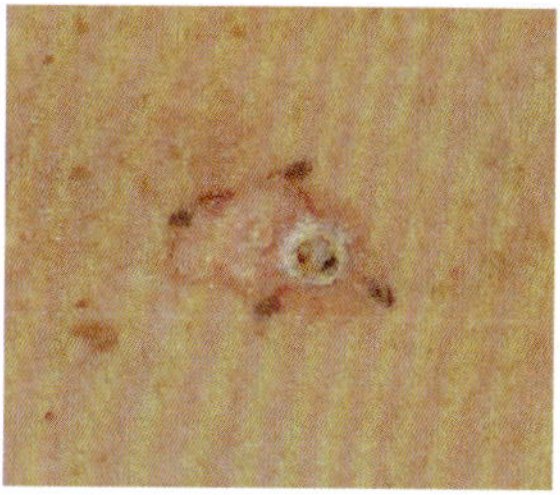

17. Squamous cell carcinoma (SCC) is the second most common type of nonmelanoma skin cancer, with approximately 300,000 cases diagnosed per year. Treatment is usually topical (ie, imiquimod, tazarotene) or destructive with cryotherapy for superficial SCCs that do not involve the entire epidermis (actinic keratoses or Bowen disease); whereas surgical excision or radiation are the most common therapies for in situ or invasive SCCs.

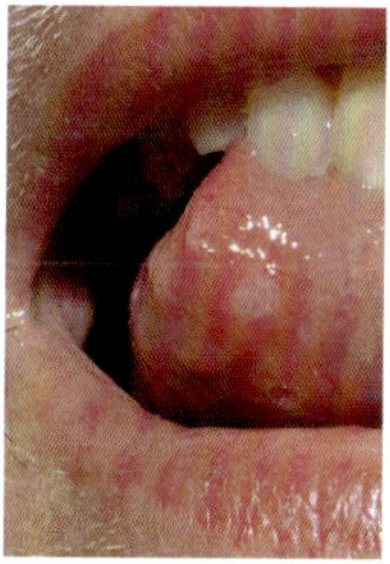

18. Oral mucositis (aphthous stomatitis-like) grade 2, related to mTOR inhibitor (temsirolimus, everolimus) therapy. Treatment consists of dexamethasone oral rinses or clobetasol ointment tid.

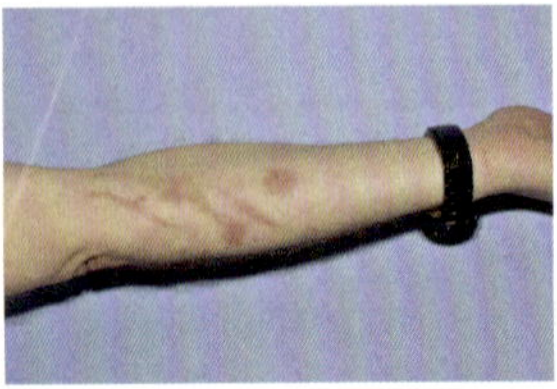

19. Extravasation reaction, grade 1, secondary to unintended leakage of doxorubicin from vasculature into perivascular tissue. Prevention through careful administration technique is key. Treatment depends on type of drug extravasated, but generally includes stopping infusion, removing venous device, elevating/demarcating affected area, and when appropriate cooling and/or neutralizing with antidote.

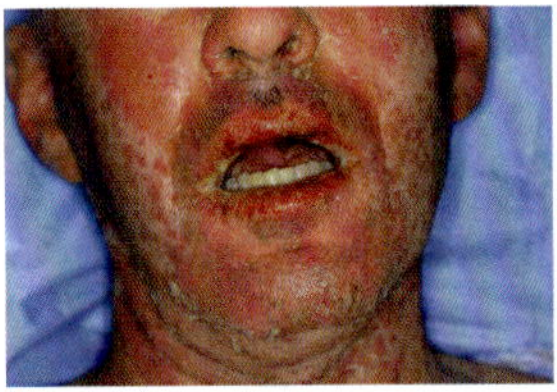

20. SJS/TEN after treatment with antiepileptic medication Zonegran while on nivolumab. Due to high mortality associated with these rashes, mainstay for treatment includes early recognition, timely removal of offending drug, + TNF-inhibition.

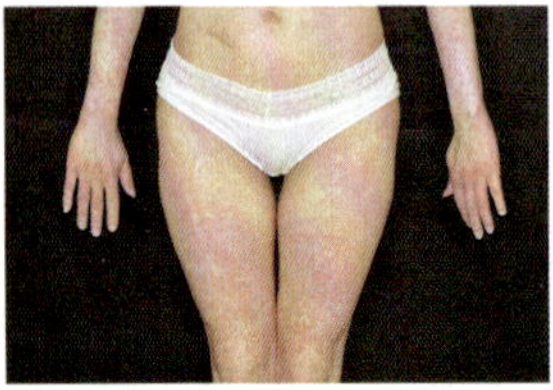

21. Acute GVHD grade 3, post stem cell transplant. Prevention with calcineurin inhibitor (cyclosporine, tacrolimus) plus a brief course of MTX. Treatment consists of high-dose systemic steroids (methylprednisolone 2–2.5 mg/kg/day) and prophylactic immunosuppression.

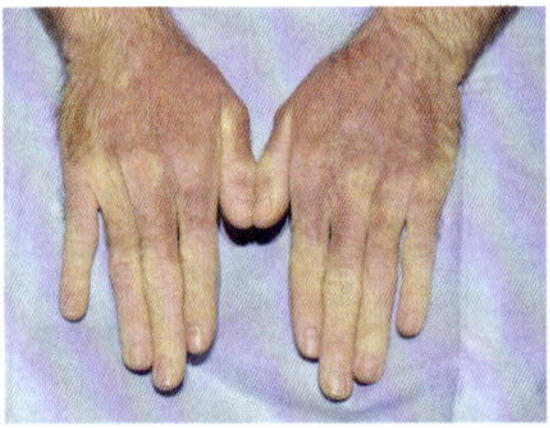

22. Photosensitivity grade 2 rash (vemurafenib, vandetanib, voriconazole). Treatment consists of triamcinolone cream bid, titanium oxide and zinc oxide sunscreen, sun avoidance, and cold compresses to alleviate symptoms.

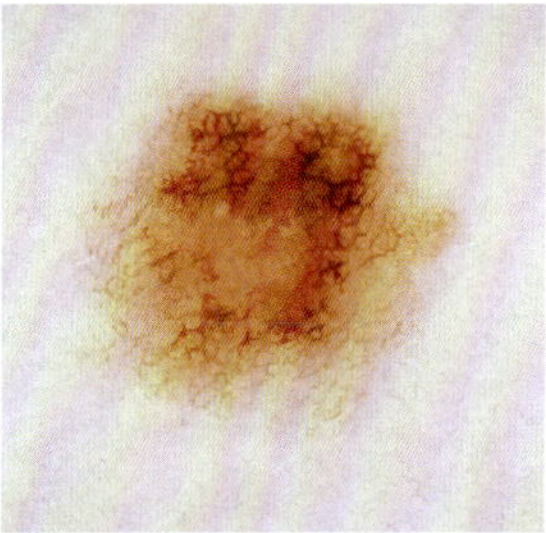

23. Development of dysplastic nevi after treatment with BRAF inhibitors (vemurafenib, dabrafenib). Close monitoring with total body skin exams by a dermatologist assisted by total-body photography and dermoscopy for new and changing lesions. Concomitant use of MEK inhibitors (cobimetinib, trametinib) will decrease the risk of atypia.

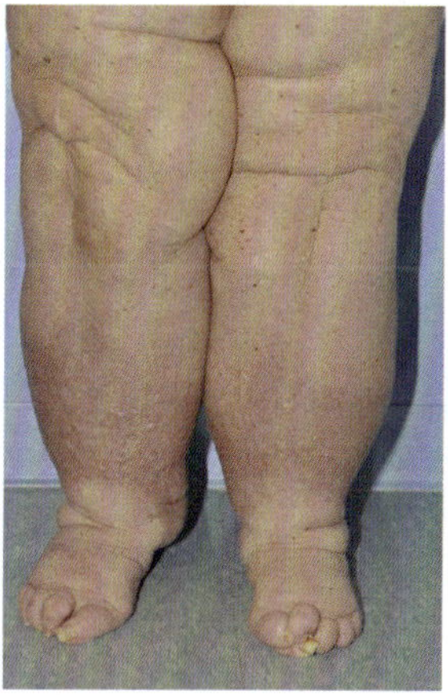

25. Peripheral edema after targeted therapy (small molecule kinase or monoclonal antibody inhibitors). Encourage leg elevation, lymphedema compression therapy if safe, and for associated skin irritation such as stasis dermatitis, use medium- to high-potency topical steroids (triamcinolone 0.1% or clobetasol 0.05%) and evaluation by a lymphedema therapist.

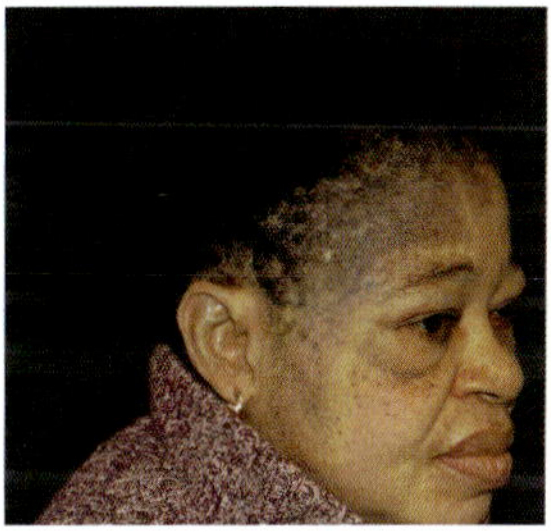

24. Hyperpigmentation grade 2 after imatinib therapy. Treat with topical triamcinolone 0.1% cream, hydroquinone 4% cream bid, sunscreen, sun avoidance.

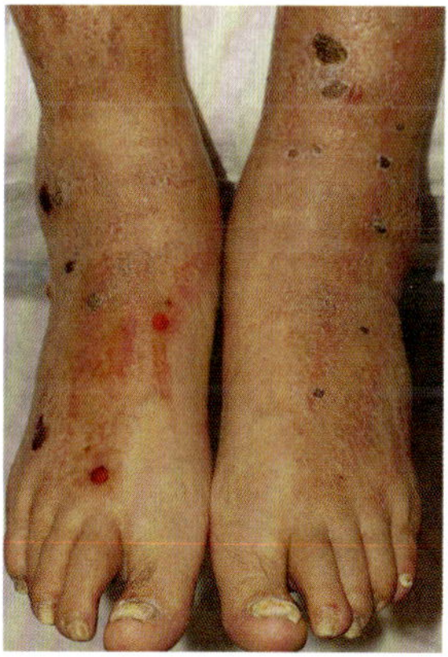

26. Immunotherapy-related bullous pemphigoid (BP) while on immune checkpoint monoclonal antibody therapy. Treatment includes temporarily or permanently withholding immunotherapy, initiation of both topical and high-dose systemic corticosteroids.

Performance scores

- Karnofsky, ECOG most common. Pt's current status –> prognostic. Can influence eligibility for tx & clinical trials. PPS for pall care, Lansky for children. Conversion between scales varies (*Eur J Cancer* 2010;46(18):3175; *World J Clin Oncol* 2018:9:140; *J Palliat Care* 2013;29:163)
- **Karnofsky:** Score runs from 100–0, where 100 is "perfect" health & 0 is death
- **ECOG** ("WHO" or "Zubrod" score): Runs from 0–5, w/ 0 denoting perfect health & 5 death

Karnofsky Performance Status Scale (KPS)	Eastern Cooperative Oncology Group Performance Status (ECOG)	Palliative Performance Status Scale Version 2 (PPSv2)					
		PPS Level	Ambulation	Activity & Evidence of Disease	Self-care	Intake	Conscious Level
100—Nl; no evidence of disease	**0**—Fully active, no restriction in predisease performance	**100**	Full	Nl activity & work; no evidence of disease	Full	Nl	Full
90—Minor s/s	**1**—Restricted in physically strenuous activity but ambulatory & able to carry out light work	**90**	Full	Nl activity & work; some evidence of disease	Full	Nl	Full
80—Nl activity w/ effort; some s/s	**1**—Restricted in physically strenuous activity but ambulatory & able to carry out light work	**80**	Full	Nl activity w/ effort; some evidence of disease	Full	Nl or reduced	Full
70—Cares for self; unable to carry on nl activity	**2**—Ambulatory; capable of all self-care but unable to work; up more than 50% of waking h	**70**	Reduced	Unable to do nl job/ work; significant disease	Full	Nl or reduced	Full
60—Occasional assistance required; capable of most self-care	**2**—Ambulatory; capable of all self-care but unable to work; up more than 50% of waking h	**60**	Reduced	Unable to do hobby/ housework; significant disease	Occasional assistance necessary	Nl or reduced	Full or confusion
50—Requires assistance, frequent medical care	**3**—Capable of only limited self-care; confined to bed/chair >50% waking h	**50**	Mainly sit/lie	Unable to do any work; extensive disease	Considerable assistance required	Nl or reduced	Full or confusion
40—Disabled; requires special care/ assistance	**3**—Capable of only limited self-care; confined to bed/chair >50% waking h	**40**	Mainly in bed	Unable to do most activity; extensive disease	Mainly assistance	Nl or reduced	Full or drowsy ± confusion
30—Severely disabled; hospital-ization indicated	**4**—Not capable of self-care; totally confined to bed/chair	**30**	Totally bed bound	Unable to do any activity; extensive disease	Total care	Nl or reduced	Full or drowsy ± confusion
20—Hospital-ization necessary; requires active supportive care	**4**—Not capable of self-care; totally confined to bed/chair	**20**	Totally bed bound	Unable to do most activity; extensive disease	Total care	Min. sips	Full or drowsy ± confusion
10—Moribund; progressing rapidly	**4**—Not capable of self-care; totally confined to bed/chair	**10**	Totally bed bound	Unable to do most activity; extensive disease	Total care	Mouth care only	Drowsy or coma ± confusion
0—Dead	**5**—Dead	**0**	Death	—	—	—	—

Adapted from *Eur J Cancer* 2010;46(18):3175; *Am J Clin Oncol* 1982;5:649; *Cancer* 1948;1(4):634–656; *J Palliat Care* 1996;9:26.

RADIOGRAPHIC RESPONSE CRITERIA

Background

- Objective response (tumor shrinkage) & progression-free survival are conventional endpoints in clinical trials, but are useful only if standard criteria are applied to assess anatomic tumor burden
- Objective response criteria standardize & objectively measure the effect of CA tx. Such measurements are used as a basis for rigorous comparison of proposed txs being evaluated in clinical trials
- Criteria used have evolved over time as clinical imaging technology/therapeutics have advanced

RECIST: Response Evaluation Criteria In Solid Tumors (version 1.1)

- **WHO** criteria (bidirectional measurements), developed in 1981, was the first published tumor response criteria
- **RECIST** 1.0 (unidimensional measurement) was developed in 2000 to further standardize & simplify response criteria, given the widespread use of adv imaging modalities (*J Natl Cancer Inst* 2000;205:216); 2009 update (RECIST 1.1) was based on evaluation of data measured according to the original RECIST criteria, including changes to the number & size of lesions evaluated, evaluation of pathologic LNs, & interpretation of PET imaging (*Eur J Cancer* 2009;228:247)
- **Measurable lesions:** 10 mm on CT or clinical exam; 20 mm on x-ray. Pathologic LNs >= 15 mm in short axis by CT. X-ray measurements discouraged
- **Nonmeasurable lesions:** <10 mm, pathologic LNs <15 mm in short axis. Leptomeningeal dz, ascites, pleural/pericardial effusions, inflammatory breast tissue, lymphangitic involvement of skin or lung, or abdominal masses on clinical exam not reproducible on imaging are nonmeasurable. Generally, previously treated lesions are nonmeasurable
- **Target lesions:** Identified lesions on the baseline scan, up to a total of 5, w/ a maximum of two per organ. These are to be followed on future scans, & the largest lesions as well as those for which reproducible measurements are expected should be prioritized

Response	Criteria
CR	Disappearance of all target lesions. Any pathologic LNs must have a short axis <10 mm
PR	≥30% ↓ in sum of diameters of target lesions compared to baseline sum of diameters
SD	Neither sufficient ↓ to qualify for PR nor ↑ to qualify for PD using the smallest sum of diameters while on study as reference
PD	New lesions or ≥20% ↑ in sum of target lesion diameters compared to smallest sum on study w/ an absolute ↑ size ≥5 mm

iRECIST: Modified RECIST 1.1 for immune-based therapeutics

- CA immunotx prompted updates to standard response criteria to account for unique patterns of tumor change, such as pseudoprogression. These updates include irRC, irRECIST, & most recently iRECIST (*Lancet Oncol* 2017;18:e143–152), which has been widely adopted in clinical trials but not yet validated for regulatory purposes
- **iRECIST** builds on RECIST 1.1 w/ addition of confirmatory scan for dz progression
- **Measurements:** Definitions of measurable & nonmeasurable lesions, target & nontarget lesions, & methods of measurement are the same as for RECIST 1.1
- **Response criteria:** Denoted w/ the prefix "i" for "immune" including iCR, iPR, iSD, iUPD (immune unconfirmed PD), & iCPD (immune confirmed PD)

Response	Criteria
iCR	As per CR for RECIST 1.1
iPR	As per PR for RECIST 1.1
iSD	As per SD for RECIST 1.1
iUPD	As per PD for RECIST 1.1 at first scan
iCPD	iCPD is assigned once iUPD is confirmed on a subsequent 4–8 wk scan showing continued progression w/ ↑ size ≥5 mm of target lesions, growth of nontarget lesions, new lesions, or progression in another lesion category. If lesions unchanged from iUPD → remains iUPD. If lesions shrink from iUPD → iCR, iPR, or iSD based on comparison to baseline

QUALITY OF LIFE ASSESSMENTS

Introduction

- **Health-related quality of life (HRQoL)** is a multidimensional concept encompassing the pt's perception of the positive & negative aspects of their sx
- Includes physical, emotional, social, & cognitive functions, as well as dz sx & s/e of tx
- HRQoL is an **important outcome measure in all CA pts,** but even more so in the met population where palliation of sx & optimization of QoL are often the main GOC
- **Patient-reported outcomes (PRO)** include HR-QOL sx & satisfaction ratings that are reported directly by pts w/o interpretation by a clinician
- Higher scores on QoL measures may be predictive of longer survival (*BMC Cancer* 2011;11:353)
- Formal QoL assessments in CA can be either **generic** (applicable across a range of CA) or **specific** (limited to a disease, site, &/or tx modality)

Generic QoL assessments

FACT-G (Functional Assessment of Cancer Therapy—General) (*J Clin Oncol* 1993;11:570)

- Includes specific subscales on physical, social, emotional, & functional well-being
- Likert scale of 0 (not at all) to 4 (very much), pts respond to statements such as "I am able to enjoy life" or "I am sleeping well"
- Higher scores indicate better QoL

EORTC QLQ-C30 (European Organization for Research and Treatment of Cancer QoL Core Questionnaire 30) (*JNCI* 1993;85:365)

- No specific subscales
- On a scale of 1 (not at all) to 4 (very much), pts respond to questions such as "Do you have any trouble taking a long walk"
- Lower scores indicate better QoL

Choosing between the FACT-G & EORTC QLQ-C30:

- FACT-G & EORTC QLQ-C30 overlap, but measure different aspects of QoL; **they are not interchangeable** (*J Clin Oncol* 1999;17:2932)

Figure APP-1 Decision tree for choosing between the Quality of Life Questionnaire Core 30 (QLQ-C30) and Functional Assessment of Cancer Therapy—General (FACT-G) for measuring QoL. *Ann Oncol* 2011;22:2179. Reprinted with permission from Elsevier.

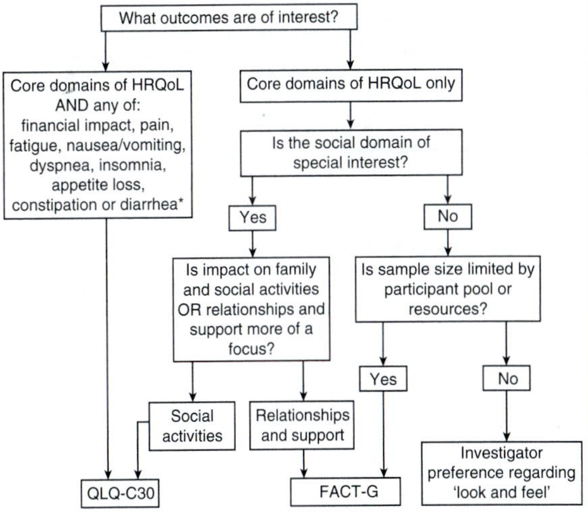

*Where cognitive functioning is an outcome of interest, researchers are encouraged to seek a dedicated questionnaire rather than rely on the scale included in the QLQ-C30.

Specific QoL assessments

- Both EORTC & FACT developed **dz-specific modules** (eg, for breast CA, EORTC-BR23, or FACT-B) which tailor questions to specific dz-related sx or tx s/e
- FACT also has **sx- & tx-specific scales**
  - 26 dz-specific sx indices (more abbreviated than dz-specific modules) to assess QoL issues specific to sx experienced commonly w/ each type of CA
  - 10 tx-specific sx indices to assess QoL issues related to types of tx (eg, taxanes) or issues related to dz &/or tx (eg, enteral feeding, neurotoxicity)
  - 17 sx-specific measures (eg, cachexia, anemia/fatigue, diarrhea)
- EORTC has specific modules to assess **pt satisfaction** w/ care/coordination/info
- HADS (Hospital Anxiety & Depression Scale) is a frequently used tool to detect anxiety & depression independent of somatic sx (*Br J Psychiatry* 1991;158:255); validated in CA pts
- COST (COmprehensive Score for financial Toxicity) measures financial distress (*Cancer* 2016;123:476); CA-related financial burden is associated w/ lower QoL

QoL & PRO assessments in clinical trials

- Varied methodologies, assessment instruments, & analyses make comparisons of trials challenging; a systematic evaluation of CA RCTs revealed that "PRO protocol content is frequently inadequate & nonreporting of PRO findings is widespread" (*JNCI* 2019;111:1170); experts/regulators are **focusing on standardization** (*Lancet Oncol* 2018;19:e267)
- NCI designed **PRO-CTCAE** converts the Common Terminology Criteria for Adverse Events (CTCAE) into a PRO measurement system of 124 items spanning 78 sx, linguistically validated in >30 languages (www.healthcaredelivery.cancer.gov/pro-ctcae)
- **CONSORT-PRO extension** provides open access international reporting guidelines for RCTs w/ PRO as primary or secondary outcomes (*JAMA* 2013;309:814)
- **SPIRIT-PRO extension** provides consensus recommendations for items to be included in trial protocols w/ PRO as key outcomes (*JAMA* 2018;319:483)
- **SISAQOL consortium** published international standards for the analysis of QoL & PRO endpoints in CA RCTs (*Lancet Oncol* 2020;21:e83)
- Semistructured interviews w/ stakeholder groups identified **barriers** to effective integration of PRO into trials (late inclusion of PRO during trial design, PROs are lower priority than survival, collection burden of PRO, & lack of staff training) (*Cancer Med* 2021;10:5475)

QoL & PRO assessments in clinical practice

Benefits of incorporating QoL/PRO assessments into routine care:

- Completion of EORTC-QLQ-C30 & HADS w/ feedback to physicians improved communication & pt well-being (*J Clin Oncol* 2004;22:714)
- A systematic review of trials to 2012 found that use of PROs incr. frequency of discussion of pt outcomes, & in some studies was associated w/ improved sx control, incr. supportive care measures, & pt satisfaction (*J Clin Oncol* 2014;32:1480)
- Self-reporting of CTCAEs w/ nurse alerts via a web-based interface by pts on chemotx for metastatic CA improved HRQoL, decr. ER visits, extended time on chemotx, & incr. survival (*J Clin Oncol* 2016;34:557; *JAMA* 2017;318:197)

Recent implementation efforts

- PRO-TECT trial w/ wkly web/telephone PRO-CTCAE in 26 community onc practices showed acceptance by pts, nurses, & oncologists (*JCO Clin Ca Inform* 2020;4:947)
- eSyM, a PRO-CTCAE management program in Epic (*JCO Clin Ca Inform* 2022;6:e2100137)
- ASyMS, an Advanced Symptom Management System in Europe (*BMJ* 2021;374:n1647)

Recommended user guides & reviews describing key implementation considerations:

- ISOQOL (International Society for QoL Research)—www.isoqol.org/resource-center
  User's Guide to Implementing PRO Assessment in Clinical Practice, 2015 & 2018
- PCORI (Patient-Centered Outcomes Research Institute)—www.pcori.org/resources
  Users' Guide to Integrating PRO in Electronic Health Records, 2017
- ASCO—www.asco.org/edbook
  Implementation of PRO in Routine Medical Care, 2018
- *Translation of PRO in Onc Clinical Trials to Everyday Practice* (*Ann Surg Oncol* 2020;27:65) summarizes key considerations (choice of instrument, method of delivery, frequency of query) & challenges (cost, resources, impact on workflow, clinician burnout)

TUMOR MARKERS

Definition

- Classically, a tumor marker is a substance measurable in blood or other body fluids that can be used as a surrogate marker for the presence of malignancy
- Some are sufficiently sensitive & specific to be used for dz screening when sufficiently elevated or can be followed to evaluate therapy response or dz recurrence
- Most are not sufficiently sensitive or specific for this purpose & must be used in conjunction w/ other sources of information (eg, imaging) to arrive at clinical dx

Current tumor markers by cancer site (alphabetical)

- **Breast**
  - CA 15-3, CA 27-29 (both tests measure the same serum antigen)
  - CEA
- **Gastrointestinal**
  - AFP (liver)
  - CA 19-9 (pancreas, colorectal, biliary, stomach)
  - CEA (pancreas, colorectal, biliary)
- **Genitourinary**
  - PAP (prostate)
  - PSA (prostate)
  - PSMA (prostate)
- **GTC**
  - AFP (ovary, testis)
  - hCG (trophoblastic dz, choriocarcinoma, ovary, testis)
  - LDH
- **Gynecologic**
  - CA 125 (ovary, uterine)
  - HE-4 (ovary)
- **Lung**
  - CA-125 (mesothelioma)
  - SMRP (mesothelioma)
- **Lymphoma**
  - B2M (multiple myeloma, lymphomas)
  - Monoclonal immunoglobulins (Waldenstrom's, multiple myeloma; blood & urine tests)
  - SFLC (multiple myeloma)
  - LDH
- **Melanoma**
  - LDH
- **Neuroendocrine**
  - Chromogranin A (carcinoid & PNET)
  - 5-HIAA (carcinoid); can be falsely elevated in consumption of serotonin-rich foods
  - Pancreatic polypeptide, insulin, pro-insulin, c-peptide, VIP, glucagon, gastrin (PNET)
  - Metanephrines, catecholamines, methoxytramine (pheo, paraganglioma)
  - IGF1, prolactin, LH/FSH, alpha subunit, TSH (FT4) (pituitary)
  - Cortisol, ACTH (Cushing syndrome; adrenal, pituitary, ectopic)
  - Renin, aldosterone (hyperaldosteronism; renal)
  - Cushing's (above); hyperaldosteronism (above); testosterone, DHEAS for androgen excess (adrenocortical carcinoma)
  - Catecholamines VMA, HVA; LDH; NSE (neuroblastoma)
- **Thyroid**
  - Calcitonin (medullary thyroid)
  - CEA (medullary)
  - Thyroglobulin, antithyroglobulin antibody

- **CA of unknown 1° (CK staining may be combined w/ the above-listed markers & add'l tissue stains to suggest a 1° tumor site)**
  - CK7+CK20– (lung, breast, thyroid, endometrial, cervical, salivary gland, pancreas adenoCAs)
  - CK7–CK20+ (colorectal, Merkel cell carcinomas)
  - CK7+CK20+ (urothelial, ovarian, pancreas adenoCAs)
  - CK7–CK20– (HCC, RCC, prostate, SCC, small cell lung carcinoma, head & neck carcinoma)

Specificity of tumor markers

The sn & sp of tumor markers is limited due to their correlation w/ other biologic processes

Tumor Marker	Nononcologic Causes for Elevation
AFP	Pregnancy
B2M	CD, hepatitis
CA 15-3	Benign breast conditions
CA 19-9	Pancreatitis, IBD
CA 125	Endometritis
Calcitonin	Pernicious anemia, thyroiditis
CEA	Hepatitis, colitis, pancreatitis, cigarette smoking
hCG	Pregnancy, testicular failure
PSA	BPH, prostatitis
PSMA	Normal ↑ w/ age
PAP	Prostatitis

References

Porter RS. *Merck Manual of Diagnosis and Therapy*. 19th ed. Merck: 2011, online edition chapter, 123.

Daniels R. *Delmar's Guide to Laboratory and Diagnostic Tests*. 2nd ed. Delmar Cengage Learning: 2010, online edition appendix C.

Lab Tests Online, http://labtestsonline.org/understanding/analytes/tumor-markers/, Accessed December 15, 2012.

American Cancer Society, http://www.cancer.org/treatment/understandingyourdiagnosis/examsandtestdescriptions/tumormarkers/index, Accessed December 15, 2012.

Pavlidis N, Fizazi K. Cancer of unknown primary (CUP). *Crit Rev Oncol Hematol*. 2005; 54(3):243–250.

DeVita VT, Lawrence TS, Rosenberg SA. *Devita, Hellman, and Rosenberg's Cancer: Principles & Practice of Oncology*. 10th ed. LWW: 2014.

PERFORMING BM BIOPSY/ASPIRATE

Selected common indications

- Cytopenias (idiopathic) or pancytopenia (MDS, AML), lymphoproliferative disorders (NHL, MM, ALL), storage (Fe, amyloidosis, Gaucher's), FUO, peripheral blood abnormalities (MPD, MDS), myelophthisis (solid tumor involvement)

Equipment

- Sterile skin preparation & sterile field equipment
- Lidocaine buffered w/ $NaHCO_3$, 25-gauge needle, & 5-mL syringe
- BM aspiration needle & BM bx needle (ie, Jamshidi™ needle)
- Two 30-mL syringes, sterile heparin sulfate, sterile gauze, & bandage

Location

- Iliac crest (posterior preferred, reached in either prone or decubitus position w/ knees flexed → anterior can be used, rarely); sternum may be used only under exceptional circumstances (aspirate only)

Steps

- Obtain informed consent; perform time-out (institution dependent)
- Position pt (prone or lateral decubitus) → Identify landmarks (posterior iliac spine) → Cleanse area (chlorhexidine or Iodine solution)
- Local anesthetic (Lidocaine 1% or 2%)
  - Slowly instill to raise a wheal & then administer in a star-like distribution to level of periosteum, to check effects of anesthesia may tap periosteum gently
- Procedure may be performed under sedation per pt/provider preference
- **Aspiration of marrow** (Illinois needle)
  - Prefilled tubes w/ anticoagulant (EDTA)
  - Inspect needle, ensure proper function, remove plastic guards if present
  - Hold needle perpendicular to surface of skin → insert at posterior iliac crest until bone is encountered → rotate needle gently using clockwise/counterclockwise motions while applying pressure → ↓ resistance may be felt when through cortex & marrow is entered
  - Remove stylet & attach 30-mL syringe (no heparin) → aspirate marrow (can be painful) → use sample to create slides (adequate if w/ presence of bony spicules), may be performed by assistant
  - Attach syringes (prefilled w/ heparin) → for diagnostic tests
  - Remove aspiration needle & apply pressure to prevent bleeding
- **Core bx** (Jamshidi™ needle)
  - Ensure proper function
  - Insert larger bx needle into same entry site as aspiration needle (may need to widen w/ small incision) → adv w/ stylet in place → remove stylet once anchored in bone
  - Continue to adv needle by 1–2 cm (a core length >1.5 cm preferred; stylet may be reinserted gently to determine length of specimen) w/ a rotating motion to obtain core → rotate 360 degrees clockwise & counterclockwise then rock back & forth to make sure core is detached from surrounding marrow → withdraw needle w/ similar rotating motion → remove specimen from needle by inserting sterile probe to push specimen out onto slide/gauze

Aspirate: Liquid Portion	
Tests	Smear, flow cytometry, molecular, misc tests, cytogenetics
Core Biopsy: Medullary Bone	
Tests	Morphology, IHC, misc tests
Special	If dry tap; consider touch prep

Videos in clinical medicine. Bone marrow aspiration and biopsy. *NEJM* 2009;361:e28.

ABBREVIATIONS

/y	Per year
2/2	Secondary to
1°	Primary
2°	Secondary
24-h	24 hour
2HG	2-hydroxyglutarate
4-1BBL	4-1BB ligand
4-PCC	4-factor prothrombin complex concentrate
5-FU	5-fluorouracil
6MP	6-mercaptopurine
9vHPV	9-valent HPV
A/S	HgA and HgS
a/w	Associated with
A2aR	Adenosine 2A receptor
aa	Amino acid
AABB	American Association of Blood Banks
Ab	Antibody
abd	Abdominal
Abnl	Abnormal
ABVD	Doxorubicin (A), bleomycin (B), vinblastine (V), dacarbazine (D)
ABW	Actual body weight
ABX	Antibiotics
AC	Anticoagulation
AC	Doxorubicin (Adriamycin) + cyclophosphamide
ACC	Adrenal cortical carcinoma
AChR	Acetylcholine receptor
ACOG	American College of Obstetricians and Gynecologists
ACS	American Cancer Society
ACT	Adoptive cell therapy
ACTH	Adrenocorticotrophic hormone
aCTLA-4	Anti-cytotoxic T-lymphocyte antigen 4
AD	Autosomal dominant
ADC	Antibody drug conjugate
ADCC	Antibody-dependent cellular cytotoxicity
add'l	Additional
AdenoCA	Adenocarcinoma
ADH	Antidiuretic hormone
ADL	Activities of daily living
ADP	Adenosine diphosphate
ADP	ALAD deficiency porphyria
ADR	adverse drug reaction
adv	Advanced
AE	Adverse event
AED	Antiepileptic drugs
AFAP	Attenuated familial adenomatous polyposis
AFP	Alpha-fetoprotein
Ag	Antigen
AHF	Antihemophilic factor
AI	Aromatase inhibitor
AI	Autoimmune
AICD	Antibody-induced cell death
AIHA	Autoimmune hemolytic anemia
AIP	Acute intermittent porphyria
AIS	Adenocarcinoma in situ
AJ	Ashkenazi Jewish
AJCC	American Joint Committee on Cancer
AKI	Acute kidney injury
AL	Light chain amyloidosis
ALA	Aminolevulinic acid
ALC	Absolute lymphocyte count
ALCL	Anaplastic large-cell lymphoma
ALD	Adrenoleukodystrophy
ALG	Anti-lymphocyte globulin
ALK	Anaplastic lymphoma kinase
alk phos	Alkaline phosphatase
ALL	Acute lymphoblastic leukemia
ALND	Axillary lymph node dissection
allo	Allogeneic
Allo-HCT	Allogeneic hematopoietic cell transplant
allo-SCT	Allogeneic stem cell transplant
ALP	Alkaline phosphatase
ALPS	Autoimmune lymphoproliferative syndrome
ALT	Alanine aminotransferase
AMKL	Acute megakaryoblastic leukemia
AML	Acute myeloid leukemia
amp	Amplification
AMPAR	α-amino-3-hydroxy-5-methyl-4-isoxazole-propionic acid receptor
AMS	Altered mental status
ANC	Absolute neutrophil count
ANG	Angiopoietin
ANG2	Angiopoietin 2
Angio	Angiogram
ANP	Atrial natriuretic peptide
Ant	Anterior
AP	Anterior posterior
AP	Antiphospholipid
AP	Accelerated phase
APAP	Acetaminophen
aPC	Activated protein C
APCC	Anaphase promoting complex/cyclosome
aPD-1	Anti-programmed death 1
aPD-L1	Anti-programmed death-ligand 1
APFAF-1	Apoptotic protease activating factor 1
APL	Acute promyelocytic leukemia
Approx	Approximately
APR	Abdominoperineal resection
APS	Antiphospholipid antibody syndrome
aPTT	activated partial thromboplastin time

AR	Autosomal recessive
AR	Androgen receptor
ARA-C	Cytarabine
ARA-G	9-beta arabinofuranosyl-guanine
ARDS	Acute respiratory distress syndrome
ARF	Acute respiratory failure
ARR	Absolute risk reduction
ASA	Aspirin
ASCCP	American Society for Colposcopy and Cervical Pathology
ASCT	Autologous stem cell transplantation
ASM	Aggressive systemic mastocytosis
assoc.	Associated
AST	Aspartate aminotransfer-ase
Asx	Asymptomatic
AT	Anti-thrombin
ATG	Anti-thymocyte globulin
ATLL	Adult T-cell leukemia/lymphoma
ATM	Ataxia-telangiectasia mutated
ATO	Arsenic trioxide
ATP	Adenosine triphosphate
ATRA	All-trans retinoic acid
ATRX	Alpha-thalassemia/mental retardation syndrome
AUA	American Urological Association
AUC	Area under the curve
Aut	Autosomal
auto	Autologous
Auto-HCT	Autologous
AutoAb	Autoantibody
avg	Average
AYA	Adolescent and young adult
AZA	Azacytidine
B-ALL	B-cell acute lymphoblastic leukemia
b-hCG	Beta human chorionic gonadotropin
B-PLL	B prolymphocytic leukemia
B7-H1	B7-homolog 1
B7-H3	B7-homolog 3
BAL	Bronchoalveolar lavage
BBB	Blood–brain barrier
BBW	Black box warning
BC	Blast crisis
BCC	Basal cell carcinoma
BCG	Bacillus Calmette-Guérin
BCMA	B-cell maturation antigen
BCNU	Carmustine
BCR	B-cell receptor
BCRP	Breast cancer resistance protein
BCS	Breast conservation surgery
BED	Biologically effective dose
BEP	Bleomycin (B), etoposide (E), platinum (P)
BER	Base excision repair
Bev	Bevacizumab
BFM	German Berlin, Frankfurt, Muenster Study Group
BH3	Bcl-2 homology domain 3
BID	Twice per day
Bilat	Bilateral
BiTE	Bispecific T-cell engager
BK	BK virus
BL	Burkitt lymphoma
BM	Bone marrow
BMA	Bone marrow aspiration
BMBx	Bone marrow biopsy
BMD	Bone mineral density
BMF	Bone marrow failure
BMI	Body mass index
bp	Base pair
BR	Bendamustine (B), rituximab (R)
BRAF	V-raf murine sarcoma viral oncogene homolog B
BRCA	Breast cancer gene
BRCA1/2	Breast cancer gene 1/2
BRIP1	BRCA1 Interacting Protein 1
BSA	Body surface area
BsAb	Bispecific antibody
BSC	Best supportive care
BSO	Bilateral salpingo-oophorectomy
BTK	Bruton's tyrosine kinase
BTKi	Bruton's tyrosine kinase inhibitor
btw	Between
b/w	Between
Bu	Busulfan
BV	Brentuximab vedotin
BWS	Beckwith–Weidemann syndrome
bx	Biopsy
C'	Compliment
c/w	Compared with
Ca	Cancer
Ca	Calcium
CA 125	Cancer antigen 125
CAD	Coronary artery disease
CAP	Chest, abdomen, pelvis
CAPD	Continuous ambulatory peritoneal dialysis
CAR	Chimeric antigen receptor
CAR-T	Chimeric antigen receptor T-cell
Carbo	Carboplatin
Cat	Category
CB	Cord blood
CBC	Complete blood count
CBE	Clinical breast exam
CBF	Core binding factor
CBU	Cord blood unit
CBV	Cyclophosphamide, carmustine, etoposide
CCL2	Chemokine (C-C motif) ligand 2
CCND1	Cyclin D1
CCNU	Lomustine
ccRCC	Clear-cell renal cell cancer/clear cell renal cell carcinoma

CCyR	Complete cytogenetic response
CD	Cluster of differentiation
CD	Collagen disease
CDA	Cladribine
CDA	Cytidine deaminase
CD40L	CD40 ligand
C. diff	Clostridium difficile
CDK	Cyclin-dependent kinase
CDKN2A	Cyclin dependent kinase inhibitor 2A
cDNA	Complementary DNA
CEA	Carcinoembryonic antigen
CEP	Congenital erythropoietic porphyria
CGD	Chronic granulomatous disease
cGVHD	Chronic graft-versus-host disease
cGy	centi-Gray
chemo	Chemotherapy
CHF	Congestive heart failure
CHOEP	Cyclophosphamide (C), doxorubicin (H), vincristine (O), etoposide (E), prednisone (P)
CHOP	Cyclophosphamide (C), doxorubicin (H), vincristine (O), prednisone (P)
Chr	Chromosome
CHR	Complete hematologic response
CID	Combined immunodeficiency
CIN	Cervical intraepithelial neoplasia
CIP	CDK interacting protein
CIS	Cisplatin
CISNE	Clinical index of stable febrile neutropenia
CIT	Chemoimmunotherapy
CIV	Continuous intravenous infusion
CKC	Cold knife cone
CLL	Chronic lymphocytic leukemia
Clo	Clofarabine
CLP	Common lymphoid progenitors
cm	Centimeter
CML	Chronic myelogenous leukemia
CML	Chronic myeloid leukemia
CMML	Chronic myelomonocytic leukemia
CMMRD	Constitutional mismatch repair deficiency syndrome
CMP	Common myeloid progenitors
CMV	Cytomegalovirus
CN	Cranial nerves
CN-H	Copy number-high
CN-L	Copy number-low
CNI	Calcineurin inhibitor
CNS	Central nervous system

coag	Coagulation
COG	Children's Oncology Group
conc.	Concentration
CoNS	Coagulase-negative staphylococci
COPD	Chronic obstructive pulmonary disorder
costim	Costimulatory
CP	Chest pain
CP	Chronic phase
CPI	Checkpoint inhibitors
CPK	Creatine phosphokinase
CPS	Combined positive score
CR	Complete response
Cr	Creatinine
CR1	First complete remission
CRC	Colorectal carcinoma
CrCl	Creatinine clearance
CRMP	Collapsin response mediator protein
CRP	C-reactive protein
CRPC	Castrate resistant prostate cancer
CRS	Cytokine release syndrome
CRT	Chemoradiation
CRTC1	CREB regulated transcription coactivator 1
CSA	Cyclosporine
CSC	Cancer stem cell
CSF	Cerebrospinal spinal fluid
CSF-1	Colony-stimulating factor 1
CSF1R	Colony-stimulating factor 1 receptor
CSI	Cranial spinal irradiation
CT	Chemotherapy
CT	Computed tomography
CTCAE	Common Terminology Criteria for Adverse Events
CTL	Cytotoxic T-lymphocytes
CTLA-4	Cytotoxic T-lymphocyte–associated protein 4
CTLs	Cytotoxic T lymphocytes
cum.	Cumulative
CV	Cardiovascular
CVA	Cerebrovascular accident
CVC	Central venous catheter
CVD	Cardiovascular disease
CVP	Cyclophosphamide (C), vincristine (V), prednisone (P)
CVT	Cisplatin (C), vinblastine (V), temozolomide (T)
CW	Chest wall
CXCL2	Chemokine (C-X-C motif) ligand 2
CXR	Chest X-ray
Cy	Cyclophosphamide
CYP	Cytochrome
cyto	Cytogenetics
D	Day
d/o	Disorder
d/t	Due to
dab	Dabrafenib

daEPOCH	Dose-adjusted etoposide (E), prednisone (P), vincristine (O), cyclophosphamide (C), doxorubicin (H)
DAH	Diffuse alveolar hemorrhage
DART	Dual-affinity retargeting protein
DAT	Direct antiglobulin test
dauno	Daunorubicin
DBA	Diamond–Blackfan anemia
DC	Dendritic cell
DCIS	Ductal carcinoma in situ
DDB2	Damaged DNA-binding protein 2
DDI(s)	Drug–drug interaction(s)
ddNTP	Dideoxynucleotide triphosphate
DDR	DNA damage repair
DDx	Differential diagnosis
decr.	Decreased
Del11q	Deletion of chromosome 11q
Del13q	Deletion of chromosome 13q
Del17p	Deletion of chromosome 17p
derm	Dermatologic
dex	Dexamethasone
Dexa	Dexamethasone
DFCI	Dana-Farber Cancer Institute
DFS	Disease-free survival
DGC	Diffuse gastric cancer
DHAP	Dexamethasone(D), high-dose Ara C (HA, cytarabine), cisplatin (P)
DI	Diabetes insipidus
DM	Diabetes mellitus
DM	Dermatomyositis
DIBH	Deep inspiratory breath hold
DIC	Disseminated intravascular coagulation
DIPG	Diffuse intrinsic pontine glioma
DKC	Dyskeratosis congenita
DLBCL	Diffuse large B-cell lymphoma
DLCO	Diffusing capacity for carbon monoxide
DLI	Donor lymphocyte infusion
DLT	Dose-limiting toxicity
DMSO	Dimethyl sulfoxide
DNA	Deoxyribonucleic acid
dNTP	Deoxyribonucleotide triphosphate
DOAC	Direct oral anticoagulant
DOR	Duration of response
DOTL1	Disruptor of telomeric silencing 1-like
DP	Dimerization partner
DP-IMRT	Dose-painted intensity-modulated radiation therapy
DRC	Dexamethasone, rituximab, cyclophosphamide
DS	Down syndrome
DSB	Double-strand break
DTIC	Dacarbazine
Dur	Duration
Dx	Diagnosis
Dx'd	Diagnosed
dz	Disease
Eg	For example
EBER	EBV-encoded
EBRT	External beam radiation therapy
EBUS	Endobronchial ultrasound
EBV	Epstein–Barr virus
ECG	Electrocardiogram
EKG	Electrocardiogram
ECHO	Echocardiogram
ECOG PS	Eastern Cooperative Oncology Group Performance Status Classification
ECP	Extracorporeal photopheresis
ed.	Edition
EDTA	Ethylenediaminetetraacetic acid
EEG	Electroencephalogram
EFS	Event-free survival
EGD	Esophagogastroduodenoscopy
EGF	Epidermal growth factor
EGFR	Epidermal growth factor receptor
ELISA	Enzyme-linked immunosorbent assay
ELN	European Leukemia Net
EMBX	Endometrial biopsy
EMG	Electromyography
EMR	Endoscopic mucosal resection
EMT	Epithelial to mesenchymal transition
EN	Extranodal
enco	Encorafenib
ENE	Extranodal extension
EOC	Epithelial ovarian cancer
EOD	Extent of disease
EOI	End of induction
EOL	End of life
eos	Eosinophils
EpCAM	Epithelial cell adhesion molecule
EPO	Erythropoetin
EPP	Erythropoietic protoporphyria
ER	Emergency room
ER	Estrogen receptor
ERCP	Endoscopic retrograde cholangiopancreatography
ERK	Extracellular signal-related kinase

ES Ewing sarcoma
ESD Endoscopic submucosal dissection
ES-SCLC Extensive stage small-cell lung cancer
ESA Erythropoiesis stimulating agent
escBEACOPP Escalated bleomycin (B), etoposide (E), doxorubicin (A), cyclophosphamide (C), vincristine (O), procarabazine (P), prednisone (P)
ESCC Epidural spinal cord compression
ESFT Ewing sarcoma family of tumors
ESHAP Etoposide (E), methylprednisone (S), high-dose cytarabine (HA), cisplatin (P)
Eso Esophageal
esp Especially
ESRD End-stage renal disease
ET Endocrine therapy
ET Essential thrombocythemia
EtOH Ethanol
ETT Epithelioid trophoblastic tumor
EUA Exam under anesthesia
EUS Endoscopic ultrasound

F Factor
F Female
F/N Fever and neutropenia
F&N Fever
FADD Fas-associated death domain
FAMMM Familial atypical multiple mole melanoma syndrome
FAP Familial adenomatous polyposis
FASL FAS ligand
Fc Fragment crystallizable region [of antibody]
FcgammaR Fc-gamma receptor
FcR Fc receptor
FDA Food and Drug Administration
FDG Fluorodeoxyglucose
FDR First-degree relative
FdUMP 5-fluorodeoxyuridine monophosphate
FE Fractional excretion
FFP Fresh frozen plasma
FFPE Formalin-fixed paraffin-embedded
FFS Failure-free survival
FGF23 Fibroblast growth factor-23
FGFR Fibroblast growth factor receptor
FH Favorable histology
FHx Family history
FIGO International Federation of Obstetrics and Gynecology
FISH Fluorescence in situ hybridization
FL Follicular lymphoma
FLAIR Fluid-attenuated inversion recovery
FLC Free light chains
FLIPI Follicular lymphoma international prognostic index
Flu Fludarabine
FNA Fine-needle aspiration
FOBT Fecal occult blood test
FOLFOX Folinic acid, leucovorin, fluorouracil, oxaliplatin
Freq Frequent
FT Fallopian tube(s)
F-UMP Fluorouridine monophosphosphate
FUO Fever of unknown origin
FVL Factor V Leiden
Fx Fraction
fxn Function

g Gram
G-CSF Granulocyte colony-stimulating factor
g/dL Grams per deciliter
G6PD Glucose-6-phosphate
Gab GRB-associated binding protein
GAD Glutamic acid decarboxylase
GAL9 Galectin-9
GBM Glioblastoma multiforme
GC Genetic counselor/counseling
GCSF Granulocyte colony-stimulating factor
GCT Germ cell tumor
GEM Gemcitabine
GemOx Gemcitabine, oxaliplatin
GERD Gastroesophageal reflux disease
GF Growth factor
GFR Glomerular filtration rate
GI Gastrointestinal
GJ Gastrojejunostomy
GIB Gastrointestinal bleeding
GIST Gastrointestinal stromal tumor
GITR Glucocorticoid-inducted TNFR-related protein
Glc Glucose
GLD Globoid cell leukodystrophy
Glu Glucose
GM-CSF Granulocyte macrophage colony-stimulating factor
GBM Glioblastoma
GMP Good manufacturing practice
GNR Gram-negative rods
GO Gemtuzumab ozogamicin
GOC Goal of care
GP Glycoprotein
gp100 Glycoprotein 100

GPA	Graded prognostic assessment
Grb	Growth factor receptor-bound protein
GT	Genetic testing
GTR	Gross total resection
GU	Genitourinary
GVD	Gemcitabine (G), vinorelbine (V), pegylated liposomal doxorubicin (D)
GvH	Graft versus host
GVHD	Graft-versus-host disease
GVL	Graft-versus-leukemia
Gy	Gray
gyn	Gynecologic
h	Hour(s)
h/o	History of
H&N	Head and neck
H&P	History and physical
H1RA	Histamine 1 receptor antagonist
H2RA	Histamine 2 receptor antagonist
HA	Headache
HAART	Highly active antiretroviral therapy
Hb	Hemoglobin
Hgb	Hemoglobin
HBcAb	Hepatitis B core antibody
HBsAg	Hepatitis B surface antigen
HBV	Hepatitis B virus
HCC	Hepatocellular carcinoma
HCL	Hairy cell leukemia
HCLc	Classical hairy cell leukemia
HCP	Hereditary corpophyria
Hct	Hematocrit
HCT	Hematopoietic cell transplantation
HCT-CI	Hematopoietic cell transplantation-specific comorbidity index
HCV	Hepatitis C virus
HD	Hemodialysis
HD MTX	High-dose methotrexate
HDAC	Histone deacetylase
HDC	High-dose chemotherapy
HDR	High-dose rate
HDT/ASCR	High-dose therapy/autologous stem cell rescue
HEENT	Head, eyes, ears, nose, throat
HELLP	Hemolysis, elevated liver enzymes, low platelet syndrome
Hep	Hepatitis
HEP	Hepatoerythropoietic porphyria
HER	Human epidermal growth factor receptor
HER-2	Human epidermal growth factor receptor 2
HGF	Hepatocyte growth factor
HGFR	Hepatocyte growth factor receptor
HGG	High-grade glioma
HGS	High-grade serous ovarian cancer
HHV6	Human herpesvirus 6
HIAA	5-hydroxyindoleacetic acid
HIF	Hypoxia inducible factor
HIPA	Heparin-induced platelet aggregation
HITT	Heparin-induced thrombocytopenia and thrombosis
HIV	Human immunodeficiency virus
HL	Hodgkin lymphoma
HLA	Human leukocyte antigen
HLA Sp	HLA-specificity
HLH	Hemophagocytic
HNPCC	Hereditary non-polyposis colorectal cancer
HNSCC	Head and neck squamous cell cancer
HoTN	Hypotension
HPT	Hyperparathyroidism
HPV	Human papillomavirus
HR	Hazard ratio
HRD	Homologous recombination deficiency
HrHPV	High-risk HPV
HRQOL	Health-related quality of life
H	Herceptin/trastuzumab
HR	Homologous recombination
HR	Hormone receptor
HRT	Hormone replacement therapy
HSC	Hematopoietic stem cells
HSCs	Hematopoietic stem cells
HSCT	Hematopoietic stem cell transplantation
HSM	Hepatosplenomegaly
HSR	Hypersensitivity reaction
HSV	Herpes simplex virus
HSV-1	Herpes simplex virus type 1
hTERT	Human telomerase reverse transcriptase
HTLV-1	Human T-lymphotrophic virus 1
HTN	Hypertension
HU	Hydroxyurea
HUS	Hemolytic uremic syndrome
HVA	Homovanillic acid
hx	History
hydrea	Hydroxyurea
hyperCA	Hypercalcemia
hyperCVAD	Hyper-fractionated
HypoNa	Hyponatremia
I-125	Iodine-135
I&D	Incision and drainage
IABP	Intra-aortic balloon bump
IBD	Irritable bowel disease
IBW	Ideal body weight
ICANS	Immune effector cell-associated neurotoxicity syndrome
ICE	Ifosfamide (I), carboplatin (C), etoposide (E)

ICI Immune checkpoint inhibitors
ICOS Inducible T-cell costimulatory
ICP Intracranial pressure
ICU Intensive care unit
ID Infectious disease
IDA Iron deficiency anemia
IDH Isocitrate dehydrogenase
IFE Immunofixation
IFLN Inguinofemoral lymph node (LN)
IFLND Inguinofemoral lymph node (LN) dissection
IFN Interferon
IFN-g Interferon gamma
IFND Inguinal femoral lymph node dissection
IFRT Involved-field radiation therapy
Ig Immunoglobulin
IGCCC International Germ Cell Consensus Classification
IgE Immunoglobulin E
IGF Insulin-like growth factor
IGFR1 Insulin-like growth factor receptor 1
IgG Immunoglobulin G
IGHV Immunoglobulin variable region heavy chain gene
IHC Immunohistochemistry
IL Interleukin
IL-6R Interleukin 6 receptor
ILD Interstitial lung disease
IMIDs Immunomodulatory drugs
ImmTAC Immune-mobilizing monoclonal TCR against cancer
IMRT Intensity-modulated radiation therapy
IMT Inflammatory myofibroblastic tumor
Incl. Including
incr. Increased
infx Infection
infxn Infection
INR International normalized ratio
Intraop Intraoperative
Invest Investigational
IO Immunotherapy
IP Intraperitoneal
IPC Indwelling pleural catheter
IPEX Immunodysregulation polyendocrinopathy enteropathy X-linked syndrome
ipi Ipilimumab
IPI International prognostic index
IPS International prognostic score
IPS Idiopathic pneumonia syndrome
IR Interventional radiology
IR Ionizing radiation
irAEs Immune-related adverse events
IRR Irradiated
ISH In situ hybridization
ISM Indolent systemic mastocytosis
IST Immunosuppressive therapy
IT Intrathecal
ITD Internal tandem repeat
ITP Immune thrombocytopenic purpura
IU International units
IUP Intrauterine pregnancy
IV Intravenous
IVB Intravenous bolus
IVE Ifosfamide (I), epirubicin (V), etoposide (E)
IVF Intravenous fluids
IVIG Intravenous immunoglobulin
IVP Intravenous push
iwCLL International Workshop on Chronic Lymphocytic Leukemia

J Joule
JAK Janus kinase
JC John Cunningham virus
Jxn Junction

K Thousand
kb Kilobase
kg Kilogram
KIP Kinase inhibitory protein
KIP2 Kinesin-like protein
KIR Killer cell immunoglobulin-like receptor
KPS Karnofsky performance status
KS Kaposi sarcoma

L Liter
LA Lupus anticoagulant
LAC Lupus anticoagulant
LAD Lymphadenopathy
LAN Lymphadenopathy
LAG3 Lymphocyte activation gene 3
LAMB Liposomal amphotericin B
LAR Low-anterior resection
LBL Lymphoblastic lymphoma
LC Local control
LCWS Low continuous wall suction
LD Low dose
LDH Lactate dehydrogenase
LDR Low-dose rate
LE Lower extremity
LEEP Loop electrosurgical excision procedure
LFS Li–Fraumeni syndrome
LHRH Luteinizing-hormone-releasing hormone
Lin– Lineage negative
LFT Liver function tests
LGG Low-grade glioma

LGL	Large granular lymphocytic
LMN	Lower motor neuron
LMS	Leiomyosarcoma
LMWH	Low–molecular-weight heparin
LN	Lymph node
LND	Lymph node dissection
LOH	Loss of heterozygosity
LP	Lumbar puncture
LPD	Lymphoproliferative disorder
LR	Leukocyte reduced
LS	Lynch syndrome
LS-SCLC	Limited stage small-cell lung cancer
LTBI	Latent tuberculosis infection
LV	Left ventricle
LVEF	Left ventricular ejection fraction
LVI	Lymphovascular invasion
LVSI	Lymphovascular space invasion
M	Male
m^2	Square meter
MΦ	Macrophage
Mab	Monoclonal antibody
MAC	Myeloablative conditioning
MAG	Myelin-associated glycoprotein
MAGE	Melanoma-associated antigen
MaGIC	Malignant germ cell Tumor International Consortium
MAHA	Microangiopathic hemolytic anemia
MALT	Mucosa-associated lymphoid tissue
MAO	Monoamine oxidase
MAP	High-dose methotrexate (M), doxorubicin (A), cisplatin (P)
MAP	Mean arterial pressure
MAP	MUTYH-associated polyposis
MAPK	Mitogen-activated protein kinase
MART-1	Melanoma antigen recognized by T-cells-1
MASCC	Multinational Association of Supportive Care in Cancer
max	Maximum
MBL	Monoclonal B-cell lymphocytosis
MC	Mast cell
MCL	Mantle cell lymphoma
M-CSF	Macrophage colony-stimulating factor
MDR	Multidrug resistance
MDS	Myelodysplastic syndrome
MDSCs	Myeloid-derived suppressor cells
MEC	Mucoepidermoid carcinoma
med onc	Medical oncology
MEK	Mitogen-activated protein kinase
Mel	Melphalan
memb	Membrane
mEq	Milliequivalents
met	Metastasis
Mets	Metastases
MF	Myelofibrosis
MFS	Metastases free survival
MG	Myasthenia gravis
mg	Milligram
mGluR1	Metabotropic glutamate receptor 1
mgmt	Management
MGMT	Methylguanine-DNA methyltransferase
MGUS	Monoclonal gammopathy of undetermined significance
MHC	Major histocompatibility complex
MI	Myocardial infarction
MIBG	Metaiodobenzylguanidine
MIPI	Mantle cell lymphoma international prognostic index
mL	Milliliter
ML-DS	Myeloid leukemia of down syndrome
mL/d	Milliliter per day
MLD	Metachromatic leukodystrophy
MLH	Mutl homolog
MLH1	MutL homolog 1 (mismatch repair system component)
MLH6	MutS homolog 6 (mismatch repair system component)
MM	Multiple myeloma
MMAE	Monomethyl auristatin E
MMF	Mycophenolate mofetil
MMG	Mammogram
MMR	Mismatch repair
MMRd	Mismatch repair deficiency
MNZ	Metronidazole
Mϕ	Macrophage
mo(s)	Month(s)
MOF	Multiorgan failure
MOGTC	Malignant ovarian germ cell tumor
MPD	Myeloproliferative disorder
MPE	Malignant pleural effusion
MPN	Myeloproliferative neoplasms
MPNST	Malignant peripheral nerve sheath tumor
MR/MRI	Magnetic resonance imaging
MRC	Medical research council
MRCP	Magnetic resonance cholangiopancreatogrpahy

MRD	Minimal residual disease
MRD	Matched related donor
MRI	Magnetic resonance imaging
mRNA	Messenger RNA
MRSA	Methicillin-resistant Staphylococcus aureus
MS	Mental status
MSC	Mesenchymal stem cells
MSH	MutS homolog
MSH2	MutS homolog 2 (mismatch repair system component)
MSKCC	Memorial Sloan Kettering Cancer Center
MSI	Microsatellite
MSI-H	Microsatellite instability-high
MSS	Microsatellite stable
MSTS	Musculoskeletal tumor society
Mt	Mutation
Mt(s)	Mutation(s)
Mut	Mutant/mutation
MTC	Medullary thyroid cancer
MTHFR	Methylene tetrahydrofolate reductase
mTOR	Mammalian target of rapamycin
MTX	Methotrexate
MUC-1	Mucin-1
MUC16	Mucine-16
MUD	Matched unrelated donor
MUGA	Multiple-gated acquisition scan
MF	Mycosis fungoides
MZL	Marginal zone lymphoma
MΦ	Macrophage
N	North
N/C	Nuclear/cytoplasmic
n/v	Nausea/vomiting
NAC	Neoadjuvant chemotherapy
nAChR	Nicotinic acetylcholine receptor
NAFLD	Nonalcoholic fatty liver disease
NASH	Nonalcoholic steatohepatitis
NB	Neuroblastoma
NBN	Nibrin
NCCN	National Comprehensive Cancer Network
NE	Neuroendocrine
neb	Nebulizer
neg	Negative
neoadj	Neoadjuvant
NER	Nucleotide excision repair
NF-1	Neurofibromatosis type 1
NFALD	Nonalcoholic fatty liver disease
ng	Nanogram
NG	Nasogastric
NGS	Next-generation sequencing
NHEJ	Nonhomologous end joining
NHL	Non-Hodgkin lymphoma
NI	Noninferiority
Nivo	Nivolumab
NK	Natural killer cell
nl	Normal
NLPH	Nodular lymphocyte-predominant Hodgkin lymphoma
NMA	Nonmyeloablative
NMDA	N-Methyl-D-aspartate
NMDAR	N-methyl D-aspartate receptor
NMDP	National Marrow Donor Program
NMSC	Nonmelanoma skin cancer
NO	Nitric oxide
NOS	Not otherwise specified
NP	Nasopharynx
NPO	Nil per os
NRM	Nonrelapse mortality
NS	Night sweats
NS	Normal saline
NSAID	Nonsteroidal anti-inflammatory drugs
NSCLC	Non–small-cell lung cancer
NSE	Neuron-specific enolase
NTRK	Neurotrophic tyrosine receptor kinase
NY-ESO-1	New York esophageal squamous cell carcinoma 1
NYHA	New York Heart Association Heart Failure classification
OB	Obstetric
OCP	Oral contraceptive pills
OFS	Ovarian function suppression
OGCT	Ovarian germ cell tumor
OKT3	Muromonab-CD3
OMAS	Opsoclonus-myoclonus-ataxia syndrome
ONJ	Osteonecrosis of jaw
OP	Oropharynx
OR	Operating room
ORR	Overall response rate
OS	Overall survival
OTR	Organ transplant recipient
OV	Oncolytic virus
OX40L	OX40 ligand
P-gp	P-glycoprotein
p/w	Presents with
PA	Posterior-anterior
PAH	Pulmonary arterial hypertension
PAI	Plasminogen activator inhibitor
PALB2	Partner and localizer of the BRCA2 gene
PAP	Prostatic acid phosphatase
PAP	Pulmonary alveolar proteinosis
PARP	Poly (ADP-ribose) polymerase
PARPi	PARP inhibitors

PAS Platelet additive solution
Path Pathology
Pathophys Pathophysiology
PAX8 Paired Box 8 gene
PB Peripheral blood
PBG Porphobilinogen
PBMC Peripheral blood mononuclear cell
PBSC Peripheral blood stem cells
PBSCT Peripheral blood stem cell transplant
PC Protein C
PCALCL Primary cutaneous anaplastic large-cell lymphoma
PCN Penicillin
PCNSL Primary central nervous system lymphoma
PCOS Polycystic ovary syndrome
pCR Pathologic complete response
PCR Polymerase chain reaction
PCT Porphyria cutanea tarda
PCV Procarbazine, lomustine and vincristine
PD Progressive disease
PD-1 Programmed cell death protein 1
Pd-103 Palladium-103
PD-L1 Programmed death ligand 1
PD-L1/2 Programmed death-ligand 1/2
PDGFRa Platelet-derived growth factor receptor alpha
PDT Photodynamic therapy
PE Physical exam
PE Pulmonary embolus
PEx Physical exam
PEG Percutaneous endoscopic gastrostomy
Pembro Pembrolizumab
perf Perforation
perm Permeability
PET Positron emission tomography
PET/CT Positron emission tomography–computerized tomography
PF24 Plasma frozen within 24 hours after phlebotomy
PF4 Platelet factor 4
PFA Platelet function analyzer
PFS Progression-free survival
PFT Pulmonary function test
PGD Preimplantation genetic diagnosis
PGT Preimplantation testing
PGE2 Prostaglandin E2
Ph Philadelphia
Pheo Pheochromocytoma
Plat Platinum
PI Prognostic index
PI3K Phosphinositide 3-kinase
PID Primary immunodeficiency disorder
PJP Pneumocystis jiroveci pneumonia
PK/PD Pharmacokinetics/pharmacodynamics
PLCg Phospholipase C gamma
PLCO Prostate, Lung, Colorectal and Ovarian Cancer Screening Trial
PLEX Plasma exchange
PLL Prolymphocytic leukemia
Plt Platelet
PMRT Postmastectomy radiation therapy
PMS2 PMS1 homolog 2 (mismatch repair system component)
PNA Pneumonia
PNET Primitive neuroectodermal tumor
PNH Paroxysmal nocturnal hemoglobinuria
PNI Perineural
PO Per os
PO4 Phosphate
POD Progression of disease
POMA Postoperative margin assessment
poss Possible
Post-op Postoperative
Post. Posterior
PPES Palmoplantar erythrodysesthesia
PPI Proton pump inhibitor
Ppx Prophylaxis
PR Progesterone receptor
PR Partial response
pRBC Packed red blood cells
pre-op Preoperative
PRES Posterior reversible encephalopathy syndrome
Prev Previous
Prog Prognosis
prot Protein
Prox Proximal
PS Performance status
PSA Prostate-specific antigen
PSMA Prostate-specific membrane antigen
PSTT Placental site trophoblastic tumor
psych Psychiatric
pt(s) Patient(s)
PT Prothrombin time
PTCL Peripheral T-cell lymphoma
PTCy Posttransplant cyclophosphamide
PTEN Phosphatase and tensin homolog
PTG Prothrombin gene
PTH Parathyroid hormone
PTHrP Parathyroid-related protein

PTLD	Posttransplant lymphoproliferative disease
PTO	Percutaneous transhepatic obliteration
PTT	Partial thromboplastin time
Pulm	Pulmonary
PUVA	Psoralen plus ultraviolet A
PV	Polycythemia vera
PV	Portal vein
PVR	Poliovirus receptor
px	Prognosis
PXA	Pleomorphic xanthoastrocytoma
q	Each (time interval)
QA	Quality assurance
QD	Daily
QoL	Quality of life
qPCR	Quantitative polymerase chain reaction
R	Rituximab
R-CHOP	Rituximab (R), cyclophosphamide (C), doxorubicin (H), vincristine (O), prednisone (P)
R-EPOCH	Rituximab (R), etoposide (E), prednisone (P), vincristine (O), cyclophosphamide (C), doxorubicin (H)
r/o	Rule out
R/R	Relapse/refractory
R0	Complete resection with negative microscopic margins
R1	Microscopically positive margins
rad onc	Radiation oncology
RAD51	RAD51 recombinase
RAD51C/D	RAD51 Paralog C or D
RANO	Response assessment in neuro-oncology
RAR	Retinoic acid receptor
RARS	Refractory anemia with ring sideroblasts
RARS-T	Refractory anemia with ring sideroblasts with thrombocytosis
RB	Retinoblastoma
RB1	Retinoblastoma protein
RBC	Red blood cell
RBE	Relative biologic effectiveness
RCC	Renal cell carcinoma
RCT	Randomized controlled trial
Rec	Recommended
Rel/ref	Relapsed/refractory
REMS	Risk evaluation and mitigation strategies
Retic-He	Reticulocyte hemoglobin equivalent
RF	Risk factor
RFA	Radiofrequency ablation
RFS	Recurrence-free survival
RIC	Reduced intensity conditioning
RMSF	Rocky mountain spotted fever
RNA	Ribonucleic acid
RNAi	RNA interference
R/o	Rule out
RP	Retroperitoneal
RPA	Recursive partitioning analysis
RR	Response rate
rrBLM	Risk-reducing bilateral mastectomy
rrBSO	Risk-reducing bilateral oophorectomy
rRNA	Ribosomal RNA
RRSO	Risk-reducing salpingo-oophorectomy
RS	Recurrence score
RS	Ring sideroblasts
RSV	Respiratory syncytial virus
RT	Radiation therapy
RT	Richter's transformation
RT-PCR	Reverse transcription-polymerase chain reaction
RTK	Receptor tyrosine kinase
RTOG	Radiation therapy oncology group
RUQ	Right upper quadrant
Rx	Therapy
rxn	Reaction
S	South
s/e	Side effect
s/p	Status post
S/s	Signs/symptoms
SABR	Stereotactic ablative radiotherapy
sBCC	Superficial BCC
SBP	Systolic blood pressure
SBE	Self-breast exam
SBRT	Stereotactic body radiotherapy
SC/SQ	Subcutaneous
SCC	Squamous cell carcinoma
SCCHN	Squamous cell carcinoma of the head and neck
SCF	Stem cell factor
scFv	Single-chain variable fragment
SCID	Severe combined immunodeficiency
SCLC	Small-cell lung cancer
SCT	Stem-cell transplantation
SD	Stable disease
SDC	Salivary duct carcinoma
SE	Side effect
Se	Sensitivity
SEGA	Subependymal giant cell astrocytoma
SERD	Selective estrogen receptor down-regulator
seq	Sequence

Sev.	Severe
Shh	Sonic hedgehog
SBDS	Shwachman–Diamond syndrome
SIADH	Syndrome of inappropriate antidiuretic hormone
SINS	Spinal instability neoplastic score
SIRP-1	Signal regulatory protein-1
SIRPa	Signal regulatory protein alpha
SIRS	Systemic inflammatory response syndrome
SLD	Single lineage dysplasia
SLE	Systemic lupus erythematous
SLL	Small lymphocytic lymphoma
SM-AHN	Systemic mastocytosis with associated hematologic neoplasm
SMA	Smooth muscle actin
SMITE	Simultaneous multiple interaction T-cell engaging
SMV	Superior mesenteric vein
SMZL	Splenic marginal zone lymphoma
Sn	Sensitivity
Sn	Sign
SNLB	Sentinel lymph node biopsy
SNP	Single nucleotide polymorphism
SNUC	Sinonasal undifferentiated carcinoma
SOC	Standard of care
SOS	Sinusoidal obstruction syndrome
Sp	Specificity
SPEP	Serum protein electrophoresis
SPTCL	Subcutaneous panniculitis-like T-cell lymphoma
SR	Standard risk
SRA	Serotonin release assay
SRE	Skeletal related events
SRS	Stereotactic radiosurgery
SS	Sézary syndrome
SSB	Single-strand break
SSM	Smoldering systemic mastocytosis
SSRI	Selective serotonin reuptake inhibitors
SSTI	Skin and soft tissue infection
STAT3	Signal transducer and activator of transcription 3
STI	Sexually transmitted infection
STIC	Serous tubal intraepithelial carcinoma
Stim	Stimulation
STK11	Serine/threonine kinase 11
STS	Soft tissue sarcoma
subop	Suboptimally debulked
SVC	Superior vena cava
Sx	Symptom
syn	Syndrome
T	Taxane
T-DM1	Trastuzumab emtansine
T-VEC	Talimogene laherparepvec
T. Bili	Total bilirubin
T(1/2)	Half-Life
T/C	Paclitaxel (T), carboplatin (C)
T/FL	Transformed follicular lymphoma
T4	Thyroxine
TACE	Transarterial chemoembolization
TAH	Total abdominal hysterectomy
TAH/BSO	Total abdominal hysterectomy/bilateral salpino-oophorectomy
Tam	Tamoxifen
TAM	Tumor-associated macrophage
TAP	Paclitaxel (T), doxorubicin (A), cisplatin (P)
TAR	Thrombocytopenia with absent radius syndrome
TARE	Transarterial radioembolization
TAT	Turnaround time
TB	Total bilirubin
TBBx	Transbronchial biopsy
TBI	Total body irritation
Tc99	Technetium-99
TCA	Tricyclic antidepressant(s)
TCGA	The Cancer Genome Atlas Program
TCR	T-cell receptor
T-Dxd	Trastuzumab deruxtecan
TEPA	Tetraethylenepentamine
TF	Transcription factor
TFT	Thyroid function test
TGFb	Transforming growth factor beta
TGs	Triglycerides
Thio	Thiotepa
TIGIT	T-cell immunoglobulin and ITIM domain
TIL(s)	Tumor-infiltrating lymphocyte(s)
TIM3	T-cell immunoglobulin and mucin-domain containing-3
TIW	Three times a week
TK	Tyrosine kinase
TKD	Tyrosine kinase domains
TKI	Tyrosine kinase inhibitor
TLS	Tumor lysis syndrome
TMA	Thrombotic microangiopathy
TMD	Transient myeloproliferative disorder
TME	Tumor microenvironment

TMP-SMX	Trimethoprim-sulfamethoxazole
TMZ	Temozolomide
TNBC	Triple-negative breast cancer
TNF	Tumor necrosis factor
TNFa	Tumor necrosis factor alpha
TNFR1	Tumor necrosis factor receptor 1
Tox	Toxicity
Toxo	Toxoplasmosis
TP53	Tumor protein p53
TPN	Total parenteral nutrition
TPO	Thrombopoietin
TPO-RA	Thrombopoietin receptor agonist
TRADD	Tumor necrosis factor receptor type 1–associated death domain
Treg	Regulatory T cells
TriKE	Trispecific killer engager
TSC	Tuberous sclerosis complex
TSEB	Total skin electron beam
TSG	Tumor suppressor gene
TSH	Thyroid-stimulating hormone
TTE	Transthoracic echocardiography
TTP	Thrombotic thrombocytopenic purpura
TVUS	Transvaginal ultrasound
Tx	Treatment
U/S	Ultrasound
UA	Uric acid
U/A	Urinalysis
Ucortisol	Urine cortisol
UFH	Unfractionated heparin
UGI	Upper gastrointestinal
UH	Unfavorable histology
UKCTOCS	United Kingdom Collaborative Trial of Ovarian Cancer Screening
ULN	Upper limit of normal
UMN	Upper motor neuron
unfav.	Unfavorable
UOP	Urine output
UOsm	Urine osmolarity
UPEP	Urine protein electrophoresis
UPS	Undifferentiated pleomorphic sarcoma
URD	Unrelated donor
URI	Upper respiratory tract infection
UROD	Uroporphyrinogen decarboxylase
US	United States
USPSTF	United States Preventive Services Task Force
usu	Usually
UV	Ultraviolet
UVA	Ultraviolet A
UVB	Ultraviolet B
VAC	Vincristine (V), dactinomycin (A), and cyclophosphamide (C)
VAF	Variant allele frequency
VAI	Vincristine (V), dactinomycin (D), and ifosfamide (I)
VCR	Vincristine
VDC/IE	Vincristine (V), doxorubicin (D), and cyclophosphamide (C) alternating with Ifosfamide (I) and etoposide (E)
VEGF	Vascular endothelial growth factor
VEGFinhib	VEGF inhibitor
VEGFR	VEGF receptor
vem	Vemurafenib
VGCC	Voltage-gated calcium channel
VGKC	Voltage-gated potassium channel
VGPR	Very good partial response
VHL	Von Hippel–Lindau
VIDE	Vincristine (V), ifosfamide (I), doxorubicin (D), and etoposide (E)
VIN	Vulvar intraepithelial neoplasia
VIP	Vasoactive intestinal peptide
VISTA	V-domain Ig suppressor of T-cell activation
VISTA-R	V-domain Ig suppressor of T-cell activation receptor
vit	Vitamin
VKA	Vitamin K antagonist
VMA	Vanillylmandelic acid
VOC	Vaso-occlusive crisis
VOD	Veno-occlusive disease
VP	Variegate porphyria
VPEFR	V (involvement of vena cava), P (portal bifurcation), E (extrahepatic contiguous extension), F (multifocal liver tumor), R (tumor rupture)
VRE	Vancomycin resistant enterococcus
VS	Vital signs
VTE	Venous thromboembolism
vWD	von Willebrand Disease
vWF	von Willebrand factor
VZV	Varicella-zoster virus
w/	With
w/c	Which can
w/in	Within
wk	Week

w/o	Without
wt	Weight
w/u	Work-up
WAGR	Wilms tumor, aniridia, genitourinary, range of developmental delays
WBC	White blood cell
WBMRI	Whole-body MRI
WBRT	Whole brain radiotherapy
well-diff	Well-differentiated
WHO	World Health Organization
Wk(s)	Week(s)
WLL	Whole lung lavage
WM	Waldenstrom macroglobulinemia
WNT	Wingless INT
wt	Weight
WT1	Wilms tumor 1 gene
XLDPP	X-linked dominant protoporphyria
XPC	Xeroderma pigmentosum complementation group C
XR	X-ray
y	Year(s)
YAP	Yes-associated protein
yo	Years old
Δ	Change
μL	Microliter

Note: Page number followed by f and t indicates figure and table respectively.

T

U

V

W

X

Y

Z